A CLASSIFIED
BIBLIOGRAPHY OF THE HISTORY OF
DUTCH MEDICINE

1900–1974

NICOLAI PARADYS

M. D. MEDICINAE IN ACADEMIA LUGDUNO-BATAVA
PROFESSORIS ORDINARII

ORATIO

DE

COGNITIONE HISTORIAE MEDICINAE MAGNO, CUM AD MEDICI IN ARTE EXERCENDA SOLERTIAM, TUM AD ARTIS AMPLIFICATIO-NEM, ADJUMENTO.

PUBLICE HABITA

A. D. XXVII. *SEPTEMBRIS* MDCCC.

QUUM

ORDINARIAM HISTORIAE MEDICINAE PRO-FESSIONEM AUSPICARETUR.

LUGDUNI BATAVORUM,
APUD HAAK ET SOCIOS,
MDCCC.

Title-page of Nic. Paradijs *Oratio de cognitione historiae medicinae* (1800)

A CLASSIFIED
BIBLIOGRAPHY OF THE HISTORY
OF DUTCH MEDICINE
1900-1974

compiled and arranged

by

Dr G. A. LINDEBOOM
F.R.C.P.
EMERITUS PROFESSOR OF MEDICINE IN THE FREE UNIVERSITY AT AMSTERDAM

with the assistance of
Miss A. A. G. HAM

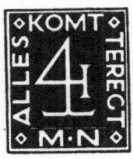

THE HAGUE
MARTINUS NIJHOFF
1975

Published with financial support from the Netherlands
Organization for the Advancement of Pure Research (Z.W.O.)

ISBN-13: 978-94-010-1699-5   e-ISBN-13: 978-94-010-1697-1
DOI: 10.1007/ 978-94-010-1697-1

Preface and Introduction

1. In some periods of the past Netherlands medicine has played a major role in the evolution of European medicine; today its history still enjoys much interest even at the other side of the Ocean. In this bibliography it has been my endeavour to compile references for all that has been written on the history of Dutch medicine in our country and elsewhere in our age.

The main concern of this work is with the medicine of the Northern Netherlands. However, before the end of the sixteenth century the Northern and Southern Netherlands were not yet divided into two separate countries; they were still politically one and for the greater part spoke the same Flemish language. So before their separation the present-day Belgium and Netherlands also had a common medical history. Therefore many entries have been included which bear on early (and sometimes later) Flemish medicine, but it has not been the intention to strive for completeness in this respect.

2. It was difficult to explain in the title of this bibliography that it has further been the endeavour to collect not only references on Dutch medicine, but also data on all articles and books bearing on medical historical topics written by Netherlands authors, in order to represent all the medical historical work done in the Netherlands. In this way the present volume covers a far greater field than just the medical past of Holland as described by Netherlands and foreign writers, for it also contains a not too small selection of the medical history of other countries as seen through the eyes of Dutch medical historians.

3. The studies whose titles are compiled in this volume appeared in the period between the year 1900 and December 31, 1974. However, the early limit has not always been strictly kept to. "Jede Konsequenz führt zum Teufel." In the nineteenth century, especially its second half, several valuable studies have been published that are still indispensable for the study of one or another subject. For example, because a modern biography of the famous Frederik Ruysch is not available, it was felt that the one of 1886, though in some respects out of

date, should be included. Likewise a nineteenth century series of articles on the Leiden Medical Faculty, written by G. C. B. Suringar, still being a rich and well documented source of information, could not be omitted.

4. Naturally the great majority of publications on Netherlands, medicine have been written in the native language, with which most English-speaking historians are not familiar. As the least that could be done, all Dutch titles of books and articles have been given an English translation in parentheses. Titles in another modern language or in Latin have not been translated.

Moreover, it should be noted that a considerable part of the references for particular topics of the Dutch medical past have been published in periodicals with only a regional, local or otherwise restricted distribution. Such items often are only available in the Netherlands and even there not without much trouble. Yet they were included as many of them offer archivistic or other data not to be found elsewhere.

5. This systematic bibliography has not the claim to be a "dictionnaire raison-né". However, in many cases, especially when a title was not very clear or even cryptic, a short note gives some information about the content. Authors having the bad habit of choosing such titles are not aware of the troubles they cause to bibliographers or to those who are especially interested in their topic. Someone who is studying the history of a particular town hospital does not learn from the title "a small sixteenth century hospital", whether that article will furnish him material, and may take much effort in vain. Whereever possible an attempt has been made to avoid such troubles for the user.

6. The collected items have been arranged in twenty-two chapters using numerous headings in order to make the search for information on a special subject easier. A few items that could not be classified under current headings were listed as "varia".

For reasons of convenience, the principle of division could not always be the same, for example chronological. Often the division had to be adapted pragmatically. All entries referring to Antiquity and Medieval Medicine have been brought together into separate chapters. For times after the Renaissance more systematic chapters have been used.

An ever-recurring difficulty was that so many articles rightfully could be listed under more than one heading. To take a fictitious example, an article on Linnaeus and nutrition in Sweden could find a place in three different chapters. To deal with this difficulty cross-references have been made as much as possible. Only a few items have been fully inserted twice.

7. Three indexes have been included: one of the historical persons, one of the (first) author and one of place-names. *All numbers in the indexes refer to the entry numbers, not to the pages.*

Perhaps someone will feel the lack of a subject index. However, in view of the three indexes just mentioned, a subject index did not seem absolutely necessary. To meet the want of it, the table of contents has been elaborated extensively. It should be consulted first whenever going in search for literature on a special topic not connected with the name of a person, a place or an author. Everyone who is consulting this bibliography on a certain subject and does not find primarily what he is looking for, is urgently advised to glance in other chapters or under other headings.

8. Although all efforts have been made for accuracy, it must be conceded that in a work such as the present volume some errors are inevitable. For any errors or mistakes that may have crept in, sincere apologies are made.

Furthermore, though it may be trusted that most of the relevant literature has been collected in this bibliography, the compiler does not indulge in the hope that the striving for completeness has been entirely successful. He can only be most grateful for notification of any omitted reference that has not come to his knowledge, or for the receipt of any reprint sent with a similar purpose.

G.A.L.

Acknowledgements

The compilation of this bibliography would not have been possible without the invaluable aid of several institutes and many persons interested in the medical past of the Netherlands.

The library of the "Rijksmuseum voor de Geschiedenis der Natuurwetenschappen" in Leiden proved to be an important source of entries completing our own collection.

To the librarians of Groningen and Utrecht Universities I am indebted for information on publications concerning their institutions.

Further I am under obligation to Dr. J. H. Sypkens Smit who showed a lively interest in the enterprise of a bibliography of Dutch medicine and supplied many poorly known references; to Dr. D. A. Wittop Koning who kindly supplied many entries on pharmacy; to Mr. A. M. van Prooyen who made up a long list of titles concerning medicinal herbs; to Drs J. Heniger who was very helpful in completing our lists of entries concerning Antoni van Leeuwenhoek; to Dr. D. de Moulin, Dr. H. M. Beumer, Dr. P. H. Brans and several other historians who furnished references of their own and others' publications. Without the help of them all the work would have remained more incomplete on several topics than it may be now.

However, first of all I am under very great obligation to Miss A. A. G. Ham, whose name is mentioned on the title-page, for her long year's of cooperation in the search of entries, in checking doubtful references, in listing the items and typing the manuscript. Also for the tedious work of typing and retyping I am highly indebted to Mrs. N. E. de Blok-Berkeveld.

List of Illustrations

Table of Contents

Biographies and Biographica

In this first chapter have been collected all entries that have a biographical character or presumably do offer some biographical data. In principle, every book or article bearing, in the title, the name of a person being relevant from a medical historical standpoint has been included. Only in a few cases an exception to this rule seemed appropiate. In such cases a cross-reference and the index may led in that direction. Physicians, surgeons, military medical officers and quacks have been listed in separate sections.

The same applies to the celebrated persons and royalties whose constitutions, illnesses or causes of death have induced medical historians to take the pen in hand.

In every section the entries are arranged alphabetically according to the names of the persons dealt with. These names are spaced when printed the first or the only time.

In some cases of biographical sketches in which the exact name of a person was not given in the title, effort has been made to identify the person dealt with. Eventually his name is mentioned in a note.

References to chemists are to be found in Chapter XIX (Pharmacy).

A. Collective Works

1 AA, A. J. van der (1852). *Biographisch Woordenboek der Nederlanden* (Biographical Dictionary of the Netherlands). 7 Vols. Haarlem. Reprint 1969, B. M. Israël, Amsterdam.

2 MOLHUYSEN, P. C. *et al.* (ed.) (1911–1937). *Nieuw Nederlandsch biografisch woordenboek* (New Dutch biographical dictionary). 10 Vols. A. W. Sijthoff, Leiden. Reprint 1974: N. Israël, Amsterdam.

3 FOKKER, A. A. (1901). *Levensberichten van Zeeuwsche medici* (Bio-

graphical notes of Zealand physicians). 200 pp. J. C. & W. Altorffer, Middelburg.

4   THIEL, Rudolf (1943). *Groote strijders tegen ziekte en dood. Uit het leven en werken van groote geneeskundigen* (Great fighters against disease and death. From the life and works of great physicians). Dutch translation by M. W. Schuurmans Stekhoven. 286 pp., H. J. Leopold, Den Haag.

5   ELOY, N. F. J. (1778, 1973). *Dictionnaire Historique de la Médecine ancienne et moderne.* 4 vols. Mons. Anastatic reprint: Culture et Civilisation, Bruxelles.

6   [Hirsch] (1962). *Biographisches Lexikon der hervorragenden Ärzte aller Zeiten und Völker.* 5 Vols. 3rd unchanged edition. Urban & Schwarzenberg, München-Berlin. [until 1880. Most of the biographies of Dutch physicians are written by C. E. Daniëls].

6¹ [Fischer] (1962). *Biographisches Lexikon der hervorragenden Ärzte aller Zeiten und Völker der letzten fünfzig Jahre* [1880–1930]. 2 Vols. 3rd unchanged ed. *Ibidem.*

7   SIGERIST, H. E. (1932, ³1954). *Grosse Ärzte. Eine Geschichte der Heilkunde in Lebensbildern.* 310 pp., ports. J. F. Lehmanns Verlag München. 3rd edition: 440 pp., ports. *Ibidem.*
    – With a.o. biographies of Vesalius, J. B. van Helmont, F. dele Boë Sylvius, H. Boerhaave, G. van Swieten, A. de Haen.

8   [   ] (1898). *Onze hoogleeraren. Portretten en biografieën* (Our professors. Portraits and biographies). 361 biographies and portraits. Nijgh & Van Ditmar, Rotterdam. 16°.

B. Physicians

A

9   JOSSELIN DE JONG, R. de (1931). Een natuuronderzoeker, die tevens een sociaal hervormer was: Ernst Abbe (1840–1905) (A naturalist, who was a social reformer too: E. Abbe. *NTG, 75,* I, 65–72; *BGG, XI,* 1–8. portr.

10 ALI COHEN, M. L. A. S. (1936). Iets over *Abu L. Kasem* en behan-

deling van varices (Something on Abu L. Kasem and the treatment of varices). *NTG*, *80*, III, 4032-9; *BGG*, *XVI*, 142-9.

11 NAPJUS, J. W. (1936). Augustinus Lollius Adama, hoogleraar in de geneeskunde te Franeker (A.L.A., professor of medicine at Franeker). *NTG*, *80*, 1478-84; *BGG*, *XVI*, 45-51.

12 KLAAUW, C. J. van der (1931). A letter of B. S. Albinus from Leiden to R. Nesbitt in London. *Janus*, *XXXV*, 217-20.

12ᵃ LEFANU, W. R. (1932). More letters from B. S. Albinus to Robert Nesbitt. *Janus*, *XXXVI*, 1-26.

13 KROON, J. E. (1923). Enkele aanteekeningen uit de geschiedenis van een beroemd Anatomengeslacht (Some notes from the history of a famous family of anatomists). *NTG*, *67*, II, 1673-5; *BGG*, *III*, 328-30; – On the Albinus family. (*See also* 4151)

14 LINDEBOOM, G. A. (1973). Mensen om Boerhaave. XII. Bernhardus Albinus de oudere (Men around B. XII. B. Albinus the elder). *GG.*, *4*, 242-3, portr.

15 [editorial] (1966). Bernard Siegfried Albinus (1697-1770) German-Dutch anatomist. *JAMA*, *196*, 910. (*See also* 456)

16 LEERSUM, E. C. van (1910). Shorthand Lecture-notes of the 17th century. *Janus*, *XV*, 273-81, ill.
– Lecture-notes of Albinus on Physiology. (Leyden University Library B.P.L. 860). (*See also* 4149)

17 HENIGER, J. (1972). Gerard Alewijnsz (*ca* 1280 – *ca* 1355), poorter van Leiden (G.A., citizen of L.). *Leids Jbk*, 29-57.

18 FEYFER, F. M. G. de (1941). In memoriam Martinus Antonie van Andel (1878-1941). *Janus*, *XLV*, 193-5. portr.

19 — (1941). In memoriam Martinus Antonie van Andel. *NTG*, *85*, II, 2735-6; *BGG*, *XXI*, 82-3.

20 RIJNBERK, G. van (1941). In memoriam Martinus Antonie van Andel. *NTG*, *85*, II, 2672. *BGG*, *XXI*, 81, portr.

21 SCHOUTE, D. (1942). Levensbericht van Martinus Antonie van Andel (Biographical note of M.A.v.A.). *Hand. Levensber. Mij Ned. Letterk.*, 38-45.
– with an extensive bibliography.

22 MOULIN, D. de (1960). Dominique Anel and his operation for aneurysm. *BHM*, *34*, 498–507.

23 SEVENSMA, T. P. (1909). Apollinaris O oder Q? *Janus*, *XIV*, 895–7.
    – Is the name Quintus Apollinaris or Offredus Appollinaris? Q.A. is the author of a small sixteenth century *Kurz Handbüchlein...viler artzneyen.*

24 MOSSEL, D. A. A. (1953). Nicolaas Appert (1750–1841). *Voeding*, *14*, 441–3, portr.
    – Appert, born in Châlons-sur-Marne, applied himself to preserving methods such as drying, pickling etc.

25 NEUBURGER, M. (1922). Leopold Auenbrugger (1722–19 november – 1922), bij den 200sten gedenkdag zijner geboorte. (— at his 200th anniversary). *NTG*, *66*, II, 2623–9; *BGG*, *II*, 367–73;
    – Lecture, held on 24 october 1922 at Bois-le-Duc.

26 KLEY, J. J. van der (1921). Auenbrugger's "Inventum novum". *NTG*, *65*, II, 711; *BGG*, *I*, 323.

27 NAPJUS, J. W. (1925). Alardus Auletius. *NTG*, *69*, II, 2559–63; *BGG*, *V*, 300–4.

28 NIJHOFF, G. C. (1922). Auletius en de hoogeschool te Franeker. (A. and the University at Franeker). *NTG*, *66*, I, 877; *BGG*, *II*, 84.
    – Letter to the editor.

29 AULETIUS, A. (1603, 1922). *Monitio de reformanda praxi medica* – with Dutch translation., *Opusc.*, *IV*, 1–35.

30 MOULIN, D. de (1970). The influence of Caelius Aurelianus on early medieval Surgery. *Atti Congr. intern. di Storia della Medicina*, E. Cossidente, Rome, 1485–8.

31 BOLK, L. (1916). Toespraak tot C. U. Ariëns Kappers ter gelegenheid van de uitreiking van de Tilanus-medaille. (Address, delivered on the occasion of the awarding of the "Tilanus"-medal to —). *NTG*, *60*, I, 112–5.
    – C. U. Ariëns Kappers (1877–1946) was a well-known neuro-anatomist.

32 BROUWER, B. (1946). In Memoriam Prof. Dr. Cornelius Ubbo Ariëns Kappers. *Psych. en Neurol. Bl.*, 16 pp., portr. Also in: *NTG*, *90* (1946), III, 944, portr.

32ᵃ VEEN, J. P. W. van der (1974). Het geslacht Baart de la Faille (The family — —). *AP*, no 16–17, 99–103.

33 VERJAAL, A. (1957). Joseph Babinski. *De geschiedenis van het pyramidebaan syndroom*. (Joseph Babinski. History of the pyramidal tract syndrome). 34 pp. portr. Bohn, Haarlem, 8°.

34 FEYFER, F. M. G. de (1909). Bijdrage tot de kennis omtrent het leven van J. de Back. (Contribution to the knowledge of the life of —). *NTG*, *53*, I, 1879–86.

35 LAKE, Bernard (1966). *A discourse of the Heart* by James de Back. *Med. Hist.*, *10*, 60–8.
    – on the work of the Rotterdam physician Jacob de Back (1594–1658), entitled *Dissertatio de Corde* and added to an edition of Harvey's *De motu cordis* (Rotterdam, 1648). The whole volume appeared in an English translation in 1653.

36 BACK, J. de (1648, 1926). *Dissertatio de corde* – with Dutch translation. *Opusc.*, *V*, 1–177. *Dissertatio de corde. Ed. Altera* (1654). *Opusc.*, *V*, 178–259. (With Dutch translation).

37 LINDEBOOM, G. A. (1951). Methode en taak der wetenschap by Francis Bacon. (Method and task of science at F.B.). *G&W*, *49*, 165–82.

38 WITTE, A. de (1959). Cornelis de Baersdorp, lijfarts van Keizer Karel, korrespondentie 1548–1561. (C.d.B., physician-in-ordinary to the Emperor Charles. Correspondence). *Sci. Hist.*, *1*, 177–90.

39 MEYER, I. de (1845). Corneille van Baersdorp. *Ann de la Soc. Méd-chir.*, *VI*, 32 pp. portr.

40 BARUCH, J. Z. (1964). *Guillaume de Baillou en zijn betekenis voor de reumatologie*. (G. de B. and his significance for rheumatology). 85 pp. "De Tijdstroom", Lochem.

41 — (1965). Guillaume de Baillou, voorloper van de moderne reumatologie. (G. de B., precursor of modern rheumatology). *NTG*, *109*, 2086–91; *BGG*, *XLV*, 27–32, portr.

42 — (1973). De betekenis van Guillaume de Baillou voor de rheumatologie (Significance of G. de B. for rheumatology). *Arts en Auto*, 39, nr. 1, 21–3.

43 VRIJER, M. J. A. de (1928). *Ds. Petrus van Balen. Medicinae et Juris Doctor, Ambassade- en Hofprediker in de gouden eeuw*. (Minister of the embassy and the court in the Golden Age). 8°, Utrecht.

44 ANDEL, M. A. van (1937). Uit het dagboek van dr. Jelle Banga, die van 1807–1870 te Franeker practiseerde. (From the diary of dr. J. B.,

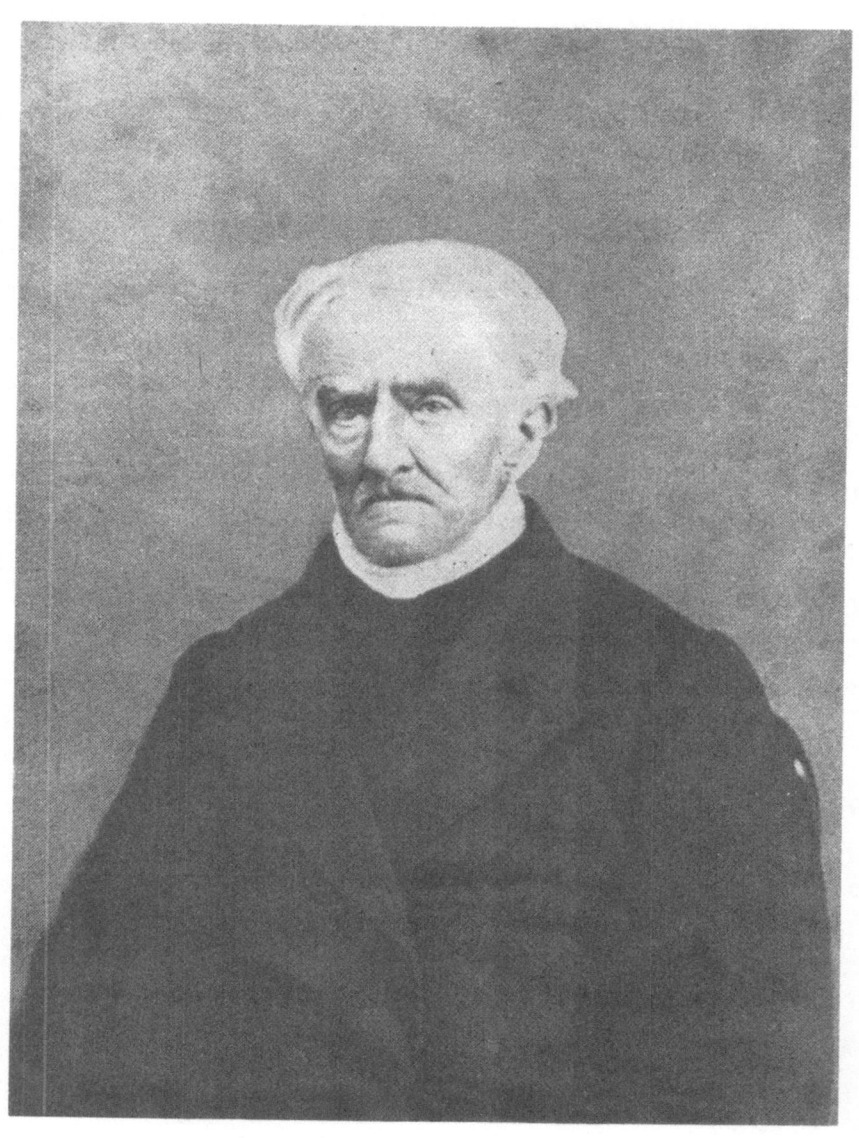

J. Banga (1786–1877)

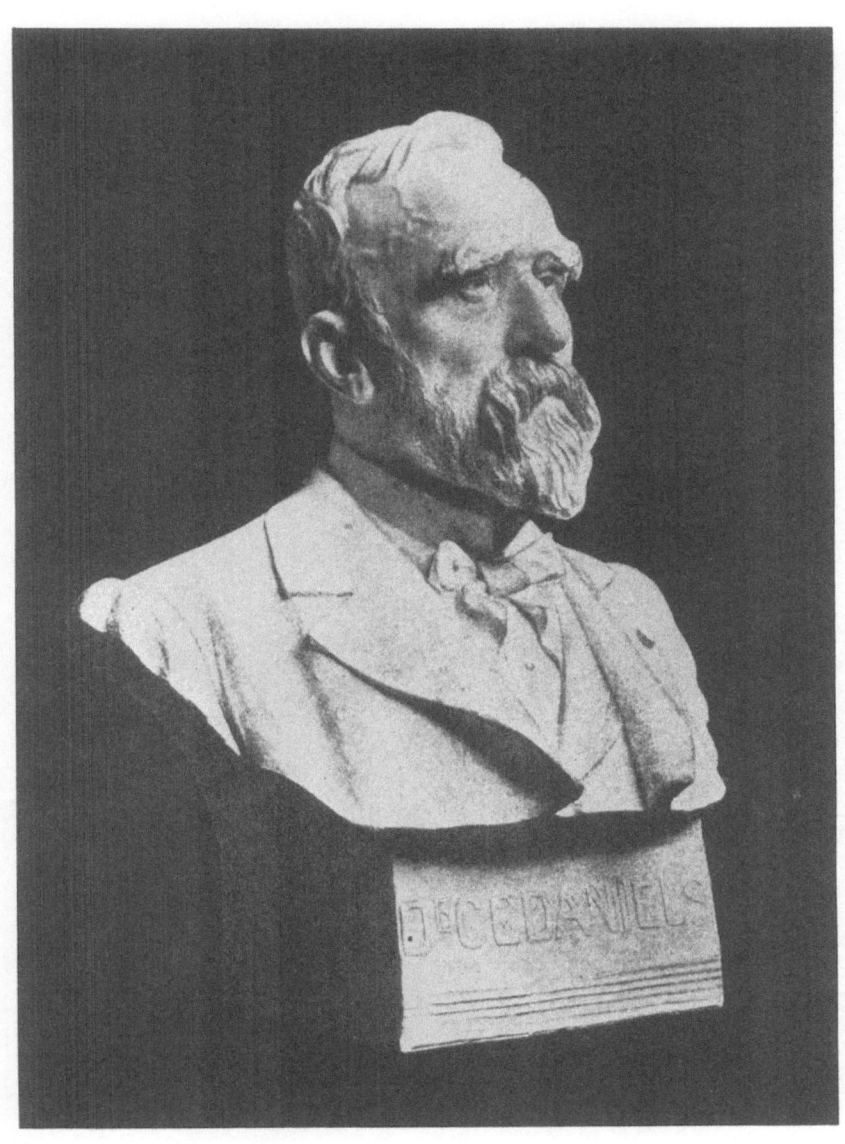

C. E. Daniëls (1839–1921)

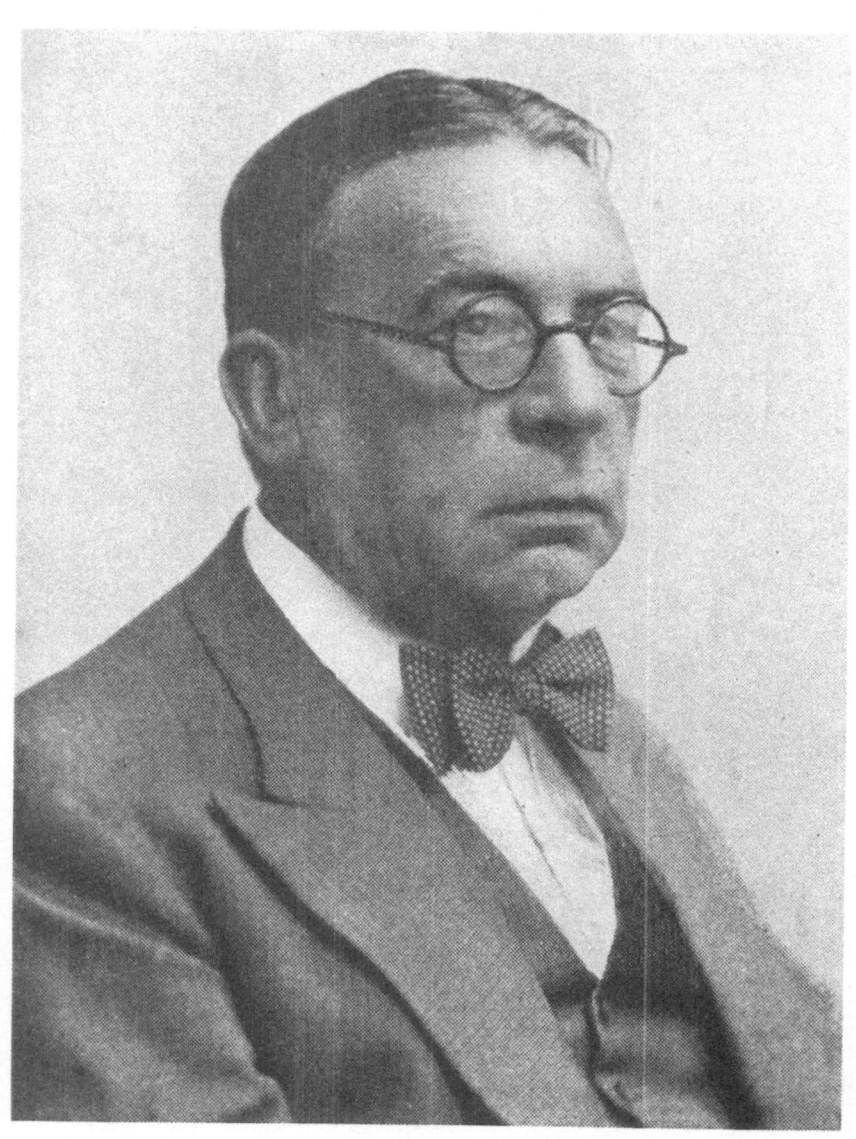

M. A. van Andel (1878–1941)

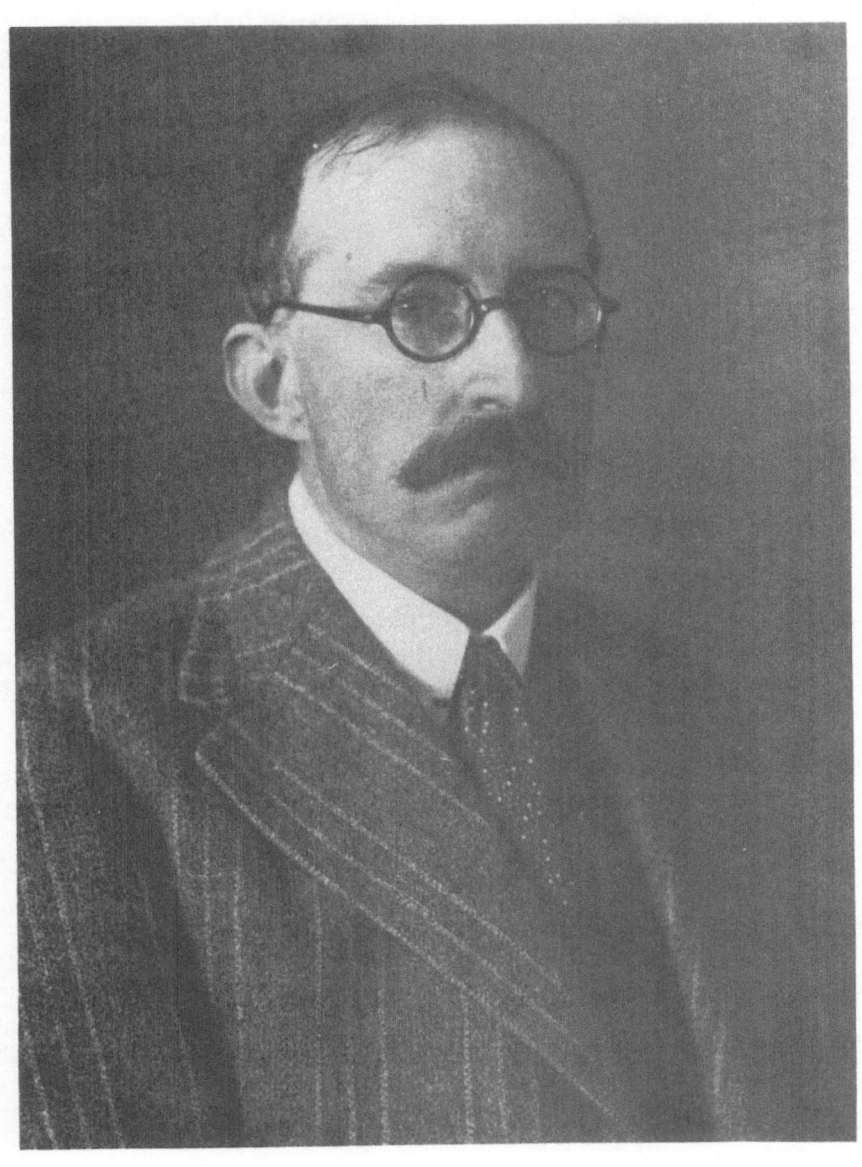

E. D. Baumann (1883–1966)

who practised from 1807–1870 at F.). *NTG, 81*, I, 41–52; *BGG, XVII*, 1–12, port.

45   Best, C. H. (1969). Frederick Grant Banting. *Voeding, 30*, 137–43, portr.
    – From: *Obituary Notices of Fellows of the Royal Society, 4* (1942), 21–6.

46   [Editorial] (1972). Het laboratorium van Banting en Best. (The laboratory of Banting and Best). *GG, 3*, 10. ill.

47   Mildner, T. (1963). Krebsmittel bei Paul Barbette. *Deutsch. med. J. 14*, 542–8.

48   Ridell, William Renvich (1927). Some cases of a noted heelmeester (Surgeon) *Med. J. and Record, 127*, 607
    – On the Amsterdam physician Paul Barbette (1629–99) and his therapeutic measures.
    See also 1595, 3227.5

49   Spronsen, J. W. van (1966). Barchusen 1666–1723. De eerste Utrechtse chemie-hoogleraar, Johann Conrad Barchusen, werd 300 jaar geleden geboren. (The first Utrecht professor of chemistry, J.C.B., born 300 years ago). *Chem. Wbl., 62*, 604–6, ill.

50   Hannaway, O. (1967). Johann Conrad Barchusen (1666–1723). Contemporary and rival of Boerhaave. *Ambix, 14*, 96–111, portr.

51   Lindeboom, G. A. (1970). Barchusen and Boerhaave. *Janus, LVII*, 30–41, ill.

52   — (1971). Barchusen, rivaal van Boerhaave?. (Barchusen, rival of Boerhaave?). *Chem. Wbl., 67*, 10–2, ill.

53   Leersum, E. C. van (1916). Thomas Bartholin. *NTG, 60*, II, 1885–9.

54   Porter, I. H. (1963). Thomas Bartholin (1616–80) and Niels Stensen (1638–86) master and pupil. *Med. Hist., VII*, 99–125, 2 portrs., 2 ill.

55   Molhuysen, P. C. (1916). Quatre lettres de Thomas Bartholin. *Janus, XXI*, 371–7.

56   Petersen, Jul. (1909). Der Kreis der Bartholiner und die Holländische Medizin. *Janus, XIV*, 457–66.

57   Rochat, G. F. (1917). De oogheelkunde van George Bartisch. (Ophthalmology of George Bartisch). *NTG, 51*, II, 1106–8.

58   Halbertsma, K. T. A. (1937). *Georg Bartisch (1535–1607) en zijn werk.* (— and his work), Delft, 8°, ill.

59 GOEMANS, M. (1951). De H. Basilius de Grote en de geneeskunde. (St. Basilius the Great and medicine). Dekker & van de Vegt, Nijmegen.
– Address.

60 ROMIJN, H. M. (1972). Libavius' mening over Basilius Valentinus. (L's opinion on —) PhW, 107, 499–502.

61 BENTHEIM JUTTING, W. S. S. and C. M. van Hoorn (1967). Oude en nieuwe gegevens over leven en arbeid van dr. Job Baster (1711–1755). (Old and new data on life and work of dr. J. B.). Arch. Zeeuwsch Gen., 29–70, 6 ill.

62 PAUW-de Veen, L. de (1964). Baten (Battus, Batin), Carel (Carolus). Nationaal Biografisch Woordenboek (Brussels), I, col. 79–82.

63 BAUMANN, E. D. (1918). Carel Baten. 36 pp. Van Loghum Slaterus & Visser, Arnhem. 8°.

64 BONTINCK, E. D. (1938). Het "secreet-boek" van Carel Baten [Ghent c. 1540-Amsterdam c. 1617] (The "Secret-book" of C.B.) MKVAW, 801–20.

65 ROOSEBOOM, Maria (1966). Dr. E. D. Baumann 1883–1966. GeWiNa, 20 (sept.). 22–3.

66 HOEVEN, J. van der (1933). De steen- en breuksnijder Jacques de Beaulieu te Rotterdam in 1699 (The lithotomist and herniotomist J. de B. at R. in 1699). Rotterd. Jbk., 24, vierde reeks, N.S. 1, 57–62, portr.
– reviewed by J. G. de Lint: NTG, 77 (1933), 4591; BGG, XIII, 237.

67 — (1936). Een onbekend portret van Jacques de Beaulieu (An unknown portrait of —). NTG, 80, I, 988–9; BGG, XVI, 40–1.

68 MOONEN, W. A. (1968). Frère Jacques de Beaulieu, een veel omstreden periodeut (1651–1714). (—, a much contested periodeut). NTG, 112, 25–32, ill.

69 SCHMITZ-CLIEVER, E. (1964). Der Bruch- und Steinschneider Jacques Beaulieu (Frère Jacques") in der Reichsstadt Aachen (1698). SA, 48, 18–26.

70 —, und Herta Schmitz-Cliever (1972). Die Ikonografie des Steinschneiders Jacques Beaulieu (1651–1714). Mediz. hist. J., 7, 84–102, 10 ill.

71 LINDEBOOM, G. A. (1953). William Beaumont. *NTG, 97*, III, 2021–7, 1 ill. + portr. *BGG, XXXIII*, 49–55. Also in: *Voeding, 17* (1956), 363–71.

72 SCHEVENSTEEN, A. F. C. van (1936). Levensschets van Goropius Becanus, geneesheer-philoloog (Biographical sketch of —, physician-philologist). *Vlaamsch Geneesk. T.* nr. 14, 3–12.

73 FREDERICKX, E. (1972). Ioannes Goropius Becanus, Arts, Linguist, Graecus (—, Physician, philologist, Graecus). *Hermèneus, 43*, 129–36, portr. – *See also* A. Ham (1973): *AP* no 11, 41.

74 KRUYTZER, E. M. (1962). Dokter Beckers honderd jaar geleden geleden geboren (Dr. —, born 100 years ago). *Natuurhist. Mbl. 51*, 95–101, portr.

75 HOEVEN, J. van der (1933). Een brief van Justinus van Assche aan Isaäc Beeckman. (A letter of J.v.A. to —). *NTG, 77*, I, 66–72; *BGG, XIII*, 17–23.

76 BEECKMAN, Isaac (1939–53). *Journal tenu de 1604 à 1634.* Publié avec une introduction et des notes par C. de Waard. 4 vol^s (I–IV) Nijhoff. The Hague, ill.

77 OOSTERHUIS, R. A. Benthem (1941). Emil von Behring 1854–1917. *Timotheus,* 5 april.

78 KLOOSTERMAN, G. J. and J. G. Stolk (1959). Inleiding tot het Dr. J. C. Beker–nummer (Introduction to the Dr. J. C. Beker issue). *NTVerl. Gyn. 59*, 81–97, portr.
    – Survey of the work of —, with bibliography.

79 HARTOG, C. den (1965). Stanley Rossiter Benedict, 1884–1936. *Voeding, 26*, 86.

80 NUYENS, B. W. Th. (1915). Ant. Benivenius van Florence. Een patholoog-anatoom uit de 15de eeuw. (A pathologist-anatomist from the 15th century). *NTG, 59*, II, 714–26.

81 OUDSCHANS DENTZ, Fr. (1942). Eenige bladzijden uit het leven van Dr. G. C. Berch Gravenhorst. (Some pages from the life of —). *NTG, 86*, II, 1430–6; *BGG, XXII*, 81–7.

82 POLAK, A. (1961). Berczeller 1855–1955). *Voeding, 22*, 594.

83 LEERSUM, E. C. van (1916). In Memoriam W. S. van den Berg. *NTG, 60*, I, 1309.

84 [   ] (1967). H. Berger, uitvinder van de EEG. (H.B., the inventor of the EEG). *T. Ziekenverpl. 20*, 560.

85 VERBIEST, H. (1964). *Claude Bernard en de functionele neurochirurgie* (— — and functional neurosurgery). 36 pp. Scheltema & Holkema, Amsterdam. Address.

86 SLUITER, E. (1955). Claude Bernard 1813–1878. *Voeding, 16*, 499–502, portr.

87 DOUMA, Sj. (1939). *Johannes Stephanus Bernard "Medicus en philoloog", 1718–1793.* (J.S.B. "Physician and philologist"). Thesis Groningen (supervisor: Groeneboom), 104 pp. Assen.
   – see on Bernard, an Amsterdam physician, also: Martin Plessner. (Bruchstücke lateinischer Übersetzungen des 18. Jahrhunderts aus Ibn Abi Usaibi'as Ärztebiographien) in *Medizingeschichte in unserer Zeit* (Festgabe E. Heischkel-Artelt und W. Artelt), Stuttgart, 1971, p. 225-6.

88 ITTERSON, G. van, L. E. Dooren de Jong and A. J. Kluyver (1940). *Martinus Willem Beijerinck. His life and his work.* XI + 192 pp., 13 pl., portr., 8°. Den Haag.

89 [Editorial] (1963). Martinus Willem Beijerinck (1851–1931). *JAMA, 185* (1), 40–1, 4 refs.

90 KLINKENBERG, G. A. van (1967). De grootvader van de chromato-grafie. De micro-analytische techniek van de geldiffusie, die pas na de tweede oorlog in gebruik is genomen, werd 80 jaar geleden al door M. W. Beyerinck (1851–1931) op grote schaal toegepast. (The grand-father of chromatography. The micro-analytical technique of gel-diffusion, which came into use after the second world-war, was em-ployed in a large way already 80 years ago by M.W.B.). *Chem. Wbl., 63*, 66–7., portr.
   – B. was the first to describe, in 1898, the mozaic virus in the tobaccoplant.

JOHAN VAN BEVERWIJCK

91 KRUL, R. (1893). Dr. Johan van Beverwijck. *NTG, 29*, I, 921–32.

92 BAUMANN, E. D. (1910). *Johan van Beverwijck in leven en werken ge-schetst.* (J.v.B., sketched in life and works). Thesis University of Am-dam (Supervisor: Ruitenga), 311 pp. J. P. Revers, Dordrecht.
   – With bibliography —.

93 — (1959). Johan van Beverwijck, 1594–1647. *Voeding, 20*, 51–7, portr.

94 GEYL, A. (1911). De promotor van van Beverwijck. (The "supervisor" of —). *NTG*, *55*, I, 1591.

95 LEERSUM, E. C. van (1911). De promotor van van Beverwijck. (The "supervisor" of —). *NTG*, *55*, I, 1591.

96 VARLEY, D. H. (1959). On the arteries of the human arm, from Johan van Beverwijck's „Wercken der Geneeskonst", Amsterdam, 1672. *Trans. Coll. phys. Surg. Gyn. S. Afr.*, *3*, 50–1, ill.

97 BEVERWIJCK, J. van (1640, 1641, 1643, 1935). *Briefwisseling tussen Joh. van Beverwijck, Descartes, V. F. Plemp, Guy Patin en Corn. van Someren.* (Correspondence between J.v.B., Descartes, Plemp, Patin and Van Someren). – with German translation. *Opusc.*, *XIII*, 121–214.
    – On heart action, circulation, renal calculi and bladder stones.

98 — (1652, 1943). *Steen-stuck.* (Treatise on the stone). – With English translation. *Opusc.*, *XVII*, 10–129.
    See also 3227.6

99 BEEKMAN, F. (1935). Bidloo and Cowper. *Ann. Med. Hist.*, n.s. *VII*, 113–29, ill., portr.

100 BROEK, A. J. P. van der (1942). Bidloo en Cowper. Een bijdrage tot de kennis van "plagiaat" en uitgeverij aan het einde van de 18e eeuw. (A contribution to the knowledge of "plagiarism" and publishing at the end of the 17th and the beginning of the 18th century). *NTG*, *86*, II, 1421–6; *BGG*, *XXII*, 72–7.

101 VASBINDER, W. (1948). *Govard Bidloo en William Cowper.* Thesis Utrecht (supervisor: J. Boeke). 248 pp. ill. Utrecht.

102 HERRLINGER, R. (1966). Bidloo's "Anatomia" – Prototyp barocker Illustration? *Gesnerus*, *23*, 40–7, 8ill.
    – The illustrations by Gerard van Lairesse in B's *Anatomia* are an utterance of the classicistic French academy-graphic art.

103 OBORIN, N. A. and A. N. (1971). Anonymous scientific advance. (History of the translation into Russian of Godfried Bidloo's "Anatomia humani Corporis" at the beginning of the 18th century. [Russian]. *Arkh. Anat. Gistol. Embriol.*, *60* (2), 91–7.

104 BIDLOO, G. (1698, 1972). *Letter to Anthony van Leeuwenhoek about the animals which are sometimes found in the liver of sheep and other beasts.* With a new English translation, an introduction and annotations by

J. Jansen. 103 pp. Dutch Classics in History of Science, nr. 18, De Graaf, Nieuwkoop.

105 — (1685, 1972). *Anatomia Humani Corporis*. Joannis à Someren, Amsterdam. Roger Dacosta, Parijs (1972). f°.

– a photostatic reprint of Bidloo's famous atlas, with a short biography and an iconography of B. by Pierre Huard.

106 BOGOIAVLENSKII, N. A. (1966). Student handwritten textbook on human anatomy from the Moscow Medical School of Nikolai Bidloo. [Russian]. *Arkh. Anat. Gistol. Embriol.*, *51*, 108–11.

– Nikolaus Bidloo (*ca.* 1674–1735) was a nephew of Govert Bidloo, who went to Russia in 1703.

107 OBORIN, N. A. (1969). The 1st manual on surgery in Russia (260th anniversary of the Moscow School of Medicine and Surgery and 255th of the 1st licensure of Russian surgeons. Nicolaus Bidloo. [Russian]. *Khirurgiya* (Mosk.), *45*, May, 148–54.

108 DANKMEIJER, J. and Th. Röell (1970). Nicolaas Bidloo and the institution of medical education in Moscow. In: G. A. Lindeboom (ed.). *Boerhaave and His Time*. Analecta Boerhaaviana VI, 165–79, 8 ill., Brill, Leiden.

109 ZIKEEV, P. D. (1973). Bidloo, Peter I's private physician. [Russian]. *Klin. Med.* (Mosk.), *51* (3), 146–9.

110 BOEREMA, I. (1956). Theodor Billroth. *NTG*, *100*, II, 1313–7; *BGG*, *XXXVI*, 31–5. portr.
also in: *Arch. chir. néerl.*, *8*, 396–400, portr.

111 FOKKER, A. A. (1865). Louis de Bils en zijn tijd. (L.d.B. and his time). *NTG*, I, II, 167-220.

112 JANSMA, J. R. (1919). *Louis de Bils en de anatomie van zijn tijd*. (L.d.B. and the anatomy of his time). Thesis Utrecht, (supervisor: J. Boeke), 115 pp., ill., Pet, Hoogeveen.

113 LAMERS, A. J. M. (1920). Lodewijk de Bils. Professor in de anatomie aan de Illustre School te 's-Hertogenbosch (1669). (Professor of anatomy at the Illustrious School at Bois-le-Duc). *Taxandria*, *27* (3de reeks, 7), 72–83.

114 ERDMAN, A. M. (1969). Max Oskar Bircher-Benner, 1867–1939. *Voeding*, *30*, 1–9, portr.

115 BOER, J. G. de (1972). Greene Vardiman Black, grondlegger van de

moderne parodontologie. (G.V.B., founder of modern parodontology). *Ned. T. Tandheelk.*, *79*, 11-6.

116 SCHIERBEEK, A. (1942). Over enkele tot heden onbekend gebleven handschriften van Stephaan Blankaart (24 Oct. 1650 - 23 Febr. 1704). (On some unknown manuscripts of —. *NTG*, *86*, 3069-75; *BGG*, *XXII*, 147-53.

117 HOFMEIER, H. K. (1966). Stephan Blancaards Ansichten über Ernährung und Aufziehen der kleinen Kinder. *Klin. Med. Monatschr.*, 356-9.

118 BLANKAART, Stefaan (1633, 1967). *De borgerlyke Tafel.* Om lang Sonder Ziekten Gesond te Leven. Waar in van yder spijse in 't besonder gehandelt werd, door —, M.D. (The Common Table. To live long and healthy without diseases. Wherein every food is dealt with). Facsimile of the 1633 edition. 8 + 192 + 16 pp., Hollandia, Baarn.

119 — (1684, 1966). *Verhandelinge van de opvoeding en ziekten der kinderen.* (Treatise on education and diseases of children) Facsimile of the 1674 edition. 352 pp., Hollandia, Baarn.
See also 699, 3227.9

120 GRENDEL, E. (1967). Dr. Bleeker en potio Bleekeri. *Ph.W. 101* (1966), 664-9; *Bull. Pharm.* no. 37, 1-5, ill.

121 BÁNKI, Ö. (1939). Het levenswerk van professor Jan Bleuland en zijn leerling en prosector *Petrus Koning*, alsmede een tentoonstelling. The life-work of professor J.B. and his pupil and prosector *P.K.* as well as an exhibition). *NTG*, *83*, III, 3838-44, ill.
– J. Bleuland (1756-1838), professor at Utrecht 1795-1826.

122 MEINERS, J. W. F. (1961). Een Utrechts hoogleraar-kunstverzamelaar in de Franse tijd. (A Utrecht professor-art collector in the French time. *Oud Utrecht*, *34*, 1-5, ill.

123 BIK, J. G. W. F. (1962). Doctor Jan Bleuland, hoogleraar te Harderwijk en Utrecht, 1756-1838. (—, professor at Harderwijk and Utrecht). *NTG*, *106*, I, 476-82; *BGG*, *XLII*, 8-14; also in: *GeWiNa*, no *10*, 13-4·

124 GILS, J. B. F. van (1941). De grafschriften van Dr. Martinus Herculanus Blonck. (The epitaphs of Dr. —). *NTG*. *85*, 3934-6; *BGG*, *XXI*, 142-4, 2 ill.

HERMAN BOERHAAVE

Biographica

125 KROON, J. E. (1916). Boerhaaviana. *NTG, 60*, II, 1745–6.

126 — (1919). Boerhaave als hoogleraar-promotor. (Boerhaave as Professor-Supervisor). *NTG, 63*, I, 87.

127 — (1918). Boerhaave as Professor-Promotor. *Janus, XXIII*, 291–311.

128 — (1922). Het "kasboek" van Boerhaave met beschrijving van Poelgeest en aankoop daarvan. (The "cash-book" of B. with description of Poelgeest and the purchase of it). *NTG, 66*, II, 559–65; *BGG, II*, 175–81.
  – B.P.L. no. 2196 Bibl. Lugd. Bat.

129 HAES, R. L. de (1918). Boerhaave als humorist. (— as a humorist). *Navorscher, LXVII*, 273.
  – with postscript of M. G. Wildeman.

130 LEERSUM, E. C. van (1912). Hoe sprak Boerhaave? (How did B. speak) *NTG, 66*, I, 657–64.

131 — (1912). How did Boerhaave speak? *Janus, XVII*, 145–52, 1 ill.

132 — (1916). Boerhaaviana. I. Een tweetal Collegelijsten van Boerhaave. (I. Two lecture-lists of Boerhaave). *NTG, 60*, II, 1480–90. II. Een proeve van Boerhaave's rijmkunst. (II. A sample of B.'s art of rhyming). *NTG, 60*, II, 1557–61. III. Uit Boerhaave's praktijk. (From B.'s practice). *NTG, 60*, II, 1712–9.
  See also 228, 1666

133 — (1916). Boerhaaviana. I. Boerhaave et la poésie. *Janus, XXI*, 445–9.

134 BISSELING, G. H. (1921). Een protest van Boerhaave. (A protest of B.). *NTG, 65*, I, 686; *BGG, I*, 100.
  – The advertisement of Boerhaave of 21 Oct. 1726 against the publishing of unauthorized editions of his works and lecture-notes.

135 EEGHEN, I. H. van (1950). Leidse professoren en het auteursrecht in de achttiende eeuw (Leyden professors and copyright in the 18th century). *Econ. Hist. Jbk., 24*, 179–208.

136 WALSEM, G. C. van (1931). Boerhaaviana. *GG, 9*, 874–7, 1 ill.

137 SCHULTE, J. E. (1938). Herman Boerhaave en de classieke vorming van

den arts. (H.B. and the classical education of the physician). *NTG*, *82*, IV, 4912; *BGG*, *XVIII*, 280.

138 PENNING, C. P. J. (1938). De promotie van Boerhaave te Harderwijk. (The graduation of — at Harderwijk). *NTG*, *82*, IV, 4895–9; *BGG*, *XVIII*, 263–7.

- Address, delivered on September 24, 1938, at Harderwijk.

139 SCHOUTE, D. (1946). Boerhaave's karakter. (B.'s character). *NTG*, *90*, I, 65–7; *BGG*, *XXVI*, 1–3.

140 SCHLICHTING, Th. H. (1955). Boerhaave als pathograaf. (B. as a writer of pathographies). *NTG*, *99*, III, 2652–9; *BGG*, *XXXV*, 77–84.

141 BLACK, D. A. K. (1959). Johnson on Boerhaave. *Med. Hist.*, *3*, 325–9.

141ª [Anonym] (1952). Een oordeel over Boerhaave uit 1712 (A judgement on — from 1712). *Amstelodamum*, *39*, 104.

142 HERMANS, A. G. J. (1962). Boerhaave en de oude Griekse Genees-kunde. (Boerhaave and the ancient Greek medicine). *NTG. 106*, I, 1201–2; *BGG*, *XLII*, 28–9.

- Letter to the editor, referring to Lindeboom's article with the same title. (*See* 151)

143 HESS, W. C. (1962). Samuel Johnson's life of Boerhaave. *Georgetown med. Bull.*, *15*, 256–8.

144 LINDEBOOM, G. A. (1955). De kijk van Busken Huet op Boerhaave. (The view of Busken Huet on B.). *T. v. Geschiedenis*, *LXIII*, 205–12.

145 — (1955). Boerhaave's ziekten. (Illnesses of B.). *NTG*, *99* 3519–30; *BGG*, *XXXV*, 93–104.

146 — (1956). Boerhaave's rijkdom. (B.'s wealth). *NTG*, *100*, I, 919–28; *BGG*, *XXXVI*, 12–21.

147 — (1956). Beter beeld van Boerhaave. (Better image of Boerhaave). *Elseviers Wbl.*, 21 january.

148 — (1957). Boerhaave als Christen. (B. as a Christian). *G&W*, *55*, 137–49.

149 — (1958). Boerhaave in het weeshuis. (B. in the orphanage). *NTG*, *102*, I, 1158–9; *BGG*, *XXXVIII*, 10–1.

149ª SCHOUTEN, J. (1974). The "mystery" illness. [Boerhaave and an epidemic of hysteria]. *JAMA*, no *227*, 324.

150 LINDEBOOM, G. A. (1961–3). Boerhaave and the ancient Greek writers on medicine. *Janus, L,* 25–37, ill.

151 — (1962). Boerhaave en de oude Griekse geneeskunde. (Boerhaave and the ancient Greek medicine). *NTG, 106,* I, 28–30; *BGG, XLII,* 1–3.

152 — (1966). Oosterse vertalingen van Boerhaave. (Oriental translations). *GeWiNa, 20,* 21.

153 — (1968–9). Boerhaave in Harderwijk. *Gelre, LXIII,* 103–17.

154 — (1972). Mensen om Boerhaave. I. Herman Boerhaave. (Men around B.). I. — *GG, 2,* 51–3, ill.

155 — (1974). Boerhaave: Author and Editor. *Bull. Med. Libr. Ass., 62,* no. 2, 137–48.

156 LEERSUM, E. C. van (1919). H. Boerhaave. *NTG, 63,* I, 1–12.

157 — (1924). Herman Boerhaave. In: *NNBW, VI,* col., 127–41.

157ᵃ WIERSUM, E. van (1932). De dure Boerhaave (The expensive Boerhaave) *Rott. Jbk,* IIIe reeks, *10,* 186.
   – on a protocol drawn up for Gommer van Bortel on the high bills sent to him by B. [Rotterdam Municipal Archive]

158 GRENDEL, E. (1968). Verslag door een tijdgenoot van een consult bij Professor Boerhaave. (Report by a contemporary of a consultation at —). *NTG, 112,* I, 42–4, 3 fig.

159 MARX, O. M. (1968). M. Boerhaave en Europe: the origins of an anecdote explained? *J. Hist. Med., 23,* 389.

160 ELAUT, L. (1969). Boerhaaviana uit 1968. (Boerhaaviana from 1968). *Sci. Hist., 11,* 84–90.

161 HOVESEN, E. (1971). Herman Boerhaave (1668–1738). *Med. Forum* (Copenh.), nr. 4, 119–26, ill, portr.
   – Kbh. Univ. med.-hist. Inst. Mus. Årsberetu, 1971.

162 LINDEBOOM, G. A. (ed.) (1970). *Boerhaave and His Time.* Papers read at the international symposium in commemoration of the tercentenary of Boerhaave's birth, Leyden 15–16 November 1968. (*Analecta Boerhaaviana VI*). 174 pp., ill. Brill, Leiden.
   – reviewed by G. B. Risse: *J. Hist. Med., 29* (1974), 432–3.

163 — (1970). De mysterieuse glans van Boerhaave's naam (The mysterious splendour of B.'s name). *Gids, 133,* 211–9.

164 — (1970). Herman Boerhaave. In: C. C. Gillispie (ed.) *Dictionary of Scientific Biography*, Vol. *II*, 224–8. Scribner's Sons, New York.

165 — (1971). Boerhaave en Descartes. *G&W*, *69*, 153–66.

166 NOVAK, Alfred (1971). Boerhaave: Three chairs to Oblivion. *Bioscience*, *21*, 479–82.

167 GUNST, J. W. 1934. *Herman Boerhaave*, 145 pp., portr., Punt. Leiden. – Dutch.

168 MÜLLER, M. (1935). Boerhaave. *Pharma-Medico*, *3*, 96–100.

169 WELLS, R. V. (1957). Hermann Boerhaave. *School Sci. Rev.*, *38*, (136), 324–34.

170 BOCHALLI, R. (1957). Hermann Boerhaave, praeceptor totius mundi. *Med. Monschr. 11*, 459–61.

171 MEURS, G. J. (1959). Herman Boerhaave. *Voeding*, *20*, 2–9, portr.

171 JONAS, [   ] (1960). Herman Boerhaave (1668–1738). *Ars Medici*, *15*, 693–6, portr.

173 KING, L. S. (1962). Herman Boerhaave. *JAMA*, *180*, 240–1. – Editorial.

174 JANSSEN, Paul (1968). *Herman Boerhaave.* Actuele Onderwerpen Reeks, nr. 1229, 16 pp., 8 ill., Stichting IVIO, Amsterdam.

175 KAISER, W. and W. Piechocki (1938). Hermann Boerhaave (1668–1738). *Med. Bild, 12* (3), 81–5, ill., portrs.

176 LINDEBOOM, G. A. (1956). Herman Boerhaave. *Therapeutische Mededelingen*, *21*, 27–31.
– Also in the French and German edition of this journal.

177 — (1968). Herman Boerhaave (1668–1738), Teacher of All Europe. *JAMA*, *206*, 2297–2301.

178 — (1968). *Herman Boerhaave. The Man and His Work.* XX + 452 pp., ill., Methuen & Co., London, 8°.
– with a foreword by E. Ashworth Underwood.

See also 858, 5124, 5407

Relatives

179 SCHIMMELPENNINCK VAN DER OYE VAN DE POLL en NYENBEEK, (1904). Boerhaave en zijn nazaten uit Oud-Geldersche geslachten. (B. and his descendants from Old-Gueldrian families). *Geldersche Volksalmanak*, 3.

180 BARGE, J. A. J. (1925). Het nakroost van Boerhaave. (The descendants of —). *Pallas Leidensis.*

181 BIJLEVELD, W. J. C. C. (1939). Boerhaave's schoonzoon. (B's son-in-law). *Leidsch Jbkje*, *31*, 157–76.
   – Count de Thoms (1696–1746).

182 DOMMELEN, J. van (1917). "Boerhaave-huis" en hervormde kerk te Voorhout bij Leiden. ("Boerhaave-house" and the reformed church at Voorhout near Leyden). *Buiten*, *11*, 268–9.

Commemorations

183 LEERSUM, E. C. van (1918). Herman Boerhaave (31 Dec. 1668–23 Sept. 1738). *Janus, XXIII*, 193–222.

184 DIERGART, Paul (1919). Zur Erinnerung an Hermannus Boerhaave (Geb. 1668 zu Voorhout bei Leiden, gest. 1738 zu Leiden). *Ztschr. angew. Chemie*, *32*, I, 58–9.

185 HUNGER, F. W. T. (1919). Boerhaave-herdenking. *Leids Jbk., XVI*, 42.

186 [Editorial] (1938). Boerhaave Bicentenary. *Ann. Med. Hist.* n.s. *X*, 458–9.

187 ARTELT, W. (1938). Herman Boerhaave. *Z. ärztl. Fortbild.*, *35*, 569–71, 4 ill.

188 ATZROTT, E. H. G. (1938). Herman Boerhaave. Das Bild des volkommenen Arztes. *DMW.*, *64*, 1882–4, 1 ill.

189 LINT, J. G. de (1929). Discours commémoratif de Boerhaave (19 juillet). *VIᵐᵉ Congrès Int. d'Hist. de la Méd. Leyde-Amsterdam 1927*, 79–81, Anvers.

190 NACHMANSON, E. (1939). Herman Boerhaave. Ett Jvåhundraårsminne. *Med. Föreningens Tidskrift*, nr. 2, 1–8.

191 OOSTERHUIS, R. A. B. (1938). Hermanus Boerhaave (1668–1738). Bij de herdenking van den 200sten sterfdag op 23 September 1938 van den beroemden geneesheer en geleerde (At the commemoration of the

200th anniversary of the dying-day, September 23, 1738 of the famous physician and scientist). *Stemmen des Tijds*, Oct., 263–88.

192 — (1938). Professor Hermanus Boerhaave, de beroemdste nederland-sche geneesheer (— the most famous Dutch physician). *Timotheus*, 5 pp., Sept.

193 PACKARD, Fr. (ed.) (1938). Hermann Boerhaave (1668–1738). The Dutch Hippocrates. *Ann. Med. Hist.*, n.s. *X*, 356–7.

194 RIJNBERK, G. van (1938). Boerhaave: *NTG*, *82*, IV, 4779–80; *BGG*, *XVIII*, 173–4.

195 — and E. Sluiter (1938). Boerhaave. (De Boerhaave-herdenking. Leiden – 23 en 24 September 1938 – Harderwijk) (commemoration). *NTG*, *82*, IV, 4779–85; *BGG*, *XVIII*, 269–77.

196 SCHOUTE, D. (1938). Boerhaave-herdenkingsrede te Leiden op 23 September 1938. (commemoration oration). *NTG*, *82*, IV, 4807–22; *BGG*, *XVIII*, 175–90.

197 SCHULTE, J. E. (1938). Herman Boerhaave herdacht. (B. commemorat-ed). *GG*, *16*, 1022–34.

198 TAMINIAU, Ph. L. M. M. (1938). Eenige historische bijzonderheden uit den tijd der oprichting van het standbeeld van Herman Boerhaave. (Some historical details from the time of the erection of the statue of —). *NTG*, *82*, IV, 4909–11; *BGG*, *XVIII*, 277–9.

199 [Various authors] (1939). *Memorialia Herman Boerhaave optimi medici.*, 133 pp., Bohn. Haarlem.
 – Addresses delivered on 23 and 24 September 1938 at Leyden and Harderwijk.

200 SIGERIST, H. E. (1939). A Boerhaave pilgrimage in Holland. *BHM*, *VII*, 1, 258–75, 14 ill.

201 HOFFMANN, K. F. (1939). Herman Boerhaave, der grosze Naturfor-scher und Arzt. *Korresp. bl. Zahnärzte*, *63*, 125–30.

202 DONGEN, J. A. van (1959). Boerhaave en zijn nagedachtenis. (B. and his memory). *NTG*, *103*, II, 1810; *BGG*, *XXXIX*, 12.
 – In this note the author joins J. E. Schulte in his appeal to restore the Caecilia Gasthuis where Boerhaave taught bedside medicine.

203 [   ] (1968). Boerhaave-Symposium, Leiden, November 14–16, 1968. *Clio Med.*, *4*, 57–8.

204 FOX, J. (1968). *Herman Boerhaave driehonderd jaar geleden te Voorhout geboren*. (B., 300 years ago born at Voorhout). Herdenking (Commemoration) te Voorhout 15 November 1968, Pamflet 4 pp., (to the cover). Publication of the Zuid-Holland Historical Association under the device "Vigilate Deo confidentes".

205 ROOSEBOOM, Maria (1968). *Herman Boerhaave 1668–1968. Tentoonstelling* 14 juni – 1 december. Rijksmuseum voor de Geschiedenis der Natuurwetenschappen Leiden 1968. Mededeling no. 136). National Museum for the History of Science, Leiden 1968. Bulletin no. 136), 54 pp., 24 ill. Leiden (Exhibition).

206 SASSEN, F. L. R. and J. Dankmeijer (1968). *Herman Boerhaave 1668–1968*. Leidsche Voordrachten, 48, 40 pp., Universitaire Pers, Leiden.
– Sassen: Het geestelijk klimaat te Leiden ten tijde van Boerhaave. (The intellectual climate at Leyden in the time of B.) Dankmeijer: Is Boerhaave's faam gerechtvaardigd? (Is B.'s fame justified?).

207 SPRONSEN, J. W. van (1968). Boerhaave 300 jaar geleden geboren; herdenking in tentoonstelling te Leiden (B. born 300 years ago; commemoration in an exhibition at Leyden). *ChemWbl.*, no. 43, 19–23.

208 UNDERWOOD, E. Ashworth (1968). Boerhaave after Three Hundred Years. *Brit. Med. J.*, IV, 820–4 (28 December).

209 [editorial] (1969). Herman Boerhaave. *Endeavour, 28*, 2.

210 FRANKL, J. (1969). Remembering Boerhaave. [Magyar]. *Orv. Hetil, 110*, 1759–61.

211 ROCCHIETTA, S. (1969). Nel 3 centenario della nascita. Contributi chimici di Hermann Boerhaave (1668–1738). *Minerva Med. 60*, 2122–3.

212 OOSTERHUIS, R. A. B. (1969). Het nieuwe boek van Prof. Dr. G. J. [sic!] Lindeboom over Hermannus Boerhaave. (The new book of Prof. L. on H.B.). *Natura Docet, 21*, no. 6, 188–96.

213 VRIEND-VERMEER, W. (1969). A Page From History – Herman Boerhaave. *Archimedes*.

214 ACHIWA, G. *et al.* (1969). *The special issue of the 300th birthday anniversary of Herman Boerhaave*. 31 pp., [In Japanese]. portr. Itan, J. Kansai Branch Jap. Soc. Med. Hist., no. 40, december.
– The contents: Portrait of Herman Boerhaave; On the beginning of the special issue of ITAN of Herman Boerhaave (1668–1738) by G. Achiwa; A short study of Boerhaave's Manhyo Chijun (transl. by Shindo Tsuboi) by S. Tsuda; Komori Tou's

"Ranpo Suki" and W. Buchan's "Huislyke Geneeskunde" (Prolog) by R. Otori; Some reasons why Goethe had an ardent admiration for Dr. H. Boerhaave by Fujimori; "Naikasoku" transl. by R. Shingu, by S. Nakayama.

215 KAISER, Wolfram and Christine Beierlein (ed.) (1969). *In Memoriam Hermann Boerhaave 1668–1738.*, 254 pp., ill., portrs. Wissenschaftliche Beiträge der Martin-Luther-Universität Halle-Wittenberg (R. 10). Halle (Saale).

216 KAISER, W. and W. Piechocki. In Memoriam Hermann Boerhaave (1668–1738). In: Kaiser u. Beierlein (ed.). (1969). *In Memoriam Hermann Boerhaave 1668–1738*, 9–27, 12 ill. See 215.

See also 5492–94

General scientific thoughts.

217 GROOT, J. V. de (1917). *Denkers over ziel en leven.* (Thinkers on soul and life). 345 pp., Bussum-Amsterdam.

– On Thomas van Aquino and the new biology; René Descartes, Boerhaave (p. 166–210)., Maine de Biran, La Cordaire.

218 deleted.

219 DELAUNAY, Paul (1927). L'évolution Philosophique et médicale du biomécanisme. De Descartes à Boerhaave. De Leibnitz à Cabanis. *Progrès Médical*, 20, 27 august, 3 September.

220 KING, Lester S. (1965). *The background of Herman Boerhaave's doctrines.* 20 pp., Series Leidse Voordrachten, no. 1, Universitaire Pers, Leiden.

– Address held on September 17th, 1964.

221 KUDLIEN, Fridolf (1966). Agrippa und Boerhaave: zwei Positionen im Ringen um die certitudo medicinae. *Gesnerus*, 23, 86–96.

222 PREMUDA, Loris (1963). La reazione metodologica di Hermann Boerhaave alla scienza cartesiana. *Atti della V Biennale della Marca e dello Studio Firunano*, Fermo 2–5 Maggio 1963, 437–47.

223 PREMUDA, Loris (1966). La filosofia anatomica di Boerhaave. *Minerva Med.*, 57, 3229–35.

224 MITARITONNA, Onofrio (1967). L'influsso di Herman Boerhaave sul pensiero scientifico del suo tempo. *Riv. Storia Med.*, 11, 206–27.

225 LINDEBOOM, G. A. (1961). Boerhaave's plaats in de wetenschap. (Boerhaave's place in science). *MKVAW*, 23, no. 2, 32 pp., 9 ill.

– As an appendix an address of Sir William Osler (1849–1919) on the same subject. (ms in *Bibliotheca Osleriana*, Mac Gill University, Montreal (Canada).

226 — (1970). Boerhaave's concept of the basic structure of the body. *Clio Med.*, *5*, 203–8.

227 — and L. J. Rather (1973). *Los grandes Sistemáticos*. In: *Historia Universal de la Medicina*, Tomo IV, 319–26, 341: Boerhaave (L.) and G. E. Stahl and F. Hoffmann (R.), 327–40., 8. ill., 3 portrs. Salvat Ed., S. A., Barcelona-Madrid-Buenos Aires.

Clinical and theoretical teaching, lecture-notes

228 LEERSUM, E. C. van (1918). Cours de Boerhaave, en particulier ses leçons cliniques. Description de l'héritage sténographique laissé par Gerard van Swieten. *Janus*, *XXIII*, 316–46, ill.

229 FISCHER, I. (1938). Herman Boerhaave als Kliniker. (Herman Boerhaave as a clinician). *NTG*, *82*, IV, 4835–40; *BGG*, *XVIII*, 203–8.

230 THERSTAPPEN, Ria (1942). *Ueber die Entstehung der klinischen Vorlesung und ihre Reform durch Herman Boerhaave*. Thesis Cologne, 52 pp., ill. no pl.

231 PROBST, Chr. (1968). Das Krankenexamen. Methodologie der Klinik bei Boerhaave und in der ersten Wiener Schule. *Hippokrates*, *39* "Heft" 21, 820–5.

232 — (1972). *Der Weg des ärztlichen Erkennens am Krankenbett*. Herman Boerhaave und die ältere Wiener medizinische Schule. Band I (1701–1787). *SA*, Beiheft 15, 235 pp., Franz Steiner Verlag, Wiesbaden.

233 LEERSUM, E. C. van (1919). Boerhaave's dictaten, inzonderheid zijner klinische lessen. Met een beschrijving van Gerard van Swieten's stenografische nalatenschap (B.'s lectures, particularly his clinical lessons. With a description of the stenographic inheritance). *NTG*, *63*, I, 50–76.

234 — (1919). Two of Boerhaave's lecture lists. *Janus*, *XXIV*, 115.

235 LINDEBOOM, G. A. (1958). Boerhaave's eerste college (Boerhaave's first lecture). *NTG*, *102*, II, 2378–82; *BGG*, *XXXVIII*, 33–7, 1 ill.

236 LEWIS, R. V. (1971). Footnote to medical history – Boerhaave, Brett and Waterhouse. *R. I. med. J.*, *54*, 157–8.

– Author locates lecture notes of B.

237   HOFMEIER, H. K. (1966). Ein Besuch in Boerhaaves Krankenhaus zu Leiden. *Mediz. Monatschr.*, *20*, 218–20, ill.

238   WALLACH, Emil (1927). Abhandlung über eine zweite tödliche und sehr seltene Krankheit (Geschwulst der Brusthöhle) von Herman Boerhaave. Atrocis rarissimique morbi historia altera conscripta ab Hermanno Boerhaave. Lugduni Batavorum 1728. Ins Deutsche übertragen von — (German translation). *Janus, XXXI*, 152–69. *See* 244.

239   DERBES, Vincent J. and Robert Edgar Mitchell (1955). Herman Boerhaave's *Atrocis, nec Descripti Prius, Morbi Historia*. The First translation of the Classic Case. Report of Rupture of the Esophagus with Annotations. *Bull. Med. Libr. Ass. 43*, 217–40, portr., ill.

240   LINDEBOOM, G. A. (1964). Herman Boerhaave. *Atrocis, nec descripti prius, morbi historia, 1724*. Facsimile of the first edition, and of the first French translation, with introduction by —. B. de Graaf, Nieuwkoop, 12°.
      – Reviewed by V. J. Derbes: *J. Hist. Med., XX* (1965), 176–7 and D. G. Bates: *BHM, XLI*, (1967), 85–6.

241   BELLONI, Luigi (1970). La rottura spontanea dell'oesofago, acquisizione monografica di H. Boerhaave. *Simposi Clinici, 7*, XXIII–XLI, ill.

242   WALLACH, Emil (1924). Hermann Boerhaave's Beschreibung einer Zerreissung der Speiseröhre. Atrocis nec descripti, morbi historia secundum medicae artis leges conscripta ab Hermanno Boerhaave. Lugduni Batavorum 1724. Mit Kürzungen ins Deutsche übertragen. *Janus, XXVIII*, 473–89.

243   BLANK, Margarete (1934). Eine Krankengeschichte Herman Boerhaaves und ihre Stellung in der Geschichte der Klinik. *SA, 27*, 51–87.

244   KING, Lester S. (1968). Description of an other dreadful and unusual disease drawn up by Herman Boerhaave. Translated by Maria Wilkin Smith. With an introductory note. *J. Hist. Med., 23*, 331–48.

245   FULTON, J. F. (1938). The influence of Boerhaave's "Institutiones medicae" on modern physiology. *NTG, 82*, IV, 4860–6; *BGG, XVIII*, 228–34.

246   COPELMAN, L. S. (1957). Herman Boerhaave. Une édition rare des "Praelectiones academicae" et un témoignage inédit dans un texte roumain du XIXième siècle. *NTG, 101*, I, 780–1; *BGG, XXXVII*, 13–4, portr.

247 LAIGNEL-LAVASTINE, M. and J. Vinchon (1929). Les Aphorismes d'Herman Boerhaave et leur traducteur la Métrie. *VIme Congrès de la Méd. Leyde-Amsterdam, 1927*, 327–9, Anvers.

248 TRZCINSKA-DABROWSKA, Z. and S. Dabrowski (1969). Hermanni Boerhaave: "Praelectiones publicae de morbis oculorum". [Polish]. *Klin. oczna. 39*, 125–8.

249 CREUTZ, R. (1938). Herman Boerhaaves akademische Antrittsrede "De commendando studio Hippokratico"; *Hippokrates, 9*, 789–95.

250 BOERHAAVE, H. (1703, 1907). *De usu ratiocinii mechanici in medicina.* – with Dutch translation. *Opusc., I*, 98–169.

251 — (1703, 1964). *De usu ratiocinii mechanici in medicina.* Oratio Habita in Auditorio Magno. XXIV. Septembris MDCCIII.
– Translation of the final part of the formal address delivered by Boerhaave, 1703, in which he designed a modern medical curriculum. Printed on the occasion of the Boerhaave conference on Medical Education, September 16–19, 1964.
Translation: Excerpta Medica, Amsterdam·
See also 132, 1666, 4146–7, 5143

Various concepts and diseases.

252 KNUTSON, S. L. and M. L. SEARS (1973). Hermann Boerhaave and the history of vessels carrying aqueous humor from the eye. *Amer. J. Ophthal., 76*, 648–54.

253 SCHULTE, B. P. M. (1959). *Hermanni Boerhaave Praelectiones de morbis nervorum 1730–1735.* Thesis Leiden (supervisor: E. A. D. E. Carp). 438 pp., ill. Brill, Leiden.
– This work has been also published as Vol. II of the *Analecta Boerhaaviana*. With list of the Boerhaaviana at Leningrad).

254 — (1961). Herman Boerhaave over zenuwziekten. (— on nervous diseases). *GeWiNa*, no. 9, 9–10.

255 — (1964). De neurologie van Herman Boerhaave. (The neurology of H.B.). *NTG, 108*, 1331–2.

256 — (1964). The neurophysiology of Herman Boerhaave, in: *Von Boerhaave bis Berger. Die Entwicklung der kontinentalen Physiologie im 18. und 19. Jahrhundert*, herausgegeben von K. E. Rothschuh, Medizin in Geschichte und Kultur, Bd 5, Gustaf Fischer, Stuttgart, 5–13, ill.

257 — (1966). *Een Mechanistische Ziekteleer van het Zenuwstelsel in de*

Eerste Helft van de 18de Eeuw. (A mechanistic pathology of the Nervous System in the First Half of the 18th Century). 14 pp., 6 ill., *MKVAW*, Klasse der wetenschappen, XXVIII, no. 7, Paleis der Academiën, Brussel.
– On Boerhaave's neurological views.

258 — (1970). The concepts of Boerhaave on physic function and pathology. In: G. A. Lindeboom (ed.) *Boerhaave and His Time*, Brill, Leiden, 93–101.

259 CAPRARIIS, E. de (1969–70). Considerazione sulle vedute neurofisiologiche di Herman Boerhaave. *Acta med. Hist. patav.*, *16*, 89–100, refs.

260 GROOT, J. V. de (1912). Boerhaave en de psychologie van zijn tijd. (B. and the psychology of his time). *NRC*. 16th March.

261 STIGTER, D. (1901). Boerhaave and epilepsy. *Janus, VI*, 140–5 and 187–95.

262 ZEEMAN, W. P. C. (1918). Boerhaave et l'Oculistique. *Janus, XXIII*, 207.

262 — (1919). Boerhaave en de oogheelkunde. (B. and ophthalmology). *NTG, 63*, I, 44.

264 MÜNCHOW, W. (1969). Hermann Boerhaave und die Augenheilkunde. In: Kaiser u. Beierlein (ed.). *In Memoriam Hermann Boerhaave 1668–1738*, 45–8.

265 HARIG, Georg (1969). Boerhaaves Ansichten zur theoretischen Pharmakologie. In: *In memoriam Hermann Boerhaave 1668–1738*, edited by W. Kaiser and Chr. Beierlein. Wissensch. Beiträge Martin-Luther Univ. Halle-Wittenberg 1969/2 (R. 10). Halle/S.

266 JARCHO, S. (1970). Boerhaave on inflammation. *Amer. J. Cardiol., 25*, 244–6 and 480–2.

267 LANGEN, C. D. de (1964). Boerhaave and the peripheral circulation; *Proc. Kon. Ned. Akad. Wet. (Biol. Med.), 67*, 1–6.

268 BELLONI, L. (1965). Leeuwenhoek, Boerhaave und Bleyswyk über Spermatozoën. *Janus, LII*, 193–217, ill.

269 [   ] (1966). Boerhaave's pregnancy date rule. *Midwives Chron., 79*, 136.

270 LINDEBOOM, G. A. (1972–1973). Boerhaave geen animalculist. (B. no animalculist). *Hermèneus*, *44*, no. 2, 101–2.

See also 3227. 10

Chemical writings and Chemistry.

271 NEVILLA, Roy, G. (1959). Boerhaave's "Elementa chemiae", 1732, *Book Collector*, *8*, 428–9.

272 — (1959, 1960). Query 159. – Boerhaave's Elementa Chemiae. A bibliographical point. *Isis*, *50*, 481; *51*, 84.

273 POYNTER, F. N. L. (1960). "Elementa chemiae", 1732. *Book Collector*, *9*, 64.
     – A bibliographical note on Boerhaave's *Elementa Chemiae*.

274 SHERBO, Arthur and F. W. Gibbs (1965–66). The translation of Boerhaave's *Elementa Chemiae*. *Ambix*, *13*, 108–17.

275 READ, John (1947). *Humour and Humanism in Chemistry*. Bell & Son, London.
     – Chapter III (124–57): Chemistry comes to the textbooks (On B.'s *Elementa chemiae*).

276 GIBBS, F. W. (1949). *The Life and Work of Herman Boerhaave with particular reference to his influence in Chemistry*. Thesis University of London, 3 parts, unpublished.

277 — (1958). Boerhaave's chemical writings. *Ambix*, *6*, 117–35.

278 — (1960). Dr. Johnson's first published work? *Ambix*, *8*, 24–34.
     – on a translation of Boerhaave's *Elementa Chemiae*.

279 — (1963). Boerhaave and the Place of Chemistry in Medicine, in: F. N. L. Poynter (ed.) *Chemistry in the Service of Medicine*, Pitman Med. Publ. Comp., London, p. 27–42.

280 COHEN, E. (1918). Herman Boerhaave und seine Bedeutung für die Chemie. *Janus*, *XXIII*, 223–90.

281 — (1919). Boerhaave als mensch en chemicus. (B. as a man and as a chemist). *NTG*, *63*, I, 13.

282 — (1919). *Herman Boerhaave en zijn Beteekenis voor de Chemie.* Met eene Vertaling van Boerhaave's Natuurwetenschappelijke Redevoeringen en Verhandelingen door Margareta Renkema (H.B. and his

significance for Chemistry. With a translation of B. Scientifical Addresses and treatises by M. Renkema). 168 pp., no. pl.

283 SPETER, Max (1929). Boerhaave. In: G. Bugge. *Das Buch der groszen Chemiker*, Bd I, Verlag Chemie, Berlin, p. 204–20.

284 KNIGHT, J. G. (1933). *The Chemical Studies of Herman Boerhaave 1668–1738*. A dissertation presented for part II of the degree of Master of Science, in the University of London, 130 pp., unpublished.
– in the University of London Library.

285 KERKER, Milton (1955). Herman Boerhaave and the Development of Pneumatic Chemistry. *Isis*, *46*, 36–49.

286 KOPP, Herman (1931). *Geschichte der Chemie*. Leipzig. (Reprint of the original edition in 4 vols of 1843–47).
– on Boerhaave: Vol. I, 197–201.

287 SCOTT, Wilson Ludlow (1955). *Some of Boerhaave's medical lectures on physics, with particular reference to the significance of these lectures to physical chemistry*. An essay submitted to the Faculty of Philosophy of The Johns Hopkins University for the degree of Master of Arts. 126 + IX pp., Baltimore, not printed.

288 JEVONS, F. R. (1962). Boerhaave's Biochemistry. *Med. Hist.*, *6*, 343–62.

289 — (1963). Boerhaave's Teaching in Relation to Beccari's Identification of Gluten as an "Animal" Substance. *J. Hist. Med.*, *18*, 174–5.

290 LIPPMANN, E. O. von (1938). Boerhaave als Chemiker. *NTG*, *82*. IV, 4867–77; *BGG*, *XVIII*, 235–45.

291 DAVIS, Tenny L. (1926). Boerhaave's Attitude Toward Alchemy. *Med. Life XXXIII*, 261–4.

292 — (1928). The vicissitudes of Boerhaave's Textbook of Chemistry. *Isis*, *10*, 33–46, 2 ill.

293 PARTINGTON, J. R. (1961, 1969). *A History of Chemistry*. Mac Millan, London. Vol. II, Chapter *XX*: Boerhaave, p. 736–68.

294 ROCCHIETTA, S. (1969). L'apporto di un medico, Herman Boerhaave (1668–1738), al progresso della chemica. *Boll. Soc. ital. Farm. osped.*, *15*, 414–8, portr.

295 BACKER, H. J. (1943). Boerhaave's ontdekking van het ureum. (B.'s discovery of urea). *NTG, 87*, III, 1274–8; *BGG, XXIII*, 55–9.

296 BLANKSMA, J. J. (1949). Boerhaave en zwaar kwik. (B. and heavy mercury). *ChemWbl., 44*, 94–6.

297 LOVE, R. (1972). Some sources of Herman Boerhaave's concept of fire. *Ambix, 19*, 157–74.

298 DIJKSTERHUIS, E. J. (1922). Van Boerhaave tot Kamerlingh Onnes. (From — till —). *Chem.Wbl., 19*, 569.

299 METZGER, Hélène (1930). *Newton, Stahl, Boerhaave et la Doctrine chimique.* 332 pp., Alcan, Paris.
   – Reviewed by J. G. de Lint: *NTG, 75* (1931), IV, 5508; *BGG, XI*, 303.

300 COHEN, I. Bernard (1955). Franklin, Boerhaave, Newton, Boyle & the Absorption of Heat in Relation to Color. *Isis, 46*, pt. 2, no. 144 (June), 99–104.

301 LINDEBOOM, G. A. (1971). Barchusen and Boerhaave. *Janus, LVII*, 30–41.

302 — (1972). Boerhaave's Impact on the Relation between Chemistry and Medicine. *Clio Med., 7*, 271–8.

303 ROUSSEAU, G. S. (1967). Smollet's "acidum vagum". *Isis, 58*, 244–5.
   – On a substance mentioned in the works of Tobias Smollet, and occurring in Boerhaave's *Elementa Chemiae* (1732): "acid, vague, volatile liquid" or "vague universal acid".

Botany

304 HUNGER, F. W. T. (1918). Boerhaave comme naturaliste. *Janus, XXIII*, 347–57.

305 — (1919). Boerhaave als natuurhistoricus. (B. as a natural historian). *NTG, 63*, I, 36.

306 — (1919). De boom van Boerhaave (The tree of —). *Buiten*, 13, 10.

307 SPRAGUE, T. A. (1938). Boerhaave as a botanist: *NTG, 82*, IV, 4891–4; *BGG, XVIII*, 259–62.

308 UITTIEN, H. (1938). Boerhaave's beteekenis voor de plantkunde. (B.'s significance for botany). *NTG, 82*, IV, 4841–51; *BGG, XVIII*, 209–19.

Also in: *Memorialia Herman Boerhaave optimi medici.* 1939, Bohn, Haarlem, 95–103. (Boerhaave et son influence sur la Botanique).

309 GIBBS, F. M. (1957). Boerhaave and the botanists. *Ann. Sci.*, *13*, 47–61.

310 HENIGER, J. (1971). Some botanical activities of Herman Boerhaave, Professor of Botany and Director of the Botanic Garden at Leiden. *Janus, LVIII*, 1–78, ill.

Letters and manuscripts

311 LEERSUM, E. C. van (1916). Boerhaaviana, II. Trois lettres de Boerhaave. *Janus, XXI*, 450–6.

312 POWER, D'ARCY (1917). The letters of Boerhaave to Cox Macro. *Proc. Royal Soc. Med.* (Section Hist. of Med.), *XI*, 21–46.

312ᵃ LEERSUM, E. C. van (1919). Een paar brieven van Boerhaave aan Cox Macro (A couple of letters from — to —). *NTG, 63*, I, 100–4.

313 MAANEN, W. van (1917). Brief van Herman Boerhaave aan Abraham Titsingh. (Letter from B. to A. Titsingh). *Wapenheraut, XXI*, 286.

314 WIEDEMANN, A. (1922). Fünf Briefe an Boerhaave. *Arch. Gesch. Mediz. XIV*, 48–55.

315 DARMSTAEDTER, Ernst (1927). *Herman Boerhaaves Briefe an Johann Bapt. Bassand in Wien.* Ausgewählt und eingeleitet von —. III. Sonderheft der Münchener Beiträge zur Geschichte und Lit. der Naturw. und Medizin, XLVI pp., München.

316 LINDEBOOM, G. A. (1957). *Boerhaave's brieven aan Bassand* (B.'s letters to Bassand)., 273 pp., portr., Bohn, Haarlem, 8°.

317 — (1957). *Boerhaave's Correspondence I and II*, 241 pp. and 471 pp., *Analecta Boerhaaviana III and IV*, Brill, Leiden.
   Vol. *I* contains letters to Cox Macro, William Sherard, Hans Sloane, Richard Mead, Cromwell Mortimer and some other English-speaking physicians. Vol. *II* contains letters to persons in Middle, East and South Europe, and all the letters to Bassand. All letters with English translation.

318 BOERHAAVE, H. (1717, 1935). Epistola X ad Joannem Baptistam Bassand – with Dutch translation. *Opusc., XIII*, 215–30.

319 LEFANU, W. R. (1934). Four letters from Boerhaave. *Janus, XXXVIII*, 70–6.

320 BLOCH, M. (1936). Unveröffentlichte Manuskripte von Boerhaave und Fahrenheits Briefe an Boerhaave. *Archeion, XVIII,* 184–5.

321 COHEN, E. (1931). Een nieuw ontdekte briefwisseling tusschen Boerhaave en Fahrenheit. (Newly discovered correspondence between Boerhaave and Fahrenheit). *NTG, 75,* II, 2990–1; *BGG, XI,* 183–4.
– included in the report of a meeting of the "Genootschap" refers to 12 letters from Fahrenheit to Boerhaave, that are present in the Leningrad collection.

322 COHEN, E. and W. A. T. Cohen-de Meester (1938). Teruggevonden manuscripten en briefwisselingen van Herman Boerhaave. (Again found manuscripts and correspondence of Herman Boerhaave). *NTG, 82,* III, 4327–30; *BGG, XVIII,* 147–50.

323 — (1939). Der vermisste Brief Antoni Leeuwenhoeks an Hermann Boerhaave vom 26. August 1717. *MKNAW,* Afd. Natuurkunde I, sectie 17, *I,* 1–25, 3 ill, 9 facs.

324 — (1941). Katalog der wiedergefundenen Manuskripte und Briefwechsel von Herman Boerhaave. *NAW,* afd. Natuurk. Tweede Sectie, Deel XL, no. 2, 45 pp., Noord-Holl. Uitg. Mij. Amsterdam.

325 WITTOP KONING, D. A. (1959). A letter from Boerhaave to Ebenezer Gilchrist. *Janus, XLVIII,* 258–63.

326 LINDEBOOM, G. A. (1956). De Russische Boerhaaviana in copie in Nederland. (Copies of the Russian Boerhaaviana in the Netherlands). *G&W, 54,* 32–3.

327 RATH, G. (1965). Unbekannte Briefe Boerhaaves und Morgagnis an Triller. *Berl. Med.,* 466–9, facs.

328 DONGEN, J. A. van (1964). Een brief van Boerhaave. (A letter from —). *MC, 19,* 198.
– To William Burton (1729), who wrote later a biography of Boerhaave.

329 MITARITONNA, O. (1968). A proposito di alcuni consulti epistolari di Boerhaave. *Med. Secoli,* Suppl. to N. 4, 14–27.

330 BELLONI, L. (1971). Contributo all'epistolario Boerhaave-Morgagni. L'edizione delle "Epistolae anatomicae duae" Leidae, 1728. *Physis, 18,* 81–109, facs. and refs.

331 LINDEBOOM, G. A. (1968). Boerhaave and his Italian correspondents *Atti XXI Congresso Internazionale di Storia della Medicina,* Siena, 22–8. Also in: *Pag. Stor. Med., 13* (1969), 49–61.

332 BELLONI, L. (1974). Aus dem Briefwechsel zwischen Herman Boer-
     haave und Johannes Jakob Scheuchzer. In: *Circa Tiliam*, 83–106.
     Brill, Leiden.

Iconography

333 MARTIN, W. (1918). Das Bildnis Boerhaave's von Aert de Gelder.
     Janus, XXIII, 366–9. portr.

334 WILDEMAN, M. G. (1918–19). Nog een portret van Boerhaave door
     Aert van Gelder. (Again a portrait of B. by Aert van Gelder). *Oude
     Kunst*, IV, 13.

335 KLEIWEG DE ZWAAN, J. P. (1919). Het portret van Boerhaave door Aert
     de Gelder. (The portrait of B. by Aert de Gelder). *NTG, 63*, I, 77.

336 LINT, J. G. de (1918). Les portraits en gravure de Boerhaave. *Janus,
     XXIII*, 358–65.

337 — (1919). Boerhaave's beeltenissen in gravuren. (B.'s portraits in
     engravings). *NTG, 63*, I, 79.

338 LEERSUM, E. C. van (1919). Bij het portret van H. Boerhaave. (At the
     portrait of H.B.) *NTG, 63*, I, 85.

339 WILDEMAN, M. G. (1918–19). Portretten van Herman Boerhaave.
     (Portraits of —). *Oude Kunst*, IV, 80.

340 LINDEBOOM, G. A. (1963). *Iconographia Boerhaavii*. 29 pp., 40 pl.,
     Brill, Leiden.
     – Reviewed by H. M. Sinclair: *Med. Hist., VIII* (1964), 384–5.

341 NIEMEYER, J. W. (1964). Een nieuwe "Iconographia Boerhaavii".
     (A new "Iconographia Boerhaavii"). *Jbk. Centr. Bur. Genealogie, 18*,
     254–60, 2 ill.
     – Notes and replenishments to G. A. Lindeboom's *Iconographia Boerhaavii* (1963).

342 REYS, J. H. O. (1938). Boerhaave en de penning. (Boerhaave and the
     medal). *GG, 16*, 1035–7.
     – Deals with B.'s picture on medals.

Foreign relations and influence

343 [Anonymous] (1959). Origin of Leyden's fame – Boerhaave – doctor
     to princes and one-man medical faculty. *World Health*, Sept–Oct., ill.,
     portr.

344 COMRIE, J. D. (1938). Boerhaave and the early medical school at Edinburgh. *NTG*, *82*, IV, 4828–35; *BGG*, *XVIII*, 196–203.

345 GUTHRIE, Douglas (1959). The Influence of the Leyden School upon
Scottish Medicine. *Med. Hist.*, *III*, 108–22.

345ª LINDEBOOM, G. A. (1974). Boerhaave's influence on British Medicine.
In: *Proc. XXIII Int. Congr. Hist. Med. London 2–9 Sept. 1972*. Vol. I,
734–8. Wellcome Institute of the History of medicine, London.

345ᵇ ASHWORTH UNDERWOOD, E. (1974). Boerhaave and the London hospitals. In: *Circa Tiliam*, 61–82. Brill, Leiden.

346 KAISER, W. and H. Krosch (1968). Leiden und Halle als medizinischen Zentren des frühen 18. Jahrhunderts. Zum 300. Geburtstag
von Hermann Boerhaave (1668–1738). *Ztsch. Ges. inn. Medizin*, *23*,
330–8. portr.

347 — (1968). Das wissenschaftliche Werk von Hermann Boerhaave
im Spiegel hallescher Universitätsschriften des 18. Jahrhunderts.
Münch. med. Wsch., *110*, 1950–60, ill.

348 DIEPGEN, P. (1938). Der Weg von Boerhaave's Medizin nach Deutschland. *NTG*, *82*, IV, 4852–60; *BGG*, *XVIII*, 220–8. Also in: *Memoralia
Herman Boerhaave optimi medici*, Bohn, Haarlem (1939), 23–31.

349 — (1939). Hermann Boerhaave und die Medizin seiner Zeit mit besonderer Berücksichtigung seiner Wirkung nach Deutschland. *Hippokrates*, *10*, 298–306 and 345–51.

350 DITTRICH, Mauritz (1969). Boerhaaves Schüler in Greifswald. Ein
Beitrag zur Medizingeschichte des frühen 18. Jahrhunderts. In:
Kaiser u. Beierlein (eds). *In Memoriam Hermann Boerhaave 1688–1738*,
29–44.

351 WENCKEBACH, K. F. (1938). Boerhaave und die Wiener medizinische
Schule. *NTG*, *82*, IV, 4899–901; *BGG*, *XVIII*, 267–9. Also in: *Memorialia*, 46–7.

352 LESKY, Erna (1958). Albrecht von Haller, Gerard van Swieten und
Boerhaavens Erbe. *Gesnerus*, *15*, 120–40.

353 SPIELMANN, I. (1968). Influenta invataturii lui H. Boerhaave in Trans-
silvania. *Revista Medic.* (Turgu-Mures), *14*, 358–361.
– Witness of Boerhaave's influence in Transsylvania: 3 manuscripts of his students.

354   VATAMANU, N. (1969). Der Einflusz der Schule Boerhaaves auf die
      Medizin der Donaufürstentfümer In: Kaiser u. Beierlein (ed.) *In
      Memoriam Hermann Boerhaave 1668-1738*, 59–62.

355   SPIELMANN, J. (1969). Der Einflusz von Boerhaaves Lehre auf die
      Medizin in Siebenbürgen. In: Kaiser u. Beierlein (ed.). *In Memoriam
      Hermann Boerhaave 1668-1738*, 63–6.

356   DUKA, N. (1972). Hermann Boerhaave and the development of medi-
      cine in Slovakia. [Slovak with Engl. abstract]. *Dej. Ved. Techn*, 5,
      18–32.

357   LINDEBOOM, G. A. (1955). Boerhaave's naam en neven in Rusland.
      (B.'s name and nephews in Russia). *Almanak Studenten Corps Vrije
      Universiteit* (Amsterdam), 274–80.

358   CASTIGLIONI, A. (1929). Boerhaave en Italie. *VIme Congrès Int.
      d'Hist. de la Méd. Leyde-Amsterdam 1927*, 74–6, Anvers.

359   BRATESCU, G. (1969). Boerhaave und La Mettrie. In: Kaiser u. Beier-
      lein (eds). *In Memoriam Hermann Boerhaave 1668-1738*, 67–8.

360   SIGERIST, H. E. (1938). Boerhaave's influence upon American medicine.
      NTG, 82, IV, 4822–8; *BGG, XVIII*, 190–6.

361   DANIËLS, C. E. (1912). La version orientale, arabe et turque des deux
      premiers livres de Herman Boerhaave. Etude bibliographique. *Janus,
      XVII*, 295–312, 1 ill.

362   — (1912). De Oostersche vertaling der twee eerste boeken van Her-
      man Boerhaave. (The oriental translation of the two first books of
      H.B.). *NTG, 66*, II, 1328–34.
      – Address "Geneeskundige Kring" Amsterdam, September 24, 1912.

363   ACHIWA, Goro (1965). A Study of Shindo Tsubor's Translation of
      Commentaria in Hermanni Boerhaave Aphorismos. *Janus, LII*, 138–
      42, ill.

364   — (1969). *Herman Boerhaave 1668-1738*. His life, thought and in-
      fluence upon Japanese medicine in the period of Dutch learning. With
      a foreword by G. A. Lindeboom, 206 pp., ill. Ogato Bookstore,
      Tokyo. [In Japanese].

365   — (1971). Herman Boerhaave's Influence upon Japanese Medicine
      in the period of Dutch Learning. In: *Rangaku in Japanese culture*,
      239–50.

Catalogues

366 HERTZBERGER, Menno (1927). *Short-title catalogue of books written and edited by Herman Boerhaave.* 27 pp., 1 portr., Hertzberger, Amsterdam.
– With the assistance of E. J. van der Linden (With a preface by J. G. de Lint.)

367 VELDE, A. J. van der (1938). Boerhaaviana. Proeve van een Bibliografie der werken van Herman Boerhaave (1668–1738) ter gelegenheid van den 200en verjaardag van zijn overlijden op 23 september 1938. (Sample of a bibliography of the works of H.B. on the occasion of the 200th anniversary of his death on september 23, 1938). *Jbk. Dodonaea,* 5, 121–165.

368 LINDEBOOM, G. A. (1959). *Bibliographia Boerhaaviana* (Analecta Boerhaaviana, I), 106 pp., Brill, Leiden, 8°.

Varia

369 LAIGNEL-LAVASTINE, M. and J. Vinchon (1929). Un chapitre du "Médecin de Machiavel" à propos de Boerhaave. *VIme Congrès Int. d'Hist. de la Méd. Leyde-Amsterdam 1927,* 77–8, Anvers.

370 LUYDENDIJK-ELSHOUT, A. M. (1970). The anatomical illustrations in the London edition (1741) of part I of Herman Boerhaave's *Institutiones Medicae.* Lindeboom, G. A. (ed.). (1970). *Boerhaave and his Time,* Leiden, 83–93.

371 NAPJUS, J. W. (1940). De hoogleeraren in de geneeskunde aan de Hoogeschool en het Athenaeum te Franeker (1585–1843). (The professors of medicine at Franeker Academy and Athenaeum (1585–1843). XIX. Godefridus Du Bois. *NTG, 84,* IV, 4809–14; *BGG, XX,* 184–9.

372 ARIËNS KAPPERS, J. (1963–64). Levensbericht van Siegfried Thomas Bok (19 maart 1892 – 4 februari 1964). (Biographical notice of —). *Jbk. KNAW.,* 407–12, portr.

373 SCHOUTE, D. (1926). Dr. Bolle en zijn werk. (Dr. B. and his work). *Arch. Zeeuwsch Gen.,* 14 pp., Middelburg.
– J. Bolle (1853–1919), became in 1879 physician at Middelburg.

374 ENDTZ, L. J. [1973]. *Dr G. C. Bolten, neuroloog aan de Gemeenteziekenhuizen van 's-Gravenhage. Bibliografie met een levensschets* (G.C.B., neurologist at the Municipal Hospitals at The Hague. Bibliography with a biographical sketch). 32 pp. Labaz BV, Maassluis.
– G. C. Bolten (1872–1940).

375 BRUINVIS, C. W. (1915). Cornelis Bontekoe, de theedoctor. (—, the Tea-doctor). *Navorscher, LXIV*, 551. also in: *Elzevier's geill. Maandschr.*, (1892).

376 BAUMANN, E. D. (1949). *Cornelis Bontekoe (1640–1685)*. *De Theedoctor*. (The Tea-doctor). 165 pp. Misset, Oosterbeek.

377 BONTEKOE, C. (1678, 1937). Tractaat van het excellenste kruyd thee. (Treatise about the most excellent herb Tea) – with English translation. *Opusc., XIV*, 118–462.

378 KROON, J. E. de (1929). Le premier professeur en médecine à l'université de Leyde. Gerard de Bont (1536–99). *VIme Congrès Int. d'Hist. de la Méd. Leyde-Amsterdam, 18–23 Juillet, 1927*, Anvers, 156–7.

379 POP, G. F. (1870). Nog iets over Jacob Bontius. (Something more on J.B.) *Geneesk. T. Zeemagt.*, 29.

380 EBSTEIN, Wilhelm (1902): Ueber die Mitteilungen von Jacob Bontius, betreffend die Dysenterie auf Java im 3. Jahrzehnt des 17. Jahrhunderts. *Janus, VII*, 288–95 and 337–45.

381 JEANSELME, E. (1929). 1. l'Oeuvre de J. Bontius. 2. Titres et frontispices gravés des éditions de J. Bontius. *VIme Congrès Int. d'Hist. de la Méd. Leyde-Amsterdam 1927, 18–23 Juillet*, 223–8, 3 ill., Anvers.

382 ANDEL, M. A. van (1931). Bontius en Piso over de dysenterie in beide Indiën. (B. and P. on dysentery in both the Indiens). *NTG, 75*, IV, 5490–7; *BGG, XI*, 285–92.

383 — (1931). Jacobus Bontius, geneesheer der O-I-Compagnie. (J.B., physician to the East-Indian-Company). *NRC*, 13 december.

384 LINT, J. G. de (1932). Een portret van Jacobus Bontius. (A portrait of —). *NTG, 76*, IV, 4669–70; *BGG, XII*, 202–3, portr. See 387.

385 RÖMER, L. A. S. M. von (1932). Dr. Jacob Bontius (1592–1631). Bijblad op het *Geneesk. T. Ned-Indië*, 33 pp., ill.

386 BONTIUS, Jac. (1642, 1931). Tropische geneeskunde. (Tropical medicine). With English translation. *Opusc., X*, 410 pp.
     – His will, index and Latin text of the six books by Bontius, lists of the plants and animals mentioned by him.

387 SCHOUTE, D. (1938). Een verzonnen beeltenis. (A made-up picture) *NTG, 82*, III, 3872–3; *BGG, XVIII*, 145–6.

– With postscript by W. A. P. Schüffner and Ch. W. F. Winckel; On a picture of Jac. Bontius, published by L. S. A. M. von Römer. *Historische Schetsen*; Batavia 1921, 28–31, ill.: V, VI and IX.

388 REDDY, D. V. S. (1963). Jacob Bontius, and his writings on Diseases and herbs of East India. *BDHM Hyderabad, I*; 118–28, portr.

With a letter of Jac. Bontius to his brother W. Bontius, who was mayor of Leyde, and an index of the first four books of Bontius.

See also 3832

389 BLANKHART, D. M. (1966). Dr. W. G. Boorsma 1867–1937. *Voeding*, *27*, 167–71, portr.

390 ANDEL, M. A. van (1924). Arnoldus Boot en de eerste beschrijving van de rachitis. (A.B. and the first description of rachitis). *NTG, 68*, I, 946–7; *BGG, IV*, 69–70.

391 — (1927). Arnoldus Boot author of one of the first descriptions of Rickets (1649). *Janus, XXXI*, 346–58.

392 BOOTIUS, A. (1649, 1926). Observationes Medicae de affectibus omissis – with Dutch translation. *Opusc., V*, 260–75.

393 GAIZO, Modestino del (1909). L'oeuvre scientifique de J. A. Borelli, étudiée dans ses rapports avec l'école Hollandaise. *Janus, XIV*, 506–11.

394 LINDEBOOM, G. A. (1960). De uitreiking van de Hijmans van den Bergh-medaille aan Prof. Dr. J. G. G. Borst, op 12 November 1960 te Leiden. (The presentation of the Hijmans van den Bergh-medal to J. G. G. Borst.). *Fol. Med. Neerl., 3*, 192–203, 2 portr., 1 ill.

395 SCHÈLE, S. [1965]. *Cornelis Bos; a study of the origins of the Netherlands grotesque*. 238 pp. Almquist & Wiksell.

– p. 149–58: Anatomical subjects.

396 BORGERS, H. A. C. (1941). *Doctor Willem Bosch en zijn invloed op de geneeskunde in Nederlands Oost-Indië.* (Doctor W.B. and his influence on medicine in the Dutch East Indies). Thesis Utrecht (Supervisor: J. Boeke), 145 pp., portr., Kemink en Zoon, Utrecht.

397 VIEYRA, D. (1937). Een pijnlijk incident tusschen prof. H. Bosscha en de stedelijke commissie van geneeskundig toevoorzicht, in 1821. (A awkward incident between H.B. and the municipal commission of medical supervision in 1821). *NTG, 81*, II, 1963–5; *BGG, XVII*, 93–5; 115–9; 139–40.

398   Es, A. J. H. van (1956). Boussingault 1802–1887. *Voeding, 17*, 41–4, portr.

399   PLATE, W. P. (1965). Van Bouwdijk Bastiaanse. *N. T. Verl. Gyn.*, *65*, 1–4, portr.

400   HOOYKAAS, R. (1942). Robert Boyle. Een studie over Natuurweten-schap en Christendom. (— —. A study on natural science and Christianity). *G&W*, special issue, 126 pp.

401   BRA, Henricus a (1594, 1935). De morbo quodam novo et incognito "Die Barenn" – with Dutch translation. *Opusc., XIII*, 107–20.

402   HARRIS, L. E. (1961). *The two Netherlanders, Humphrey Bradley and Cornelis Drebbel.* 227 pp., Brill, Leiden.

403   VERMEULEN, H. (1943). Een reizend geestelijke geneesheer. (A travelling priest-physician). *NTG, 87*, IV, 1711; *BGG, XXIII*, 94.
– On Jan Brikkenaar (1688–1760), priest and eye-surgeon.

404   MEURS, G. J. van (1962). Anthelme Brillat-Savarin. *Voeding, 23*, 651–61 and 868.

405   BEUMER, H. M. (1972). Willem Bronkhorst (1888–1960). Een pionier der longziekten. (A pioneer of lung-diseases). *GG., 3*, 400–3, 3 ill.
– with reference to articles in journals and minor periodicals.

406   — (1972). *Leven en werken van Willem Bronkhorst (1888–1960).* (Life and works of W.B.) 72 pp., portr., ill. De Tijdstroom, Lochem.

407   WEVE, H. (1960). Levensbericht van W. Bronkhorst (26 juni 1888 – 29 april 1960). (Biographical notice). *KNAW*, 1959/60, 288–94. Amsterdam.

408   SETERS, W. H. van (1953). Prof. Johannes Brosterhuysen (1596–1650). Stichter en Opziener van de Medicinale Hof te Breda. (Founder and Inspector of the medicinal garden at Breda). *Jbk. Breda "De Oranjeboom", VI*, 106–51, ill.

409   LINDEBOOM, G. A. (1955). François Joseph Victor Broussais (1772–1838). *NTG, 99*, I, 955–63; *BGG, XXXV*, 17–25, 2 ill., portr.

410   — (1955). De leer van Broussais in Nederland. (The doctrine of B. in the Netherlands). *NTG, 99*, II, 1240–5; *BGG, XXXV*, 36–41.

411   — (1957). L'influence de Broussais dans les Pays-Bas. *Scalpel* n° 44, 2 November.

412 PRICK, J. J. G. (1949). A la mémoire du Prof. Dr. B. Brouwer. *Foliq Psych. Neurol. et Neurochir. Neerl.*, no. 5, portr.

413 DROOGLEEVER FORTUYN, J. (1959). In Memoriam Bernardus Brouwer 1881–1949. *Monthly Rev. Psychiatr. and Neurol.*, *119*, no. 2.

414 BIEMOND, A. (1950). In Memoriam Prof. Dr. B. Brouwer. *NTG, 94*, I, 711–5, portr.

415 — (1961). Bernardus Brouwer: Dutch neurologist (1881–1949). *Cereb. Pas. Bull.*, *2*, 292–4, portr.

416 ESSO BZN, I. van (1935). "Praten als Brugman" (Talking as Brugman). *NTG, 79*, III, 4287; *BGG, XV*, 200.

– The saying "talk as Brugman" does not refer to S. J. Brugmans (1753–1819), as suggested in the *BioLex*, but to father Johannes Brugman (1400–73), a Minorite.

417 LINDEBOOM, G. A. (1963). In Memoriam Doctor Jan Willem Bruins *G&W, 61*, 61–2, portr.

– J.W.B. (1904–63) was one of the founders of the "Nederlandse Anthropogenetische Vereniging" (1949), and at the time of his death Governor of the Free University at Amsterdam.

418 TREUB, Hector (1905). C. L. van der Burg. In Memoriam (Obituary). *Janus, X*, 617.

419 WOLFF, J. W. (1955). Dr. C. L. van der Burg 1840–1905. *Voeding, 16*, 403–5, portr.

420 BURGER, H. (1930). *Uitgezochte opstellen en toespraken.* Bijeengebracht door vrienden en vereerders bij de herdenking van zijn vijfentwintig-jarig Hoogleeraarsambt aan de Universiteit van Amsterdam op 5 october 1930 (Selected essays and addresses. Collected by his friends and admirers at the commemoration of his 25th anniversary of his professorate at the University of Amsterdam, on October 5, 1930). X + 538 pp., portr. De Bussy, Amsterdam.

– Contains a.o. obituaries of A. A. G. Guye, D. van Haren Noman, P. H. Eykman and N. van Rijnberk.

421 PRAKKEN, J. R. (1957). Professor H. Burger† *NTG, 101*, 2409.

422 GERLINGS, P. G. and J. J. van Loghem (1954). Prof. Dr. Hendrik Burger 90 jaar (The 90th anniversary of —). *NTG, 98*, IV, 3278–81, portr.

423 SCHOUTE, D. (1940). Cornelis Helenus Burgersdijk (1803–1840). *NTG, 84*, I, 826–34; *BGG, XX*, 41–9.

424 CITTERT-EYMERS, J. C. van (1968). C. H. D. Buys Ballot (1817–1890). *Sci. Hist.*, *10*, 145–53, fig.

C.

425 FEYFER, F. M. G. de (1933). Jan Steven van Calcar (Johannes Stephanus) 1499–1546. *NTG*, *76*, III, 5562–80; *BGG*, *XIII*, 177–194.
See also 5216, 5217

PETRUS CAMPER

Biographica

426 DANIËLS, C. E. (1880). *Het leven en de verdiensten van Petrus Camper* (Life and merits of P.C.) 149 pp., Utrecht. 8°

427 OOSTERHUIS, R. A. B. (1939). Petrus Camper (1722–1789). *Timotheus*, nr. 29.

428 — (1939). Petrus Camper (1722–1789). De wereldvermaarde geleerde uit de gesmade 18e eeuw. (Petrus Camper (1722–1789) (The world-famous scientist from the defamed 18th century). *Timotheus*. April, 2 pp.

429 KAPLAN, E. B. (1956). Peter Camper, 1722–1789. *Bull. Hosp. Jt. Dis.* (N.Y.), *17*, 371–85, portr., ill.

430 LINDEBOOM, G. A. (1971). Petrus Camper. In: C. C. Gillispie, ed. *Dictionary of Scientific Biography*, vol. III, 37–8. Scribner's Sons, New York.

431 [Editorial]. (1964). Peter Camper (1722–1789). *JAMA*, *166*, 14 sept., 158–9.

432 WURFBAIN, J. W. (1913). Fragment-genealogie Camper (Fragment-genealogy of —). *Ned. Leeuw*, *31*, kol., 299–300.

433 [Anonym] (1927). Over de spelling van de naam Camper (On the spelling of the name of C.) *Ned. Leeuw*, *45*, kol. 90. See also: kol. 58–59.

434 [Anonym] (1939). Levensschets van Petrus Camper (Biographical sketch). *GG*, *17*, 400–3.

435 HARTING, P. (1878). Pieter Camper in zijn leven en werken geschetst (P.C. sketched in his life and works). *Alb. Nat.*, 1–24.

436 OOSTERHUIS, R. A. B. (1939). De zekerheid der geneeskunde. Inaugurele rede van Petrus Camper (The certainty of medicine. Inaugural oration by Petrus Camper 22 June 1758, translated by —). *NTG, 83*, II, 2085–2102; *BGG, XIX*, 86–103.

437 — (1939). Petrus Camper. De beroemde 18de eeuwsche chirurg, zoöloog en vergelijkend ontleedkundige bij de herdenking van zijn 150-ste sterfjaar (The famous surgeon, zoologist and comparative anatomist of the 18th century, at the 150th anniversary of his death). *Stemmen des Tijds, 28*, 844–60.

438 — (1939). Petrus Camper en Amsterdam. De wetenschappelijke loopbaan van Camper en de wederzijdsche culturele betrekkingen van 1755 tot 1761 (P.C. and Amsterdam. The scientific career of C., and the cultural interrelations from 1755 till 1761). *GG, 17*, 403–19, 1 ill.

439 BOELES, P. C. J. A. (1932). Uit den frieschen tijd van Prof. Petrus Camper (From the Frisian period of —). *Vrije Fries, 31*, 104–8.

440 VISSER, R. P. W. (1972). Petrus Camper nummer. *Doc. bl. Werkgr. 18e eeuw*, nr. 17 (sept.), 1–34, portr.
– This issue contains a chronology, and inventory of P.C.'s correspondence. With a bibliography of 147 items, among which many of the XVIIIth and XIXth century.

441 ENGELHARD, J. L. B., G. van Rijnberk and D. Schoute (1939). Petrus Camper, April 7 – 1789 – 150th anniversary of the death of Petrus Camper. *Isis, 30*, 510–1. Also in: *Ann. Med. Hist.*, s. 3, *I*, 200.

442 GALLAS, Th. (1939). Herdenking van den sterfdag van Petrus Camper (7 April 1789) te Groningen, 29–30 april 1939 (Commemoration P.C.'s death). *NTG, 83*, II, 2147–9; *BGG, XIX*, 149–51.

443 NUYENS, B. W. Th. (1939). Petrus Camper, herdenkingsrede op 29 april 1939 (Commemorative oration). *NTG, 83*, II, 2073–83; *BGG, XIX*, 75–85.

444 RIJNBERK, G. van (1939). Petrus Camper † 7 april 1789 (Obituary) *NTG, 83*, II, 2039; *BGG, XIX*, 73.

445 GOSLINGS-LIJSEN, J. A. (1939). Van twee vroolijke medici (On two merry physicians). *NTG, 83*, I, 1028–31; *BGG, XIX*, 57–60.
– On Petrus Camper and Jacob Ploos van Amstel.

446 SCHIERBEEK, A. (1922). Van Aristoteles tot Pasteur. XV. Petrus Camper ... *Levende Nat.*, 26, nr. 9, 225–9.

– Also in: A. Schierbeek. *Van Aristoteles tot Pasteur. Leven en werken van grote biologen*, (1923). Amsterdam, 231–5.

447   NIJHOFF, G. C. (1931). Iets over Petrus Camper. 1722–1789 (Something on P.C.). *Natuur en Mensch*, 129–31.

448   OLDEKAMP, J. (1948). Onbekende nakomelingen van Dr. Petrus Camper (Unknown descendants of Dr. P.C.) *Gens nostra, 3*, nr. 4, 58–61. *See also* 5408

Letters

449   DONGEN, J. A. van (1971). Een brief van Martinus van Marum aan Petrus Camper (A letter from M. van M. to P.C.). *MC, 26*, 19–20.

450   — (1971). Een brief van Petrus Camper aan Paulus de Wind (A letter of Petrus Camper to P. de Wind) *MC, 26*, 79–80.

451   — (1971). Een brief van Wouter van Doeveren aan Petrus Camper (A letter of W. van D. to P.C.), *MC, 26*, 133.

452   — (1971). Een brief van Matthias van Geuns aan Petrus Camper (A letter of M. van G. to P.C.). *MC, 26*, 253–4.

453   — (1971). Een brief van Emanuel Haller aan Petrus Camper (A letter of A. E. Haller to P.C.). *MC, 26*, 414.

454   — (1971). Een brief van Adriaan Gilles Camper aan Petrus Camper (A letter of A.G.C. to P.C.) *MC, 26*, 1272.

455   — (1972). Een brief van A. Balla aan Petrus Camper (A letter of A. Balla to P.C.) *MC, 27*, 44.

456   — (1972). Een brief van Bernhard Siegfried Albinus aan Petrus Camper (A letter of B. S. Albinus to P.C.). *MC, 27*, 172–3.

457   GRÜNSTEIN, L. (1904). Goethe, Merck und Camper (Aus ungedrückten Briefen Mercks an Peter und Adrian Camper). *Neue Freie Presse*, Morgenblatt, 18 Sept., nr 14392, 36–7.

458   BOOY, J. de (1957). Sur une lettre de Diderot à Pierre Camper. *Rev. d'hist. litt. d.l. France, 57*, 411–5.

459   GEYL, A. (1908). Briefwisseling tusschen Petrus Camper en Albert Titsingh over "regt" en dwars geklemde hoofden (Correspondence between P.C. and A.T. on "straight" or transversely pinched heads). *NTG, 52*, II, 228–47.

459ᵃ VERKROOST, C. M. (1974). Enkele brieven van Petrus Camper aan Paulus de Wind (Some letters from — to —). *MC, 29*, 1285-6.

459ᵇ VISSER, R. P. W. (1974). Een brief van Petrus Camper aan Frans Hemsterhuis (A letter from — to —). *Doc. bl. 18e eeuw*, no 25, october, 13-23.

460 CAMPER, P. (1770, 1771, 1934). *Brief aan D. van Gesscher en brief aan Prov. Justitie Kamer van Stad en Lande en antwoord van Prins van Oranje, 18 juni en 5 augustus 1770.* (Letter to D. v. G. and a letter to the Provincial Court of Justice of Town and Country and the answer from the Prince of Orange, June 18 and August 5, 1770). *Opusc. XII*, 1-33.
– Letter of P.C. on symphysiotomy.

461 — (1777, 1943). Brief aan de heeren Martens, van Gesscher, Zwagerman en Van Hussem, zeer kundige en zeer beroemde heelmeesters te Amsterdam over "het Steensnyden in twee reizen" (Letters to Mrs — — —, —, very able and very famous surgeons at A. on the Cutting for the stone in two stages). – with English translation. *Opusc., XVII*, 346-59.

462 — (1780, 1935). *Consilium de Comtissa de Randwyck viro clarissimo D. C. Velse.* – with Dutch translation. *Opusc., XIII*, 259-64.

463 DANIËLS, C. E. and H. C. Rogge (1881). *Catalogue de manuscrits de Pierre Camper et de lettres inédites ... qui se trouvent dans la Bibliothèque de la Société Néerlandaise pour le Progrès de la Médecine. Amsterdam. 8°.*

Voyages

464 [Anonym] (1939). Ein holländischer Arzt (Petrus Camper) besucht Friedrich den Groszen. *Z. ärt. Fortbild., 36*, 439-40.

465 NUYENS, B. W. Th. (1939). Reis van Petrus Camper naar Berlijn in het jaar 1730, zijn audiëntie bij den koning van Pruisen, Frederik de Groote, en wat daar gebeurde. (Voyage of P.C. to Berlin in the year 1730, his audience at the king of Prussia, Frederick the Great, and what happened there). *NTG, 83*, II, 1922; *BGG, XIX*, 145-9.

466 RIJNBERK, G. van (1939). *Opusculum* XV. *Petrus Camper's* reizen naar Engeland (*P.C.'s* voyages to England). *NTG, 83*, II, 1922; *BGG, XIX*, 74.

467 GUTHRIE, D. (1948). The travel journals of Peter Camper (1722-1789). *Edinb. Med. J., 55*, 338-53.

468 [   ] (1748–49, 1939). Campers reisjournalen (Camper's travel
     journals). With English translation. *Opusc.*, *XV*, 264 pp.
     – With biographical notes.

469 SCHULTE, J. E. (1939). Petrus Camper en de studie der menschenras-
     sen (P.C. and the study of the human races). *GG*, *17*, 441–9.

470 REYS, J. H. O. (1909). Goethe en Camper als voorloopers van Dar-
     win (G. and C. as precursors of Darwin). *Vrag. Dag*, *XXIV*, 540.

471 SCHIERBEEK, A. (1922). Petrus Camper en George Cuvier. *Levende
     Natuur*, *XXVI*, (1 Jan.), 225.

472 SCHAMELHOUT, G. (1943). Petrus Camper (1722–1789). Zijn verdien-
     sten als geneeskundige, natuuronderzoeker en anthropoloog. Een her-
     denking 220 jaar na zijn geboorte (His merits as a physician, investiga-
     tor of natural science and anthropologist. Commemoration 220 years
     after his birth). *Verh. Kon. Vl. Acad. Geneesk.*, *5*, nr. 2, 41–86.

473 THOMSEN, W. (1939). *Petrus Campers Abhandlung über die beste Form
     der Schuhe.* 105 pp. 9 ill., J. A. Barth, Leipzig, 8°.

474 VOS, J. J. Th. (1939). Petrus Camper als ziektekundige (Petrus Camper
     as a pathologist). *NTG*, *83*, II, 2124–8; *BGG*, *XIX*, 126–30.

475 WESTER, J. (1939). Petrus Camper en de geneeskunde der dieren
     Petrus Camper and veterinary medicine). *NTG*, *83*, II, 2138–40;
     BGG, *XIX*, 140–2.

476 BURLET, H. M. de (1939). Petrus Camper als anatoom (P.C. as an
     anatomist). *NTG*, *83*, II, 2111–20; *BGG*, *XIX*, 113–22.

477 VARIOT, G. (1927). L'anatomiste Pierre Camper et son doctrine sur
     l'éducation physique des enfants. Une aberration de J. J. Rousseau.
     Bull. Soc. Fr. Hist. Méd., *XXI*, 134–45.

478 — (1929). Quelques souvenirs historiques sur l'anatomiste Pierre
     Camper. Son oeuvre en hygiene infantile. *VIme Congrès Int. Hist. de
     la Méd. Leyde-Amsterdam*, *1927*, 362–5, Anvers.

479 SCHIERBEEK, A. (1939). Camper en Goethe over het tusschenkaaks-
     been (C. and G. on the intermaxillary bone). *NTG*, *83*, II, 2128–33;
     BGG, *XIX*, 130–5.

480 HEUVEL, A. J. van den (1883). *Petrus Camper als chirurg beschouwd*
     (— Considered as a surgeon). Thesis Amsterdam.

481 EERLAND, L. D. (1939). Petrus Camper als heelkundige (— As a surgeon). *NTG*, *83*, II, 2120–4; *BGG, XIX*, 122–6.

482 DOETS, C. J. (1948). *De heelkunde van Petrus Camper, 1722–1789* (The surgery of Petrus Camper, 1722–1789). Thesis Leyden. (Supervisor: J. A. J. Barge), 300 pp., ill. Eduard Ydo N.V., Leiden.

483 ANDEL, M. A. van (1939). Petrus Camper en de "Steensnijding in twee reizen" (P.C. and the "lithotomy in two stages"). *NTG*, *83*, II, 2134–8; *BGG, XIX*, 136–40.

484 NUYENS, B. W. Th. (1930). Petrus Camper (1722–1789) als verloskundige (As an obstetrician). *NTG*, *74*, I, 38–60; *BGG, X*, 1–23, 3 ill.

485 ENGELHARD, J. L. B. (1939). Petrus Camper als verloskundige (as an obstetrician). *NTG*, *83*, II, 2106–11; *BGG, XIX*, 108–13.

486 KLEY, J. J. van der (1939). Petrus Camper (1722–1789) en zijn verdiensten voor de verloskunde en voor de inenting der kinderpokken (P.C. and his merits for obstetrics and for the vaccination of smallpox). *GG*, *17*, 430–40.

487 CAMPER, P. (1783, 1934). *Verhaal van de konstbewerking der doorsnede van de schaambeenderen, gedaan door J. C. Damen.* (Account of the operation of symphysiotomy, performed by J. C. Damen). *Opusc.*, *XII.*, 149–74.

488 ROCHAT, G. F. (1939). Petrus Camper als oogheelkundige (P.C. as an ophthalmologist). *NTG*, *83*, II, 2101–6; *BGG, XIX*, 103–8.

489 BURGER, H. (1913). Peter Camper's leerboek der oogheelkunde (P. C.'s textbook of ophthalmology). *NTG*, *57*, I, 1615–8.

490 DOESSCHATE, G. ten (1962). Petrus Camper. *Optical dissertation on vision 1746.* Facsimile of the original Latin text. With a complete translation and an introduction by —. Dutch Classics on History of Science III, 29 + 34 + 31 pp. 1 pl. B. de Graaf, Nieuwkoop.

491 CAMPER, P. (1913). De Oculorum Fabrica et Morbis – with German translation. *Opusc.*, *II*, 411 pp.

492 FEYFER, F. M. G. de (1939). Petrus Camper als teekenaar (As a drawer). *NTG*, *83*, II, 2140–3; *BGG, XIX*, 142–5.

493 TERPSTRA, P. (1940). Petrus Camper's samling mineralen. *It Beaken 2*, nr. 2, 35–7. [Frisian].

494 TONELLI, G. (1956). Le dottrine estetiche di Piter Camper. *Giorn. crit. d. Filos. Italiana*, 35, 79–85.

495 NYÈSSEN, D. J. H. (1927). Petrus Camper en zijne tijdgenoten (P.C. and his contemporaries). *Mensch en Maatsch.*, *3*, 73–5.

496 COURTNEY, C. P. (1962). Edmund Burke and Petrus Camper. *Engl. Studies*, *43*, 467–75.

497 BRÄUNING OKTAVIO, H. (1912/13). Johann Heinrich Merck und Petrus Camper. *Arch. Gesch. Naturw. u. Techn.*, *4*, 270–306, 306–88.

498 SCHIPPERS, H. K. (1964). Petrus Camper op 'e tekst over seare teannen (PC. on a text on sore toes). *De Strikel*, *7*, nr, 3, 43–4. [Frisian].

499 REYS, J. H. O. (1939). Petrus Camper en de penning (P.C. and the medal). *GG*, *17*, 422–3, 3 ill.

500 ROOSEBOOM, M. (1954). Wedgwood Medallion of Petrus Camper. *BHM, XXVIII*, 553, 1 ill.

See also: 3227.13, 5482

501 ZANEN, G. E. van (1969). *David Ricardo Capriles. Student-genees-heer-schrijver. Curaçao 1837–1992* (D.R.C. Student-physician-author. Curaçao). 232 pp., portr. Van Gorcum, Assen.
– With a postscript by Cola Debrot.

502 PRICK, J. J. G. (1955). Prof. Dr E. A. D. E. Ca rp, 25 jaar hoogleraar in de Psychiatrie te Leiden (— Carp, 25 years professor of Psychiatry at L.). *Fol. Psych. Neurol. Neurochir.*, *58*, no 5/6, 4 pp., port.

503 SCHULTHEISS, E. (1960). Joannes Antonius Cassonoviensis, Humanist und Arzt des Erasmus. *Gesnerus*, *17*, 117–22.

503ᵃ GEIST-HOFMAN, A. M. (1973). Iets over Ce lsus en diens gedachten betreffende rationalisme en empirie (Something on — and his thoughts concerning rationalism and empiricism). *AP*, no 10, 11–4.

504 DOESSCHATE, G. ten (1959). Was Cézanne a forerunner of Luneburg? *Ophtalomologica* (Basel), *138*, 456–8.

505 BOERMA, N. J. A. F. (1941). Iets over het tweede verblijf van Peter Chamberlain III in Holland (Something on the second stay of P.C. III in Holland). *NTG*, *85*, III, 3245–50; *BGG, XXI*, 89–94.

506 REITH, J. F. (1953). Gaspard Adolphe Chatin 1813–1901. *Voeding 14*, 489–91.
- Chatin was professor of botany. He made investigations on iodine in the food.

507 WICKESHEIMER, Er. (1909). Une version en bas-Allemand de Guy de Chauliac. *Janus, XIV*, 486–90. *See also* 3451, 3452,

508 LAAGE, R. J. C. V. ter (1970). Reflections on Johann Ludwig Choulant and his medico-historical Bibliographies. In: *Essays in Biohist.*, Utrecht, 115–32, 1 ill.

509 NAPJUS, J. W. (1936). De geneeskundige hoogleeraren aan de Franeker Hoogeschool en het Athenaeum 1585–1843. Raphaël Clingbijl (The professors of medicine at Franeker University and the Athenaeum R.C.) *NTG, 80*, II, 2612–5; *BGG, XVI*, 85–8.

CAROLUS CLUSIUS

510 BOEYNAEMS, P. (1959, 1961). Le séjour de Charles de l'Ecluse à Montpellier (1551–1554). *Compt. rend. XVIe Congr. int. Hist. Méd., Montpellier 1958*, I, 71–4. Bruxelles 1959.
also in: *Le Scalpel* (1961), *114*, 941–5.

511 ELAUT, L. (1958). De brieven van de arts Raphaël Thorius (uit Londen) naar C. Clusius (Leiden) (The letters of the physician Raphaël Thorius (London) to C. Clusius (Leyden). *Jbk. Dodonaea, 26*, 168–77.
- Raphaël Thorius (van Thoor, born *ca* 1565) studied at Leyden, and wrote letters to Clusius from London from 1597 till 1607.

512 HUNGER, F. W. T. (1927, 1943). *Charles de l'Ecluse, Carolus Clusius. Nederlandsch Kruidkundige, 1526–1609*, 2 vols. (Dutch medical botanist).
I (1927) XVIII + 445 pp., 119 ill., 4 portr.
II (1942) IX + 466 pp., 2 portr. 130 ill.
Martinus Nijhoff, The Hague, 8°.
- Vol. I reviewed by Sudhoff, in *Janus* (1928), XXXII, 383–8. Vol. II contains 195 Latin letters (1573–98) to Joachim II Camerius (1534–98).

513 — (1925). Acht brieven van Middelburgers aan Carolus Clusius (Eight letters of Middelburgerians to C.C.) *Arch. Zeeuwsch Gen.*, 110–35.

514 GUGLIA, O. F. (1972). Carolus Clusius. Burgenland und "der berühmteste Botaniker seiner Zeit". *Biblos, 21*, 145–51, ill. portr.

515 GUÉDÈS, M. (1972). Notules de bibliographie botanique V–VIII. *J. Soc. Bibliog. nat. Hist.*, *6*, 174–80, facs. refs.
– on Carolus Clusius.

516 HUNGER, F. W. T. (1941). Nieuwe gegevens omtrent Clusius (New data on —). *NTG*, *85*, IV, 4546–7; *BGG*, *XXI*, 155–6.
– review of an address, communicated by Burger.

517 — (1927). Charles de l'Ecluse (Carolus Clusius), 1526–1609. *Janus*, XXXI, 139–51.
– Address at the commemoration of Clusius' 400th birthday.

518 — (1926). Charles de l'Ecluse (Carolus Clusius) 1526–1609. *NTG*, *70*, II, 1856–63; *BGG*, *VI*, 281–8.

519 JONG, M. de and D. A. Wittop Koning (ed.) (1963). *Carolus Clusius Aromatum et simplicium aliquot medicamentorum apud Indos nascentium historia. 1567. étant la traduction latine des Coloquios dos simples e drogas e cousas medicinais da India de Garcia da Orta.* Facsimile avec une introduction du Dr. Wittop Koning. Dutch Classics on History of Science VI, ill. 64 + 250 pp. B. de Graaf, Nieuwkoop

520 MUNTENDAM, P. (1926). Clusius-herdenking (Clusius commemoration) *NTG*, *70*, II, 1882–3; *BGG*, *VI*, 280.
– Short note on the commemoration of Clusius (Charles de l'Ecluse, 1526–1609). at Leyden on 19 October 1926.

521 — (1926). De Clusius-herdenking te Leiden. 19 october 1926. (The commemoration of Clusius). *NTG*, *70*, II 1882; *BGG*, *VI*, 307.

522 NUYENS, B. W. Th. (1926). Een kort levensbericht met een portret ter herinnering aan Carolus Clusius (A short biography in memory of C.C., with a portrait). *NTG*, *70*, I, 979–81; *BGG*, *VI*, 59–61, portr.

523 OPSOMER, Joseph E. (1966). Note sur deux ouvrages portugais de botanique tropicale du XVIᵉ siècle. *Bull. Séances Acad. royal Sci. d'Outre-Mer*, 786–95, 2 facs.
– A.o. on the work of Clusius.

524 WALTER, J. and M. Alves (ed.) (1964). Orta, G. de. *Aromatum et simplicium aliquot medicamentorum apud Indos nascentium historia, de C. Clusio.* Versao Portuguesa do epitome latino dos Coloquios dos simples. Introd. e versao portuguesa de —. Junta de Investig. do Ultramar, Lisboa.

525 SMIT, P. (1972). Clusius und die Leidener Universität. In: *Kurzfassungen d. Vortr. Dtsch. Gesell. f. Gesch. Mediz.*, Jahrestagung Sept. 1972, Göttingen, *22*, (2): 32.

526 — (1973). Clusius und die Leidener Universität. In: *Burgenländische Forschungen*. Herausgeg. vom Burgenländischer Landesarchiv, Sonderheft *V*. Clusius Festschrift, 232–52. *See also* 530.

526[a] — (1973). Carolus Clusius and the beginning of botany in Leiden University. *Janus, LX*, 87–92; also in: *Acta Septimi conventus*, 87–92. Amsterdam 1974.

526[b] — (1974). Carolus Clusius en Güssing. *Vakbl. Biol., 54*, 49–53.

527 THEUNISZ, Joh. (1939). *Carolus Clusius. Het merkwaardige leven van een pionier der wetenschap* (— —. The remarkable life of a pioneer of science). 178 pp., Patria-Reeks XVII. Van Kampen, Amsterdam.

528 VANDEWIELE, L. J. (1960). Carolus Clusius en Gent (C.C. and Ghent). *Sci. Hist., 2*, 19–20;

529 — (1972). Welke uitgaaf van het Ricettario Fiorentino lag er aan de basis van het Antidotarium van Clusius? (Which edition of the — — was the basis of the Antidotarium of C.?). *Bull. Pharm.*, no 44., 41–8, 2 ill.

530 HENIGER, Joh. (1973). Clusius und die Ungarischen und Österreichischen Pflanzen im Leidener Universitätsgarten. In: *Festschrift anläszlich der 400jährigen Wiederkehr der wissenschaftlichen Tätigkeit von Carolus Clusius (Charles de l'Ecluse) im pannonischen Raum*, 149–67. Burgenländische Forschungen, Sonderheft V. Eisenstadt.

531 JARRY, D. (1967). A propos d'un ouvrage d'Ogier Cluyt de la Bibliothèque de la Faculté de Médecine de Montpellier. *Monspeliensis Hippocrates, 10*, no. 38, 27–9, ill.

– On Cluyt's book *De Nuce medica/De Hemerobio*, Amsterdam 1634. Augerius Cluyt (1578– after 1636, son of Dirck Outgaertszoon Cluyt (*d.* 1598), worked for the Leyden Botanical Garden as an assistant of Clusius, became inspector of the Hortus in 1636.

532 ANDEL, M. A. van (1921). In Memoriam Alfons de Cock. *NTG, 65*, I, 1854–5; *BGG, I*, 145–6.

– de Cock was a writer on Flemish Folkmedicine: *Volksgeneeskunde in Vlaanderen*, 1891.

533   BIEMOND-KAM, M. J. (1972). Een vrouw van verdienste (A woman of merit). *Ons Amsterdam*, *24*, 85-7, 3 portr.

– On Freia Coenen (1899–1949), paediatrician and family doctor at Amsterdam from 1918–1949. Also on the family Coenen, a family of physicians.

VOLCHER COITER

534   ADELMANN, H. B. (ed.). (1933). (Coiter, Volcher, 1534–1600). The "De ovorum gallinaceorum generationis primo exordio progressuque, et pulli gallinacei creationis ordine" of Volcher Coiter. *Ann. Med. Hist.*, *5*, 327–41, 2 ill. and 444–57.

– Translated and edited with notes and introduction by Howard and Adelmann.

535   DANIEL, W. B. Mac. (1938). Notes on the "Tractatus de Ossibus Foetus" of Volcher Coiter. *Ann. Med. Hist.*, n.s. X, 189–90.

536   BRUINS, L. H. (1964). Een brief van de geleerde dokter Folkert Koiter (1534–1576) (A letter of the learned physician — —). *De Hogelandster*, *42*, no 29 (17 Juli), no 30 (29 Juli), no 31 (31 Juli and no 32 (7 Augustus). 12 pp.

537   HERRLINGER, Robert (1952). *Volcher Coiter 1534–1576*. 147 pp., ill., portr. Nürnberg.

538   – (1957). News on Coiter. *J. Hist. Med.*, *12*, 78–80, ill.

539   NUYENS, B. W. T. and Schierbeek, A. (1955). *Volcher Coiter*. (in 546).

540   — (1933). Doctor Volcher Coiter, 1534–1576. Een Noord-Nederlandsch geleerde uit de 16e eeuw (A scientist of the Northern Netherlands from the 16th century). *NTG*, *76*, 5383–401; *BGG, XIII*, 251–69.

541   — (1931). Volker Coiter als anatoom (V.C. as an anatomist). *NTG*, *75*, 5909–10; *BGG, XI*, 329–30.

542   — (1935). De laatste tien jaren van Volcher Coiter's leven (The last ten years of V.C.'s life). *NTG*, *79*, II, 2653–9; *BGG, XV*, 125–31.

543   SCHIERBEEK, A. (1957). Volcher Coiter (1534–1576). *Jbk. Dodonaea*, 148–56.

544   — (1957). Volcher Coiter (1534–1576). *GeWiNa*, *2*, 17–21.

545   SETZER, Irmgard (1958). *Coiters Tabellen der äusseren Körperteile (1564) übersetzt und mit Anmerkungen versehen*, 34 pp., ill. Würzburg.

546 COITER, V. (1572, 1955). Externarum et internarum principalium corporis partium Tabulae (MDLXXII). – With English translation. *Opusc.*, *XVIII*, 263 pp.

See also 1972, 5496

547 OOSTERHUIS, R. A. B. (1969). Comenius en de geneeskunde. (C. and medicine). *Natura docet*, *21*, no 10, 245–9.
– J. A. Comenius (1592–1670) lived from 1656–70 in Holland.

548 ROOD, Wilhelmus (1970). *Comenius and the Low Countries.* Some aspects of Life and Work of a Czech Exile in the seventeenth century. Thesis Utrecht. Van Gendt & Co., Amsterdam.
– Chapter 3: Comenius and Descartes, 118–162.

549 WITTOP KONING, D. A. (1957). Ein drittes Exemplar der ersten Ausgabe des Dispensatoriums von Valerius Cordus. *Z. Gesch. Pharm.*, *9*, 11.

550 BERGINK, A. H. (1962). Samuel Senior Coronel 1827–1892. *Voeding*, *23*, 473–7, portr.

551 — (1960). *Samuel Senior Coronel, zijn betekenis voor de sociale geneeskunde in Nederland* (S.S.C., his significance for social medicine in the Netherlands). Thesis Leyden (Supervisor: P. Muntendam), 237 pp., portr. Van Gorcum, Assen.
– Also published as a monograph with an introduction by P. Muntendam, 6 + 237 pp. Van Gorcum, Assen.

552 BRUIN, M. P. de (1959). Dr. Coronel en zijn tijd. Pionier van de sociale geneeskunde (Dr. C. and his time. Pioneer of Social Medicine). *Zeeuwsch T.*, *9*, 29–37.

553 — (1966). Samuel Senior Coronel. *Zeeuwsch T.*, *16*, 41.

554 HES, J. P. (1968). Samuel Senior Coronel (1827–1892) Portuguese Jewish physician, pioneer of social medicine in Holland. *Koroth*, *4*, 791–3 [Hebrew].

555 HAMMES, Th. (1950). *Dr. Samuel Coster en zijn betekenis voor de cultuurgeschiedenis van Amsterdam* (Dr. S.C. and his significance for the cultural history of Amsterdam). 87 pp., portr. J. H. de Bussy, Amsterdam.
– With an introduction on physicians who acquired fame in other fields. (*See also* 4235a)

556 NUYENS, B. W. Th. (1935). Martin Jansz. Coster, burgemeester

van Amsterdam en eerste voorlezer der Anatomie aldaar (M.J.C., mayor of Amsterdam and first praelector anatomiae there). *NTG*, *79*, II, 2109–11; *BGG*, *XV*, 121–2.

– included in the report of a meeting of the "Genootschap", made up by M. A. van Andel.

557   — (1936). Burgemeester doctor *Martin Jans-zoon Coster*, genaamd *Martinus Aedituus*, eerste voorlezer der anatomie te Amsterdam, een schets van zijn leven en van zijn bibliotheek (Mayor doctor *M.J.C.*, called *Martinus Aedituus*, first praelector of anatomy at A., a sketch of his life and of his library). *NTG*, *80*, II, 2604–11; *BGG*, *XVI*, 77–84.

558   KLAAUW, C. J. van der (1942). Twee brieven van Georges Cuvier aan Jan van der Hoeven (Two letters of G. Cuvier to J.v.d.H.). *NTG*, *86*, IV, 2473–5; *BGG*, *XXII*, 127–9.

559   NAPJUS, J. W. (1939). De geneeskundige hoogleeraren aan de Franeker Hoogeschool en het Athenaeum (1585–1843). (The medical professors at Franeker Academy and Athenaeum).
XII. Abraham Cyprianus. *NTG*, *83*, I, 70–6; *BGG*, *XIX*, 8–14, portr.
XIII, idem *NTG*, *83*, II, 2625–31; *BGG*, *XIX*, 159–65, ill.

560   WOOD, S. (1954). Abraham Cyprian's operation for full-time tubal pregnancy in 1694. *J. Obst. Gyn.*, *61*, 777–80.

561   GEYL, A. (1893). Hoe ongeveer een college zou hebben kunnen luiden van den in het laatst der 17e eeuw, in Franeker gevestigden professor A. Cyprianus (How a lecture given by the 17th century Franeker professor A.C. could nearly have run). *NTVerl. Gyn.*, *4*, 272–6.

D

562   BURGER, H. (1909). C. E. Daniëls 1839 – 4 juni – 1909. *NTG*, *53*, I, 1869–75. Also in: H. Burger (1930). *Uitgezochte opstellen en toespraken*, 512–8.

563   BURGER, C. P. Jr. (1921). *C. E. Daniëls als bibliothecaris* (— as a librarian). port. no. pl.

564   GEYL, A. (1909). Dr. Carel Eduard Daniëls (Juni 1839–Juni 1909). *Janus*, XIV, 273–86.

– on the occasion of Daniëls' 70th anniversary; with a bibliography of —.

565 LEERSUM, E. C. van (1921). In Memoriam C. E. Daniëls. *NTG*, *65*, I, 647–9; *BGG*, *I*, 61–3.

565ᵃ LUYENDIJK-ELSHOUT, A. M. (1974). In memoriam Prof. Dr. Johan Dankmeijer, 26 oktober 1907 – 12 september 1973. *AP*, no. 14, 21–3.

566 HUBRECHT, A. A. W. (1909). Darwin and the Descent of Man. *Janus*, *XIV*, 862–75.

567 VRIES, Hugo de (1909). Darwin's visit to the Galapagos-islands. *Janus*, *XIV*, 854–61.

See also 690, 2832–35

567ᵃ MULDER, R. D. (1957). Dr Michiel Dassen H. J. zn., een veelzijdig Drents medicus, 1809–1852 (Dr. M.D., a many-sided physician in Drenthe). *Nwe Drentse Volksalm.*, *75*, 5–41; *76*, 23–56.

568 [R.v.R.] (1961). Petrus Dathenus, predikant en... geneesheer (— —, preacher and ... physician). *Periodiek*, *16*, 196–7.
– Dathenus was an enthusiastic protestant preacher, but practised as a physician at the end of his life. He died in 1588 at Elburg, where the epitaph on his tombstone runs "doctor theologiae et medicinae".

569 HAMPE, J. F. (1966). In memoriam Prof. Dr H. T. Deelman. *NTG*, *110*, 322–3, port.

570 SLUITER, E. (1944–'47). Isaac van Deen 1804–1869. *Arch. Néerl. Physiol. de l'homme et des animaux, XXVIII.*

571 — (1947). Isaac van Deen, 1804–1869. *NTG*, *91*, II, 946–51; *BGG*, *XXVII*, 14–9.
See also 669, 670

572 DEEN, I. van (1838–39, 1922). Over de voorste en achterste strengen van het ruggemerg (On the anterior and posterior tracts of the spinal cord). *Opusc. IV*, 341–62.

573 BAUMANN, E. D. (1919). Frederik Dekkers. *Janus*, *XXIV*, 233–52.

574 DOCK, W. (1922). Some Early Observers of Albuminuria. *Ann. Med. Hist.*, s. 1., *IV*, 287–90, 2 ill., 2 ports.
– This article deals a.o. with Frederik Dekkers (+portrait).

575 LINDEBOOM, G. A. (1973). Mensen om Boerhaave. VIII. Frederik Dekkers (men around B. VIII). *GG*, *4*, 58–60, portr.

RENÉ DESCARTES

Biographica

576   SERRURIER, C. (1930). *Descartes. Leer en leven* (Doctrine and Life).
295 pp., portr. Martinus Nijhoff, the Hague.
– reviewed by F. M. G. de Feyfer in: *NTG, 76,* (1932), I, 74–5; *BGG, XII,* 15–6.

577   VLEESCHAUWER, H. J. de (1937). *René Descartes, levensweg en wereld-beschouwing* (R.D., path of life and world-view), 281 pp., Antwerpen-Nijmegen.

578   OEGEMA VAN DER WAL, Th. (1960). *De Mens Descartes* (The man D.)
A. Manteau, Brussel.

579   DIJKSTERHUIS, E. J. (1950). *De mechanisering van het wereldbeeld*
(The mechanization of the world picture), 590 pp., Meulenhoff, Amsterdam.
– On Descartes: 444–60. English edition (1961, 1969): *The mechanization of the world picture,* 537 pp., Oxford University Press London, Oxford – New York.

580   DIJKSTERHUIS, E. J., C. Serrurier, P. Dibon, H. J. Pos, J. Orcibal, C. L.
Thyssen-Schoute, G. Lewis (1950). *Descartes et le cartésianisme hollandais, études et documents.* 309 pp. Presses Universitaires de France,
Ed. franç. d'Amsterdam, Paris-Amsterdam.

581   FONTAINE VERWEY, H. de la (1950). Descartes en Amsterdam. *Amstelodamum, 37,* 17–21.

Works and Ideas

582   DESCARTES, René (1637, 1950). *Vertoog van de Methode* (The Discourse
on Method). Wereld-Bibliotheek, Amsterdam-Antwerpen.
– The "Discours de la Méthode", translated into Dutch by Miss H. C. Pos, with
introduction by Prof. H. J. Pos.

583   HALL, T. S. (1970). Descartes' physiological method: position, principles, examples. *J. Hist. Biol., 3,* 53–79.

583[a] SPIELMANN, I. (1973). Elements of Cartesian physiology in S. Enyedi's
manuscript "Physica seu philosophia naturalis". *Rev. Med.* (Turgu-Mures), *19,* 396–400; also in: *Orv. Szle, 19,* 392–6.
– [Ruman & Hung. with Engl., French & Russ. abstr.]

584   DANKMEIJER, J. (1951). *De biologische studies van René Descartes*
(The biological studies of René Descartes), 23 pp., Leidse Voordrachten, 9. Universitaire Pers, Leiden.

585 — (1951). Les travaux biologiques de René Descartes (1596–1650). *Arch. int. d'Hist. Sci.*, no. 16, 675–80.

586 SCHLICHTING, Th. H. (1958). Descartes over voorwaardelijke reflexen en onbewuste complexen (D. on conditional reflexes and unconscious complexes). *NTG, 102*, II, 1758; *BGG, XXXVIII*, 22.

587 ZWAN Jr., A. van der (1958). Descartes en de geneeskunde (D. and medicine). *NTG, 102*, II, 2382–6; *BGG, XXXVIII*, 37–41.

588 MOOK, P. van (1955). Descartes en de psycho-somatische geneeskunde (D. and psycho-somatic medicine). *NTG, 99*, III, 2233; *BGG, XXXV*, 76.
– A short note.

Relations

589 WALLACH, E. (1928). Descartes und Harvey. *Arch. f. Gesch. Med., XX*, 301–6.

590 PELSENEER, Jean (1932). Gilbert, Bacon, Galilée, Kepler, Harvey et Descartes: leurs relations. *Isis, 17*, 171–208.

591 CHAUVOIS, L. (1955). Un "colloque"; Harvey, Riolan, Descartes. *Presse méd., 63*, 129–30, ports.

592 GUERDULT, Martial (1970). Etudes sur Descartes, Spinoza, Malebranches et Leibniz. *Studien und Materialen zur Geschichte der Philosophie, 5*, 290 pp. Olms, Hildesheim.
— *see also* 1426–31 (Regius)

Letters/Influence

593 WAARD, C. de (1931). Une lettre inédite de Mersenne à Descartes. *Archeion, XIII*, 175–86.

594 — (1933). Une lettre inédite de Descartes à Huygens. *Archeion, XV*, 177–80.

595 — (1953). Un entretien avec Descartes en 1634 ou 1635. *Arch. Int. d'Hist. Sci., 6*, (XXXII), 14–6.

595ᵃ LINDEBOOM, G. A. (1971). De vroege invloed van Descartes op het geneeskundig denken in Nederland (The early impact of Descartes on medical thought in the Netherlands). *G&W, 69*, 207–16.

596   — (1971). The impact of Descartes on seventeenth century medical thought in the Netherlands. *Janus, LVIII*, 201–6.

   – Paper read at the XIIIth Congress of the History of Sciences, Moscow, 18–24 August 1971.

597   — (1972). Descartes en de kerk (D. and the Church). *Serta Historica, III*, 53–105, Kok, Kampen.

   – also published as a monograph, 64 pp., portr., J. H. Kok, Kampen 1973.

598   MEYER, W. (1916). Over Descartes' leven na den dood (On D.'s life after death). *Tijdspiegel, 73, II*, 226.

599   — (1911). Het leven na den dood van René des Cartes (The life after death of R. des C.). *Tijdspiegel, 68, IIIe deel*, 372–84.

600   — (1917). Wat er met het vermeende overschot van Descartes is geschied (What happened to the reputed mortal remains of —). *Tijdspiegel, 74, IIe deel*, 135–7.

HENDRIK VAN DEVENTER

601   WARTENA, B. (1882). *Het leven van Hendrik van Deventer en zijne verdiensten als verloskundige* (The life of — and his merits as an obstetrician). Thesis University of Amsterdam. 79 pp., 8°, Amsterdam.

602   KOUWER, B. J. (1912). Hendrik van Deventer. *Janus, XVII*, 425–42 and 506–24.

603   KRUL, R. (1903). Bij de woning van Hendrik van Deventer (At the residence of —). *Die Haghe*, 140.

604   LAMERS, A. J. M. (1946). *Hendrik van Deventer. Medicinae Doctor 1651–1724. Leven en werken* (Life and works). Thesis Leiden (Supervisor: J. A. J. Barge), 267 pp., ill. 4°. Van Gorcum, Assen.

   – with bibliography.

605   — (1951). Hendrik van Deventer geboren (born) 16 maart 1651 te Leiden, gestorven (died) 12 december 1724 te Voorburg. *NTG, 95, I*, 859–63; *BGG, XXXI*, 10–4, 3 ill., portr.

606   LINT, J. G. de (1924). Hendrik van Deventer. *NTG, 68, II*, 2870–7; *BGG, IV*, 299–306.

607   GEYL, A. (1908). Het bezoek van Hendrik van Deventer in Denemarken met eenige opmerkingen over beunhazerij in die dagen. (The visit

of H. van D. to Denmark with some remarks on dabbling in those days). *Geneesk. Crt*, 9, 16 en 23 May, reprint, 48 pp.,

608 HEILBRUNN, B. (1887). *Heinrich von Deventer und seine Anschauungen über die verkehrten Lagen der Gebärmutter*. Thesis Würzburg.

609 HODEL, C. and M. L. Portmann (1968). Hendrik van Deventer (1651–1724), ein Pionier der modernen Geburtshilfe. *Gynaek. Rundschau* 6, 307–12.

610 HODEL, C. (1967). Hendrik van Deventer (1651–1724) und die Anfänge moderner Geburtshilfe. *Gynaecologia* (Basel), *164*, 114–34.

611 KOUWER, B. J. (1912). Rede bij den herstelden grafsteen van Hendrik van Deventer (Address at the repaired tombstone of —). *NTG, 66*, I, 96.

612 — (1912–13). Rede, uitgesproken ter gelegenheid van de onthulling van den vanwege de Nederlandsche Maatschappij tot Bevordering der geneeskunst herstelden grafsteen van Hendrik van Deventer (Address, delivered on the occasion of the unveiling of the tombstone of H. van D. repaired by the Dutch Society for the promotion of medicine). *Med. Wbl. 19*, 174.

613 ROGGE, C. W. L. (1964). De promotie van Hendrik van Deventer (Graduation of — —). *N.T. Med. Stud., 10*, 124–6.

614 VAUBEL, E. (1969). Die Anatomie des Dr. Joan Deyman. *Grünenthal Waage, 8*, 175–8, ill.

615 HALBERTSMA, K. T. A. (1942). Dieffenbach (Johann Friedrich), 1792–1847. *NTG, 86*, 1707–13; *BGG, XXII*, 88–94.

615ᵃ HOUTZAGER, H. L. (1974). Driehonderd jaar geleden overleed IJsbrand van Diemerbroeck (Three hundred years ago died — —). *Oud-Utrecht, 47*, no 8, 69–71, port.

616 MENDES, J. C. (1964). Teria Diemmerbroeck conhecido com rigor a anatomia da árvore traquebronquica? *Arq. Anat. Antrop.* (Lisboa), *32*, 251–3, ill.

617 POSTHUMUS, S. (1960). Evart van Dieren en de aetiologie der beri-beri, 1861–1940 (Evart van Dieren and the aetiology of beri-beri, 1861–1940). *Voeding, 21*, 139–47, portr.

618 FREUDENTHAL, Hans (1965). Prof. E. J. Dijksterhuis. *Nature, 208,*
     1258–9.

     – E.J.D. (1892–1965), scientist, writer of "De mechanisering van het wereldbeeld",
     Amsterdam, 1950. (590 pp.). *See* 579.

619 HOOYKAAS, R. (1966). Eduard Jan Dijksterhuis (1892–1965). *Rev.
     d'Hist. Sci., 19,* 177–9.

620 SCHIMANK, Hans (1965). Eduard Jan Dijksterhuis † *Nachr. Deutschen
     Gesell. der Med.,* no. 26, 77–81.

621 SMEUR, A. J. E. M. (1965). In memoriam Prof. Dr. E. J. Dijksterhuis.
     Sci. Hist., 7, 163–6.

622 SETERS, W. H. van (1950). In Memoriam Dr. Clifford Dobell, F.R.S.
     (1886–1949). *NTG, 94,* II, 1274–6; *BGG, XXX,* 9–11, portr.

     – Dobell is the author of the well-known book *Antonie van Leeuwenhoek and his
     little "animals",* Swets en Zeitlinger, Amsterdam, 1932. Reprint New York 1956.

REMBERTUS DODONAEUS

623 HUNGER, F. W. T. (1923). Sur l'année de naissance de Rembertus Do-
     donaeus. *Janus, XXVII,* 213–8. ill.

624 — (1912). Over het geboortejaar van Rembertus Dodonaeus (On the
     year of birth of R.D.), *NTG,* 67, I, 1883–8; *BGG, III,* 116–21.

625 KROON, J. E. (1918). De geboorteplaats van Dodonaeus (The birth-
     place of —). *NTG, 62,* II, 100.

626 HUNGER, F. W. T. (1918). De geboorteplaats van Dodonaeus (The
     birth-place of —). *NTG, 62,* II, 340.

627 LINT, J. G. de (1917). De geboorteplaats van Dodonaeus (The birth-
     place of D.) *NTG, 61,* 325 and 510.

628 BLOK, P. J. (1917). Rembert Dodoens protestant. *Janus, XXII,* 269.

629 LINT, J. G. de (1917). De portretten van Rembertus Dodonaeus (The
     portraits of —). *NTG, 61,* I, 2126.

630 — (1917). Les portraits de Rembertus Dodonaeus. *Janus, XXII,* 174–
     81.

631 DOORSLAER, G. van (1930). Rembert Dodoens, au début de sa carrière.
     Janus, XXXIV, 132–41, 1 ill.

632 — (1926). *Glanes Nouvelles sur Rembert Dodoens*. Malines.

633 ANDRIES, R. (1917). *Rembertus Dodoens. Zijn leven en werken 1517–1585* (— —. His life and works). Antwerpen.

634 DODONAEUS, Rembert (1554), (1971). *Cruydeboeck*. In den welcken die gheheele historie, dat es Tgeslacht, tfatsoen, naem, natuere, cracht ende werckinghe, van den Cruyden, niet alleen hier te lande wassende, maer oock van den anderen vremden in der Medecijnen oorboorlijck, met grooter neersticheyd begrepen ende verclaert es,... J. Bander. Antwerpen. (In which the whole history ... of the plants ... indispensable for medicine is comprised and explained). 38 + 818 pp. Anastatic reprint, De Forel, Nieuwendijk (introduction by Wittop Koning).

635 LOUIS, A. (1954). Over het leven en het botanisch werk van Rembert Dodoens (1517–1585). bij de viering van de 400ste verjaardag van het verschijnen van Dodoens' *Cruydeboeck* (On the life and botanical work of R.D. on the occasion of the 400th anniversary of the publication of Dodoens' *Cruydeboeck*). *Jbk. Dodonaeus, 21*, 235–80.

636 ELAUT, L. (1954). Het Cruydeboeck van Rembertus Dodoens vierhonderdjarig (The "Cruydeboeck" of R.D., four hundredth anniversary). *Vlaamse Gids, 38*, 411–6.

637 HUNGER, F. W. T. (1917). Dodonaeus als kruidkundige (D. as a herbalist). *NTG, 61*, I, 2118.

638 — (1917). Dodonée comme botaniste. *Janus, XXII*, 153–62.

639 SCHIERBEEK, A. (1954). *Bloemlezing uit het Cruydt-Boeck van Rembert Dodoens* (Anthology from the Herbal of D.R.). 166 pp. ill., sec. ed. "De Hofstad", Den Haag.

640 SIRKS, M. J. (1917). Het Cruydeboeck van Rembert Dodoens (The Herbal of R.D.). *Gids, III*, 156.

641 — (1917). Rembert Dodoens en zijn Cruydtboek. (R.D. and his Herbal). *Vrag. Dag, XXXII*, 417–37.

642 VETH, J. (1917). De prenten in het Cruydtboeck van Dodonaeus. (The prints in the "Cruydtboeck" of —). *Gids, III*, 161.

643 SIRKS, M. J. (1917). L'herbier Flamand de Rembert Dodoens. *Janus, XXII*, 182–204.

644 ANDEL, M. A. van (1917). Dodonaeus en zijn invloed op de Holland-
     sche en Vlaamsche volksgeneeskunst (D. and his influence on Dutch
     and Flemish Folk-medicine). *NTG, 61*, I, 2131–9.

645 ANDEL, M. A. van (1917). Rembertus Dodonaeus and his influence
     on Flemish and Dutch Folk-medicine. *Janus, XXII*, 163–73.

646 HUNGER, F. W. T. (1923). Een tot dusver onuitgegeven brief van Rem-
     bertus Dodonaeus (A hitherto inedited letter of —). *NTG, 67*, II, 1652–
     3; *BGG*, III, 306–7.

647 ANDEL, M. A. van (1917). Rembertus Dodonaeus and his influence on
     Flemish and Dutch folk-medicine. *Janus, XXII*, 163–73.

648 SCHIERBEEK, A. (1919). Dodonaeus. *Levende Natuur XXIV* (1 Nov.),
     193.

649 RIJNBERK, G. van (1917). Bij het Dodonaeusnummer (At the D.-
     issue). *NTG, 61*, I, 2107.

650 LEERSUM, E. C. van (1917). Rembert Dodoens. *NTG, 61*, I, 2108.

651 — (1917). Rembert Dodoens (29 juin 1517 – 10 mars 1585). *Janus,
     XXII*, 141–52.

652 HUNGER, F. W. T. (1917). Rembertus Dodonaeus. *Amsterdammer*
     (Wbl. v. Ned.), 30 juni and 28 july.

653 DENIS, L. J. (1968). Dodonaeus (1517–1585). *Invest. Urol., 5*, 1420–1.
     See also 5491

654 ZWAAG, P. van der (1970). Wouter van D o e v e r e n (1739–1783).
     Leven en werken van een 18e eeuws hoogleraar in de geneeskunde (Life
     and works of an 18th century professor of medicine). Thesis Free
     University Amsterdam (Supervisor: G. A. Lindeboom), 190 pp.,
     portr., Van Gorcum, Assen.
     See also 4151

FRANCISCUS CORNELIS DONDERS

Biographica

655 LEERSUM, E. C. van *et al.* (1932). *Het levenswerk van Franciscus Cor-
     nelis Donders* (The life-work of —). 408 pp., portr., Bohn, Haarlem.
     8°.

656 DOESSCHATE, G. ten (1951). De persoonlijkheid van Franciscus Cornelis Donders (The personality of F.C.D.). *NTG*, *95*, IV, 3421–41;
BGG, *XXXI*, 66–86.

657 JONGBLOED, J. (1953). Prof. Dr. F. C. Donders 1818–1889. *Voeding*, *14*,
357–9, portr.

658 [   ] (1964). Franciscus Cornelis Donders 1818–1889 [English].
Triangle, *6*, 127, portr.

659 FISCHER, F. P. and G. ten Doesschate (1958). *Franciscus Cornelis Donders* (met een woord vooraf van Prof. Dr. H. J. M. Weve) Uitgegeven
ter gelegenheid van het eeuwfeest op 6 november 1958 van het Nederlandsch Gasthuis voor behoeftige en minvermogende ooglijders, gevestigd te Utrecht (Memorial volume on the occasion of the 100th
anniversary of the Dutch hospital for poor and indigent eye-patients
at Utrecht, with an introduction of H. J. M. Weve). Ill. Van Gorcum,
Assen, 223 pp. 4°.

660 DUKE-ELDER, Sir S. (1959). Franciscus Cornelis Donders. *Brit. J.
Ophtalm*, *43*, 65–8.

661 CITTERT-EYMERS, J. G. van (1969) Een beroepsprocedure in 1848 (On
the procedure of a call). *Universiteit en Hogeschool*, *14*, 580–1.
– On a call of F. C. Donders (1818–1889) by the Groningen University.

622 HERWERDEN, M. A. van (1918). De vriendschap tusschen Donders en
von Graefe (The friendship between D. and Von G.). *De Gids*, *II*, 500.

663 — (1918). Die Freundschaft zwischen Donders und von Graefe, *Janus*,
XXIII, 81–94.

664 WEVE, H. J. M. and G. ten Doesschate (1935). Die Briefe Albrecht
von Graefe's an F. C. Donders (1852–1870). Herausgegeben und mit
Bemerkungen versehen von —. Beilagsheft zu *Klin. Monatsbl. Augenheilk.*, Bd 95, 102 pp., 8°. Ferd. Enke, Stuttgart.

665 VOS, T. A. (1973). Geschiedkundige bijdragen. II. De rol van brieven
in de geneeskunde (Historical contributions. II. The role of letters in
medicine). *Arts en Wereld*, *6*, no. 4, 39–48, 2 portrs., 1 ill.
– on letters of Alb. von Graefe to F. C. Donders.

666 HERWERDEN, M. A. van (1941). Brieven van F. C. Donders aan Wil-
liam Bowman. Uitgegeven en van enkele aantekeningen voorzien
(Letters of F.C. D. to W.B. Edited and provided with some notes)
NTG, *85*, II, 1474–81; *BGG*, *XXI*, 39–46.

667 LESKY, Erna (1961). Aus dem Nachlass von Arlts im Wiener medizin-
     historischen Institut. *Klin. Monatsbl. Augenheilk.*, *139*, 847–56.
     – with some letters of F. C. Donders and of Ernest Fuchs (1851–1930).

668 VINKEN, P. J. (1963). Donders en Lamarck (D. and L.). *KNAW*, serie
     C, *vol. 68*, no. 3. N-Hollandsche Uitgeversmij., Amsterdam.

669 HERWERDEN, M. A. van (1914). Een vriendschap tusschen drie phy-
     siologen (A friendship between three physiologists). *De Gids, I*, 448.
     – Donders, Moleschott, van Deen.

670 — (1915). Eine Freundschaft von drei Physiologen. *Janus, XX*, 174–
     201 and 409–36.
     – Donders, Moleschott and Van Deen.

671 COLENBRANDER, M. C. (1958). Franciscus Cornelis Donders and his
     time. *Opusc., XIX*, p. IX–XV.

672 DONDERS, F. C. (1958). Rede uitgesproken te Utrecht op 28 Mei ter
     gelegenheid van de aanbieding van de oorkonde der Donders-Stich-
     ting (Address delivered at Utrecht on May 28, 1888 on the occasion
     of the Presentation of the Charter of the Donders Foundation).
     – With English translation. *Opusc., XIX*, 270–1.
     See also 5409

Commemorations

673 [Commissie] (1889). Het jubileum van Professor F. C. Donders ge-
     vierd te Utrecht op 27 en 28 Mei 1888. Gedenkboek uitgegeven door
     de Commissie. 210 pp. (The jubilee of professor F.C.D., celebrated
     at Utrecht, May, 27 and 28, 1888. Memorial volume edited by the
     Committee). 210 pp. Van de Weyer, Utrecht.

674 DANIËLS, C. E. (1893). Information on the erecting of a memorial
     for F. C. Donders. *NTG, 29*, [2de reeks *37*,] I, 456–61.

675 BURGER, H. (1911). Een gedenksteen voor Donders (A memorial stone
     for —). *NTG, 55*, II, 1853.

676 ROOSENBURG, D. L. [1915]. *Oproep aan de Nederlandsche geneeskun-
     digen.* no pl., no d.
     – Summons to contribute to a fund for the foundation of a monument to F. C.
     Donders. A circular letter.

677 RIJNBERK, G. van (1918). In memoriam F. C. Donders. *NTG, 62*, II,
     1493.

678 ENGELMANN, Th. W. (1918). In memoriam F. C. Donders. *NTG*, *62*, I, 1494.

679 PEKELHARING, C. A. (1919). Franciscus Cornelis Donders. Address held in the University of Utrecht on May 27th 1918. *Janus*, *XXIV*, 57–76.
   – Address held at the centenary of Donders' birthyear. Due to the previous war the planned monument was not yet ready.

680 [Editorial] (1969). In memoriam F. C. D[onders] *Acta psychol.* (Amst.), Jan., 23–8.

681 FISCHER, F. P. and G. ten Doesschate (1958). *Franciscus Cornelis Donders*. 223 pp., portr., ill. Van Gorcum, Assen.
   – Published on the occasion of the centenary of the "Ned. Gasthuis voor ooglijders" at Utrecht, on november 6, 1958.

Works and Ideas

682 ESSEN, J. van (1940). F. C. Donders als pionier der experimentele psychologie (As a pioneer of experimental psychology). *NTG*, *84*, I, 49–51; *BGG*, *XX*, 16–8.

683 BROZEK, Jozef (1970). Contributions to the history of psychology XII: Wayward history; F. C. Donders (1818-1889) and the timing of mental operations. *Psychol. Rep. 26*, 563–9.

684 GOODMAN, E. S. (1971). Citation analysis as a tool in historical study: a case study based on F. C. Donders and mental reaction times. *J. Hist. behav. Sci.*, 7, 187–91.

685 DONDERS, F. C. (1845, 1926). Blik op de stofwisseling van het epitellu-rische leven als bron der eigene warmte van planten en dieren (Notes on metabolism of life on the earth as a source of Natural Heat of Plants and Animals). – With English translation. *Opusc.*, V, 276–381

686 — (1845–46, 1942). Grondvormen en weefsels (Primitive forms and tissues). Physiologische en pathologische aanteekeningen van gemeng-den aard (Physiological and pathological notes of a mixed character). – With German translation. *Opusc.*, *XVI*, 60–121.

687 — (1848, 1907). De harmonie van het dierlijke leven. De openbaring van wetten (The harmony of animal life. The revelation of laws). *Opusc.*, *I*, 229–65., portr.
   – Inaugural address, 28 january 1848; Reprint 1971. Oosthoek, Utrecht.

688   — 1851–52, 1942). De vorm, de samenstelling en de functie der ele-
mentaire deelen, in verband met hunnen oorsprong (The form, composition and the function of the elementary parts, in connection with
their origin). – With German translation. *Opusc. XVI*, 142–219.

689   JOSSELIN DE JONG, R. de (1930). Donders als patholoog-anatoom (As
a pathologist-anatomist). *NTG*, *74*, I, 1064–83; *BGG, X*, 53–72.

690   DOESSCHATE, G. ten (1959). Donders als voorloper van Darwin ten
aanzien van de evolutieleer (As the precursor of Darwin in view of the
theory of evolution). *NTG, 103*, 1264–5; *BGG, XXXIX*, 5–6.

691   COLENBRANDER, M. C. (1942). Het optische werk van F. C. Donders
(The optical work of —). *NTG, 86*, IV, 3186; *BGG, XXII*, 99.

692   LAMMERTS VAN BUEREN, A. (1958). Een eeuw oogheelkunde. Prof. Dr.
Franciscus Donders herdacht (A century of ophthalmology. D. commemorated). *Goed Zicht* (ed. by Foundation "Beter Zien"), 3 pp., no. 6,
ill.

693   TANNEBAUM, S. (1967). Frans Cornelis Donders – the revolution in
ocular refraction. *J. Am. Optom. Ass., 38*, 970.

694   DONDERS, F. C. (1864, 1963). On the anomalies of accomodation and
refraction of the eye. The New Sydenham Society, London 1864.
Abridged version introd. by M C. Colenbrander. XV + 294 pp., 3 ill.,
Bohn Haarlem. In the series: *Opusc.* Vol. XIX.
– Reviewed by E. Clarke: *Arch. Int. Hist. Sci., 17* (1964), 364.

695   [Editorial] (1972). Dr. J. A. van Dongen overleden. Sinds 1949 bibliothecaris van Maatschappij Geneeskunst (Dr. J. A. van D. died.
Since 1949 librarian of the Society of Medicine). *M.C., 27*, 335, portr.
– J. A. van Dongen (1888–1972), gynaecologist at Amsterdam, was many years
librarian of the Library of the Ass. for the promotion of Medicine.

696   BAREN, J. van (1909). Jacob Elisa Doornik, een vergeten Nederlander (1777–1837) (A forgotten Dutchman). *Jbk. Gesch. Oudhk. van Leiden en Rijnland, 6*, 29 pp.
– Doornik (a philosopher, who wrote some philosophical works), studied and graduated in medicine at Leyden, practised at Amsterdam, became medical officer in
the Dutch East Indies, died at New Orleans.

697   STRUIK, D. J. (1965). William Douglass, M.D. Utrecht 1712, *J.
Hist. Med. XX*, 166.
– On W. Douglass (*c.* 1691–1752), who probably graduated at the University of
Utrecht on Feb. 6, 1712. He was a well-known Boston physician.

698 LINDEBOOM, G. A. (1972). Mensen om Boerhaave. III. Charles Drélincourt (Men around Boerhaave. III.) *GG.*, *2*, 144–6.
See also 4144

699 LINT, J. G. de (1918). Geneeskundige mededeelingen van een Gorkum-
se geneesheer uit de laatste helft der 17e eeuw (Medical communications of a Gorkum physician from the last half of the 17th century).
NTG, *62*, II, 1631.
– On Johan van Dueren, a friend and correspondent of Stephen Blankaart (1650–
1702).

E

700 LEERSUM, E. C. van (1909). Wilhelm Ebstein (1859 – 11 juillet – 1909).
Janus, *XIV*, 529.

701 WALSUM, G. C. van (1930). Dr. Frederik van Eeden. *GG*, *8*, 304–5.

702 ELAUT, L. (1961). Het medisch proefschrift van Frederik van Eeden
(The medical thesis of F. van E.) *Vlaamsche Gids*, *XLV*, 480–5.

703 WALSEM, G. C. van (1930). Op de receptie bij Van Eeden op "Walden"
(On the reception at —). *GG*, *8*, 378.
– Walden was a kind of commune near Hilversum where Van E. lived for some-
time.

704 EERLAND, L. D. (1970). *Het scalpel en de kaars* (The Scalpel and candle).
139 pp., portrs., ill., pr. pr.
– An autobiography of E. (1897–   ), professor of surgery at Groningen.

705 WATERMAN, N. (1954). Ehrlich als canceroloog. Bij zijn 100e geboortedag, 14 maart (Ehrlich as a cancerologist. On his 100th anniversary, March 14). *NTG*, *98*, II, 1103–4.

WILLEM EINTHOVEN

706 HOOGERWERF, S. (1946). Willem Einthoven. In: T. P. Sevensma (ed.)
Nederlandsche helden der wetenschap. Levensschetsen van negen Nobelprijswinnaars (Dutch heroes of science. Biographical sketches of
nine winners of the Nobel Prize)., 239–298. Kosmos, Amsterdam.

707 [Editorial] (1965). Willem Einthoven (1860–1927). *JAMA*, *191*, 494–5.

708 GAMBAROGHI, K. (1963). Willem Einthoven (1860–1927). [Russian].
Klin. Med. (Moskou), *41*, 154–6.

709 WIGGERS, C. J. (1961). Willem Einthoven (1860–1928): some facets of his life and work. *Circulation Res.*, *9*, 225–34, ill., portr.

710 JONGH, C. L. de (1954). Het levenswerk van Einthoven (The lifework of —). *NTG*, *98*, I, 270–3.

711 WAART, A. de (1957). *Het levenswerk van Willem Einthoven (1860–1927)*. (The life-work of —). XII + 258 pp. portr., 77 ill. Bohn, Haarlem, 8°.

712 [   ] (1965). Willem Einthoven. Biography (preceded by his Nobel lecture on December 11, 1925). In: *Nobel Lectures. Physiology Medicine 1922–1941*, 94–111, 112–4. Elsevier Publ. Cy, Amsterdam-London-New York.

713 WILLIUS, Frederick A., and Thomas J. Dry (1948). Willem Einthoven (1860–1927) in: *A History of the Heart and the Circulation*, 338–40, portr., Saunders, Philadelphia & London.

714 HOOGEWERF, S. (1955). *Leven en werken van Willem Einthoven, grondlegger van de electro-cardiografie* (Life and works of —, founder of electrocardiography). 93 pp., portr., "West-Friesland" Hoorn, 8°.

715 SNELLEN, H. A. van and H. Hartman (1961). Developments of phono-cardiography. *Am. Heart J.*, *61*, 347–51, ill.
     – Discussion of the contribution of some Dutchmen (W. Einthoven, M. A. H. Geluk en P. I. Battaerd) and others.

716 BURCH, G. E. (1961). Development in clinical electrocardiography since Einthoven. *NTG*, *105*, 1594–1606, ill.

717 [   ] (1960). Willem Einthoven, de grondlegger van de electro-cardiografie (Founder of electrocardiography). *GG*, *38*, 223.

718 SULEK, N. K. (1967). The Nobel price 1924 for Willem Einthoven for the discovery of the mechanism of the electrocardiogram [Polish]. *Wiadomosci Lekarskie*, *20*, 2072.

719 BRODY, D. A. (1972). Einthoven, G. J. Burch, and the capillary electrometer. *Am. Heart J.*, *84*, 280–1.

720 HERLES, F. (1968). Elektrokardiografie a vektorkardiografie 40 let po Einthovenove smrti. *Vnitrni Lek.*, *14*, 437–41.

721 GIRAUD, G. (1961). Willem Einthoven, prix nobel de médecine. *Montpellier méd.* *104*, 189–94.

722 [Editorial] (1960). Willem Einthoven – a tribute. *Canad. med. J.*, *83*, 915.

723 LEVINE, S. (1961). Willem Einthoven: some historical notes on the occasion of the centenary celebration of his birth. *Am. Heart J.*, *61*, 422–3.

724 JONKERS, J. E. (1961). Einthoven commemoration address. *Am. Heart. J.*, *61*, 366–8, ill.

725 GOTTLIEB, L. S. (1961). Willem Einthoven, M.D., Ph.D., 1860–1927. Centenary of the Father of electrocardiography. *Arch. Int. Med.*, *107*, 447–9, portr.

726 GRIGORYAN, N. A. V. (1960). Einthoven, his 100th birthday [Russian]. *Vest. Akad. med. Nauk.*, *15*, 86–8.

727 — (1960). Willem Einthoven (1860–1927). *Orv. Hetil*, *44*, 1578–9, ill., portr.

728 BURCH, G. E., H. A. SNELLEN and A. de WAART (1961). Einthoven-Symposium. Held on June 25th 1960 at Leiden University in commemoration of the birth of Willem Einthoven (1860–1927). *NTG*, *105*, II, 1594–1616.
   – Addresses delivered by G. E. Burch: Development in clinical electrocardiography since Einthoven; H. A. Snellen: Developments in phonocardiography; A. de Waart: Einthoven-Commemoration and M. Regnier: Commémoration d'Einthoven.

729 WAART, A. de (1961). Einthoven commemoration. *Am. Heart J.*, *61*, 357–60.

730 REGNIER, M. (1961). In memory of Einthoven. *Am. Heart J.*, *61*, 361–5.

731 EEKELEN, M. van (1961). In Memoriam Dr. Ir. A. Emmerie. *Voeding*, *22*, 51–2, portr.

732 BENTHEIM JUTTING, W. S. S. van (1968). Dr. Hendrik Engel, zoologist and historian, curator and professor. *Beaufortia*, *15*, no. 179, 1–5.

733 VEEN, B. van der (1968). List of scientific publications of professor Dr. H. Engel. *Beaufortia*, *15*, no. 180, 7–14.

ERASMUS

General

734   SCHULTHEISZ, E. (1967). Desiderius Erasmus Roterodamus. *Horus, 7,* 605–8, portr.

735   VLOEMANS, A. (1937). *Erasmus. Een levensbeeld met een keuze uit zijn brieven* (Erasmus. A Biography with a choice of his letters) 172 pp., 's-Gravenhage.

736   LINDEBOOM, G. A. (1935). Erasmiana. *Wbl. Reformatie,* 25 Jan., 9 and 16 Febr.

737   — (1936). Erasmiana medica. *NTG, 80,* III, 3164–70; *BGG, VI,* 108–14.

738   — (1936). Erasmus in zorgen (E. worried). *Hermèneus, 8,* no. 10. 167.

739   — (1936). Erasmus van Rotterdam. *Calvin. Wbl.,* 26 June and 3.

740   — (1936). Erasmus. *Stemmen des Tijds,* 25 July, 1–33 pp.

741   — (1947). Erasmus. Serie: *Getuigen van Christus.* Ten Have. Amsterdam.

Erasmus and medicine (c.q. dentistry)

742   GYSEL, C. (1968). Erasmus, de tijdgeest en de geneeskunde (E., timespirit and medicine). *Ned. Tandartsenbl., 23,* 385–94, ill.

743   — (1968). Erasmus, het humanisme en de geneeskunde (E., humanism and medicine). *Ned. Tandartsenbl., 23,* 404–12, ill.

744   — (1970). Erasme, la médecine et la France. *Rev. franç. Odonto-Stomat., 17,* 947–56.

745   — (1968). Erasmus, zijn actualiteit en de geneeskunde (E., his actuality and medicine). *Ned. Tandartsenbl., 23,* 261–7, ill.

746   — (1966). Erasme, la médecine dentaire et l'ergonomie. *Revue belge Méd. dent., 21,* 509–17.

747   — (1969). Erasme, son humanisme et l'orthodontie. *Orthodont. franç., 40,* 119–26.

748   O'MALLEY, C. D. (1971). Desiderius Erasmus. The spirit and the Flesh. *JAMA, 216,* 66–70.

749 NUYENS, B. W. Th. (1936). Erasmus en de geneeskunde (E. and medicine). *NTG*, *80*, III, 3157–63; *BGG*, *XVI*, 101–7.

750 ELAUT, L. (1950). *Een betoog over de lof van de Geneeskunde door Erasmus van Rotterdam.* Vertaald naar de oorspronkelijke uitgave. (An argument on the praise of Medicine by —. Translated from the original edition). 28 pp. Standaard boekhandel, Antwerpen.

751 — (1958). Erasme, traducteur de Galien. *Bibliothèque d'Humanisme et Renaissance, 20,* 36–43, ill.

752 HAJDUKIEWICZ, L. (1960). Im Bücherkreis des Erasmus von Rotterdam, aus der Geschichte der bibliophilen Beziehungen zwischen Polen und Basel im 16. Jahrhundert. *Kwart. Hist. Nauki Techn. 5,* Sonderheft 2, 49–102, ill., portr.

753 SCHULTE, J. E. (1936). Erasmus en de eugenetische gedachte (E. and eugenetic thought). *NTG, 80,* III, 3572; *BGG, XVI,* 132.

754 JENNY, Ed. (1937). Hygiene und Kinderpflege bei Erasmus von Rotterdam. *Schweiz. med. Wschr.,* 67, no. 41, 979–81.

755 ERASMUS, Des. (1518, 1907). Encomium artis medicae – With Dutch translation. *Opusc., I,* 1–44.

756 — (1526, 1943). Epistolae ad Guilhelmum Copum Medicum pars prima. Epistola ad Franciscum Medicum – With English translation *Opusc., XVII,* 2–9.

Erasmus and contemporaries

757 BOEYNAEMS, P. (1959). Afinus een Lierse arts en vriend van Erasmus (A., a Lier physician and friend of —). *Land van Ryen, 9,* 3–13.

758 KERNER, D. (1959). Ein Brief des Paracelsus an Erasmus von Rotterdam. *Grünenthal Waage, 1,* 146–9, portr., facs.

759 MURRAY, W. A. (1958). Erasmus and Paracelsus. *Bibliothèque d'Humanisme et Renaissance, 20,* 560–4.

760 STOCKI, E. (1966). Polish physicians, friends of Erasmus of Rotterdam. [Polish]. *Wiad. lek., 19,* 77–81.

761 KRIVATSKY, Peter (1973). Erasmus' medical milieu. *BHM, XLVII,* 113–54.

762 LINDEBOOM, G. A. (1936). Calvijn en Erasmus (C. and E.) *Geref. apol. T.* "*Horizon*", Nov.

See also 503, 2016–2025, 2257.

763 HOEVEN, J. van der (1931). Eenige brieven van prof. F. Z. Ermerins en prof. G. J. Loncq aan prof. C. Pruys van der Hoeven (Some letters from F.Z.E. and G.J.L. to C.P.v.d.H.) *NTG*, *75*, IV, 5911–2; *BGG*, *XI*, 331–2.
– included in the report of a meeting of the "Genootschap"; The letters, present in a family archive, refer to Pruys van der Hoeven's book *Anthropologische onderzoek*.

764 — (1932). Zes brieven van prof. F.Z. Ermerins en vier brieven van prof. dr. C. Pruys van der Hoeven (Six letters from F.Z.E. and four letters from C.P.v.d.H.). *NTG*, *76*, I, 1115–28; *BGG*, *XII*, 45–58.

765 KLEY, J. J. van der (1918). De werken van Bartholinus Eustachius. (The works of —). *NTG*, *62*, II, 1913

CHRISTIAAN EYKMAN

766 LINDEBOOM, G. A. (1971). Eykman, Christiaan. In (C. C. Gillispie, editor): *Dictionary of Scientific Biography*, *IV*, Charles Scribner's Sons, New York, 310–2.

767 JANSEN, B. C. P. (1959). *Het Levenswerk van Christiaan Eykman (1858–1930)* (The life-work of — (1858–1930). VII + 205 pp., portr., Bohn, Haarlem, 8°.

768 POSTMUS, S. (1953). Christiaan Eykman 1858–1930. *Voeding*, *14*, 317–9, portr.

769 — (1958). Christiaan Eykman 1858–1930. *Pharm. J.*, *181*, 92.

770 GRIJNS, C. (1931). In Memoriam Prof. Dr. Chr. Eykman. *Ned. T. Hyg. Microbiol. en Serol.*, *V*, 109–17, portr.

771 BAART DE LA FAILLE, J. M. (1946). Christiaan Eykman. In: T. P. Sevensma (ed.) *Nederlandsche helden der wetenschap*. Levensschetsen van negen Nobelprijswinnaars (Dutch heroes of Science. Biographical sketches of nine winners of the Nobel Prize), 299–332. Kosmos, Amsterdam.

772 — (1965). Christiaan Eykman. Biography (Preceded by his Nobel lecture (1929). In: *Nobel lectures. Physiology or Medicine 1922–1941*, 199–207, 208–10. Elsevier Publ. Cy, Amsterdam-London-New York.
See also 861–69 (Grijns), 994

773 ROEKEL, G. van (1939). Een priester-arts op het einde van de 14e eeuw (A Priest-physician at the end of the 14th century). *NTG, 83*, IV, 5291–2; *BGG, XIX*, 252–3.
– On Evert van der Eze (?–1404), physician at Deventer. Afterwards priest and founder of a monastery.

F

774 KRUL, R. (1898). Arnoldus Fey. *Tijdspiegel*, 2, 53–62.

775 NAPJUS, J. W. (1930). Arnoldus Fey. *NTG, 74*, II, 4431–44; *BGG, X*, 237–50.

775ᵃ SCHOUTE, D. (1950). In Memoriam Dr. F. M. G. de Feyfer. *NTG, 94*, IV, 3618–9. (not in *BGG*)

776 ELAUT, L. (1964). Het dieetboekje van J. B. Fiera (1498) en zijn betekenis als voorloper van de geneeskundige renaissance. (The diet book of J.B.F. (1498) and his significance as precursor of medical renaissance). *Sci. Hist.*, 6, 169–77.
– Giovanni-Battista Fiera (1469–1538), a physician from Mantua.

777 ESSO, Bzn., I. van (1940). Jean Charles August Fischer. *NTG, 84*, I, 435; *BGG, XX*, 39.

778 [Anonymous] (1965). Willem Godschalk van Focquenbroch. Laatzeventiende-eeuws medicus-dichter (Late 17th century physician-poet. *MC*, 20, 226–7.
– W. G. Focquenbroch (ca. 1630–75).

778ᵃ NOLTE, M. (1974). De dichter-arts Willem Godschalk Focquenbroch (The poet-physician —). *AP*, no 19, 19–20.

778ᵇ SIJMONS, B. (1907). Prof. Dr A. P. Fokker (8 Juli 1840–8 October 1906). *Gron. Volksalm.*, 18, 130–42.

779 SCHOUTE, D. (1946). *Het leven van Prof. Dr. A. P. Fokker* (1840–1906) (The life of —). Swets & Zeitlinger, Amsterdam.

PETRUS FORESTUS (Pieter van Foreest)

780 MEUNIER, L. (1902). Un Grand praticien du XVIe siècle. Le Hollandais Pierre van Foreest (Petrus Forestus), 1522–1595. *Janus, VII*, 307–12; 365–9; 466–9; 505–8; 586–9 and 617–21.

781   KLEIJ, J. J. van der (1924). Een Hollandsche dokter en zijn praktijk in de tweede helft der zestiende eeuw (A Dutch doctor and his practice in the second half of the 16th century). *NTG*, *68*, II, 1259–70; *BGG*, *IV*, 222–33.
– on Pieter van Foreest.

782   HALBERTSMA, K. T. A. (1940). Petrus Forestus (1522–1597). *NTG*, *84*. II, 1713–20; *BGG*, *XX*, 80–7.

783   JONAS, [   ] (1957). Pieter van Foreest 1521–1597. *Ars medici* (Gand), *12*, 7–9, portr.

784   LINDEBOOM, G. A. (1960). *Pieter van Foreest, 1522–1597.* 27 pp., portr. Pieter van Foreestkliniek, Amsterdam, pr. pr.

785   GEIST-HOFMAN, A. M. (1965). Doctor Pieter van Foreest. *NTG*, *109*, II, 1251–3; *BGG*, *XLV*, 15–7, portr.

786   KROON, J. E. (1929). *Le premier professeur en médecine à l'université de Leyde.*, 2 pp. De Vlijt, Antwerpen. also in: *Communication faite au Sixième Congrès Int. d'Hist. de la Méd. Leyde-Amsterdam 18–23 juillet 1927.*
– on Pieter van Foreest.

787   SCHUWIRTH, P. (1923). The dentistry of Petrus Forestus. *Med. Life 30*, 349, 428 and 448.

787ᵃ SOUTENDAM, J. [*ca* 1890]. Uittreksel uit de opera omnia van Petrus Forestus, betreffende Delft, Delvenaars, Delftsche toestanden, enz., loopende over de jaren 1558–1596 (Abstract from the opera omnia of P.F., referring to Delft, citizens and situations of Delft, etc., covering the years 1558–1596). *Nijhoffs Bijdr. Vaderl. Gesch. en Oudheidk.*, IIIde reeks, Vol. V, 251.

788   FORESTUS, P. (1558, 1935). *De Scorbuto* – with Dutch translation. *Opusc.*, *XIII*, 17–94.

789   — (1589, 1626, 1929). *De incerto, fallaci urinarum iudicio* – with Dutch translation, based upon the Latin text from 1589 and the Dutch translation from 1626. *Opusc.*, *VIII*, 138–313.

790   ANDEL, M. A. van (1919). J. H. Francken, een reizend meester in de 18de eeuw (A travelling master in the 18th century). *Med. Wbl.*, *26*, 349–56, 361–8 and 373–81.

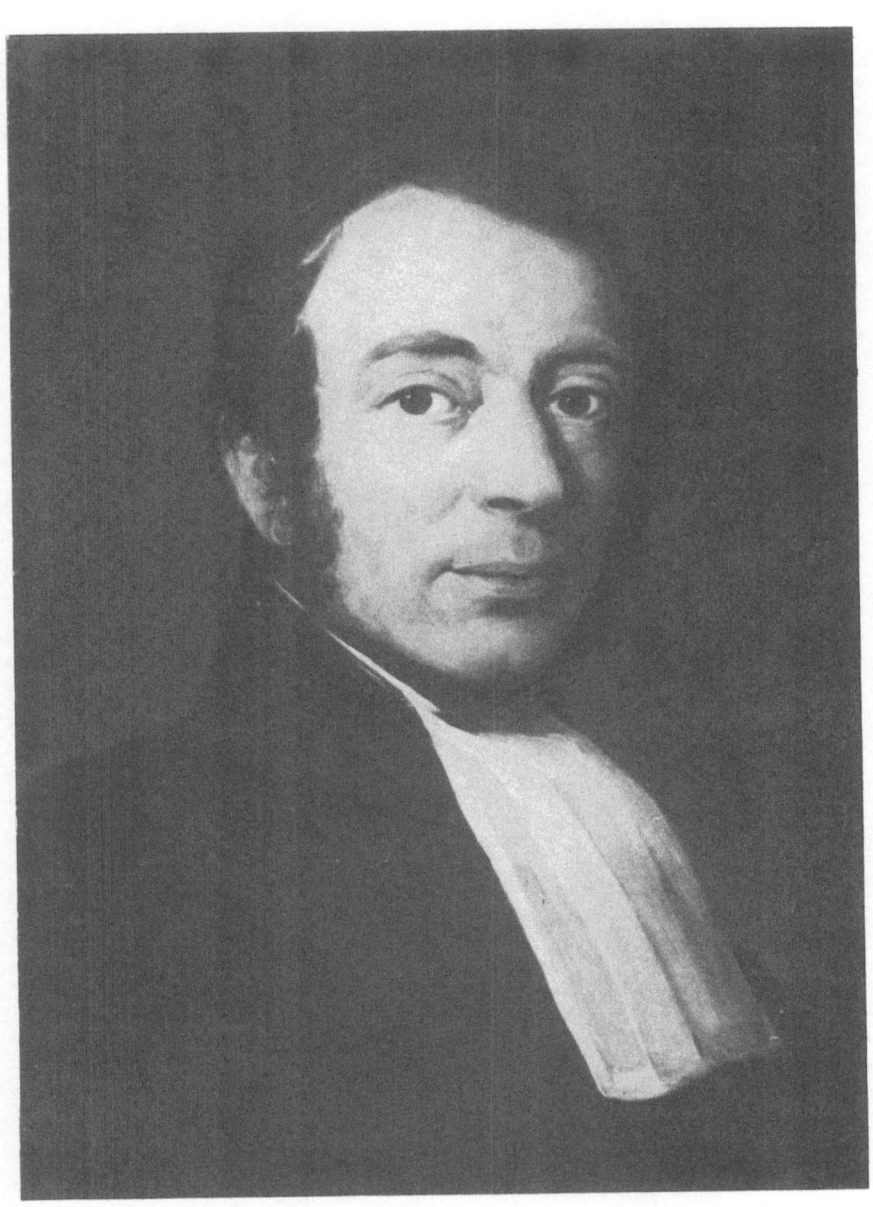

F. Z. Ermerins (1808–1871)

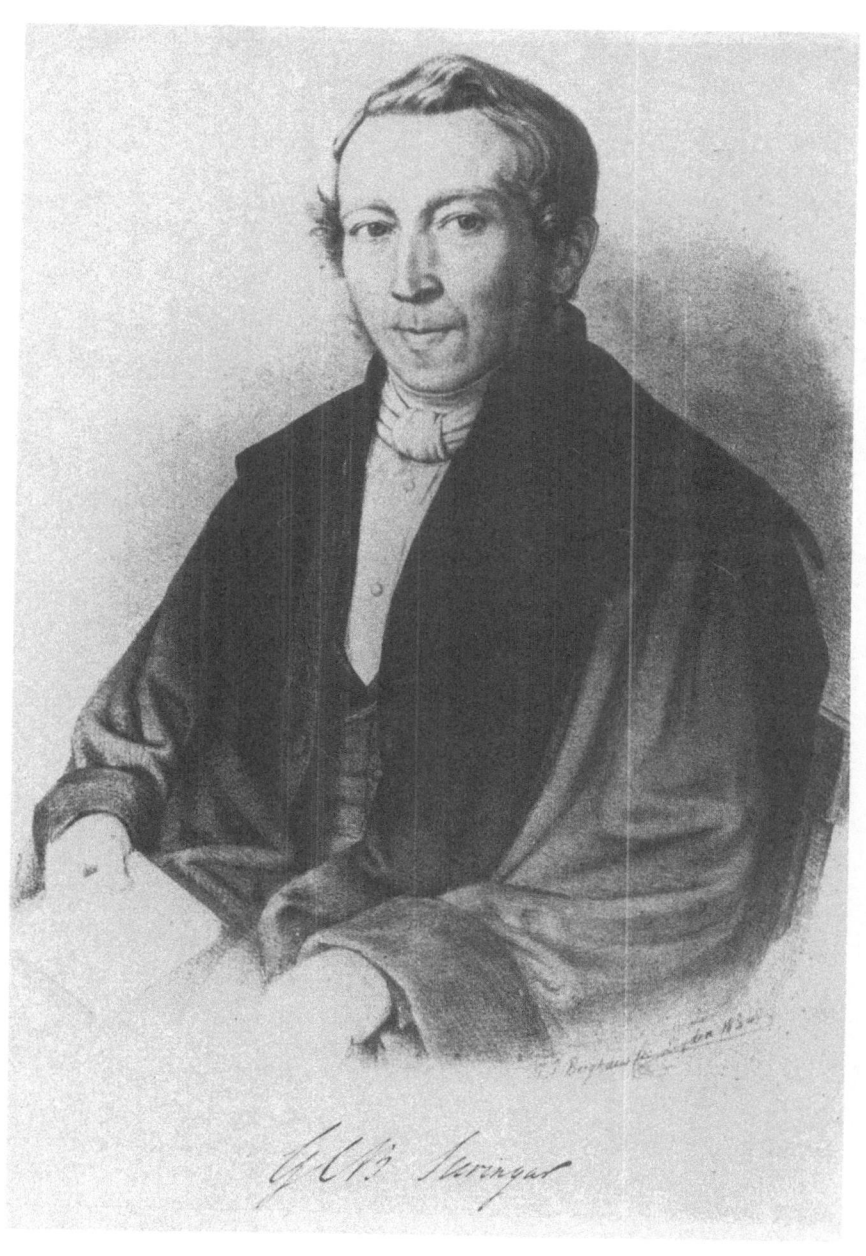

G. C. B. Suringar (1802–1874)

791 PUTTO, J. A. (1964). Johann Peter Frank (19-3-1745 – 24-4-1821). *GG*, *42*, 43.

792 BAUMANN, E. D. (1912). Frederick de Groote en de geneeskunst (Frederick the Great and medicine) *Med. Revue*, *12*, 450-79.

793 SLEESWIJK, J. G. (1924). Frederik de Groote en de Geneeskunde (Frederick the Great and medicine). *NTG*, *68*, I, 948-9; *BGG*, *IV*, 71-2. *See also* 2123-26

794 NAPJUS, J. W. (1937). De hoogleeraren in de geneeskunde aan de Hoogeschool en het Athenaeum te Franeker (1585-1843): Joachim Frencelius (The medical professors at Franeker Academy and Atheneum: J. Frencelius). *NTG*, *81*, III, 4262-7; *BGG*, *XVII*, 154-9, portr.

795 SCHULTS VAN KLOOSTERHUIS, E. (1933). *Freud als ethnoloog* (As an ethnologist). Thesis Amsterdam (Supervisor: Steinmetz). Amsterdam.

796 WESTERMAN HOLSTIJN, A. J. (1956). Sigmund Freud 1856 – 6 mei – 1956. *NTG*, *100*, II, 1317-20; *BGG*, *XXXVI*, 35-8.

797 NOOTEN, S. I. van (1971). Contributions of Dutchmen to the early history of film technology. *Janus*, *LVIII*, 81-100, ill.
– a.o. on Gemma Frisius (1508-55), who published the oldest known illustration of a *camera obscura*.

798 MEURS, G. J. van (1959). Casimir Funk en zijn Vitamine "hypothese" (C.F. and his "hypothesis" on Vitamines). *Voeding*, *20*, 305-11, portr.

G

799 FABBRI Jr., R. (1966). Dr. Paul-Ferdinand Gachet: Vincent van Gogh's last physician. *Trans. Stud. Coll. Phys. Philad.*, *33*, 202-8.

800 LINT, J. G. de (1926). David Henry Gallandat. *NTG*, *70*, II, 651-61, portr.; *BGG*, *VI*, 181-91.

801 BURGER, H. (1905). Een honderdjarige (A hundred years old man). *NTG*, *41*, I, 717-9.
– on Manuel Garcia, born 17 March 1805, the inventor of the laryngoscope.

802 SASSEN, Ferd. (1960). *De reis van Pierre Gassendi in de Nederlanden (1628-1629)* (The journey of P.G. in the Netherlands). 47 pp. *MKNAW*, afd. Letterkunde, Nieuwe Reeks, deel 23, no. 10. Noord-Holl. Uitg. Mij, Amsterdam.
– Gassendi, philosopher and physicist, correspondent of Descartes, visited also some Dutch physicians.

H. D. GAUBIUS

803   BETT, W. R. (1955). Hieronymus David Gaub (1705–80) physician and chemist. *Chem. and Drugg.*, *163*, 207.

804   RATHER, L. J. (1960). Gaub on psychosomatic medicine. *Stanf. med. Bull.*, *18*, 111–9, facs.

805   — (1965). *Mind and Body in Eighteenth Century medicine. A Study on Jerome Gaub's De regimine mentis.* Wellcome Hist. med. Libr., London. XII + 275 pp.
    – Reviewed by: P. Huard in *Arch. Int. d'Hist. des Sci.*, *19*, (1966) 309–10.

806   [editorial] (1969). Gaubius on hypotheses in pathology. *Bull. N.Y. Acad. Med.*, *45*, 238–9.

807   JARCHO, S. (1970). Gaubius on inflammation II. *Amer. J. Cardiol.*, *26*, 406–8.

808   MEYER-STEINEG, Th. (1923). Hieronymous Dav. Gaub über die "natürlichen Heilkräfte". *Arch. Gesch. Mediz.*, *XV*, 114–20.

809   ROCCATAGLIATA, G. (1971). G. D. Gaubio's Vitalistic psychopathology. *Arch. Psicol. Neurol. Psichiat.*, *32*, 473–80.

810   GAUB, H. D. (1731, 1907). *Oratio inauguralis qua ostenditur chemiam artibus academicis jure esse inserendam* – with Dutch translation. *Opusc.*, *I*, 170–228.

811   — (1747, 1932). *De regimine mentis, orationes duo* – with German translation, *Opusc.*, *XI*, 89–281.

                           See also 942, 3358, 3360, 3362, 4148

812   GILS, J. B. F. van (1941). Gaudanus (Theodoricus Gerardus). *NTG*, *85*, I, 449–53; *BGG*, *XXI*, 12–6.

813   HAMERS, N. A. (1959). De la Genesse, geslacht verbonden met de beide blindeninrichtingen te Grave (—, a family related to the two blind-institutions at Grave). *Numaga*, *6*, 52–94, 187–8, ill.
    – Two blind-institutions were founded by a member of the De la Genesse family. For one and a half century a member of this family practised as physician at Grave.

814   SCHIERBEEK, A. (1920). Konrad Gesner en Marcello Malpighi. *Levende Natuur*, *XXIV*, (1 febr.), 289.

815   DURR, K. (1965). Arnold Geulincx and the classical logic of the 17th century. [German]. *Stud. gen.* Berlin *18*, 520–41.

JACOB, JAN EN MATTHIAS VAN GEUNS

816 JORISSEN, W. P. (1914, 1915, 1919). Jan van Geuns en zijn ontdekking van het vulcaniseren van caoutchouc (J. van G. and his discovery of vulcanizing caoutchouc). I–IV.
I. *ChemWbl. XI* (1914), 852
II. *ibid. XII* (1915), 799
III–IV *ibid. XVI* (1919), 527 and 1014
also in: *T. Tandh. XXVI* (1919), 498 and 581.

817 STOKVIS, B. J. (1882) *Levensschets van Jan van Geuns* (Sketch of the life of —) 45 pp. Joh. Müller, Amsterdam.
– with a bibliography of—

818 KÜHLER, K. P. (1953). *Jan van Geuns. Zijn betekenis voor de geneeskundige wetenschap en het geneeskundig onderwijs* (J.v.G.: His significance for medical science and medical teaching). 142 pp., portr. Thesis Amsterdam (Supervisors: J. J. van Loghem and A. C. Ruys), de Jong, Leiden.

819 HOEVEN, J. van der (1940). Een brief van dr. J. van Geuns aan prof. dr. C. Pruys van der Hoeven (A letter of J. van G. to C.P.v.d.H.). *NTG, 84,* II, 1318–21; *BGG, XX,* 65–8.

820 EEGHEN, I. H. van (1969). *Meniste Vrijage. Jakob van Geuns (1769–1832) Gronings dokter, Amsterdams "Kassier"* (Mennonite courtship. J.v.G. a Groningen physician, Amsterdam "casher"). 277 pp., 3 ill. Tjeenk Willink, Haarlem.

820ᵃ NIEUWENHUYZEN, H. J. W. A. van (1943). De delicate hoogleraarsbenoeming van professor Mathias van Geuns te Utrecht, 1791 (The delicate appointment of professor — — at U., 1791). *Jbk. Oud-Utrecht,* 85–93.

821 SYPKENS SMIT, J. H. (1953). *Leven en werken van Matthias van Geuns, M. D. 1735–1817* (Life and works). Thesis Groningen (Supervisor: J. J. Th. Vos). 613 pp., ill. 4°. Van Gorcum, Assen.
– also as a monograph.

822 [   ] [1964]. Een Hooggeleerde Vader (A very learned Father). *Organorama, I,* 17–20.
– concerns letters of Matthias van Geuns to his son.

823 GEUNS, M. van (1770, 1935). *Brief aan Petrus Camper* (Letter to P. Camper) with French translation. *Opusc., XIII,* 239–48.

824   [P.J.B.] (1914). In Memoriam Dr. A. Geyl. *Janus, XIX*, 333.

825   SCHOUTE, D. (1946). Ter herdenking van Joh. Bapt. Franc. van Gils (Commemoration J.B.F. van G.) *NTG, 90*, IV, 1315–6; *BGG, XXVI*, 34–5.

826   JORISSEN, W. P. (1918). Iets over Glauber's Amsterdamsche tijd. (On G's Amsterdam period). *Chem. Wbl., XV*, 268.

827   WITTOP KONING, D. A. (1950). J. R. Glauber in Amsterdam. *Jbk. Amstelodamum, 44*, 1–6.

828   — (1950). J. R. Glauber en zijn Pharmacopoea Spagyrica (J.R.G. and his Pharmacopoeia Spagyrica). *Ph W, 85*, 273–83.

829   PANSE, F. and H. J. Schmidt (1971). De opkomst van nieuwe realiteiten bij twee grote Europeanen: 2. Hugo van der Goes (1420/30–1482) (The rise of new realities with two great Europeans: 2. H. van der Goes) *Image*, no. 44, 5–16, 10 ill.

830   DALDERUP, L. M. (1962). Joseph Goldberger 16 juli 1874 – 17 januari 1929. *Voeding, 23*, 325–9, portr.

831   NOYON, I. (1924). Twee oogheelkundige vrienden van Goethe. (Two ophthalmological friends of —). *NTG, 68*, I, 2628–31; *BGG, IV*, 123–6.
      – On: J. H. J. Jung (-Stilling), (1740–1817) and Joh. Fr. Lobstein (1736–84).

832   OOSTSTROOM, S. J. (1961). David de Gorter en de Nederlandse Botanie (D. de G. and Dutch Botany). *GeWiNa*, no *10*, 12–3.

833   TIMMERMAN, W. Aeg. (1968). Johannes de Gorter. Een schets van zijn leven en werk (A sketch of his life and work). *NTG, 112*, 35–41.

834   GENTILI, P. (1969). L'epidemia influenzale del 1733 in uno scritto di Giovanni de Gorter (1688–1762) (With Italian translation of text). *Med. nei Secoli, 6* (3), 54–79, facsism.
      See also 5184a

834ª PÜSCHEL, E. (1973). Dictata von Johannes de Gorter (1689–1762) zu seinen Werken "Compendium medicinae" und "Praxis medicae systema". Bericht über einen Fund. *GeWiNa*, no. 32, 9–10.

REINIER DE GRAAF

835 CATCHPOLE, H. R. (1940). Regnier de Graaf, 1641–1673. *BHM, XIV*, 1261–1300, ill.

836 BEYDALS, Petra (1941). Reynier de Graef (1641–1673). *NTG, 85*, III, 3250–3; *BGG, XXI*, 94–7, portr.

837 SAKAI, H. (1971). Über den Vornamen de Graafs. *Nihon Ishigaku Zasshi, 17*, 347–53. With Japanese abstract.

838 MEUNIER, L. (1901). Regnier de Graaf, 1641–1673. L'ovulation démontrée au XVIIe siècle par l'anatomie normale, par l'anatomie pathologique et par l'expérimentation. *Janus, VI*, 524–30.

839 SPEERT, H. (1956). Obstetric-gynecologic eponyms. Reinier de Graaf and the Graafian follicles. *Obstet. Gynec., 7*, 582–8, portr., ill.

840 HERINGA, G. C. and J. I. H. Mendels (1936). Regnier de Graaf's onderzoekingen over follikel en corpus luteum (R. de G.'s investigations on the follicle and the corpus luteum). *NTG*, 80, IV, 5034–40; *BGG, XVI*, 184–90, portr., ill.

841 TUR, J. (1930). Regnerus de Graaf, der letzte Embryologe ohne Mikroskop. *Arch. Hist. i. Filoz. Med., 10*, 242–57 [Polish].

842 [   ] (1943). De Graaf, Regner. On the female testes or ovaries. Chapter XII of *De mulierum organis generationi inservientibus*. (Leyden: 1672). Translated by George W. Corner. *Essays in Biology in honor of Herbert M. Evans*, 121–37, 3 ill., portr. University of California Press.

843 BARGE, J. A. J. (1941). Regnerus de Graaf herdacht (1641–1673) (R.d.G. commemorated). *NTG, 85*, IV, 4544–5; *BGG, XXI*, 153–4. – short review of an address (communicated by Burger).

844 — (1942). Reinier de Graaf 1641–1941. *MNAW*, afd. Letterkunde, Nieuwe Reeks, 5, no. 5, 25 pp., portr. Noord-Holl. Uitg. Mij, Amsterdam.

845 LINDEBOOM, G. A. (1973). *Reinier de Graaf. Leven en werken.* (— —. Life and works). 143 pp., 10 ill., port. Elmar, Delft. – reviewed by D. de Moulin: *Clio Med., 9* (1974), 253.

846 — (1973). Reinier de Graaf en de biologie (— — and biology). *Vakbl. Biol., 53*, 232–7, 2 ill. port.

847   — (1973). Reinier de Graaf en de Koninklijke Sociëteit te Londen (R. de G. and the Royal Society at London). *NTG*, *117*, 1049–55, portr., facs.

847[a]   — (1974). Reinier de Graaf (1641–1673). *NTG*, *118*, 789–95, port., 2 ill.

848   HOUTZAGER, H. L. (1973). Reinier de Graaf. *Spiegel Historiael*, *8*, 420–3, ill.

849   — (1973). Reinier de Graaf. *Organorama*, *10*, no. 5, 28–31, 2 ill., portr.
– also in the French, English, German and Spanish edition of this periodical.

850   — (1973). Reinier de Graaf, Tercentenary Symposium. *NTG*, *117*, 1658.

850[a]   — (1973). Delftse figuren rond Reinier de Graaf (Delft figures around — —). *AP*, no 11, 36–40, port.

851   GRAAF, R. de (1671, 1927). *Tractatus anatomico-medicus de Succi Pancreatici natura et usu* – with Dutch translation. *Opusc.*, *IV*, 160–213.

852   BROCKBANK, W. and O. R. Corbett (1954). De Graaf's "Tractatus de clysteribus". *J. Hist. Med.*, *IX*, 174–90, 8 ill., portr.

853   GRAAF, R. de (1673, 1922). *De mulierum organis generationi inservientibus tractatus novus* – with Dutch translation. *Opusc.*, *IV*, 160–213.

854   DONGEN, J. A. van (1965). *Reinier de Graaf. De mulierum organis generationi inservientibus*. Facsimile with an introduction by —. Dutch Classics on Hist. of Science, XIII, 84 pp. + facs; 20 + 358 pp., 27 ill. B. de Graaf, Nieuwkoop.
– Reviewed by E. C. Roosen-Runge in: *J. Hist. Med.*, *XXI* (1966) 321; by J. G. Bearn in: *Med. Hist. X*, (1966), 297–9, 2 ill.

855   JOCELYN, H. D. and B. P. Setchell (1972). *Regnier de Graaf on the Human Reproductive organs*. An annotated Translation of *Tractatus De virorum organis generationi inservientibus* (1668) and *De Mulierum organis generationi inservientibus Tractatus novus* (1672). 222 pp., 27 pl. Blackwell Scientific Publ. Oxford-London-Edinburgh-Melbourne. (= Suppl. no. 17 of *J. of Reproduction and Fertility*).

856   KLEIN, Marc (1959, 1962). Histoire et actualité de l'iconographie de l'ouvrage: *De mulierum organis generationi inservientibus* (1672) de R. de Graaf. *Compt. rend. XVIe Congrès int. Hist. Méd. Montpellier 1958*, Bruxelles, 1959, I, 316–20. *Le Scalpel*, *115* (1962), 109–13.
See also 3528, 5479

857 Vos, T. A. (1973). Geschiedkundige bijdragen. III. Biografie van Albrecht von Graefe. (Historical contributions. III. Biography of A.v.Gr.). *Arts en Wereld*, *6*, no. 5, 26–49, 7 ill.

857ᵃ VERKROOST, C. M. (1974). De Delftsche Wonderdokter – Jacob Janszoon Graswinckel (The Delft quack – — —). *AP*, no 14 10–3.
– on the principal person in the 19th century Dutch novel of A. L. G. Bosboom-Toussaint: *De Delftsche Wonderdokter* (Amsterdam, 1870; many later editions).

858 KNAPPERT, L. (1908). Les relations entre Voltaire et 's-Gravesande. *Janus*, *XIII*, 249–57.
– With Voltaire's judgement on Boerhaave.

859 BEYDALS, Petra (1141). Cornelis Isaacz. 's-Gravesande, stadsanatomicus (city-anatomist). *Delftsche Courant*, 2 december.

860 GREIDANUS, S. (1908). *De dagen van olim; herinneringen van een geneesheer* (The days of yore; memories of a physician). Amsterdam, 8°.
– Autobiographical notes of S. Greidanus.

GERRIT GRIJNS

861 POSTMUS, S. (1955). Gerrit Grijns 1865–1944. *Voeding*, *16*, 3–4, portr.

862 REITH, J. F. (1971). Christiaan Eijkman en Gerrit Grijns (C.E. and G.G.) *Voeding*, *32*, 180–95.

863 KIK, M. C. (1957). Gerrit Grijns (May 28, 1865 – November 11, 1944). *J. Nutr.*, *62*, 3–12, portr.

864 [   ] (1936). Prof. Dr. G. Grijns. *Almanak Wageningsch Studentencorps*, 63–5.

865 BROUWER, E. (1932). Prof. Dr. G. Grijns, *Landbouwk. T.*, *44*, no. 531, 3 pp., portr.

866 SWELLENGREBEL, N. H. (1941). Toespraak tot Prof. Grijns (An address to —). *NTG*, *85*, I, 120–2.
– on the occasion of the conferring of the Swammerdam-medal on prof. Grijns; included in a report of a meeting of the "Genootschap ter bevordering der Natuur-, Genees- en Heelkunde" at Amsterdam, 13 November 1940.

867 GRIJNS, G. W. (1941). Rede (Address). *NTG*, *85*, I, 122–3.

868 [   ] (1935). *Prof. Dr. G. Grijns' Researches on Vitamins 1900–1911 and his Thesis on the Physiology on the N. opticus translated and reedit-*

ed bij a Committee of Honour on the occasion of his 70th birthday, 6 pp. J. Noorduyn & Zn., Gorichem.

869 JANSEN, B. C. P. (1946). In Memoriam Prof. Dr. G. Grijns. *NTG*, 90, 240–1, portr. *See also* 766–72 (Chr. Eykman), 994.

870 ANDEL, M. A. van (1933). Geert Groote en de kwakzalverij (G. G. and quackery). *NTG*, *76*, III, 3985–7; *BGG*, *XIII*, 212–4.

871 HEEREN, Jac, (1959). De oud-Helmondse doktersfamilie van den Grootenacker (The old-Helmond family of physicians: V.v.d.G.). *De Brabantse Leeuw*, *8*, 28–32 and 36–8.

872 HELLINGA, G. (1942). Een pamflet uit de 17e eeuw tot klaarheid gebracht (A pamflet from the 17th century cleared up). *NTG*, *86*, IV, 3077–81; *BGG*, *XXII*, 155–9.
– On the Amsterdam physician Petrus Guenellon Jr. (1650–1722).

873 [   ] (1905). In Memoriam A. A. G. Guye. *Janus*, *X*, 58.

874 SCHULTHEISS, and L. Tardy (1964). Paul Gyongyossi, ein vergessener Boerhaave-Schuler. *Janus*, *51*, 152–9, ill.
– Gyongyossi, the son of a Hungarian emigrant; studied first theology and philology, later medicine at Leyden, graduated at Harderwijk (1753), whereafter he departed for Russia, where he became, at last, court-physician. G.'s contribution to the spread of Boerhaave's doctrine in Russia.

H

875 SMIT, P. (1967). Ernst Haeckel and his "generelle Morphologie": an evaluation. *Janus*, *LIV*, 236–52, ill.
See also 2840

ANTON DE HAEN

876 BIJLEVELD, W. J. J. C. (1942). Prof. Dr. Antoni de Haen. *NTG*, *86*, II, 845; *BGG*, *XXII*, 55.

877 BOERSMA, J. (1961–3). Antonius de Haen 1704–1776; Life and Work. *Janus*, *L*, 264–307.

878 — (1963). *Antonius de Haen (1704–1776). Leven en Werk* (Life and Work). Thesis Free University Amsterdam (Supervisor: G. A. Lindeboom). 154 pp., ill. Van Gorcum, Assen. Also as a monograph: Van Gorcum's Historische Bibliotheek no. 71.

879 — (1964). Een tweetal medische verklaringen van Antonius de Haen (1704–1776) (Two medical certificates of —). *NTG, 108*, II, 1491–3; *BGG, XLIV*, 26–8, ill.

880 SCHULTE, J. E. (1942). Antoni de Haen te Weenen (A. de H. at Vienna). *NTG, 86*, II, 1097–8; *BGG, XXII*, 70–1.

881 WYKLICKY, H. (1958). Zur Kenntnis des Wiener Klinikers Anton de Haen. *Wiener med. Wschr., 108*, 596–8, ill.

882 JANTSCH, Marlene (1955). Anton de Haën und der Beginn des klinischen Unterrichtes in Wien. *Wiener Klin. Wschr., 67*, N.F. *10*, 1–3, ill.

883 NEUBURGER, M. (1913). Anton de Haën und Maximiliaam Stoll als Neuropathologen. *Wiener med. Wschr.*, no. 17 en 18, 11 pp.

884 ESSO, Bzn., I. van (1940). A. de Haen en G. van Swieten. *NTG, 84*, 4825; *BGG, XX*, 200.

885 CICHON, Dieter (1971). *Antonius de Haens Werk "De Magia" (1775). Eine Auseinandersetzung mit der Magie und ihre Bedeutung für die Medizin in der Zeit der Aufklärung.* Thesis Münster (Supervisor: K. E. Rothschuh). 101 pp., 1 portr., 5 ill. Münstersche Beiträge zur Geschichte und Theorie der Medizin, nr. 5, Münster.

886 HECKER, J. F. C. (1839). *Geschichte der neueren Heilkunde.* 614 pp. Verlag Enslin, Berlin. Zweites Buch: *Die Wiener Schule*: II Klinischer Unterricht: De Haen, 397–428.

887 JARCHO, S. (1973). Anton de Haen, Louis Odier, and the inoculation controversy. *Bull. N.Y. Acad. Med., 49*, 236–40.

888 DOOREN, L. (1936). De familierelaties van Dr. Hermannus van der Hagen, stadsgeneesheer te Arnhem (1588–?) (Family-relations of —, city-physician at Arnhem). *GG, 14*, 727–30.

889 OOSTERHUIS, R. A. B. (1943). Hahnemann, de ontdekker der homoeopathie, als mensch en geleerde. Zijn beteekenis voor verleden, heden en toekomst (1755–1843) (H., the discoverer of homoeopathy, as a man and a scientist. His importance for the past, present and future). *T. Artsenijkunde*, nos. 33, 34 and 35 (14, 21, 28 August), 19 pp., portrs.

890 LOGHEM, Sr. J. J. van (1958). Een biografie van Hahnemann (A biography of —). *NTG, 102*, I, 237.

891 BOLHUIS, J. J. van (1963–64). Klaas Tjalling Agnus Halbertsma 19
Jan. 's-Gravenhage – 8 juni 1963. *Jbk. Mij. Ned. Letterk.*, 47–52.
– K. Tj. A. Halbertsma was a well-known ophthalmologist at The Hague.

892 LEERSUM, E. C. van (1913). Stephen Hales and the mensuration of
blood-pressure. *Janus, XVIII*, 333–40, 1 ill.

893 MOULIN, D. de (1972). Stephen Hales 1677–1761. *Hart Bulletin, 3*,
63–4, portr. *See also* 2846

894 KNEGTEL, A. P. C. H. (1970). Een studiereis naar Parijs in 1822. (A
study tour to Paris in 1822). *NTG, 114*, 24–8.
– On H. C. van Hall (1801–74), who kept a diary of his studytour to Paris.

895 — (1970). Extraits du journal de Van Hall. A propos d'un voyage à
Paris en 1822. *Hist. Sci. Méd.*, Juillet–Décembre, 143–4.

ALBRECHT VON HALLER

896 SCHIERBEEK, A. (1956). Albrecht von Haller. *Jbk. Dodonaea, 23*, 348–
81.

897 LINDEBOOM, G. A. (1958). *Haller in Holland. Het dagboek van Albrecht von Haller van zijn verblijf in Holland (1725–1727).* Ingeleid
en geännoteerd door — (The diary of A. von H. of his stay in Holland
(1725–1727) with introduction and annotation by —). 106 pp., ill.
Kon. Ned. Gist- en Spiritusfabriek, Delft.

898 — (1963). Von Haller à Leyde. *Médecine et Hygiène, XXI*, no. 606, 4
September.

899 LESKY, Erna (1959). Albrecht von Haller und Anton de Haen im Streit
um die Lehre von der Sensibilität. *Gesnerus, 16*, 16–46.

899ᵃ LAMMERS, J. W. J. (1974). Johan Ham, de ontdekker van de zaad-
diertjes (J. H., discoverer of the spermatozoa). *NTG, 118*, 784–8, 3 ill.

900 BROUWER, E. (1967). H. J. Hamburger (1859–1924). *Voeding, 28*,
483–9, portr.

PIETER HARTING

901 VINKEN, P. J. (1963). Pieter Harting en de afstamming van de mens
(P. H. and the descent of the human). *Proc.KNAW*, serie C, 66, 383–9.

902 GEYL, A. (1961). Pieter Harting. Het geleerdenwereldje van een eeuw geleden (The world of scientists a century ago). *Vrij Nederland*, 27 mei, p. 11.

903 HARTING, P. (1961). *Mijne Herinneringen. Autobiografie* (Memories. Autobiography) edited by J. G. van Cittert-Eymers and P. J. Kipp. 148 pp. + 80 pp. appendices, 3 ill. Noord-Holl. Uitg. Mij., Amsterdam.

– P. Harting (1812–85), professor of botany, chemistry and pharmacy at Franeker (1841), since 1843 at Utrecht. Reviewed by J. A. van Dongen in: *NTG, 106* (1962), I, 30–1; *BGG, XLII*, 3–4.

904 — (1839, 1942). *Bijdragen tot de mikroskopische kennis der zachte dierlijke weefsels* (Contributions to the microscopical knowledge of the soft animal tissues) – with German translation. *Opusc., XVI*, 2–59.

WILLIAM HARVEY

905 SCHIERBEEK, A. (1920). William Harvey. *Levende Natuur, XXIV* (1 jan.), 262.

906 FEYFER, F. M. G. de (1928). William Harvey (1578–1657). *NTG, 72*, I, 2196–2220; *BGG, VIII*, 119–43.

907 LEERSUM, E. C. van (1913). William Harvey and the haematoma. *Janus, XVIII*, 332.

908 LINDEBOOM, G. A. (1964). Harvey legt zijn hand op het kloppend mensen hart (H. puts his hand on the beating human heart). *NTG, 108*, I, 42–3; *BGG, XLIV*, 24–5.

909 — (1957). William Harvey en zijn ontdekking van de bloedsomloop (W. H. and his discovery of the circulation of the blood). *NTG, 101*, II, 2209–15; *BGG, XXXVII*, 34–40.

909[a] SCHOUTEN, J. (1974). Hoe kwam William Harvey tot de ontdekking van de bloedsomloop? (How came — — to the discovery of the circulation of the blood?). In: *Circa Tiliam*, 292–7. Brill, Leiden.

910 PAGEL, W. (1967). Harvey and Glisson on Irritability with a note on van Helmont. *BHM, XLI*, 497–514.

911 FEYFER, F. M. G. de (1909). Bemerkungen zu Harvey's *Exercitatio Tertia De Circulatione Sanguinis ad Joannem Riolanum Filium. Janus, XIV*, 335–46.

– also on de Wale and de Back.

912 LINDEBOOM, G. A. (1957). William Harvey. *Elsevier's Wbl.*, 1 June.

913 RATHER, L. J. (1965). Old and New Views of the Emotions and Bodily changes: Wright and Harvey versus Descartes, James and Cannon. *Clio Med.*, *1*, 1–25.

914 LINDEBOOM, G. A. (1957). William Harvey (1578–1657). *GeWiNa*, 2, 9.

915 HOEVEN, J. van der (1928). Harvey herdenking (Commemoration of H.) *NTG*, *72*, I, 2682–4; *BGG*, *VIII*, 166–8.

916 FRANCIS, W. W. (1957). On the death of Harvey. A premature threnody by Nikolaas van Assendelt. Dutch text with English translation. *J. Hist. Med.*, *12*, 254–5.

917 MOULIN, D. de (1972). Ita cor principium vitae et sol microcosmi (W. Harvey). *Hart Bulletin*, *3*, 34–5, portr., 1 ill.
see also 2993–97, 3000, 3002–04 (circulation of the blood)

918 HARTOG, C. den (1965). J. Haverschmidt 1862–1938. *Voeding*, *26*, 41–3, portr.

919 HOEVEN, J. van der (1938). Albertus de la Haye, med. doctor (1655–1774). *NTG*, *82*, III, 4331–2; *BGG*, *XVIII*, 151–2.

920 ELAUT, L. (1956). De Limburger Hendrik de Heer en de bronnen van Spa (The Limburger H. de H. and the sources of Spa). Repr. from *Limburg*, *35*, 141–51.

921 MAN, J. C. de (1905). *Antonius de Heide, Med. Doctor te Middelburg, ontdekker der later zoo beroemd geworden trilhaarbeweging* (A. de H., Med. Dr. at M., discoverer of the motion of the vibrissae of such fame later on). 69 pp., D. G. Kröber Jr., Middelburg.
– Reviewed by C. E. Daniëls: *NTG*, *41* (1905), 704–6 and by V.d.B.: *Janus*, *X* (1905), 1605.

J. B. VAN HELMONT

922 STRUNZ, Fr. 1907). *Johann Baptist van Helmont (1577–1644). Ein Beitrag zur Geschichte der Naturwissenschaften.* 66 pp., Leipzig-Wien.

923 PARTINGTON, J. R. (1936). Joan Baptista van Helmont. *Ann. Sci.*, *I*, 359–84.

924 FEYFER, F. M. G. de (1947). Johan Baptist van Helmont als arts (J. B. van H. as a physician).

I. *NTG, 91*, III, 1807–14, portr.; *BGG, XXVII*, 20–7.

II. *NTG, 91*, III, 2205–12; *BGG, XXVII*, 34–47, (II en III).

III. *NTG, 91*, III, 2525–32.

925 HIERONYMI, E. (1957). Johann Baptist van Helmont und sein System der Krankheitslehre im Rahmen der Barockmedizin. *Tierärtzl. Umschau, 12*, 261–4.

926 MOON, R. O. (1931). Van Helmont, Chemist, Physician, Philosopher and Mystic. *Proc. Royal Soc. Med., 25*, 23–8; *Sect. Hist.Med.*, 1–6.

927 RATTANSI, P. M. (1964). The Helmontian-Galenist controversy in Restoration England. *Ambix, XII*, 1–23.

928 MULTHAUF, R. P. (1955). J. B. van Helmont's Reformation of the Galenic Doctrine of Digestion. *BHM, XXIX*, 154–63.

929 WAELE, Henri de (1947). *J. B. van Helmont.* 78 pp., portr., Lebèque & Cie, Bruxelles.

930 PAGEL, W. (1930). *Joh. Bapt. van Helmont.* Einführung in die philosophische Medizin des Barocks. VIII + 224 pp., 1 portr., 1 ill. Julius Springer, Berlin, 8°.

931 — (1944). The Religious and Philosophical Aspects of van Helmont's Science and Medicine. *Suppl. BHM.*, no. 2, *IX*, 44 pp.

932 — (1949). J. B. van Helmont, de Tempore, and biological time. *Osiris, 8*, 405.

933 — (1955). J. B. van Helmont's reformation of the Galenic doctrine of digestion – and Paracelsus. *BHM, XXIX*, 563–8.

934 — (1956). Van Helmont's ideas on gastric digestion and the gastric acid. *BHM, XXX*, 524–36.

935 — (1972). Van Helmont's concept of disease – to be or not to be. The influence of Paracelsus. *BHM, 46*, 419–54.

936 NÈVE MÉVERGNIES, Paul de (1935). *Jean Baptiste van Helmont philosophe par le feu.* 232 pp. Bibl. de la Fac. de Philosophie et Lettres de l'université de Liège; Fasc. LXIX, Paris, Librairie E. Droz.

937 HOWE, H. M. (1965). A Root of van Helmont's Tree. *Isis, 56*, 408–19.

938 NIEBYL, P. H. (1971). The Helmontian Thorn. *BHM, 45*, 570–95.

939 HOFF, H. E. (1964). Nicolaus of Cusa, van Helmont, and Boyle: The

First Experiment of the Renaissance in Quantitative Biology and Medicine. *J. Hist. Med.*, *19*, 99–117, 1 ill.

940   RETI, L. (1969). Van Helmont, Boyle and the alkahest. In: *Some aspects of seventeenth century medicine and science*, 1–19. William Andrews Clark Memorial Library, Los Angeles.

941   NIEBYL, P. H. (1971). Sennert, Van Helmont, and medical ontology. *BHM, XLV*, 115–37.

942   PAGEL, W. (1944). J. B. van Helmont (1579–1644). *Nature, 153*, 675.

943   RADIN, H. T. (1924). Van Helmont. *Med. Life, 31*, 397–405.

944   FLORKIN, M. (1945–6). Pour saluer Van Helmont. *Bull. de l'Acad. r. d. Méd. de Belgique, 10*, 355–72, 1 ill.

945   FISCHER, H. (1945). Erinnerung an Johann Baptista van Helmont (1579 bis 1644) zu seinem 300. Todesjahr. *Gesnerus, 2*, 45–6.

946   VANDEVELDE, A. J. J. (1929). Helmontiana III. *MKVAW*, 857–79.

947   HELMONT, Jan Baptist van (1648, 1966). *Opuscula medica inaudita.* Ed. 2a. Amsterdam 1648. (Impression anastatique). Culture et Civilisation, Brussels.

948   — (1660, 1944). *Dageraad ofte Nieuwe Opkomst der Geneeskonst, in verborgen grond-regulen der Nature.* Tot Rotterdam. Bij Joannes Naeranus. Anno 1660. Facsimile Reprinted by Standaard Boekhandel, Antwerp-Brussels, Gent, Louvain.

949   — (1648, 1966). *Ortus medicinae. Ed. F. M. van Helmont.* Amsterdam 1648. (Impression anastatique). 800 pp. Culture et Civilisation, Brussels.

950   — (1648, 1683, 1932). *Archeus Faber, Spiritus vitae* – with German translation. *Opusc., XI*, 45–88.
    See also 5410

HELVETIUS (Schweitzer)

951   KRUL, R. (1893). Haagsche en Amisfoortse krukkendans. Bijdrage tot het leven van Johann Friedrich Schweitzer (Helvetius). (The Hague and Amersfoort "crutch dance". Contribution to the life of — —). *Haagsch Jbk., 5*, 4–32.

952 — (1896–97). Jean-Frédéric Helvetius et sa famille. *Janus, I,* 564–71.
– on J. F. Schweitzer (Helvetius), 1639–79. *See also* 1582.

953 VIEYRA, D. (1936). De Hollandsche geneesheer (Adriaan) Helvetius
legt in Frankrijk groote eer in (The Dutch physician — gained great
honour in France). *NTG, 80,* III, 4046; *BGG, XVI,* 156.
– a short note on A.H. (1661–1727), son of J. F. Helvetius.
See also 4624

954 NAPJUS, J. W. (1939). De hoogleeraren in de geneeskunde aan de Hoo-
geschool en het Athenaeum te Franeker (1585–1843): Johannes
Hemsterhuis (The professors of medicine at Franeker Academy and
Athenaeum: J.H.). *NTG, 83,* III, 4320–6; *BGG, XIX,* 211–7.

955 BEYERMAN, J. J. (1957). Dr. W. Hendriksz, 1857. *NTG, 101,* II,
1944.

956–965: deleted

966 RAEMAKERS, Ch. L. (1962). Marcus Ulpius Heracles de eerste Nijmeegse oogarts (— —, the first Nijmegen ophthalmologist). *Numaga,
IX,* 49–62, 9 ill.

967 OUDSCHANS DENTZ, F. (1930). Dr. Constantin Hering en Johannes
Hering. *West-Indische Gids,* Juli-Aug.
– Reviewed by de Feyfer in: *NTG, 74* (1930), II, 5396; and in *BGG, X* (1930), 296;
C. Hering practised 6 years in Surinam and introduced homeopathy in North
America.

968 SMIT, Pieter (1969). Paul Hermann (1646–1695). Ein Vertreter der
niederländischen Botanik des 17. Jahrhunderts. In: Kaiser u. Beierlein (ed.) *In Memoriam Hermann Boerhaave 1668–1738,* 69–88. See
also in: *Wiss. Beiträge Martin-Luther Univers. Halle-Wittenberg* (2),
69–88.

969 LINDEBOOM, G. A. (1972). Mensen rond Boerhaave. VI. Paulus Hermann (Men around Boerhaave. VI. P. Hermann). *GG, 2,* 290–2, ill.

970 KARSTEN, M. C. (1963). Heurnius and Hermans, the earliest known
plant collectors at the Cape. *J. South Afr. Bot., 29,* 25–32, ill.
– On Justus Heurnius, a missionary, who collected plants at the Cape in 1624, and
on Hermans.

970ᵃ SCHRIJVER, F. (1935). Dr Maria Anna van Herwerden. *Erfelijkheid
bij de Mens, 1,* 13–36, port. (with chronological list of publications).

971 HERWERDEN, C. A. B. van (1948). *Marianne van Herwerden (16 Fe-*

bruari 1874 – 26 Januari 1934). 240 pp., port. W. L. en J. Brusse, Rotterdam.

– with chronological list of publications; M. van Herwerden was reader (lector) of cytology at Utrecht University (1927); letters from Wenckebach to M.v.H., see: G. A. Lindeboom (1965). *Karel Frederik Wenckebach*, Bohn, Haarlem, 106–16.

972 STERRENBURG, F. A. S. [1972]. Henri Ferdinand van Heurck, maecenas, geleerde en leek (H. F. van H., maecenas, scientist and layman). *Organorama*, *9*, no 3, 24–7, 3 ill.

– H. F. van Heurck (1838–1909) was born at Antwerp, he was a self-taught man, botanist (he re-organized the Botanical Garden at Antwerp), microscopist. He wrote some books a.o. *Traité des Diatomées* (1899).

973 ELAUT, L. (1961). Een brief van Brucaeus uit Rostock naar Jan van Heurne te Leiden (1590). (A letter of — from Rostock to — at Leyden). *Sci. Hist.*, *3*, 21–4.

JAN PIETER HEYE

974 QUERIDO, A. (1964). Jan Pieter Heije 1809–76. *T. Soc. Geneesk.*, *42*, 893–8.

975 DANIËLS, C. E. (1909) Dr. J. P. Heye. Wat hij deed voor zijn vaderland als geneeskundige. Rede uitgesproken bij de herdenking van Heye's 100sten geboortedag, op 1 Maart 1909. (What he did for his country as a physician. Address held on the occasion of the 100th anniversary of his birthday). *NTG*, *53*, I, 729–43.

976 VRIES, J. de (1909). Dr. Jan Pieter Heye. Geboren 1 Maart 1809 (Dr. J. P. H. Born March, 1, 1809). *Eigen Haard*, XXXV, 117.

977 PIJZEL, E. D. (1909). De Heye-herdenking te Amsterdam en elders (The Heye-commemoration at Amsterdam and elsewhere). *EigenHaard* XXXV, 120.

978 BURGER, H. (1909). Jan Pieter Heye 1809 – 1 Maart 1909. *NTG*, *53*, I, 617–24.
Also in: H. Burger (1930). *Uitgezochte opstellen en toespraken*, 519–24. cf: *T. Ned. Mij. Geneesk.*, *VI* (1855), 39 en *VII* (1856), 18.

979 HORST, L. van der (1957). Het centenarium van G. J. Heymans (Centenary of —). *Ned. T. Psychol.*, N.R. *XII*, 153–8, port.
– Professor of psychology at Groningen (1890–1927).

980 BOOTH, C. C. (1963). William Hillary, a pupil of Boerhaave. *Med. Hist.*, *VII*, 297–316, 2 ill.

981 HILLE, Ph. van (1967). De familie van Hille in Nederland (The family
— in the Netherlands). *Vlaamse Stam*, *3*, 17–21. ill.
–a.o. on M. van Hille, author of *Toneel der chirurgie* (sec. ed. 1726, Antwerp).

982 LUDEMAN, J. C. (1741, 1935). *Horoscoop van Claes Hinloop en* (Horos-
cope of —) - with German translation. *Opusc.*, *XIII*, 231–8.

983 ESSO Bzn., I. van (1954). Thomas Hodgkin. *NTG*, *98*, III, 2526–8;
BGG, *XXXIV*, 78–80, 2 ill., portr.

984 KLAAUW, C. J. van der (1932). The scientific correspondence between
Jan van der Hoeven and professor Richard Owen. *Janus*, *XXXVI*,
327–51, 2 portrs.
– J. van der H. (1801–68) was professor of zoology at Leyden, R. Owen (1804–
92), a comparative anatomist. (see: *The life of Richard Owen* by his grandson the
Rev. Richard Owen, M.A., 2 vols., London, 1894).

985 — (1931). Een brief van den theologischen hoogleeraar Clarisse aan
zijn leerling in de natuurlijke historie den lateren hoogleeraar Jan van
der Hoeven (A letter of the professor of theology — to his pupil in
biology the later professor J. van der H.). *NTG*, *75*, III, 4561–4; *BGG*,
XI, 253–6.

986 LINT, J. G. de (1934). Frederick Hoffmann's Man as a Machine.
Med. Life, *41*, 169–76.

987 DANIËLS, C. E. (1908). In memoriam J. J. Homoet 18 Nov. 1818–16
Febr. 1908, *NTG*, *52*, I, 581.

988 LEERSUM, E. C. van (1913). Robert Hooke and artificial respiration.
Janus, *XVIII*, 341–7.

JOHAN VAN HOORN

989 DANIËLS, C. E. (1916). Bijdrage tot de geschiedenis der verloskunde.
III (Contribution to the history of obstetrics. III). *NTG*, *60*, I, 1365–73.
– on Johan van Hoorn (1661–1724), born of Dutch parents, at Stockholm, the
founder of obstetrics in Sweden.

990 DJURBERG, Vilhelm (1942). *Läkaren Johan van Hoorn, Förlossnings*
konstens grundläggare i Sverige. Efterlämnat manuskript utgivet ge-
nom Lärdomshistoriska Samfundet, Med. ett. Förord av. O. T. Hult.
319 pp., 16 ill., Almquist en Wiksell, Uppsala (Lychnos-Bibliotek, 4).

991 MÖLLER, W. (1962). Till Johan von Hoorns bibliografien hittils okänd
tysk upplaga av "Siphra och Pua". *Nord. Med. Hist. Årsbok*, 9 pp.

992　Kock, W. (1963). Mågra Glintar ur obstetrikens och Gynekologiens i Stockholm Historia (With English abstract). *Nord. Med. Hist. Arsbok*, 17 pp., ports.

– Föredrag vid Svensk Gynekologisk Förenings sammanträde den 14–10–1959; with a portrait of Johan van Hoorn and a title page of one of his books (1697).

992ª HOUTZAGER, H. L. (1974). Nederlandse arts in Zweden: Johan van Hoorn (Dutch physician in Sweden, — —). *Spiegel Historiael*, 9, 546– 9, 7 ill.

933　SLUITER, E. (1953). Sir Frederic Gowland Hopkins 1861–1947. *Voeding*, *14*, 277–9, portr.

994　SCHOORL, P. (1962). Axel Horst. 6 September 1860 – 26 april 1931. *Voeding*, *23*, 436–40, portr.

– Horst was a Norwegian, who made studies on the dietetics of Grijns and Eykman.

995　LINDEBOOM, G. A. (1973). Mensen om Boerhaave. IX. Petrus Hotton (Men around B. IX. P.H.). *GG*, *4*, 102–4, 2 ill.

996　DOOREN, L. (1939). Adriaen van Houtenborch, aangesteld als lijfarts van het Hof van Gelderland (1570) (Appointed as court-physician to the Court of Gelderland (1570)). *NTG*, *83*, I, 530–2; *BGG*, *XIX*, 35–7.

997　SLEESWIJK, J. G. (1910). Hufeland. *NTG*, *54*, I, 525–8.

998　STRAUB, M. (1908). Eine bisher nicht veröffentlichte Schrift von Christian Huygens über das Auge und das Sehen. *Klin. Monatsbl. Augenheilk.*, *46*, 295.

999　ZAAYER, F. (1894). Joseph Hyrtl. Toespraak bij de opening der Academische lessen op den 15den October 1894 (Address on the occasion of the beginning of the Academic lessons, October, 15, 1894). *NTG*, *40* (*32*), 707–20.

I and *J*.

JAN INGENHOUSZ

1000　GODEFROI, M. J. (1875). Het leven van dr. Jan IngenHousz (The life of — —). *NTG*, *11*, (19), II, 285–302.

1000ª WIESNER, J. (1905). *Jan Ingen-Housz. Sein Leben und sein Wirken als Naturforscher und Arzt.* 252 pp., port. Carl Konegen, Wien.
– with a complete bibliography of I.

1001 REED, Howard S. (1949). Jan Ingenhousz, plant physiologist. With a History of the Discovery of Photosynthesis. *Chron. Botan., 11*, no. 5/6, 291–393, portrs. Chron. Botanica Co., Mass. U.S.A.
– review in *Centaurus*, 2 (1951–53), 259–60.

1002 HOFF, H. E. (1962). Jan Ingen-Housz and the cover-slip. *BHM, 36*, 365–8.

1003 PAS, P. W. van der (1963). The Ingenhousz-Jenner correspondence. *Congr. int. Hist. Sci.* 1962; *Bull singal. Hist. Sci. Tech., 17* (1), no. 7824 Abstr. Also in: *Actes dixième Congrès int. Hist. Sci. Ithaca*, 1962, II, 957–60, Hermann, Paris. And in: *Janus, LI* (1964), 202–20.

1004 FOREGGER, R. (1956). Jan Ingen Housz and Joseph Priestley on carbon dioxide absorption. *Anaesthesiology, 17*, 511–22, ill.

1005 SCHIERBEEK, A. (1921). Ingen-Housz, Senebier, de Saussure. *Levende Natuur, XXVI*, (1 oct.), 129.

1006 — (1954). Een tot heden niet gepubliceerde brief van de eerste markies van Lansdowne over de laatste levensdagen van Jan Ingenhousz en een oproep om te komen tot het aanbrengen van een gedenksteen in de kerk te Calne (An up to the present inedited letter from the first marquis of Lansdowne on the last days of the life of — and a call for placing a memorial stone in the church at Calne). *NTG, 98*, III, 2521–5; *BGG, XXXIV*, 73–7.

1007 SCHUSTER, J. (1923). Ein Brief von Jan Ingen Housz an Benjamin Franklin aus dem Jahr der Amerikanischen Unabhängigkeitserklärung. *Arch. Gesch. Mediz., XV*, not printed.

1008 SCHIERBEEK, A. (1957). An Ingen-Housz memorial at Calne. *Arch. int. Hist. Sci., 10*, (39), 195–7.

1009 DANIËLS, C. E. (1884). Levensschets van Dr. A. H. Israëls (Sketch of the life of —). *NTG, 20* (2de reeks), 881–903 and 913–27.
– with a list of his publications.

1010 ZEEMAN, J. (1883). In memoriam Prof. A. H. Israëls. *NTG, 19*, 72–4.

1011 SUDHOFF, K. (1934). Bibliographie Isaaks und Johann Isaaks, der "Holländer". *S.A.*, *27*, 45–50.

– Isaaks and his son, called the "Holländer" were two Dutchmen, known in the early history of chemistry.

1012 HULSMAN, G. and A. Zwaveling (1965). Jan Egens van Iterson, chirurg, uit twee werelden (surgeon from two worlds). *NTG*, *109*, I, 33–8; *BGG*, *XLV*, 6–11, portr.

1013 MENDELS, J. I. H. (1938). Holger Jacobaeus' reizen in Holland (H. J.'s journeys in Holland). *NTG*, *82*, III, 4333–44; *BGG*, *XVIII*, 153–67.

– H. Jacobsen (Jacobaeus, 1650–1701) visited Holland several times. The article is based on: Vilhelm Maar (1910). *Holger Jacobaeus' Rejsebog (1671–1692)*. Copenhagen.

1014 ELAUT, L. (1956). Jan-Corneel Jacobs, promotor van een nieuwe behandeling der gonorroe (Promotor of a new treatment of gonorrhoea). *NTG*, *100*, III, 1994–8; *BGG*, *XXXVI*, 44–8.

1015 WIBAUT, F. P. (1972). Dr. Aletta Jacobs begon 90 jaar geleden met geboortenregelingsadviezen (Dr. A. J. began 90 years ago with birth-control advices). *NTG*, *116*, 533.

B. C. P. JANSEN

1016 SLUYTER, E. (1954). Prof. Dr. B. C. P. Jansen 70 jaar (The 70th birth-day of —). *NTG*, *98*, IV, 2970–1, portr.

1017 WESTENBRINK, H. G. K. (1962–63). Levensbericht van Barend Coenraad Petrus Jansen (1 april 1884 – 18 october 1962) (Biographical notice). *Jbk. KNAW*, 387–400, portr.

1018 EYS, J. van (1970). Barend Coenraad Petrus Jansen – a biographical sketch (1884–1962). *J. Nutr.*, *100*, 485–90.

1019 BERGH, S. G. v. d. (1964). Levensschets van B. C. P. Jansen (Biographical sketch). *Folia Civitatis*, 20 June.

– Jansen, originally vitamin chemist, isolated with Donath the crystalline Vitamin B (aneurin). From 1928–54 he was professor of physiological chemistry in the Medical Faculty of the University of Amsterdam.

1020 LINT, J. G. de (1935). Edouard Jeanselme. *NTG*, *79*, II, 2108; *BGG*, *XV*, 120, portr.

– Ed. Jeanselme (1858–1935), was an expert on syphilis, framboesia and lepra, as well as a medico-historian.

1021 CARP, E. A. D. E. (1942), *Jelgersma. Leven en werken van een ver-dienstelijk Nederlander* (Life and Work of a deserving Dutchman), 124 pp., ill. serie: Nederlandsche Monographieën, *3*, De Tijdstroom, Lochem.

– Rev. by B. Brouwer in: *Psych. en Neurol. Bladen*, 1944, no 1/2.

1022 ANDEL, M. A. van (1929). In Memoriam Dr. J. W. S. Johnsson. *Janus*, *XXXIII*, 49–51.

1022ᵃ JOSSELIN DE JONG, R. de (1927). In Memoriam Prof. Dr D. A. de Jong (1865–1925). *Versl. Tuberculose-Studie-Commissie*, no. 1, 7–11, port.

1023 BILIKIEWICZ, Tadeusz. (1930). Johann Jonston (1603–1675) und seine Tätigkeit als Arzt. *Arch. Gesch. Mediz.*, *23*, 357–81, portr.

– Jonston, born in Poland, studied also in Holland under Heurnius and Schrevelius. Probably he influenced Dele Boë Sylvius. Several of his works were printed in Holland.

1024 — (1931). *Jan Jonston (1603–1675) zywot i dzialalność lekarska* (Leben und ärztliches Wirken). 233 pp. 4 ill., 8°. Warszawa [Polish].

1024ᵃ HELSDINGEN, R. J. van (²1974). *C. G. Jung.* 140 pp., Kruseman, Den Haag.

– C. G. Jung (1875–1961).

1025 WORMSER, C. W. [1943]. *Frans Junghuhn.* 244 pp. W. van Hoeve, Deventer.

– Serie: *Bouwers van Indië*, Vol. V. *See also NNBW* IV, col. 820–4.

K

1026 HALBERTSMA, K. T. A. (1941). Engelbert Kaempfer (1651–1716). *Janus*, *XLV*, 40–55.

1027 VERBRUGGEN, F. (1972). Immanuel Kant (1724–1804) en de scheikunde op het einde van de achttiende eeuw (I.K. and chemistry at the end of the 18th century). *Sci. Hist.*, *14*, 1–16.
See also 2137

1028 BELDEROK, B. (1965). Johan Rudolf Katz, 1880–1938, en zijn onderzoekingen over het oudbakken worden van brood (his investigations on stale bread). *Voeding*, *26*, 485–92.

1029 GLODEN, A. (1955). Un éminent professeur de chimie de l'athénée de

Luxembourg: le Hollandais Petrus-Johannes-Jacobus van Kerck-hoff, 1813–1876. *Bull. Pharm.*, nov., no. 12, portr.

– Extrait de la Biographie Nationale du Pays de Luxembourg, fasc. 6, 1954.

1030 BROUWER, B. (1949). In Memoriam Prof. Dr. A. P. H. A. de Kleyn. *NTG, 93,* II, 1658–61.

– De Kleyn (1883–1949) was professor of otorhinolaryngology at the University of Amsterdam.

1031 SALTET, R. H. (1891). Robert Koch. *Mannen van betekenis*, afl. 3, portr.

1032 NIEMANDSLAND, N. [pseudonym] (1948). *Arbeid. Uit het leven van een zenuwarts* (Work. From the life of a neurologist), 190 pp. F. van Rossem, Amsterdam.

– Autobiography Dr. S. Koster, a psychiatrist at Amsterdam.

1033 SWELLENGREBEL, N. H. and J. J. van Loghem (1954). Willem Kouwenaar 28 juli 1891 – 5 september 1954. *NTG, 98,* III, 2646–50, portr.

1034 HONIG, C. J. (1942). In Memoriam Dr Rijk Kramer. *G&W*, 43–7.

– Dr. R. Kramer (11 April 1870 – 24 May 1942), an Amsterdam physician.

1035 NICOLAÏ, C. (1903). Johannes Leonardus Arnoldus Kremer (1758–1867), predikant te Heeze en Leende (Noord-Brabant) als oogarts (Clergyman at Heeze and Leende (Northern-Brabant), as an ophthalmic surgeon). *NTG, 39,* II, 953–60.

1036 Kruif, Paul de (1963). *Brausender Wind. Die Geschichte meines Lebens.* Orell Füssli, Zürich.

– Translation from American into German by S. Ullrich.

1037 LEERSUM, E. C. van (1923). Levensbericht van Dr. R. Krul. 20 pp. Reprint of: *Levensber. Mij. Ned. Letterk. te Leiden 1922–23.* E. J. Brill, Leiden.

– with bibliography.

1038 BROWN, A. C. (1961). Prof. B. J. Krijgsman 1901–1961; Physiologist. *Nature* (London), *190,* 1057–8.

1039 STOKVIS, B. J. (1900). In Memoriam Willi Kühne (1837–1900). *NTG, 36,* (2de reeks), I, 1157–62.

1040 LINDEBOOM, G. A. (1955). *Kuyper over de geneeskunde* (K. on medicine). 20 pp., J. H. Kok, Kampen. Also in :*G&W, 53* (1955), 17, 35. (*See also* 2075)

L

LAENNEC

1041 LINT, J. G. de (1919). Laënnec. *NTG*, *63*, II, 372.

1042 HIJMANS VAN DEN BERG, A. A. (1927). Laennec. *Feestbundel Klinkert* p. 221–8, Brusse, Rotterdam.

1043 KNEGTEL, A. P. C. H. [1965] Laennec's methodiek in pathologie en kliniek (— methods in pathology and clinical medicine). *Organorama*, *2*, 13–6.

1044 — (1966). *Laennec*. 217 pp., portrs., ill. Historische Bibliotheek no. 77, Van Gorcum, Assen.

1045 — [1966]. Biografische notities over Laennec (Biographical notices on —). *Organorama*, *3*, 10–2.

1045ᵃ — (1974). Iconografie van Laennec (Iconography of —). *AP*, no 14, 1–9, port.

1046 METS, A. de (1938). Le Docteur Pierre Joseph Lambrechts 1795–1889. Médecine d'Hier et de Demain. *L'Art méd.*, nr. 8, 113–28.

1047 BROUWER-FROMMANN, H. M. (1959). Professor Dr. Cornelia de Lange 1871–1950. *Voeding*, *20*, 101–5, portr.

C. D. DE LANGEN

1048 HULST, L. A. (1953). Bij het afscheid van prof. dr. C. D. de Langen als clinisch hoogleeraar (At the retirement of — as clinical professor). *NTG*, *97*, II, 862–5, portr.

1049 SWELLENGREBEL, N. H. (1967). Levensbericht van Cornelis Douwe de Langen (10 september 1887 – 12 april 1967) (Biographical note of —). *Jbk. KNAW 1966–67*, 353–7, portr.

1050 OOMEN, H. A. P. C. (1967). Cornelis Douwe de Langen, 1887–1967 *Trop. and Geogr. Med.*, *19*, 358.

1051 [Editorial] (1967). In memoriam Prof. Dr. C. D. de Langen. *Voeding*, *28*, 221–3.

J. D. LARREY

1052 WINTERS, V. M. E. (1933). *Jean Dominique Larrey. Een biographie* (— —. A biography) Van der Marck's Drukkerij, Heerlen.

1053 VERAART, B. A. G. (1953). Dominique Jean Larrey, de legerchirurg van Napoleon (The army surgeon of Napoleon). *NTG*, 97, I, 611–21; *BGG, XXXIII*, 1–11,
– cf: a short note: *NTG, 96* (1952), IV, 3209–10; *BGG, XXXII* (1952), 46–7.

1054 HALBERTSMA, K. T. A. (1942). Jean Dominique Larrey (1766–1842). *GG, 20*, 709–18; portr. 725–33.

1055 NAPJUS, J. W. (1938). De hoogleraren in de geneeskunde aan de Hoogeschool en het Athenaeum te Franeker (1585–1843): Petrus Latané (The professors of medicine at Franeker Academy and Athenaeum). *NTG, 82*, IV, 5759–64; *BGG, XVIII*, 307–12.

1056 Es, A. J. H. van (1956). John Bennet Lawes (1814–1900) en Joseph Henry Gilbert (1817–1901). *Voeding, 17*, 81–4, portr.

1057 ANDEL, M. A. van (1939). In Memoriam Prof. Dr. E. C. van Leersum, Febr. 12, 1862 – Febr. 15, 1938. *Janus, XLIII*, 81–3.

ANTONI VAN LEEUWENHOEK

Biographies and general

1058 DOBELL, Clifford (1932,[2] 1960). *Antoni van Leeuwenhoek and his "Little Animals"*. Being some account of the father of protozoology and bacteriology, and his multifarious discoveries in these disciplines. 435 pp., ill. Swets & Zeitlinger, Amsterdam;Dover Publ. Inc. New York.

1059 SCHIERBEEK, A. (1920). Anthoni van Leeuwenhoek. *Levende Natuur, XXV*, (Aug.-Sept.), 81.

1060 — (1929). Neues aus dem Leben Leeuwenhoeks. *VIme Congrès Int. d'Hist. Méd. Leyde-Amsterdam 1927*, 82–7, Anvers.

1061 — (1930). Een paar nieuwe bijzonderheden over Van Leeuwenhoek (Some new details on —). *NTG, 74*, II, 3891–9; *BGG, X*, 209–17, 2 ill.

1062 — (1932). Leven en werken van Anthony van Leeuwenhoek (Life and works of — —). *NTG, 76*, IV, 5149–63; *BGG, XII*, 209–23.

1063 — (1950–51). *Antoni van Leeuwenhoek. Zijn leven en zijn werken.* (His life and his works). 2 vols. pp. 1–278 and 279–526., port. De Tijd-stroom, Lochem.

1064 — (1959). *Measuring the invisible World. The life and works of Antoni van Leeuwenhoek FRS.* With a biographical chapter by Maria Roose-boom PhD. 223 pp., 27 pl. Abelard-Schurman, London and New York.

– An abridged English version of S's. two volumes book on L. (1950–51) in Dutch.

1065 SETERS, W. H. van (1929). La vie et les oeuvres de Van Leeuwenhoek. *VIme Congrès Int. d'Hist. Méd. Leyde-Amsterdam, 1927,* 88–90. An-vers.

1066 TEUNISSEN, R. (1944). *Uit leven en werken van Antony van Leeuwenhoek* (From the life and works of — —). III pp., ill. Spectrum, Utrecht.

– Reviewed by K. de Jong: *GG, 22* (1944), 168.

1067 KUYER, J. H. (1915). Antoni van Leeuwenhoek. *Eigen Haard, XLI,* 202.

1068 BOEKE, J. (1923). Anthony van Leeuwenhoek. 24 October 1632–17 Augustus 1723. *Vragen des Tijds, 49,* 317–32.

1069 ROOSEBOOM, Maria (1959). Antoni van Leeuwenhoek vu dans le milieu scientifique de son époque. *Arch. int. Hist. Sci., 12,* 27–46.

1070 — (1959). Loevenguk, fils de sa nation et de son temps. [Russian]. *Voprosy Istorii Estetvoznaniia i Tekhniki, 8,* 74–81.

– Communication du Musée de l'Histoire des Sciences naturelles à Leyde. (cf. 1069).

1071 — (1968). Antoni van Leeuwenhoek, zijn ontdekkingen en het denken van zijn tijd (A. v. L., his discoveries and the thought of his time). *Spiegel Historiael, 3,* 13–21, ill.

1072 BLOOM, V. (1956). Antoni van Leeuwenhoek, man and scientist. *Univ. Mich. med. Bull., 22,* 39–44.

1073 ARNIM, S. S., (1962). Antony van Leeuwenhoek – the first periodontist. *Acad. Rev.* (Calif. Acad. Periodont), *10,* 57.

1074 SETERS, W. H. van (1968). Van Leeuwenhoek's tweede huwelijk (V. L.'s second marriage). *NTG, 112,* 1258–61, ill.

1075 SERVAAS van ROOYEN, A. J. (1904). Anthoni van Leeuwenhoek door Leuven's hoogeschool gehuldigd (A. v. L. honoured by Louvain University). *Alb. Nat.,* 380.

1076   SCHUUR, J. A. (1962). Een groot Delfts burger (A great Delft citizen). *Natuur en Techniek*, *30*, 371–4, ill.
     – Antoni van Leeuwenhoek.

1076ᵃ   BARTLOW, R. M. (1972). Antony van Leeuwenhoek: symbol of modern science's childhood. *Aesculapius* (Chicago), *1*, 4–6, ill., port.

1077   [Anonym] (1961). The Bedellus of Delft [Ant. van Leeuwenhoek]. *JAMA*, *177*, 860–1.

1078   BEYDALS, Petra (1933). Twee testamenten van Antoni van Leeuwenhoek (Two last wills of — —). *NTG*, *77*, I, 1021–33; *BGG*, *XIII*, 67–79.

1079   BRIM, C. J. (1932). Anton van Leeuwenhoek *Med. Life*, *39*, 425–38, 6 ill., ports.
     – Commemoration of the 300th anniversary of his birth.

1080   KLEIN, K. (1933). Zum Andenken an den 300. Geburtstag van Leeuwenhoecks. *Münch. med. Wschr.*, *80*, 159.

1081   LINDEBOOM, G. A. (1973). Antoni van Leeuwenhoek (1632–1723) à l'occasion du 250ᵉ anniversaire de sa mort. *Méd. et Hygiène*, *31*, 1177–80, 4 ill., port.

1082   HOUTZAGER, H. L. (1973). Anthonie van Leeuwenhoek 1632–1723. Enkele notities bij de herdenking van zijn 250ste sterfdag (Some notes to the memory of the 250th anniversary of his death). *AP*, no 13 (october), 78–82.

1083   MOULIN, D. de (1973). In tenui labor at tenuis non gloria. *Arch. Chir. Neerl.*, *XXV*, 331–3, 2 ill.
     See also 2987, 5480.

Instruments

1084   SETERS, W. H. van (1933). Leeuwenhoeck's microscopen, praepareer- en observatiemethodes (L.'s microscopes, preparation- and observation methods). *NTG*, *77*, III, 3059–60; *BGG*, *XIII*, 174–5.
     – Report of a lecture, held for the "Genootschap"; also in: *NTG*, *77*, IV, 4571–89, ill.; *BGG*, *XIII*, 217–35.

1085   — (1956). Leeuwenhoeks aalkijker-modellen (L.'s eel-viewer models). *NTG*, *100*, I, 175–7, ill.; *BGG*, *XXXVI*, 9–11.

1086   SCHIERBEEK, A. (1947). Van Leeuwenhoek's schenking van 26 micro-

copen aan de Royal Society (V.L.'s gift of 26 microscopes to the — —).
NTG, *91*, I, 708–9; *BGG*, *XXVII*, 7–8.

1087 — (1948). Een en ander over de vergroting van Leeuwenhoek's microscopen en zijn verhouding tot een microscopiserende Amsterdamse burgemeester (Something about the magnification of L.'s microscopes
and his relation to an Amsterdam burgomaster). *NTG*, *92*, I, 44; *BGG*,
XXVIII, 3.
– Burgomaster Joh. Hudde (1628–1704); included in a report of a meeting of the
"Genootschap".

1088 BISSELING, G. H. (1921). Leydse Courant Ao 1747, no 28 and Leydse
Courant Ao 1747, no 61. *NTG*, *65*, I, 1899–1900; *BGG*, *I*, 190–1.
– Two advertisements on the estate of L. (containing some 600 magnifying-glasses).

1089 LINDBERG, J. Antony van Leeuwenhoek – 1600-talsmikroskopisten
och mikroskoptill verkaren. *Nord. Med. Hist. Årsbok*, 17 pp., ill.,
port.

1089ᵃ FALUDY, A. (1973). Antoni van Leeuwenhoek and the simple microscope. [Magyar]. *Orv. Hetil.*, *114*, 2429–31.

Views on circulation, digestion and other topics

1090 MEYER, A. W. (1937). Leeuwenhoek as experimental biologist. *Osiris*,
III, 103–22.

1091 OYE, E. L. van (1952). Anthoni van Leeuwenhoek en het bloed (A.v.
L. and the blood). *MKVAW*, *14*, no 10.

1092 SCHIERBEEK, A. (1960). Antoni van Leeuwenhoek over de spijsverte-
ring (L. on digestion). *Voeding*, *21*, 231–6, ill.

1093 — (1939). Leeuwenhoek en zijn globulentheorie (L. and his theory on
globules). *Natuurwtsch. T.*, *21*, 185–9.

1093ᵃ — (1963). *Antoni van Leeuwenhoek en zijn voornaamste ontdekkingen*
(— — and his most important discoveries). 140 pp., ill. Kruseman, Den
Haag.
– Serie: Helden van de Geest, 26.

1093ᵇ KLUYVER, A. J. (1954). *The Discovery of Unicellular Life*. Excerpts
from Communications by Antoni van Leeuwenhoek to the Royal
Society of London (September 7, 1674 & October 9, 1676). 15 pp.,
ill. (Keepsake issued by the editors of *Chronica Botanica*).

1094 LEEUWENHOEK, Ant. van (1688, 1962). *On the circulation of the blood.*
Latin text of his 65th letter to the Royal Society (Sept. 7th 1688).
Facsimile with an introduction by A. Schierbeek. Serie: *Dutch Classics
on History of Sci.*, *II*, 34 + 27 pp., ill. B. de Graaf, Nieuwkoop.

1095 — (1688, 1907). *Den waaragtigen Omloop des Bloeds* (The real circulation of the Blood). *Opusc.*, *I*, 45–68, ill.

1096 (1695, 1966). *Arcana Naturae* Detecta Ab Antoni van Leeuwenhoek.
Delphis, Apud Henricum a Krooneveld, 1695. (Impression anastatique). 591 pp., 28 pl. Culture et Civilisation, Bruxelles.

1097 — (1697, 1966). *Continuatio Arcanorum Naturae detectorum, Qua con-
tinentur Quicquid hactenus ab Auctore lingua Vernacula editum, & in
linguam Latinam transfusum non fuit.* Delphis Batavorum, Apud
Henricus a Kroonevelt. (Impression anastatique). Culture et Civilisation, Bruxelles.

1098 SCHLICHTING, Th. H. (1951). Waarom vond van Leeuwenhoek geen
navolging? (Why did L. have no followers?). *NTG*, *95*, IV, 3887–91
BGG, *XXXI*, 96–101.

Letters

1099 SCHIERBEEK, A. (1960). *De Van Leeuwenhoek brief van 9 oktober 1676,
de geboorte van de microbiologie, met een inleiding* (The letter of —
of October 9, 1676, the birth of microbiology, with an introduction).
22 + 31 pp., 6 pl. Kon. Ned. Gist- en Spiritusfabriek, Delft.
– Reviewed by M. Rooseboom: *Arch. int. Hist. Sci. 15* (1962), 439–40.

1100 RIJNBERK, G. van (1934). Lijst van gezochte brieven van Leeuwenhoek (List of letters of — looked for). *NTG*, *78*, IV, 5467–70; *BGG*, *XIV*,
219–22.

1101 BEYDALS, P. (1933). Leeuwenhoeck-brief No 27 en andere gegevens
(Leeuwenhoeck-letter nr 27 and other data). *NTG*, *77*, I, 522–7; *BGG*,
XIII, 31–6.

1102 SERVAAS van ROOYEN, A. J. (1906). Brieven van Anthony van Leeuwenhoek (Letters from —). *Alb. Nat.*, 57.

1103 SIRKS, M. J. (1909). Brieven van Antony van Leeuwenhoek (Letters
from —). *Alb. Nat*, 317–21.

1104 VANDEVELDE, A. J. J. (1922–1932). De Send-brieven van Antoni van Leeuwenhoek (The letters from —).

1104.1 I. *MKVAW* (1922), 323–59

1104.2 II. De Brieven 28 tot 52 van —. *MKVAW* (1922), 645–90

1104.3 III. De Brieven 53 tot 75 van —. *Ibid.*, 1019–56.

1104.4 IV. De brieven van 76 tot 107 van —. *Ibid.*, 1093–1132.

1104.5 De Brieven van 108 tot 146 van —. *Ibid.* (1923), 1–33.

1104.6 VI. Bijdrage tot de studie over de geschriften van den Stichter der micrographie (Contribution to the study on the writings of the Founder of micrography). *Ibid.* (1923), 350–400.

1104.7 VII. De 2e en 3e Engelsche reeksen der brieven van — (The second and third English series of the letters from —). *Ibid.* (1924). 130–48.

1104.8 VIII. Over eenige handschriften der brieven van — — (On some manuscripts of the letters from —). *Ibid.*, (1924), 285–300.

1104.9 IX. (and W. H. van Seters). Over eenige handschriften der brieven van — (On some manuscripts of the letters from —). *Ibid.*, (1925), 3–35.

1104.10 X. (and Ir. Vandekeere). Leeuwenhoekiana. *Ibid.* (1932), 209–45.

1105 LEEUWENHOEK, A. van (1692, 1943). Uit de 69ste missive van den 4den January 1692 aan de Royal Society te Londen (A part of the 69th letter of January 4th, 1692 to the Royal Society in L.) *Opusc.*, *XVII*, 176–83.

1106 COHEN, Ernest and W. A. T. COHEN-de MEESTER (1939). Der vermisste Brief Antoni Leeuwenhoeks an Herman Boerhaave vom 26. August 1717. *MKNAW*, afd. Natuurkunde, 1e sectie, deel *XVII*, no 1. 1–25, ill. Noord-Holl. Uitg. Mij., Amsterdam.

1107 RIJNBERK, G. van (1933). Een verloren brief van Leeuwenhoeck teruggevonden! (A lost letter of L. found again). *NTG*, 77, I, 478–9; *BGG*, *XIII*, 29–30.

1108 — and M. van RIJNBERK (1934). Leeuwenhoeck-brieven Een oproep. (Letters of L.). *NTG*, 78, IV, 5463–6; *BGG*, *XIV*, 215–8.

1109 RIJNBERK, G. van et al. (1674–78, 1930). *Veertien tot heden geheel onuitgegeven brieven van Anthony van Leeuwenhoek uit de jaren 1674–1678*

(Fourteen hitherto totally unpublished letters of — from the years —).
With English translation. *Opusc.*, *IX*, LXXV + 145 ill.

1110   RIJNBERK, G. van (1931). Het negende *Opusculum*. Veertien tot heden
       geheel onuitgegeven brieven van Anthoni van Leeuwenhoek uit de
       jaren 1674–78 (The ninth *Opusculum*. Fourteen hitherto totally unpub-
       lished letters of — from the years —). *NTG*, *75*, IV, 4972–5; *BGG*, *XI*,
       261–4.
       – a review of the previous item.

1111   — (1938). Alle de brieven van Antoni van Leeuwenhoek (The collected
       letters of —). *NTG*, *82*, II, 2279–80; *BGG*, *XVIII*, 80–1.

1111.1 — (1939). Alle de brieven van Antoni van Leeuwenhoek, deel I, 1673–
       1676 (The collected letters of — —, Vol. I, —) *NTG*, *83*, IV, 4826–7;
       BGG, *XIX*, 233–4.
       – a short note

1112   LEEUWENHOEK, Antoni van (1939–   ). *Alle de brieven van Antoni
       van Leeuwenhoek* (The collected letters of — —). Annotated. Swets &
       Zeitlinger, Amsterdam.

1112.1 Vol. *I* (1939): letters no 1–21 (28 April 1673 – 22 Febr. 1676).
       – Reviewed by F. J. Cole: *Nature*, *144* (1939), 956–8; and by P. H. van Cittert:
       Ned. T. Natuurkunde, *VII* (1939), 366–7.

1112.2 Vol. *II* (1941): letters no 22–42 (21 April 1676 – 21 Febr. 1679).

1112.3 Vol. *III* (1948): letters no 43–69 (25 April 1679 – 28 July 1682).
       – Rev. by: G. Sarton: *Isis*, *41* (1950), part 1, no 123, 116–7. by P. H. van Cittert:
       Ned. T. Natuurk., *15*, 284; F. J. Cole: *Nature*, *163* (1949), 192; O. T. Hult: *Lychnos*
       1948/49), 428–9.

1112.4 Vol. *IV* (1952): letters no 70–81 (22 Jan. 1683 – 25 July 1684).
       – Rev. by H. Engel: *NTG*, *97* (1953), III, 2028; by P. H. van Cittert: *Ned. T. Na-
       tuurk.*, *XX* (1954), 20; by F. J. Cole: *Nature*, *172* (1953) 696–7; by I. Bernard Cohen:
       Isis, *46* (1955), part 2, 183–4.

1112.5 Vol. *V* (1957): letters no 82–89 (5 January 1685 – 22 January 1686).
       – Rev. by David E. Wolfe: *BHM*, *XXXVI* (1962), 578–80; by F. J. Cole: *Nature*.
       181 (1958), 1753–4; by I. B. Cohen: *Isis*, *50* (1959), 278–9.

1112.6 Vol. *VI* (1961): letters no 90–101 (2 April 1686 – 11 July 1687).
       – Rev. by L. Buchheim: *SA*,*46* (1962), 88–9; by L. A. Harvey: *Nature*, *193* (1962),
       913; by H. Engel: *NTG*, *106* (1962), 31; by F.N.L.P. [oynter]: *Med. Hist.*, *6* (1962),
       198; by J. Lorch: *Isis*, *54* (1963), 424–6; and in: *Science*, 135 (1962), 662.

1112.7   Vol. *VII* (1964): letters no 102–109 (6 August 1687 – 24 August 1688).
– Rev. by H. Engel: *NTG, 109* (1965), 1261.

1112.8   Vol. *VIII* (1967): letters no 110–119 (7 September 1688 – 7 March 1692).
– Rev. by Frank N. Egerton: *Epistème, 3* (1969), 267–8.

1112.9   Vol. *IX* (in the press): letters no 120–133 (22 April 1692 – 24 February 1694).
See also 104, 1094

Special topics

1113   RIJNBERK, G. van (1923). Anthonie van Leeuwenhoek, de ontdekker der konijnen-coccidiën (A. v. L., the discoverer of the rabbit coccidia). *NTG, 67*, I, 1883; *BGG, III*, 121.
– Review of an article by Clifford Dobell in: *Parasitology, 4* (1922) 342–8.

1114   COLE, F. J. (1937). Leeuwenhoek's zoological Researches. Part I and II + Index to the published letters. *Ann. of Sci., II*, 1–46 and 185–235.

1115   EGERTON, Frank N. (1968). Leeuwenhoek as a founder on animal demography. *J. Hist. Biol., I*, 1–22.

1116   LINDSAY, L. (1929). Worms in the teeth. *VIme Congrès int. d'Hist. Méd. Leyde-Amsterdam, 1927*, 280–5. Anvers.
– Largely apropos of L.

1117   HOFMEIER, M. (1964). Leeuwenhoek's Erforschung der Bakterien flora des Mundes. *Zahnärztl. Mitt.*, Heft 23.

1118   RING, M. E. (1971). Anton van Leeuwenhoek and the toothworm. *J. Am. dent. Ass., 83*, 999–1001.

1119   MCCARTY, D. J. (1970). A historical note – Leeuwenhoek's description of crystals from a gouty tophus. *Arthr. and Rheum., 13*, 414–8.

1120   CHAPMAN, A. C. (1931). "The yeast cell: what did Leeuwenhoek see?". *J. Inst. Brewing, 37*, 433–6.

1121   SVIHLA, G. (1967). "The yeast cell: what did Leeuwenhoek see?" *The Microscope and Crystal Front, 15*, 289–300. Brighton, Sussex.

1122   [Anonym] (1962). Leeuwenhoek e i suoi "piccoli animali". *Castalia, 18*, 166–71.

1123   CASTELLANI, Carlo (1963). La scoperta degli spermatozoi e gli studi di A. van Leeuwenhoeck sullo sperma maschile. *Riv. Storia Medic.*, *VII*, 18–43.

1123ᵃ — (1973). Spermatozoan biology from Leeuwenhoek to Spallanzani, *J. Hist. Biol.*, *6*, 37–68.

1124 BELLONI, Luigi (1966). Appunti per una storia pre-Leeuwenhoekiana degli "animalcula". *Gesnerus*, *23*, 13–22.

Criticism

1125 RIJNBERK, G. van (1924). Kritiek op Leeuwenhoek's ontdekkingen (Criticism on the discoveries of —). *NTG*, *68*, II, 1274–5; *BGG*, *IV*, 237–8.
– Review of an article of De Toni on the Italian scientist Giaconto Cestoni, who studied L.'s letters accurately: *Arch. di Storia della Scienza*, *4*, no 3.

Friends and Correspondence

1126 LEERSUM, E. C. van (1913). Marcello Malpighi, Anthony van Leeuwenhoek and the capillary circulation. *Janus*, *XVIII*, 357–62, 4 ill.

1127 BOEKE, J. (1920). Leeuwenhoek en Mendel. *Vragen des Tijds*, *II*, 303.

1128 RIJNBERK, G. van (1924). Joblot en Leeuwenhoek. *NTG*, 68, II, 1274; *BGG*, *IV*, 237.
– Review of an article by C. Dobell in: *Parasitology*, *15*, no 3.

1129 RIJNBERK, M. van (1937). De briefwisseling tusschen Leeuwenhoeck en Magliabechi (The correspondence between L. and M.). *NTG.* *81*, III, 3147–59; *BGG*, *XVII*, 126–38.

1130 SCHIERBEEK, A. (1943). Leeuwenhoek, Malpighi en Swammerdam, een bijdrage tot de geschiedenis der entomologie (Cecidologie en Schneumonidae) (L., M. and S., a contribution to the history of entomology). *Jbk. Dodonaea*, *10*, 71–6. De Sikkel, Antwerpen.

1131 BEYDALS, P. (1944). Een geromantiseerde ontmoeting tusschen Leibniz en Leeuwenhoek (A romanticized meeting between L. and L.). *NTG*, *88*, II, 490–2; *BGG*, *XXIV*, 5–7.

1132 BELLONI, L. (1963). Leeuwenhoek, Boerhaave e Bleyswyk sugli spermatozoi. *Physis*, *5*, 327–32.

1133 FRACASTORO, G. (1971). Da Gerolamo Fracastoro ad Athanasius

Kircher ed Antony van Leeuwenhoek. *Fracastoro, 64,* 196–228, ports.

1134 SETERS, W. H. van (1935). Leeuwenhoeck-ceramiek (Leeuwenhoeck-ceramics). *NTG, 79,* II, 1583–7; *BGG, XV,* 70–4, ill.

1135 HOFMEIER, H. (1960). Eine wenig bekannte Gedenkmedaille des Antoni van Leeuwenhoek. *Neue Ztschr. ärztl. Fortbild., 12,* 896–7, ill.

Language

1136 RIJNBERK, G. van (1933). De taal van Leeuwenhoek (The language of —). *NTG, 77,* II, 2508–10; *BGG, XIII,* 133–5.

1137 DAMSTEEGT, B. C. (1965). Syntaktische verschijnselen in de taal van Antoni van Leeuwenhoek (Syntactic phenomena in the language of —). *T. Ned. Taal & Lett., 81,* 161–94.

1138 HOORN, C. M. van (1966). Levinus Lemnius. *Zeeuws Tijdschr., 16,* 58–60.

1139 — (1968). Dr. Lieven Lemse (Levinus Lemnius) 1505–1568. *GeWiNa,* no. 24, sept. 9–13.

1140 — (1971). Levinus Lemnius en Willem Lemnius. Twee zestiende-eeuwse medici (Levinus and Willem L. Two physicians from the 16th century). *Arch. Zeeuws Gen.,* 37–86. 4 portrs., 1 ill.

1140ª CLAES, F. (1974). Levinus Lemnius, een Zeeuwse bron van Kiliaan (— —, a Zealand source of —). *T. Ned. Taal- en Letterk., 90,* 132–49.

1141 LAAGE, R. J. C. V. ter (1969). Louis Lewin en zijn opvattingen over Cannabis Indica (and his views on Cannabis Indica). *Ph. W., 104,* nr. 27, 91–8.

1142 VRIES, K. A. de (1953). Justus von Liebig 1803–1873). *Voeding, 14,* 529–31, portr.

1143 DEELNAM, H. T. (1954). Prof. Dr. G. O. E. Lignac 1893 – 5 september 1954, *NTG, 98,* III, 2650–1, portr.

1144 ROEKEL, G. van (1939). Een sociaal geneesheer op het einde van de 16de eeuw (A social physician at the end of the 16th century). *NTG, 83,* IV, 4865; *BGG, XIX,* 229–30.
– On dr. Petrus Lijsselius, town-physician at Nijmegen. Leprologist and fighter against quackery.

1145 WEITS, J. (1954). James Lind 1716–1794. *Voeding, 15,* 477–9, portr.

1145ª MEER, C. van der, J. V. MEININGER, J. SCHOUTEN (eds) (1974). *Circa Tiliam. Studia Historiae Medicinae Gerrit Arie Lindeboom septuagenario oblata,* 302 pp., ill., ports. E. J. Brill, Leiden.
– with a short biography, a bibliography of G. A. L. and 13 medico-historical articles.

J. A. VAN DER LINDEN

1146 NAPJUS, J. W. (1936). Joh. Ant. van der Linden. I: *NTG, 80,* III, 4317–24; *BGG, XVI,* 163–70. II: *NTG, 80,* IV, 5436–46; *BGG, XVI,* 209–19.

1147 — (1937). Bijzonderheden omtrent de voorouders van Johannes Antonides van der Linden en in het bijzonder omtrent zijn vader Antonius van der Linden (Details about the forefathers of — and particularly about his father Antonius van der L.) *NTG, 81,* III, 3844–7; *BGG, XVII,* 141–4.

1148 — (1937). Onderzoek in Engeland en Frankrijk naar een opvolger van Johannes Antonides van der Linden als medisch hoogleraar te Leiden (Investigation in England and in France into a successor of — as professor of medicine at Leyden). *NTG, 81,* II, 2640–4; *BGG, XVII,* 99–102.

1149 — (1937). Notulen van de vroedschap van Utrecht omtrent de benoeming van J. A. van der Linden tot hoogleraar aldaar in 1649 (Minutes of the town council of Utrecht about the appointment of — as professor in 1649 there). *NTG, 81,* II, 2654–6; *BGG, XVII,* 113–5.

1150 SARTON, George (1953). Johannes Antonides van der Linden (1609–1664) medical writer and bibliographer. In: E. Ashworth Underwood (ed.) *Science, Medicine and History,* Oxford, University Press, London, New York, Toronto, 1953, vol. II, 3–20.

1151 NIJHOFF, G. C. (1924). Drie Enkhuizer professors in de Geneeskunde (van der Linden, Bakker, Hendriksz) (Three Enkhuizer professors of medicine Van der L., B., H.). *NTG, 68,* II, 2257–61; *BGG, IV,* 294–8.
– On J. A. van der Linden (1609–64, Leiden), Gerard Bakker (1771–1828, Groningen), and Petrus Hendriksz (1779–1845, Groningen (surgery)). *(See also* 4141)

1152 PREISER, G. (1969). Zur Hippokratesauffassung des Johannes Antonides van der Linden. *Mediz. Hist. J., 4,* 305–13.

1153 DONGEN, J. A. van (1962). In memoriam E. J. van der Linden. *NTG*, *106*, I, 482; *BGG, XLII*, 14.

– E. J. v. d. L. (1885–1961) was assistant of the librarian of the library of the Dutch Association of Physicians during more than half a century. He had no academical education, published nothing, but was a friend and source of information for several Dutch medical historians.

CAROLUS LINNAEUS

1154 BEUKERS, P. G. (1907). *Het leven van Linnaeus* (The life of Linnaeus). De Bussy, Amsterdam.

1155 HOFF, J. J. (1907). Carolus Linnaeus. 23 Mei 1707 – 10 Jan. 1778. *Vrag. Dag, XXII*, 353.

1156 KERBERT, C. (1907). Carolus Linnaeus 1707–1778. *Eigen Haard*, 311.

1157 LEERSUM, E. C. van (1907). En souvenir du jour de naissance de C. Linné (23 mai 1707). *Janus, XII*, 313–8, facs.

– two letters of Linnaeus (one to Boerhaave and one to Joh. Burman).

1158 LOTSY, J. P. (1907). *Carolus Linnaeus. Een en ander over zijne betee-kenis, vooral ten opzichte van het soortsbegrip. Rede ter herdenking van zijn 200sten geboortedag* (Something about his significance, particularly with respect to the concept of species. Address to the memory of his 200th anniversary of his birthday) 32 pp. Erven Loosjes, Haarlem.

1159 SURINGAR, J. Valckenier (1908). *Linnaeus*, 's-Gravenhage. 8°.

1160 HAGBERG, Knut (1944). *Carl Linnaeus, de bloemenkoning* (The King of the Flowers), ill. Amsterdam, 8°.

– Translated from Swedish into Dutch by Marie Vos.

1161 NIEUWENHUIS-VON UEXKÜLL, M. (1909). *Karl von Linné's Bedeutung als Naturforscher und Arzt*. Schilderungen herausgegeben anläsz-lich der 200-jährigen Wiederkehr des Geburtstages Linné's. Jena, Gustav Fischer 1909. *Janus, XIV*, 828–34.

1162 SCHIERBEEK, A. (1920). Carolus Linnaeus. *Levende Natuur, XXV* (1 Nov. and 1 Dec.), 148 and 177.

1163 PULLE, A. A. (1935). *Carolus Linnaeus*. Rede ter gelegenheid van de herdenking van den dag, waarop Linnaeus voor twee honderd jaar aan de Academie van Harderwijk den graad van doctor in de geneeskunde behaalde, uitgesproken in de Raadszaal te Harderwijk op 24 Juni 1935 (Address, delivered in the Harderwijk Council-room on the two hundredth anniversary of L.'s medical graduation at Harderwijk Academy). 20 pp., Oosthoek, Utrecht.

1164 HUNGER, F. W. T. and C. P. J. Penning (1937). Het borstbeeld van Linnaeus in het Hortustorentje te Harderwijk en de beeldhouwer, die deze buste maakte (The bust of — in the tower of the Hortus at H. and the sculptor who made this bust). *NTG, 81*, II, 1955–61; *BGG, XVII*, 85–91, 2 portrs.

1165 BOERMAN, A. J. (1953). *Carolus Linnaeus als middelaar tussen Zweden en Nederland* (As a mediator between Sweden and the Netherlands). Thesis, Utrecht, Supervisor: H. J. M. Weve, 208 + XXIII pp. Pressa Trajectina, Utrecht. 8°.

1166 UGGLA, Arvid HJ. (1957). *Linnaeus.* 19 pp., portr., ill. Almqvist & Wiksell, Uppsala.
    – Translated into Dutch by A. J. Boerman.

1167 ENGEL, H. (1957). Linnaeus. *Bull. Neth. University Foundation for Int. Co-operation* I, (3), 22–4.

1168 ROOSEBOOM, Maria (1957). Linnaeus 1707–1957. *GeWiNa, 2*, 23.

1169 [   ] (1957). *Linnaeus commemorated* 1707 – May 23rd – 1957. Addresses delivered at the Academic Session on the 23rd of May, 1957 in the Ridderzaal of the Town Hall, Haarlem. *Communication no. 103.* National Museum for the History of Science, Leiden.

1170 LAM, H. J. (1957). Carolus Linnaeus (1707–1778). *NRC*, 18 May.

1171 LAGRANGE, E. (1970). A la découverte de Linné, médecin-naturaliste. *Scalpel* (Brux.), *123*, 57–62.

1172 LINDEBOOM, G. A. (1957). Linnaeus and Medecine. In: *Linnaeus Commemorated*, 23–32. (See no. 1169).

1173 — (1958). Linnaeus en de Geneeskunde (L. and medicine). *NTG, 102*, I, 22–5; *BGG, XXXVIII*, 1–4.

1174 — (1957). Linnaeus and Boerhaave. *Janus, XLVI*, 264–74.

1175 — (1958). Linnaeus en Boerhaave. *GG, 36*, 96.

1176 — (1957). Linnaeus als Christen (As a Christian). *G&W, 55*, 177–85.

1177 EBSTEIN, W. (1903). Carl von Linné als Arzt. *Janus*, *VIII*, 115–22, 2 portrs.

1178 KETEL, B. A. van (1903). Linnaeus als geneesheer. (L. as a physician). *PhW*, *40*, 677–89.
– Address, held on July 12, 1903 at Zwolle for the Association of the History of Natural Science.

1179 BRYK, F. (1919). *Linnaeus im Auslande. Jugendschriften autobiographischen Inhaltes 1732–1738.* 298 pp., Stockholm.

1180 BOERMAN, A. J. (1971). Linnaeus en de voedingsleer (L. and the dietetics). *Voeding*, *32*, 230–42.

1181 ENGEL, H. (1950). Linnaeus in Holland. *Vakbl. Biol.*, *30*, 29–32.

1182 — (1957). Carolus Linnaeus in Holland. In: *Linnaeus Commemorated*, 11–22. (See n°. 1169).

1183 GRAAF-SCHOTEL, N. de and F. de Graaf (1957). In het voetspoor van Linnaeus door Lapland (Following the track of L. through Lapland). *Levende Natuur*, *60*, 97–104, ill.

1184 ENGEL-LEDEBOER, M. S. J. and H. Engel (1964). *Carolus Linnaeus Systema Naturae 1735*, Facsimile of the first edition. With an introduction and a first English translation of the "Observationes" by —. Dutch Classics on Hist. of Science, VIII, 32 + 16 pp. 2 pl. portr. B. de Graaf, Nieuwkoop.
See also 1484

1185 RADHAKRISHNA, P. A. (1965). A Dutch physician of the XVI century on Indian drugs. *Bull. Dept. Hist. Med. Hyderabad*, *III*, 173–83 (port. of Paludanus) (Osmania medical college).
– Linschoten's (1563–1633) account of spices and drugs of India supplemented and annotated by Dr. Bernardus Paludanus.
See also 1328

1186 GILS, J. B. F. van (1936). In memoriam Dr. Jan Gerard de Lint. *NTG*, *80*, III, 4311–2; *BGG*, *XVI*, 157–8, portr.

1187 TRICOT-ROYER, J. J. G. (1938). Jean Gerard de Lint, Historien de la médecine (1867–1936). *Archeion*, *19*, 51–5.
See also 2281

JOSEPH LISTER

1188   SCHULTE, J. E. (1965). Lister de grootste weldoener van de negentien-de eeuw? (The greatest benefactor of the nineteenth century?). *NTG, 109*, II, 1262; *BGG, XLV*, 26.

1189   ESSED, W. F. R. (1927). *De honderdste geboortedag van Josephus baron Lister 1827 – 5 april – 1927* (The hundredth anniversary of the birthday of L.) Semarang.
– commemorative lecture.

1190   VERAART, B. A. G. (1927). Joseph Lister 5 april 1827 – 5 april 1927. *NTG*, 71, I, 1832–3; *BGG, VII*, 322–3.

1191   — (1929). Paper in commemoration of Lister. *VIme Congrès Int. d'Hist. de la Méd., Leyde-Amsterdam, 1927*, p. 300–1, Anvers.

1192   MOULIN, D. de (1966). Honderd jaar geleden in Glasgow (Hundred years ago at G.). *NTG, 110*, 906–7; also in: *GeWiNa*, no. *19*, 7.
– On Joseph Lister (1872–1912).
See also 1545

1193   LOUIS, Armand (1966). De Obel (de Lobel, Lobelius, Matthias. *Nat. Biogr. Woordenboek (Brussels)*, vol. 2, col. 643–8.

1194   LECLAIR, E. (1968). Matthias de Lobel, médecin et botaniste Lillois (1538–1616). *Monspeliensis Hippocrates, 11*, no. 41, 11–20, ill.

1195   WITTOP KONING, D. A. (1951). Mathias de l'Obel en zijn betekenis voor de pharmacie (Mathias de l'Obel and his significance for pharmacy). *Ph. T. België, 28*, 36–41; *Bull. Pharm., I*, 1–6.

1196   DEWHURST, Kenneth (1961–3). John Locke's Medical Notes during his Residence in Holland (1683–1689). *Janus, L*, (1961–63), 176–92.

1197   TAUSK, M. (1973). Otto Loewi en zijn werk. Een eeuwfeest (O. Loewi and his work). *NTG, 117*, 1620–1. (ill. of stamp.)
– A centenary, held at Graz, to the commemoration of Loewi (1873–1961).

1198   WIERINGA, K. T. (1964). In memoriam Dr. Maria P. Löhnis. *Antonie van Leeuwenhoek J. of Microb. and serol., 30*, 337–42, portr.

1199   BAUMANN, E. D. (1920). Jodocus Lommius Buranus. *Arch. Gesch. Mediz., 22*, Heft 1, 60–71.

1200   — (1927). Josse Lommen uit Buren (— from Buren). *Vlaamsch Geneesk. T.*, no. 51 and 52, 909–15 and 929–39.

1201 LOMMIUS, J. (1560, 1732, 1929). *Observationum medicinalium Liber I* (The Latin text from 1560, with English translation), *Opusc.*, *VIII*, 76–137.

1202 MAGNUS, O. (1967). To the memory of A. M. Lorentz de Haas (30th september 1911 – 4th october 1967). *Epilepsia*, *8*, 218–22. also in: *Fol. Psych. Neurol. Neurochir.*, *70*, 423–6, ill.

1203 BRUINVIS, C. W. (1903). Een recept van doctor Ludeman (A prescription of doctor —) *Navorscher*, *LIII*, 551.

1204 LUDEMAN, J. C. (1741). (1935). Horoskop des Herrn Claes Hinloopen. *Opusc.*, *XIII*, 231–8.
– with German translation.

1205 THIJSSEN-SCHOUTE, C. L. (1960). Hermannus Lufneu, stadarts te Rotterdam (city-physician at Rotterdam). *Rotterdams Jbk.*, 6de reeks, *8*, 180–227, ill.
– Lufneu (1657–1744).

1206 ANDEL, M.A. van (1939). In memoriam H. J. Lulofs. *NTG*, *83*, I, 512–3; *BGG*, *XIX*, 17–8.

1207 MEURS, G. J. van (1956). Graham Lusk 1866–1932. *Voeding*, *17*, 121–5, portr.

1208 SETERS, W. H. van (1962). *Pierre Lyonet 1706–1789. Sa vie, ses collections de coquillages et de tableaux, ses recherches entomologiques.* Translated from the Dutch by Louis Laurent. XIII + 227 pp. 13 ill. Martinus Nijhoff, The Hague. 8°.
– Lyonet, a lawyer, was an experienced entomologist. He wrote also a defence of a quack (Jacques Reynaud) who pretended to be able to cure cancer. Reviewed by A. Schierbeek in : *NTG*, *107*, (1963), 965; *BGG*, *XLIII*, 7.
See also 5207

M

1209 MEURS, G. J. van (1955). François Magendie 1783–1855. *Voeding*, *16*, 311–4, portr.

1210 BIJLSMA, U. G. (1969). Magnus as scientist and teacher. *Acta Physiol Pharmacol. Neerl.*, *15*, 111–6.
– On Rudolf Magnus (1873–1927); from 1908–1927 professor of pharmacology at Utrecht.

1211 MAGNUS, O. (1969). Rudolf Magnus, Personal reminiscences. *Acta Physiol. Pharmacol. Neerl.*, *15*, 117–22.

1212   HOEVEN, A. J. van der (transl.) (no. d.). *Andrea Majocchi. Chirurg.*
343 pp. A. M. C. Stok. Z-H. Uitg. Mij, Den Haag. 9th ed.
– Autobiography (translated by A. J. van der Hoeven) of the Italian surgeon A.
Majocchi (20th century).

MAIMONIDES

1213   HOOG, P. H. van der (1938[?] *Rabbi Mozes ben Maimon.* 211 pp., ill.
Zuid-Holl. Uitg. Mij, The Hague.

1214   REISEL, M. (1963). *Maimonides.* Series: Helden van de Geest. Kruseman, Den Haag, 78 pp.

1215   BARUCH, J. Z. (1952). Bij het graf van Maimonides (At the grave of —).
NTG, 96, II, 1543–5; *BGG, XXXII,* 29–31.

1216   — (1969). Maimonides as a physician. *Janus, LVI,* 248–59. Also in:
NTG, 113, 1196–1201.

1217   — (1971). De betekenis van Maimonides als geneesheer (The importance of — as a physician). *Arts en Auto, 37,* 1583–5.

1218   LINDEBOOM, G. A. (1971). Het (aan Maimonides toegeschreven) och-
tendgebed van een arts (The morning-prayer of a physician (attributed
to M.)). *NTG, 115,* 924–7, ill.

J. C. DE MAN

1219   DANIËLS, C. E. (1909). In Memoriam J. C. de Man, 20 sept. 1818 –
2 jan. 1909. *NTG, 53,* I, 133.

1220   GEYL, A. (1909). Dr. J. C. de Man geb. 20 Sept. 1818, gest. 2 Jan. 1909.
Janus, XIV, 1–3.

1221   SCHOUTE, D. (1915). Het wetenschappelijk leven van Dr. J. C. de Man
(The scientific life of —). *Arch. Zeeuw Gen.,* I.

1222   — (1936). Auto-suggestie? Uit een nagelaten geschrift door dr. J. C.
de Man te Middelburg (Self-suggestion? From a posthumous writing
of —). *NTG, 80,* II, 1923–30; *BGG, XVI,* 63–70.

1223   NUYENS, B. W. Th. (1937). Brieven van dr. J. C. de Man aan zijn vader.
Relaas van zijn studiereis naar Parijs en Weenen 1842 (Letters of —
to his father. Story of his study-tour to Paris and Vienna 1842). *NTG,*
81, II, 1447–51; *BGG, XVII,* 68–72.

1224 POLMAN KRUSEMAN, W. (1910). *Ter herinnering aan Dr. J. C. de Man*
(To the memory of —). 92 pp., portr., J. C. Altorffer, Middelburg.

1225 CLARK, G. (1971). Bernard Mandeville, M. D. and eighteenth
century ethics. *BHM, 45,* 430–43.
– B.M. was the great-grandson of Michaël de Mandeville.

1225ᵃ ROUSSEAU, G. S. (1974). Mandeville and Europe: medicine and philosophy. In: *Proc. XXIII Int. Congr. Hist. Med. London, 2–9 Sept. 1972,*
Vol. I, 739–47. Wellcome Institute of the History of Medicine, London.
– on Bernard Mandeville (*b.ca* 1670).

1226 [Editorial] (1962). De Doctorsbul van Michael de Mandeville (The
doctor's diploma of — —). *Numaga, IX,* 44–6.
See also: 5044.

1227 WEITS, J. (1964). Ernst Mangold, 1879–1961. *Voeding, 25,* 406–7.
– Mangold was a physiologist, director of the "Tierphysiologisches Institut" at
Berlin. He wrote a.o. a book on dietetics.

1228 MC BRYDE, Bruce (1970). Rediscovery of G. Marcgrave's Brazilian
collections. *Taxon, 3,* 349.
– Brief account of the existence of a herbarium of George Marcgrave, recently
found at Copenhagen, entitled *Herbarium vivum Brasiliense Plantarum et fructuum
in Brasiliana insula singulari studio collectarum et observatarum.*
It contains part of the collection used for the text of "the only illustrated work on
Brazilian natural history untill the 19th century" written by G. Marcgrave and William Piso in 1648, following explorations and collections in North-eastern Brasil.

MARTINUS VAN MARUM

1229 FORBES, R. J. (ed.) (1969–1973). *Martinus van Marum. Life and Work.*
Vol. I: XII + 415 pp., 36 ill.; Vol. II (1970): 401 pp., 64 ill.; Vol. III
(1971): 386 pp., 35 ill.; Vol. IV (E. LEFEBVRE and J. G. de BRUYN,
eds., 1973): 401 pp., XVII plates and 312 fig. Tjeenk Willink, Haarlem.
Vol. IV: Noordhoff International Publ. formerly Tjeenk Willink).
– with descriptive catalogue of Van Marum's instruments in Teyler's Museum,
Haarlem. Vols. V. and VI are forthcoming; not yet published.

1230 — (1966). Een reis naar Londen in 1790 van Dr. Martinus van Marum
(A voyage to London in 1790 of —). *Olie, 19,* 242–6, 8 ill.

1231 — (1966). Met Van Marum door Zuid-Nederland en Rijnland (1782)
(With — through the Southern Netherlands and the Rhineland).
Sci. Hist., 8, 135–51.

1232 VEEN, H. (1938). Martinus van Marum (20 Maart 1750 – 26 December 1837) en zijn beteekenis voor de geneeskunde (and his significance for medicine). *NTG*, *82*, I, 42–66; *BGG, XVIII*, 1–25.

1233 LEVERE, T. H. (1966). Martinus van Marum (1750–1837). The introduction of Lavoisier's chemistry into the Low Countries. *Janus, LIII*, 115–34, portr., ill.

1234 DAS, H. A. (1966). De introductie van de moderne scheikunde in Nederland. Het werk van Martinus van Marum (The introduction of modern chemistry into the Netherlands. The work of—). *Chem Wbl.*, *64*, 11–27, 29.

1235 LEVERE, T. H. (1970). Friendship and influence, Martinus van Marum, F.R.S. *Not. Rec. Royal Soc. London*, *25*, 113–20, ill., portr.

1236 BOSSCHA, J. (1905). *La correspondance de A. Volker et M. van Marum*, ill., facs. Leyden 1905.

1237 HACKMANN, W. D. (1972). The researches of Dr. Martinus van Marum (1750–1837) on the influence of electricity on animals and plants. *Med. Hist.*, *16*, 11–26, ill.

1238 — (1971). The design of the triboelectric generators of Martinus van Marum, F.R.S. A case history of the interaction between England and Holland in the field of instrument design in the eighteenth century. *Not. Rec. Royal Soc. London*, *26*, 163–81, ill.

ANTONIUS MATHIJSEN

1239 COOYMANS, J. (1940). Antonius Mathijsen (1805–1878), een beroemde Nederlander (— — a famous Dutchman). *Dymphna, 5*, no. 2.

1240 BEERSTECHER, H. J. P. (1964). Antonius Mathijsen *NedMGT, 17*, 118–20, port.

1241 BEELAERTS VAN BLOKLAND, Jhr. H. (1951). Dr Antonius Mathijsen. *Ned. MGT., 4*, 329–35.

1242 SNORRASSON, E. (1963). Antonius Mathijsen. *Nord. Med. Hist. Arsbok, 70*, 971.

1243 SPOELSTRA, Dirk (1970). *Dr. Antonius Mathijsen uitvinder van het gipsverband. 1805–1878.* Leven en werken van een Nederlandse officier van gezondheid met als achtergrond de militaire geneeskundige dienst in zijn tijd (— inventor of the plaster of Paris bandage. Life and works of a Dutch medical officer against the background of the military service in his time). Thesis Utrecht (Supervisor: R. Hornstra). XVII + 475 pp., portrs., facs. Van Gorcum, Assen.

1244 [Editorial] (1965). [Antonius Mathijsen]. New method for application of plaster of Paris bandage. *Clin. Orthopaedics*, *38*, 3–8.

1245 MEYERDING, H. W. and J. van Assen (1948). Dr. Antonius Mathijsen de uitvinder van het gipsverband (— — the inventor of the plaster of Paris bandage). *NTG*, *92*, 3211–5; *BGG*, *XXVIII*, 14–8.

1246 BEUMER, H. M. (1972). De promotie van Antonius Mathijsen in 1837. (The graduation of —). *Ned. MGT.*, *25*, 98–100, 1 ill.

1247 BETT, W. R. (1955). Anthonius Mathijsen (1805–1878): inventor of the plaster of Paris bandage. *Med. Press*, *234*, 237.

1248 BREMER, G. J. (1962). *Antonius Mathijsen. The plaster of Paris bandage Its invention by Antonius Mathijsen and its first applications*. Two facsimiles (1852 and 1854) with an introduction by —. 21 + 22 + 90 pp. Dutch Classics on History of Science, Vol. IV. B. de Graaf, Nieuwkoop.

1249 LECLERQ, Jacques (1962). Les origines des bandes plâtrées dans le traitement des fractures: le docteur Antoine Mathijsen. *Acta Belg. de arte medic. at pharmac. milit.*, *115*, 597–623, ill.

1250 WONDRÁCK, E. (1963). Zur Geschichte der Fixationsverbände in der Traumatologie. Die Entdeckungen und das Schicksal des Gipsverbandes (Czech with Russ. and Ger. abstr.) *Acta Univ. palack. olomuc. Fac. med.*, *32*, 85–97, ill., portr.
– also on Mathijsen.

1251 POZZI, L. (1968). Il bendaggio gessato di Antonius Mathijsen. *Arch. Ortop.* (Milano), *81*, 413–24.

1252 SMETS, J. (1939). Dokter A. Mathijsen en het gipsverband (A.M. and the plaster of Paris bandage). In: *Verzamelde opstellen*, *XV*, no. 1 and 2. Hasselt.

1253 WILKENS, J. Th. (1951). Dr. Antonius Mathijsen 1805–1878. *NMGT*, *4*, 315–9.

1254 [Anonym] (1951). Dr. Antonius Mathijsen, *NMGT*, *4*, 320–8.

1255 MATHIJSEN, A. (1870, 1935). Lettre à Félix Hippolyte Larrey, sur le bandage plâtré. *Opusc., XIII*, 303–7,
See also: 3431, 4372a

1256 NAPJUS, J. W. (1938). De hoogleeraren in de geneeskunde aan de Hoogeschool en het Athenaeum te Franeker (1585–1843): Philippus Mattheus Jr. (The professors of medicine at Franeker Academy and Athenaeum —). VIII: *NTG, 81* (1937), IV, 1490–7; *BGG, XVII*, 169–76. IX: *NTG, 82*, I, 656–63; *BGG, XVIII*, 27–34, 2 ill. X: *NTG, 82*, II, 1591–6; *BGG, XVIII*, 62–7.

1257 MAYER, J. (1970). André Mayer, 1875–1956. *Voeding, 31*, 229–38. Also in: *J. of Nutrition, 99* (1969), 1–8.

1258 BAUMANN, E. D. (1923). Job van Meekren. *NTG, 67*, I, 456–79; *BGG, III*, 25–48.

1259 POLL, C. N. van de (1896). Ter herinnering aan Prof. G. H. van der Meij Jr. (To the memory of —) *N.T. Verl. Gyn., VII*, 1-24, portr.

1260 SCHULTE, J. E. (1965). Honderd jaar Mendel (Hundred years M.). *NTG, 109*, II, 1260–1; *BGG, XLV*, 24–5.

1261 — (1967). Gregor Mendel, ein Drama im 19. Jahrhundert. *Janus, LIV*, 107–8.

1262 SCHOLTENS, M. (1958). *Antoine Menjot, docteur en médecine, ami de Pascal, réformé au temps des persécutions. Etudes historiques et psychologiques.* Portr., 3 facs., 136 pp. Van Gorcum, Assen.

1263 DANIËLS, C. E. (1907). Lettre de Friedrich Anton Mesmer à Mme Cardon, à Moersberg le 14 nov. 1803. *Janus, XII*, 475. Also in: *NTG, 51*, I, 1540.

1264 MEURS, G. J. van (1964). Elie Metchnikoff 1845–1916, *Voeding, 25*, 351–6.

1265 ESSO Bzn, I. van (1937). Doktor Lodewijk Meyer. *Revue Osé.*

1266 THIJSSEN-SCHOUTE, C. L. (1954). Lodewijk Meyer en diens verhouding tot Descartes en Spinoza (— — and his relation to Descartes and Spinoza). *Meded. Spinozahuis, XI*, 20 pp., Brill, Leiden.

1267 HABERLING, W. (1932). Der Amsterdamer Arzt Johan Georg Mezger, der Begründer der wissenschaftlichen Massage. *Janus, XXXVI*, 212.
– short report. Appeared extensively in *Medical Life, 39* (1932), 191–207 (Translation by Emile Recht).

1268   KOSTELIJK, P. J. (1972). *Dr Johann Georg Mezger 1838–1909 en zijn tijd*
       (— — and his time). 112 pp., 16 ill. Universitaire Pers, Leiden.
       - Reviewed by J. R. Prakken: *NTG, 116* (1972), 1145.

1269   HAM, A. A. G. (1974). Het achterhoedegevecht van de Groninger
       hoogleraar H. W. Middendorp (1843–1918) tegen de tuberkelbacil
       (The rear-guard action of the Groningen professor — — against the
       tubercle bacillus). *AP*, no 14, 14–6.
       - Prof. Middendorp never did accept the bacillus of Koch as the causative agent
       of tuberculosis. This resulted in a conflict with the Faculty and, finally in his
       resignation.

1270   STAFLEU, F. A. (1966). F. A. W. Miquel. Netherlands Botanist.
       Wentia, 16, 1–95 (with a complete bibliography of M.).

1271   — (1970). The Miquel-Schlechtendal correspondence: a picture of
       European botany, 1836–1866. In: P. Smit and R. J. C. V. ter Laage
       (eds) (1970). *Essays in biohistory*, 295–341. Utrecht.

1272   DEURMAN, W. Chr. (1966). In memoriam Prof. Dr Emile Jan Moeys.
       NTG, 110, 408–9, port.
       - Moeys (1918–65), first professor of surgery at Nijmegen.

JACOB MOLESCHOTT

1273   HAAN, R. E. de (1883). Jacob Moleschott. In: N. C. Balsem. *Mannen
       van beteekenis in onze dagen.*, 235–302, Tjeenk Willink, Haarlem, 8°.

1274   PEKELHARING, C. A. (1893). In Memoriam. Jacob Moleschott *NTG, 29*,
       I, 741–3.

1275   ESSO Bzn., I. van (1949). Jacob Moleschott. *NTG, 93*, I, 34–44; *BGG,
       XXIX*, 1–11.

1276   MEURS, G. J. van (1953). Jacob Moleschott 1822–1893. *Voeding, 14*,
       237–40, portr.

1277   — (1953). Jacob Moleschott. Ingezonden stukken. De benoeming
       van den Heer Halbertsma aan de hoogeschool te Leiden (Letters to
       the editor. The appointment of Mr. H. in the University of Leyden).
       NTG, 97, II, 1409–11; *BGG, XXXIII*, 43–5.
       - On the disappointment of Moleschott on the appointment of H. Halbertsma as
       extra-ordinary professor of anatomy and physiology at Leyden – with the text of
       the letters to the editor by —.

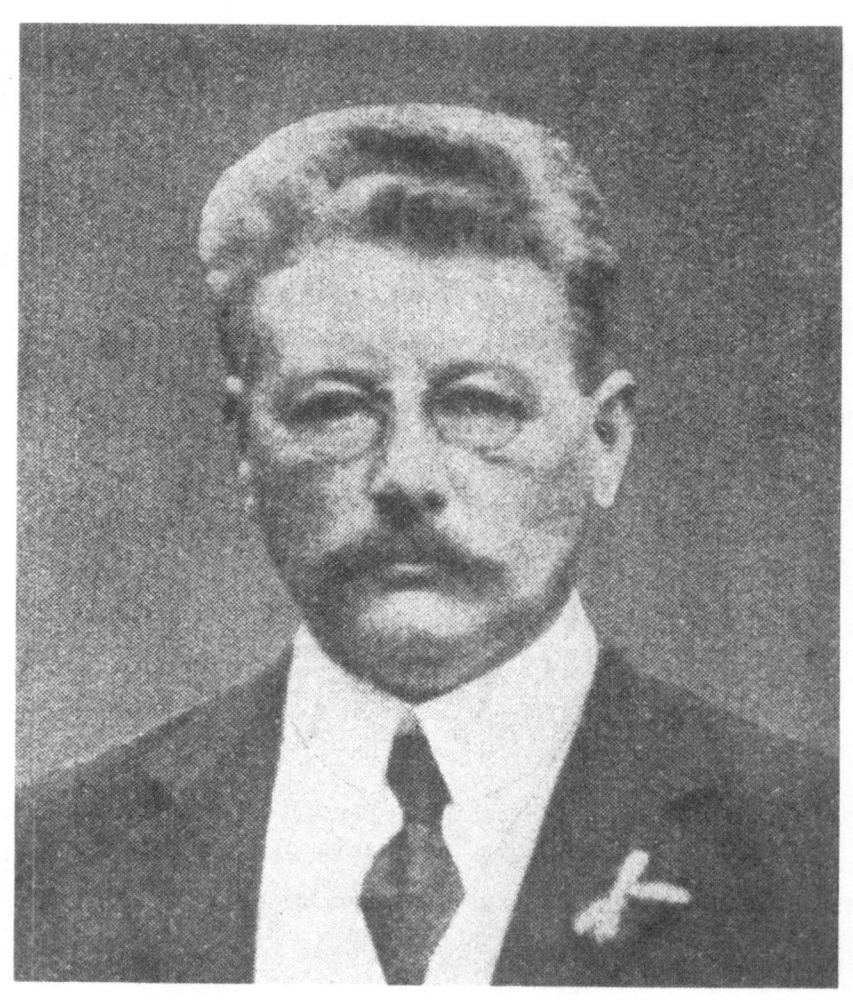

H. J. Lulofs (1871–1939)

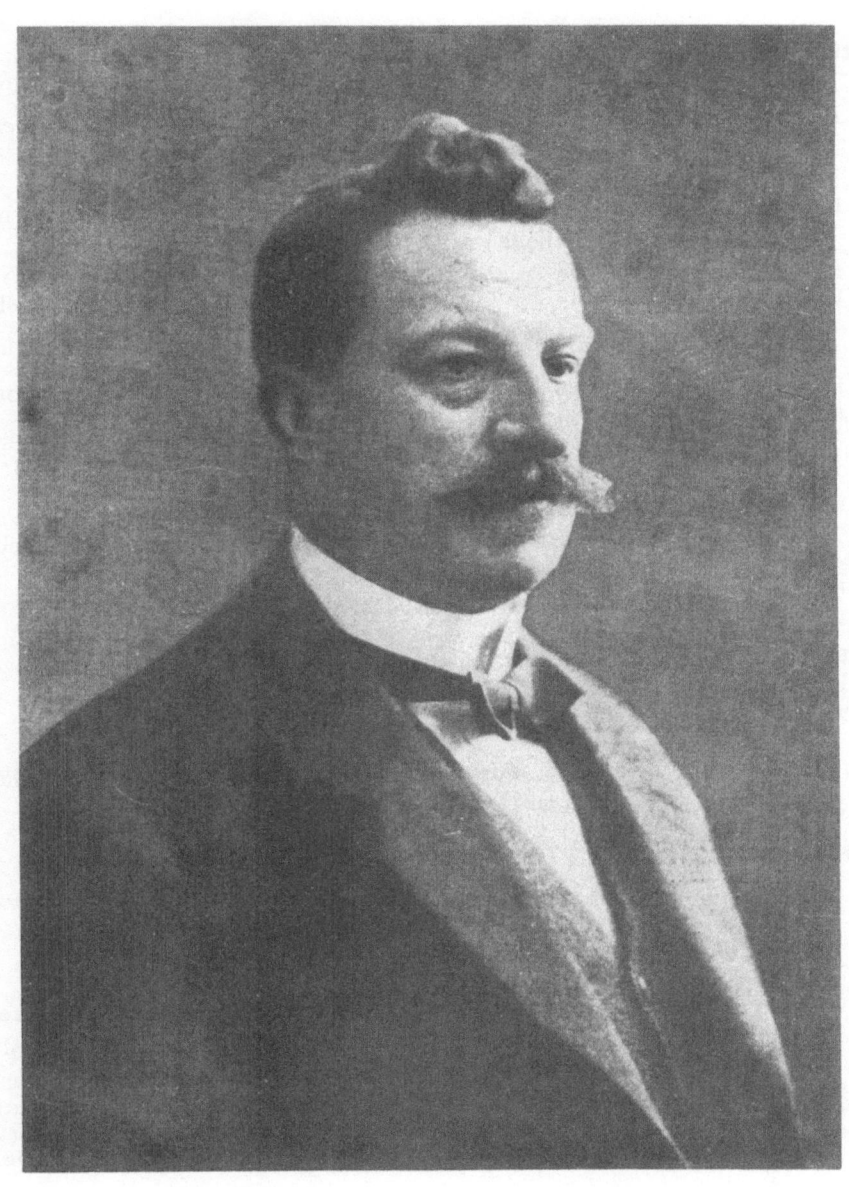

J. G. de Lint (1867–1936)

1278 BETTICA, R. (1938). D'annuncio discepolo di Moleschott? *Atti e Mem. Accad. Stor. Arte Sanit.* (2. ser.), *4*, 254–7.

1279 BAZZI, F. (1971). S. Tommasi, J. Moleschott, orsi e la pretesa riforma della medicina italiana. *Med. Secoli, 8* (4), 12 pp.

1280 DAGLIO, P. (1961). Fisiologia e filosofia nell'opera di Jacopo Mole- schott. *Pag. Stor. Med., 5*, 3–11.

1281 — (1967). Il progresso della fisiologia nell'ottocento e la concezione materialistica. *Pag. Stor. Med., 11*, no. 3, 27–35.
– on Jacob Moleschott (1822–1893).

1282 MOSER, Walter (1967). *Der Physiologe Jakob Moleschott (1822–1893) und seine Philosophie.* 54 pp. Zür. Medizingesch. Abhandlungen. Neue Reihe no. 43. Juris Verlag, Zürich.
– Thesis Zürich (Supervisor: E. H. Ackerknecht).

1283 O'HARA-MAY, J. (1971). Measuring man's needs. *J. Hist. Biol., 4*, 249–73.
– On J. Moleschott (1822–1893).

1284 STOKVIS, B. J. (1892). Jacob Moleschott Bij zijn 70-en verjaardag (At his 70th birthday). *De Gids,* no. 8.

1285 MOLESCHOTT, Jac. (1845–46, 1942). *De overgang der chylbolletjes in bloedlichaampjes* (The change of chyloid corpuscula into blooed cor- puscula). With German translation. *Opusc., XVI,* 122–41.
See also 669, 670, 2986

1286 MONCHY, S. de (1776, 1935). Brief aan Wouter van Doeveren (Letter to W. van Doeveren). With English translation. *Opusc., XIII,* 249–58.
S. de Monchy (1716–94) studied at Leiden, received his doctor's degree on 23 june 1739 on a treatise: *De opio,* and became town doctor at Rotterdam. He took much interest in inoculation; was one of the founders and first director of the "Bataaf- sche Genootschap" at Rotterdam. This letter deals with inoculation. (*See also* 3970a)

1287 WINTGENS, E. (1879). *Johannes Monnikhoff en zijn legaat* (J. M. and his legacy). Thesis Amsterdam. 120 pp., portr., Leiden.
– J. Monnikhoff (1707–87), surgeon at Amsterdam. Under his last will a fund for the promotion of the knowledge of surgery was founded (it amounted to ƒ22.000,—)

1288 SCHULTE, J. E. (1963). Giovanni Battista Morgagni. *NTG, 107,* I, 961–2; *BGG, XLIII,* 3–5.

1289 BERGINK, A. H. (1968). J. J. R. Moquette 1873–1945. *Voeding, 29.* 401–6, portr.

1290 LINDEBOOM, G. A. (1973). Mensen om Boerhaave. X. Jacobus Le Mort (Men around B. X. —). *GG, 4,* 144–6.

GERRIT JAN MULDER

1291 LABRUYÈRE, W. (1938). *G. J. Mulder (1802–1880).* Thesis Leiden. Supervisor: Blanksma. 148 pp. Leiden.

1292 BROUWER, E. (1952). Gerrit Jan Mulder (1802–1880). *J. of Nutrition, 46,* 3–11, portr.

1293 CITTERT-EYMERS, J. G. van (1966). Gerrit Jan Mulder 1802–1880. *PhW, 101,* 407–11.

1294 BROUWER, E. (1946). Iets over Gerrit Jan Mulder en zijn beteekenis voor de volksvoeding (Something about G.J.M. and his significance for the national nutrition). *Voeding, 7,* 53–67.

1295 ROOSEBOOM, M. (1967). Gedachten over gisting en cholera in een brief van Gerrit Jan Mulder uit 1867 (Thoughts on fermentation and cholera in a letter of G.J.M., 1867). *Sci. Hist., 9,* 1–16.

1296 LIEBURG, Jr., M. J. van (1973). Gerrit Jan Mulder: docent der Clinische School te Rotterdam (G.J.M.: teacher in the Clinical School at R.) In: J. van Herwaarden (ed.) (1973). *Lof der historie. Opstellen over geschiedenis en maatschappij,* 213–40.
– Essay written on the occasion of the opening of the Erasmus University at Rotterdam on november 8, 1973.
See also 3030

1297 BOLSMAN, T. W. (1969). In memoriam Prof. Dr. J. D. Mulder. *Arch. chir. Néerl., 21,* 183–4, portr.
– J. D. Mulder was an orthopedist, extra-ordinary professor of orthopedy at Leyden.

1298 MULDER, Neeltje (1926). *Uit den goeden ouden tijd, ruim 60, 70 jaar geleden. Jeugdherinneringen van Neeltje Mulder, wed. Jacob Honig Jansz. junior* (From the good old days, a good 60, 70 years ago. Youth memories of Neeltje Mulder, widow of Jacob Honig Jansz. junior), 3rd ed. P. Out, Koog a/d Zaan.

1299 ELAUT, L. (1959i). Ncolaas Mulierus uit Brugge, de eerste medische hoogleraar te Groningen (1564–1630). (— — from Bruges, the first professor of medicine at G.) *Sci. Hist.*, *1*, 3–13

1300   HALBERTSMA, K. T. A. (1959). Johannes Müller (1801–1858). *GeWiNa* no. *5*, 11–2.

1301   WILDEMAN, M. G. (1916). Een oude catalogus van instrumenten (An old catalogue of instruments). *NTG*, *60*, II, 1958–60.
       – Instrument Joh. van Musschenbroek (1687–1748).

1302   MEYER, Friedrich Albert (1961). Petrus van Musschenbroek. Werden und Werk und seine Beziehungen zu Daniel Gabriel Fahrenheit. Pinselstriche zum Charakterbild eines groszen Duisburger Hochschullehrers. *Duisburger Forschungen*, *5*, 1–51, 3 pl.
       – Musschenbroek (1692–1761) was professor at Duisburg (1719–23), Utrecht (1723–39) and Leiden (since Dec. 1739). He is the discoverer of the Leiden jars.

1303   ROOSEBOOM, M. (1970). Petrus van Musschenbroek's "Oratio de sapientia divina". In P. Smit en R. J. Ter Laage (ed.). *Essays in biohistory*, 177–90. Utrecht.
       – P. van Mussenbroek (1692–1761); 1715 Med. Dr.; 1723 professor at Utrecht; 1740 professor at Leiden. (*See also* 4148)

1303ᵃ HOOYKAAS, R. (1956). The zoogeography of Abraham van der Mijle *Arch. int. Hist. Sci.*, *9* (35), 125–32.

1304   NAPJUS, J. W. (1939–1940). De hoogleeraren in de geneeskunde aan de Hoogeschool en het Athenaeum te Franeker (1585–1843): Wijer Willem Muys (The professor of medicine at Franeker Academy and Athenaeum). XV: *NTG*, *83*, IV. 5282–8; *BGG*, *XIX*, 243–9.
       XVI: *NTG*, *84* (1940), I, 834–8; *BGG*, *XX*, 49–53.
       XVII: *NTG*, *84*, II, 1706–12; *BGG*, *XX*, 73–9.
       XVIII: *NTG*, *84*, II, 2042–8; *BGG*, *XX*, 97–103

N

1305   ENST, W. van (1954). In Memoriam Prof. Dr W. Noordenbos. *NTG*, *98*, III, 2563–5, port.
       – Noordenbos (1875–1954) was professor of surgery at the University of Amsterdam.

1306   NIVARD, R. J. F. (1960). In memoriam Professor Dr E. C. H. J. Noyons. 26 juli 1900 – 18 maart 1960. *Chem. Wbl.*, *56*, 245–6, port.

1307   HOFFMAN, K. F. (1954). Zahnärztliches bei Antonius Nuck (1650–1692). *Öst. Z. Stomatol.*, *51*, 608–9.

1308 LINDEBOOM, G. A. (1972). Mensen rond Boerhaave. IV. Anton Nuck (Men around B. IV. Anton Nuck). *GG*, *2*, 192–4, ill.

1308ª LUYENDIJK-ELSHOUT, A. M. (1974). Antony Nuck (1650–1692), The "Mercator" of the Body Fluids. A review of his anatomical and experimental studies. In: *Circa Tiliam*, 150–64, ill. Brill, Leiden.
See also 4144

1309 [   ] (1945). *Twee eeuwen medische traditie. Een stukje familiege-schiedenis.* Aanteekeningen verzameld bij gelegenheid van het veertig-jarig artsjubileum van Wilhelmus Johannes Franciscus Nuyens (Two centuries of medical tradition. A short family-history. Annotations collected on the occasion of the 40 years jubilee as a (practizing) physician). pr. pr. Maastricht.
– In the Nuyens family there Was a doctor for two centuries.

1310 HAMMES, Th. (1946). Nuyens en onze Maatschappij (N. and our Society). *NTG*, *90*, 266–8; not in *BGG*.
– On B. W. Th. Nuyens (1865–1945), librarian of the Dutch Medical Society. cf: letter to the editor (by J. E. Schulte): *NTG*, *90*, 632–3; *BGG*, *XXVI*, 24–5.

O and P

1311 BÜHLER, H. V. (1935). Das Ärztegeschlecht der Occo. Ein Beitrag zur Geschichte des Collegium medicum Augustanum. *SA 28*, 14–42, 14 ill.
– also on the relatives of the Amsterdam family Occo.

1312 THIESSEN, J. W. (1958). Julien Offray de la Mettrie. Geneesheer en satiricus (1709–1751) (Physician and satirist). *NMGT*, *11*, 269–75.

1313 METZ, W. (1960). Julien Offray de la Mettrie. *Janus*, *XIL*, 235–72.

1314 SMIT, P. (1964). Lorenz Oken – Een tijdsbeeld (Lorenz Oken – A picture of the time). *Sci. Hist.*, *6*, 66–88.

1315 — (1968). Lorenz Oken (1779–1851). *Sci. Hist.*, *10*, 100–5.

1315ª — (1972). Lorenz Oken und die Versammlungen Deutscher Natur-forscher und Ärzte: Sein Einflusz auf das Programm und eine Analyse seiner auf den Versammlungen gehaltenen Beiträge. In: H. Querner u. H. Schipperges (ed.) *Wege der Naturforschung 1822–1972 im Spiegel der Versammlungen Deutscher Naturforscher und Ärzte*, 101–24. Springer-Verlag, Berlin-Heidelberg-New York.

Ort

1316   ORT, D. H. (1848, 1935). Brieven aan C. B. Tilanus (Letters to —).
– with English translation. *Opusc.*, *XIII*, 265–86; D. H. Ort (1819/20–1904), at first a surgeon and accoucheur. Later studied medicine at Leiden and graduated there on a treatise: *Casus gastrotomicae* (1853).

1317   JONG, M. de (1964). Inleiding tot het werk van Garcia da Orta (Introduction to the work of —). *Sci. Hist.*, *6*, 16–24.
(See also 524)

1318   JANSEN, B. C. P. (1954). Thomas Burr Osborne 1859–1929 en Lafayette Benedict Mendel 1872–1935. *Voeding*, *15*, 229–31, portrs.

1319   PUTTO, J. A. (1964). Sir James Paget (1814–1899). *GG*, *42*, 232.
– a short note.

JAN PALFIJN

1320   BROECKAERT, Arthur (no. d.). *Jan Palfijn. 1650 – Een levensbeeld – 1730* (J.P. – a biographical sketch). 264 pp., Cultura, Brugge.

1321   BRUNN, W. von (1940). Jan Palfijn, der Arzt aus Kortrijk. Ein Wohltäter der Menschheit. *Brüsseler Ztg.*, nr. 154, 1–12, 1 ill.

1322   ELAUT, L. (1950). Jan Palfijn. Driehonderd jaar na zijn geboorte (Kortrijk 1650 – Gent 1730) (J.P. Three hundredth anniversary of his birth). *Dietsche Warande & Belfort*, November nr., 14 pp.

1323   RAES, A. (1970). Het leven en het werk van Jan Palfijn (Life and work of —). *De Gidsenkring*, *7*, nr. 3, 24–30.

1323ᵃ HALLEMA, A. (1963). Johannes Henricus van der Palm, 1763 – 17 July – 1963. *Ziekenhuiswezen*, *36*, 126–8.
– V.d.P. (1763–1840), a theologian and statesman, made, under the French occupation, instructions for the introduction of medical supervision by the state).

BERNARDUS PALUDANUS

1324   HUNGER, F. W. T. (1928). Bernardus Paludanus (Berent ten Broecke). 1550–1633. *NTG*, *72*, II, 5450–8; *BGG*, *VIII*, 325–33. Also in: *Janus*, *XXXII* (1928), 353–4, portr.

1325   SLUITER, E. (1928). Paludanus herdenking te Enkhuizen 29 Oct. 1928 (Commemoration of P. at E.). *NTG*, *72*, II, 5481; *BGG*, *VIII*, 356.

1326   THEUNISZ, Joh. (1933). Het honorarium van Paludanus als stadsgeneesheer van Enkhuizen (The fee of — als city-physician of Enkhuizen). *NTG*, *77*, IV, 4593–4; *BGG*, *XIII*, 239–40.

1327 — (1936). *Het ontoegankelijk hart. De roman van Bernardus Paludanus* (The inaccessible heart. The novel of —). 's-Gravenhage. 8°.
- Reviewed by J. B. F. van Gils: *NTG*, *80*, III, 4045–6; *BGG*, *XVI*, 155–6.

1328 RADHAKRISHNA, P. A. (1965). Dutch physicians of the XVI century on Indian drugs. Linschoten's account of spices and drugs of India supplemented and annotated by Dr. Bernardus Paludanus. *BDHM Hyderabad*, *3*, 173–83, portr.

1329 ENGEL, H. (1966). Bernardus Paludanus 1550–1633. *GeWiNa*, *19*, 10–2.

1330 MULLER, H. A. L. (1967). Denis Papin 1647–1714. *Voeding*, *28*, 631–2, portr.
- translation of an article by E. N. Todhunter: Denis Papin. Bibliographical notes from the history of nutrition. *J. Amer. diet. Ass.*, *51* (1967) 45.
See also 1185

PARACELSUS

1331 ENGLERT, Ludwig (1941?). *Paracelsus. Mensch en arts* (Man and physician). From the German translated into Dutch by Jhr. R. H. G. Nahuys. 152 pp. "Atlanta", Amsterdam.

1332 FEYFER, F. M. G. de (1941). *De levende gedachten van Theophrastus Paracelsus* (The living ideas of —). 190 pp., portr. Servire, Den Haag.

1333 — (1941). Theophrastus Paracelsus met portret (— with portrait). *NTG*, *85*, IV, 3923–31; *BGG*, *XXI*, 131–9.

1334 — (1941). Paracelsus (1493–1541). *NTG*, *85*, IV, 4545–6; *BGG*, *XXI*, 154–5.
- Summary of an address, communicated by Burger.

1335 — (1941). Theophrastus Paracelsus. Portrait. *Janus*, *XLV*, 196–207.

1336 HOOG, P. H. van der (1941). *Paracelsus*. 259 pp. Ad. M. C. Stok, Zuid-Holl. Uitg. Mij., den Haag, no. d., 3rd ed.

1337 MEURS, G. J. van (1962). Paracelsus 1493–1541. *Voeding*, *23*, 862–7.
- on the article: Paracelsus, ein Wegbereiter der Ernährungsphysiologie in: *Ernährungsforschung*, *6*, (1961), (5), 611–42.

1338 ORTT, Felix (1973). De verhouding tussen lichaam en geest bij Paracelsus (The relation between body and mind at —). *Natura Docet*, *24*, 164–7.

1339   OOSTERHUIS, R. A. B. (1937). *Paracelsus en Hahneman, essentieele geneeskunst en homeopathie* (essential medicine and homeopathy). Thesis Leiden (Supervisor: J. A. J. Barge), 300 pp., portr., Sijthoff, Leiden.

> – also as a monograph entitled: *Paracelsus en Hahnemann, een renaissance der geneeskunde* (P. and H., a renaissance of medicine). Sijthoff, Leiden. Reviewed by van Andel: *NTG*, *81* (1937), II, 1962–3; *BGG*, *XVII*, 92–3.

1340   — (1939). Paracelsus over de toekomst van Europa (on the future of Europe). *GG*, *17*, 1185–9 and 1203–7.

1341   — and B. C. J. Lievegoed (1941). *Paracelsus herdacht 1493–1541* (P. commemorated). With a foreword by J. G. Sleeswijk. 1. Oosterhuis, Paracelsus als hervormer der geneeskunde en als synthetische denker (P. as a reformer and as a synthetic thinker), 9–31. 2. Lievegoed. Hippocrates – Paracelsus Goethe, 32–55. Portr., 55 pp., Van Stockum, den Haag.

1342   — (1942). Paracelsus und die Niederlande. *Hippocrates*, Heft 8, 150–5.

1343   KERNER, D. (1959). Ein Brief des Paracelsus an Erasmus von Rotterdam. *Grünenthal Waage*, *I*, 146–9, portr., facs.

1344   RIETEMA, S. P. (1924). De beteekenis van Paracelsus voor de geneeskundige wetenschap (The significance of — for medical science). *NTG*, *68*, I, 52–6; *BGG*, *IV*, 18–22.

1345   HOOYKAAS, R. (1935). Die Elementenlehre des Paracelsus. *Janus*, XXXIX, 175–87.

> – with a summary in English.

1346   — (1940). Paracelsus, de Luther Medicorum. *G&W*, 98–110.

1347   — (1939). Die chemische Verbindung bei Paracelsus. *SA*, *32*, 166–75.

1348   BARUCH, J. Z. (1964). Paracelsus en tijdgenoten over enkele beroepsziekten (P. and contemporaries on some occupational diseases) *T. Soc. Geneesk.*, *42*, 153–9.

1349   — (1965). Paracelsus als pionier van de bedrijfsgeneeskunde (P. as pioneer of occupational medicine). *Sci. Hist.*, *7*, 33–41.

1350   LINDEBOOM, G. A. (1942). Paracelsus en Paracelsus-literatuur (P. and literature on P.), *Stemmen des Tijds*, *31*, 173–81.

1351 HELSDINGEN, R. J. van (1967). Paracelsus en Jung. *NTG, III*, 1210.
See also 758–9, 1970.

1352 deleted

1353 ROGGE, C. W. L. (1973). *De betekenis van Ambroise Paré (1510–1590)*, *mens, leermeester en chirurg* (A.P., The man, the teacher and the surgeon), Thesis Groningen (Supervisor: P. J. Kuijjer). 251 pp., 87 ill. Jan Haan, Groningen.

1354 SCHULTE, B. P. M. (1968). James Parkinson, neuroloog, paleontoloog en pamfletschrijver (J. P., neurologist, paleontologist and writer of pamflets). *Sci. Hist., 10*, 94–9.

1355 VELDE, A. J. J. van de (1937). Antonie Augustin Parmentier en zijn voorgangers (A.A.P. and his predecessors). *MKVAW*, October.

1356 MEURS, G. J. van (1956). De aardappel en Antonie Augustin Parmentier 1737–1813 (The potato and —). *Voeding, 17*, 210–5, portr., ill. *See also* 3017, 3018

LOUIS PASTEUR

1357 COHEN, E. (1922). Louis Pasteur (1822–1922). *NTG, 66*, II, 2490–2507; *BGG, II*, 323–40, 3 ill., portr.

1358 CALMETTE, A. (1922). L'oeuvre de Pasteur. Son influence sur les progrès de la civilisation. *NTG, 66*, II, 2480–9; *BGG, II*, 313–22.

1359 GROOT, J. V. de (1910, ²1918). *Denkers van onzen tijd* (Herb. Spencer, Em. du Bois-Reymond, L. Pasteur, Ferd. Brunetière, Joh. Henr. Newman). (Thinkers of our time). 328 pp., 8°, Amsterdam. Sec. revised edition: 1918, Bussum–Leiden, 8°.

1360 PELLE, J. C. (1905). Het leven van Louis Pasteur (Life of —). *Alb. Nat., 83*, 113.

1361 SCHIERBEEK, A. (1923). Louis Pasteur. *Levende Natuur, XXVII* (1 jan. and 1 febr.) 261 and 289.

1362 VERMEULEN, P. (1922). *Louis Pasteur herdacht in het honderdste jaar na zijn geboorte* (L.P. commemorated on the 100th anniversary of his birth). 79 pp., 1 fig., S. C. van Doesburgh, Leiden.

1363 SCHLICHTING, Th. H. [1937]. *Louis Pasteur, een schets van zijn leven en werken* (— —, a sketch of his life and works). 95 pp., Het Spectrum, Utrecht no. d.

1364   MOSSEL, D. A. A. (1955). Louis Pasteur 1812–1895. *Voeding*, *16*, 695–8, portr.

1365   SANDERS, J. (1923). De Pasteur-feesten te Straatsburg (The Pasteur-festivities at Strasbourg). *NTG*, *67*, I, 2681.

1366   LOGHEM, J. J. van (1922). Louis Pasteur 1822–1922. *Gids*, *86*, IV, 323–53.

1367   — (1922). De Nederlandsche herdenking van Louis Pasteur (The Dutch commemoration of —). *NTG*, *66*, II, 2442; *BGG*, *II*, 275.

1368   KOCH, H. (1922). Ook een Pasteurherdenking (Also a commemoration of —). *NTG*, *66*, II, 2973.

1369   CALCAR, R. P. van (1923). Pasteur herdacht (P. commemorated). *Vragen Tijds*, *I*, 191.

1370   ROUX, E. (1898). Het medische werk van Pasteur (The medical work of —). *Gen. Bl.*, *V*, 211–38.

1371   SPRONCK, C. H. H. (1922). De beteekenis van Louis Pasteur voor de medische wetenschap (Significance of — for medical science). *NTG*, *66*, II, 2466–79; *BGG*, *II*, 299–312; also in: *Chem. Wbl.*, *XIX*, 527.

1372   JAEGER, F. M. (1922). Pasteur's eerste onderzoekingen en hunne beteekenis voor de moderne chemie (P.'s first investigations and their significance for modern chemistry). *NTG*, *66*, II, 2447–56; *BGG*, *II*, 280–9.

1373   KLUYVER, A. J. (1922). Pasteur, de grondlegger der algemeene en toegepaste microbiologie (P., founder of general and applied microbiology). *NTG*, *66* II, 2457–65; *BGG*, *II*, 290–8.

1374   SCHULTE, J. E. (1963). Pasteur et les Pays-Bas. *Méd. France*, no. 140, 13–4, 48.

1375   HEYMANS, C. (1952). Une lettre autographe de Louis Pasteur. *Arch. Int. d'Hist. Sci.*, *5*, (XXXI), 65.
       See also 2847, 2848, 5384

1376   PRINSEN Izn., J. (1905). Eenige brieven van professor Pieter Pauw aan Orlers (Some letters of professor P.P. to O.). *Oud-Holland, XXIII*, 167.

1377   CATE, J. ten (1955). Iwan Petrowitsch Pawlow 1849–1936. *Voeding*, *16*, 845–7, portr.

1378 [ ] (1918). Livre jubilaire en l'honneur de C. A. Pekelharing. *Arch. néerl. de physiol. de l'homme et des animaux*, Tom, II. 4.

1379 WESTENBRINK, H. G. K. (1953). Cornelis Adrianus Pekelharing 1848–1922. *Voeding*, *14*, 198–9, portr.

1380 ERDMAN, A. M. (1964). Cornelis Adrianus Pekelharing; biographical sketch, July 19, 1848 – September 18, 1922. *J. Nutr.*, *83*, 3–9.

1381 BAART DE LA FAILLE, Joh. M., H. G. K. Westenbrink and P. Nieuwenhuijse (1948). *Leven en werken van Cornelis Adrianus Pekelharing 1848–1922* (Life and work of C.A.P.), 217 pp., Utrecht, portr. and pl.

1382 [Anonym] (1967). Grandes Vultos da nutrologia: Cornelis Adrianus Pekelharing. *Arq. bras. Nutr.*, *23*, (1), 3–4, portr.

1382ᵃ EEGHEN, I. H. van (1974). Anthonie van den Hout en Pieter Klases Pel, of de opleiding in de genees-, heel- en verloskunde (— — and — —, or education in medicine, surgery and obstetrics). *Amstelodamum*, *61*, 1–5.
 – Autobiographical notes of P. K. Pel (1797–1878), physician at Drachten, who received his medical education at Amsterdam (under A. van den Hout and W. Vrolijk).

1383 VEN, A. J. van de (1962). De twee artsen Pelt te Utrecht in de 17de eeuw (The two physicians — at Utrecht in the 17th century). *Jbk. "Oud-Utrecht"*, 125–8.

1384 MEURS, G. J. van (1954). Max von Pettenkofer 1818–1901. *Voeding*, *15*, 321–4, portr.

1385 LEERSUM, E. C. van (1916). Een drietal brieven van J. C. Peyer (Three letters of —). *NTG*, *60*, I, 889–909, 2 ill.

1386 — (1916). Trois lettres de Jean Conrad Peyer. *Janus*, *XXI*, 111–28. (*See also* 2924)

1387 GUYE, A. P. (1904). In Memoriam Dr. H. F. A. Peypers 1853–1903. *Janus*, *IX*, 1.

1388 PROOSDIJ, B. van (1959). Matériaux pour l'histoire dess ciences du temps moderne rassemblés par — X. Le docteur H. F. A. Peypers et *Janus*, *Janus*, *XLVIII*, 1–4.

1389 CATE, J. ten (1963). Eduard Friedrich Wilhelm Pflüger 1829–1910. *Voeding*, *24*, 401–5.

1390 POST, J. H. J. van der (1959). Bij de 300ste geboortedag van de Abbé
de Saint Pierre (Projets pour perfectionner la Médecine). (At the
300th birthday of — —). *Rott. Jbk.*, 6 de reeks, 7, 239–43.

1391 RIJNBERK, G. van (1929). Een medisch journalistiek jubileum (A medical journalistic jubilee). *NTG*, 73, 989.
– Refers to the jubilee of H. Pinkhof (1863–1943).

1392 HAMMES, Th. (1945). Dr. Hermannus Pinkhof. Een levensschets (a
sketch of his life). *NTG*, 89, (noodnr. XXII), 251–2.

1393 Esso Bzn., I. van (1948). In Memoriam Herm. Pinkhof. *MC.*, 3, 770–1.

1394 HUITEMA, W. (1936). *Clemens Pirquet*. Thesis Leiden (Supervisor:
Gorter), portr. ill. *See also* 3748a.

WILLEM PISO

1395 ANDEL, M. A. (1924). Willem Piso, een baanbreker der tropische geneeskunde (W.P., a pioneer of tropical medicine). *NTG*, 68, II, 1731–
46; *BGG*, *IV*, 239–54, 3 ill.

1396 — (1937). Dr. Willem Piso. *NRC*, 23 January.

1397 VOS, T. A. (1959). De geneeskunde, in het bijzonder de oogheelkunde,
bij Willem Piso (Medicine, particularly ophthalmology, in —). *NTG*,
103, II, 1805–10; *BGG*, *XXXIX*, 7–12.

1398 PIES, E. (1971). Wilhelm Piso. Ein Pionier der Tropenmedizin. *Die
Waage*, *10*, 193–6, 3 ill.

1399 PISO, W. (1658, 1937). *De indiae utriusque re naturali et medica.*
With English translation. *Opusc.*, *XIV*, 4–35.
see also: tropical medicine (3828–9), 3832

ARCHIBALD PITCAIRNE

1400 HALBERTSMA, K. T. A. (1953). Archibald Pitcairne (1652–1713). *NTG*,
97, II, 1150–1; *BGG*, *XXXIII*, 32.
– short note, included in the report of a meeting of the "Genootschap", 15 and 16
Nov. 1952.

1401 LINDEBOOM, G. A. (1963). Pitcairne's Leiden interlude, described from
the documents. *Ann. Sci.*, *19*, 273–84, ill., portr.

1402 — (1966). Pitcairne in Leiden. *NTG*. *110*, 20–6.

1403 — (1972). Mensen rond Boerhaave. V. Archibald Pitcairne (Men a-round B. V. A.P.). *GG*, *2*, 236–8, ill.

1404 TRICOT, ROYER, J. J. G. (1922). Drukker Plantijn en de geneeskundige wetenschappen (The printer — and medical sciences). *NTG*, *66*, I, 84–8; *BGG*, *II*, 37–41.
   – Lecture held on October 19, 1921 at Gorinchem (meeting of the Association of the History of Medicine etc.).

1405 — (1932). *L'imprimeur Plantin et les Sciences médicales.* Progrès médical, Rue des Ecoles 41, Paris.
   – Reviewed by F. M. G. de Fefer: *NTG*, *76*, (1932), IV, 5583–4; *BGG*, *XII*, 261–2.

1406 VOET, L. (1961). *Het Plantijnse huis te Leiden.* De bedrijvigheid van het drukkersgeslacht Raphelengius en zijn betrekkingen met Antwerpen (The Plantin house at Leyden. The activity of the printersfamily Raphelengius and its relations with Antwerp). 28 pp., no pl.
   – Also in: *Bijdr. Med. Hist. Gen.,* *75* (1961), 10*–36*. Groningen.
   – Raphelengius, son-in-law of Plantijn, was professor of Hebrew at Leyden and continued there the printing-office of his father-in-law.

1407 GULIK, E. van and H. D. L. Vervliet (1965). *Een gedenksteen voor Plantijn en Van Raphelingen te Leiden,* waarin opgenomen de *Catalogus librorum residuorum Tabernae Raphelengianae* (A memorial tablet for — and — at L., with the — —), 35 pp., facs. E. J. Brill, Leiden.
   – with a foreword by F. C. Wieder Jr.

1408 KEISER, E. (ed.) (1968). *Thomas Plater. Beschreibung der Reisen durch Frankreich, Spanien, England und die Niederlande 1595–1600.* 2 vols., Schwabe, Basel und Stuttgart.
   – Thomas II Plater (Platter), 1547–1628; 1614 professor of anatomy and botany, 1625 professor of practical medicine at Basel.

1409 GLESINGER, L. (1956). La naissance de Vopiscus Fortunatus Plempius. *Bull. Mém. Soc. Hist. Méd.,* *II*, 20–5, portr.

1410 ZWAVELING, A. and G. Hulsman (1965), Machiel Polano, laatste heelmeester van het oude tijdperk (M.P., last surgeon of the old period). *NTG*, *109*, II, 2091–5; *BGG*, *XLV*, 32–6, portr.

1411 TANIGUCHI, M. and J. Z. Bowers (1965). Pompe van Meerdervoort (1829–1909) and the first Western medical School in Japan. *J. Med. Education,* *40*, 448–54.

1412 WITTERMANS, Elizabeth and John Z. Bowers (1970). *Doctor on Desima.*

Selected chapters from Jhr. J. L. C. Pompe van Meerdervoort *Vijf Jaren in Japan* (Five years in Japan (1857–1863), translated and annotated by —. 144 pp., Publ. by Sophia University, Tokyo.

1413   OTAKI, Toshio (1971). Pompe van Meerdervoort and Japanese Medicine. In: *Rangaku in Japanese culture*, 292–303 (Japanese with English summary).
   See also Japan (5175, 5190)

1413ᵃ   MOULIN, D. de (1973). J. L. C. Pompe van Meerdervoort and his "Vijf jaren in Japan". *Janus, LX*, 129–35; also in: *Acta Septimi conventus*, 129–35. Amsterdam, 1974.

1414   WENTINK, L. (1937). Joannes Baptista Porta als physiognomicus J.B.P. as a physiognomist). *NTG, 81*, IV, 5817–33; *BGG, XVII*, 203–19.
   – abbreviated in a report of a meeting of the "Genootschap", 17–18 April, 1937; *NTG, 81*, II, 1967; *BGG, XVII*, 97.

1415   HOEVEN, J. van der (1931). 21 Brieven van Dr. Joh. Knockers van Oosterzee te Kaapstad aan Prof. Dr. C. Pruys van der Hoeven (21 letters of — at Cape Town to —). *NTG, 75*, II, 1779–90; *BGG, XI*, 102–13, portr.
   See also 763, 764, 819

1416   WOUDSTRA, D. (1969–70). Meinard Simon Du Pui (1754–1834) stadsmedicus te Kampen (1780–1788) en te Alkmaar (1788–1791). Eerste Leidse hoogleraar in de praktische chirurgie en verloskunde (1791–1826) (M. Du P., city-physician at K. and at A. First professor of practical surgery and obstetrics at L.) *Kamper Almanak*, 233–87, 4 portrs., 3 ill. Nutsspaarbank. Kampen.
   (*See also* 4152)

1417   MOULIN, D. de (1972). Johannes Evangelista Purkinje 1787–1869. *Hart-Bulletin, 3*, 91, portr.

Q and R

1418   OPSOMER, J. E. (1961). Un botaniste trop peu connu: Willem Quakelbeen (1527–1561). *Bull. Soc. Roy. Bot. Belg., 93*, 113–30, ill.

1419   [Anonym] (1968). Community mental health in the Netherlands: The story of Dr. Arie Querido. *J. Psychiat. Nurs., 6*, 101–5.

1420   SANDIFORT, J. A. (1931). *Rabelais. Verzamelde werken.* Volledige uitgave met de prenten van Gustav Doré en A. Robida, uit het Fransch vertaald door — (Collected Works. Complete edition with engravings by Gustave Doré and A. Robida, translated from the French by —). 2 vols., A. G. Schoonderbeek, Laren, 4°.

1421 RAMAER, J. N. (1848, 1935). Brieven aan C. B. Tilanus (Letters to —) - with German translation. *Opusc., XIII*, 287–302.

– J. N. Ramaer (1817–87), studied at Utrecht. He graduated at Groningen on a treatise: *De aethiopica generis humani varietate* (1839). Became director of the lunatic asylums at Zutphen and Delft. This letter deals with a case of gastrotomy.

1422 LEUFTINK, A. E. (1969). Bernardino Ramazzini (1633–1714). *T. Soc. Geneesk.*, 47, 293–8.

1423 KRANENBURG, W. R. H. (1933). Bernardus Ramazzini, 1633–1933. *NTG*, 77, III, 3581–5; *BGG, XIII*, 196–200, port. ill.

1423ª LINDEBOOM, G. A. (1973). Mensen om Boerhaave. XI. Johann Jacob Rau (Men around B. XI. — —). *GG, 4*, 198–9., ill.

1424 ELAUT, L. (1961). P. Rayer en de pathologische anatomie van de urine-afvoerwegen (P.R. and the pathological anatomy of the urinary ducts). *NTG, 105*, I, 33–5; *BGG, XLI*, 1–3.

1425 MIEREMET, C. W. G. (1923). In memoriam Prof. Dr. Rutger Adolf Reddingius. 1857–1923. *NTG*, 67, 1386–9.

– R. was appointed professor of pathology at Groningen in 1894 and taught dermatology from 1914 till 1921.

1426 VRIJER, M. J. A. de (1917). *Henricus Regius. Een "Cartesiaansch" hoogleeraar aan de Utrechtsche Hoogeschool* (A "Cartesian" professor at Utrecht University). 221 + XXII pp., portr. Martin Nijhoff, Den Haag.

– Reviewed by F. M. G. de Feyfer: *NTG, 66* (1922), 1660–3; *BGG, II*, 246–9.

1427 DECHANGE, Klaus (1966). *Die frühe Naturphilosophie des Henricus Regius (Utrecht 1641)*. Inaugural Dissertation, 65 pp. Münster.

1428 ROTHSCHUH, Karl E. (1968). Henricus Regius und Descartes. Neue Einblicke in die frühe Physiologie (1640–1641) des Regius. *Arch. int. Hist. Sci.*, 21, 39–66.

1429 — et K. Dechange (1971). La tradition et le progrès dans la *Physiologia* (1641) de Henricus Regius et ses relations avec les idées de Descartes. In: *International Congress for the History of Science, Paris 1968, Actes* 3B: 109–12.

1430 LINDEBOOM, G. A. (1972). In de ochtendschemering van de moderne fysiologie: Henricus Regius' *Physiologia* (1641) – en een eigentijds oordeel daarover (In the day-break of modern physiology: H. Regius' *Physiologia* (1641) – and a contemporary judgment on it). *NTG, 116,* 1124–9.

1431 — (1972). Nóg een exemplaar van Henricus Regius' *Physiologia* (1641) (Another copy of H. Regius' *Physiologia* (1641), *NTG, 116,* 1750.

1432 BRUINS, L. H. (1951). *Geert Reinders. Leven en werken van de grondlegger der immunologie.* (Life and Works of the founder of immunology). Thesis Groningen. Supervisor: A. B. F. A. Pondman. 200 pp. "De Marne", Leens.

1433 SASSEN, F. [L.R.] (1941). *Henricus Renerius, de eerste "Cartesiaensche" hoogleeraar te Utrecht* (H.P. the first "Cartesian" professor at U.). *MKNAW,* afd. Letterk., n.r., deel 4, no. 20. Noord-Holl. Uitg. Mij., Amsterdam, 50 pp.

1434 ROEKEL, G. van (1939). Een stadsdokter in the 16e eeuw (A town-physician in the 16th century). *NTG, 83,* IV, 5672–3; *BGG, XIX,* 270–1.
– On Dr. Johan van Rheyt, town-physician at Deventer, before at Louvain (request of increase of salary).

WILLEM TEN RHIJNE

1435 DORSSEN, J. M. H. van (1897–98). Dr. Wilhelm ten Rhijne and leprosy in Batavia in the 17th century. *Janus, II,* 252–60 and 355–64

1436 — (1911). Willem ten Rhijne (geb. te Deventer 1617, overl. te Batavia I Juni 1700) (W.t.R. (b. at Deventer 1617, died at Batavia June 1, 1700). *Geneesk. T. Ned.-Indië, LI,* 134–228.
– An extensive monograph on Ten Rhijne (in Dutch), also as reprint. Reviewed by F. M. G. de Feyfer in: *Janus, XX,* 509–11.

1437 STEIFVATER, E. (1955). *Die Akupunktur des Ten Rhyne.* Ulm.

1438 OTSUKA, Yasuo (1971). Willem ten Rhijne in Japan. In: *Rangaku in Japanese Culture,* 251–9.
– Japanese with an English summary. Rangaku "Dutch learning", is the Japanese word for western medicine.

1438ª CARRUBBA, R. W. and John Z. BOWERS (1974). The Western World's First Detailed Treatise on Acupuncture: Willem ten Rhijne's *De Acupunctura. J. Hist. Med.,* 29, 371–97, 6 ill.

1439 RHYNE, W. ten (1687, 1937). *Verhandelinge van de asiatise melaatsheid* (Treatise on the Asiatic Leprosy) – with English translation. *Opusc.*, *XIV*, 36–117.

1440 LAMERS, A. J. M. (1952). Jan van Riebeeck als chirurgijn (J.v.R. as a surgeon). *NTG, 96*, II, 816–8; *BGG, XXXII*, 1–3, portr.

1441 PENNING, C. P. J. (1934). Jan Anthonisz van Riebeeck en zijn dagboek (J.A.v.R. and his diary). *NTG, 78*, II, 2488–501; *BGG, XIV*, 103–16.

1442 (Limburg, Rob.) [no d.]. Jan van Riebeeck. In: *Nederlanders in den vreemde*, 126–46. Servire, Den Haag.
– Popular biography.

1443 GODÉE MOLSBERGEN, E. C. (1943). *Jan van Riebeeck en zijn tijd* (J.v.R. and his Time), 173 pp., 2 portr., 12 ill. 2nd ed. Patria Reeks III, P.N. van Kampen en Zn., Amsterdam.

1444 HUFFMANN, J. W. (1969). Jan van Riemsdyk, medical illustrator extraordinary. *JAMA, 208*, 121–4, 7 April.

1444ª COOMANS, H. E. (1974). *Life and malacological work of Hendrik Elingsz. van Rijgersma (1835–1877). A Dutch physician and scientist on St. Martin, Netherlands Antilles.* Thesis University of Amsterdam (Ph.D. Supervisor: J. H. Stock). 214 pp., 17 ill. Ponsen & Looijen, Wageningen Also in: *Bijdr. Dierk., 44* (1974), no 2.
(See also 3869)

1445 BERG, C. van den (1971). *H. B. J. van Rijn, burgemeester van Venlo, pioneer der milieuhygiëne* (H. B. J. van Rijn, burgomaster of Venlo, pioneer of environment hygiene), 171 pp., 10 ill. Maaslandse Monografieën. Van Gorcum, Assen.
– Rev. by M. F. Polak: *NTG, 116* (1972), 612.

G. A. VAN RIJNBERK

1446 SCHOUTE, D. (1938). Professor doctor G. van Rijnberk. Patronus Studiorum Historiae medicinae Neerlandicae. (1 Juli 1913 – 1 Juli 1938). *NTG, 82*, III, 3339–40; *BGG, XVIII*, 114–5.

1447 KOUWENAAR, W. (1953). Prof. Dr. G. A. van Rijnberk. *NTG, 97*, IV, 2642, portr.

1448 DUYFF, J. W. (1953). In Memoriam Prof. Dr. G. A. van Rijnberk. *NTG, 97*, IV, 2643–4.

1449 DEELMAN, H. T. (1953). Herinnering aan Prof. Dr. G. A. van Rijnberk
      (Memories of —). *NTG, 97*, IV, 2644–5.

1450 ELAUT, L. (1954). De Bibliotheca Occulta van Prof. Dr. G. van Rijn-
      berk. *Wetensch. Tijdingen, 14*, 101.

      – G. van Rijnberk (1875–1953), professor of physiology in the University of Amster-
      dam, for many years chief editor of the *Nederlands Tijdschrift voor Geneeskunde*,
      took a keen interest in occultism.

1451 RINGELING, J. H. A. (1959–1960). Geneesheer op Schokland. Hendrik
      Ringeling 1804–1873 (Physician on Schokland). *Kamper Almanak*,
      192–203.

1452 NAPJUS, J. W. (1941). De hoogleeraren in de geneeskunde aan de Fra-
      neker Hoogeschool en het Athenaeum 1585–1843: XXII. Johannes
      Jacobus Ritter (The professors of medicine at Franeker Academy and
      Athenaeum. XXII. J.J.R.). *NTG, 85*, III, 2965–9; *BGG, XXI*, 84–8.

1453 VOS, T. A. (1965). Herinneringen aan Prof. Dr. G. F. Rochat.
      (Memories of —). *Gron. Universiteitsblad, 15*, 111–7.

1454 HOEVEN, J. van der (1929). E. K. Rodschied. Een West-Indisch
      tropenarts uit het einde der 18de eeuw (A West-Indian tropical phy-
      sician from the end of the 18th century). *NTG, 73*, I, 1101–7; *BGG,
      IX*, 61–7.

      – On C. Roelants, *see* 1469.

                         BOUDEWIJN RONSSE

1455 HUNGER, F. W. T. (1930). Boudewijn Ronsse 1525?–1597. *NTG, 74*,
      I, 2887–2905; *BGG, X*, 145–63.

1456 BUWALDA, J. M. and E. O. Buwalda-Prey (1942). Boudewijn Ronsse
      en de opleiding van de chirurgijns (B.R. and the education of surgeons).
      NTG, 86, II, 1093–7; *BGG, XXII*, 66–70.

      – See also J. B. F. van Gils (same title), letter to the editor. *NTG, 86*, II, *1436*;
      BGG, XXII, 87.

                    WILHELM CONRAD RÖNTGEN

1457 NEHER, F. L. (1944). *Röntgen. De roman van een onderzoeker* (R. The
      novel of an investigator). 283 pp. Uitgevers-Mij. "West-Friesland",
      Hoorn.

      – a popular biography.

1458 WYLICK, W. A. H. van (1966). *Röntgen en Nederland. Röntgens betrekkingen tot Nederland en de opkomst der Röntgenologie hier te lande* (R. and the Netherlands. R's relations with the Netherlands and the rise of roentgenology in this country). 255 pp., ill. Thesis Free University Amsterdam (Supervisor: G. A. Lindeboom), J. Hoeijenbos, Utrecht.
– also as a monograph.

1459 — (1967). Twee Nederlandse brieven van Wilhelm Conrad Röntgen (Two Dutch letters of —). *NTG, 111*, 1219–20.
– To H. Kamerlingh Onnes (Jan. 18, 1899) and to H. A. Lorentz (Dec. 22, 1901).

1460 — (1968). Was Wilhelm Roentgen a German or a Dutchman? What was his relation to the Netherlands? *Thorax, 23*, 676–82, 2 portrs., 1 ill.

1461 — (1970). De ontdekking van de Röntgenstralen 75 jaar geleden (The discovery of the X-rays 75 years ago). *NTG, 114*, 1869–70.

1462 — (1970). Röntgen's Nederlandse moeder, Charlotte Constance Frowein (Roentgen's Dutch mother, C.C.F.) *NTG, 114*, 22–4.

1463 — (1973). Het door Röntgen afgewezen Utrechts professoraat (The Utrecht professorship declined by R.). *GeWiNa*, no. 31, 4–5.

1464 — (1970). Wilhelm Conrad Röntgen. *Gamma, 20*, 256–88, portr., ill.

1465 — (1971). Feestelijke bijeenkomst te Würzburg ter herdenking van de ontdekking van de Röntgenstraling (Festal meeting at W. in commemoration of the discovery of the X-Rays.) *NTG, 115*, I, 713–4.

1466 — (1971). W. C. Roentgen and the early days of X-rays. *Medicamundi, 16*, 1–8, portr., 9 ill.

1467 [Editorial] (1966). Zeventig jaar geleden gaf Wilhelm Conrad Röntgen de mensheid een stralend geschenk (70 years ago W.C.R. gave mankind a radiant gift). *T. Ziekenverpl., 19*, (januari), 19.

1468 SCHULTE, J. E. (1968). Röntgen en zijn ontdekking (R. and his discovery). *NTG, 112*, 530. With a note of S. v. Creveld: *NTG, 112*, 628.

1468ª HAGA, H. (1921). Röntgen-stralen (X-rays). *NTG, 65*, I, 1104–11, port.

1468ᵇ WERTHEIM SALOMONSON, J. K. A. (1921). De Röntgenstralen in de geneeskundige wetenschap (X-rays in medical science). *NTG, 65*, I, 1112–19.
– on the occasion of the discovery of X-rays by R. 25 years ago.

1469 SUDHOFF, Karl (1909), Die Schrift des Cornelis Roelants von Me-
cheln über Kinderkrankheiten. *Janus, XIV,* 467–85, ill.

1470 COHEN, E. J. and C. F. van Duin (1926). Zeventig jaar uit het leven
van Pieter van Romburgh (Seventy years of the life of P.v.R.)
Chem. Wbl., XXIII, 3.

1480 BOCKSTAELE, Paul (1961). Adriaan van Roomen, "medicus et mathematicus". Bij het vierde eeuwfeest van zijn geboorte (A.v.R. "medicus
et mathematicus". The fourth anniversary of his birthday). *Sci. Hist.,*
3, 169–78.
   – v.R. (1561–1615), a Belgian, was professor of medicine at Louvain and became
   the founder of medical education at the University of Würzburg.

1481 BAUMANN, E. D. (1922). Hendrick van Roonhuyse. *NTG, 66,* I,
856–74; *BGG, II.* 63–81. (see also R's secret: 3579–86).

1482 ELAUT, L. (1937). In Memoriam Prof. Dr. A. H. M. J. van Rooy.
Vlaams Geneesk. T., 953–6.

1483 VIEYRA, D. (1935). Een krasse Italiaanse geneesheer uit het jaar 1758
(A vigorous Italian physician from 1758). *NTG, 79,* III, 3760; *BGG,*
XV, 184.
   – On Joshephus Jacobus Rota, Italian physician, still active at the age of 111
   years.

1484 [   ] (1970) Johann Stensson Rothman (1684–1763). med' dr. i.
Harderwijk 1713, provinsialläkare i Kronobergs län 1718, logices et
physices lektor i växjö 1720. R. har karakteriserats som "en lärd,
vitter och mycket förtjänt läkare. *Nord. Med. Hist. Årsbok,* suppl.
III, 86.
   – J.S.R. who graduated at Harderwijk was one of the teachers of Linnaeus in his
   earlier years.

1485 NUYENS, B. W. Th. (1942). Dr. Cornelis Henricus à Roy (Haarlem
1750 – Amsterdam 1833). *NTG, 86,* II, 1083–7; *BGG, XXII,* 56–60,
portr.

1486 BIJLEVELD, W. J. J. C. (1942). Nadere gegevens over Dr. C. H. à Roy
(more details on —). *NTG, 86,* IV, 3081–2; *BGG, XXII,* 159–60.

1487 — (1947). Nogmaals de familie van dr. Cornelis Henricus à Roy (a-
gain the family of dr. C. H. à R.) *NTG, 91,* III, 2532–4; *BGG, XXVII,*
48–50, portr.

1488 VOLLGRAF, J. A. (1913). Pierre de la Ramée (1515–1572) et Willebrord Snel van Royen (1580–1626). *Janus, XVIII*, 595–625, 15 ill., portr.

1489 MEURS, G. J. van (1954). Max Rubner 1854–1932. *Voeding, 15*, 517–9, portr.

1490 SCHOUTEN, J. (1966). Doctor Jacob van Ruisdael, schilder en genees-heer (Dr. Jac. van Ruisdael, painter and physician). *Specimina Specia*, 7, nr. 33, 1–6.

1491 [Anonym] (1932). Dr Jacob van Ruisdaal, landschapsschilder en me-dicus (1629–1682), naar het manuscript van H. F. Wijnman (Dr — — —, landscape-painter and physician (— —), after the ms by — —). *Amstelodamum, 19*, 40–2.

1492 PRICK, J. J. G. (1967). Levensbericht van Henricus Cornelis Rümke (16 januari 1893 – 22 mei 1967) (Biographical notice of —). *Jbk. KNAW 1966–67*, 358–63, portr.

1493 BALLINTIJN, G. (1944). *Rumphius, de blinde ziener van Ambon* (Rum-phius, the blind seer of Ambon). 189 pp., ill., Utr. Utrecht, 8°.
– R., not a physician, was the writer of the (posthumously published) 12 volumes work: *Het Amboinsch Kruidboek* (1705) (The Amboyna Herbal).

FREDERIK RUYSCH

1494 SCHELTEMA, Pieter (1886). *Het leven van Frederik Ruysch* (Life of —). Thesis Leyden (Supervisor: T. Zaaijer), 115 pp., Luijt, Sliedrecht.

1495 TERNOWSKY, W. N. (1929). "Fredericus Ruysch". Aus dem anato-michen Institut der Universität in Kasan. *VIme Congrès Int. d'Hist. Méd. Leyde-Amsterdam 1927*, 333–8, Anvers.

1496 LUYENDIJK-ELSHOUT, A. M. (1970). Death enlightened. A study of Frederik Ruysch. *JAMA, 212*, 121–7.

1497 LEENDERS, E. and W. K. Sieber (1970). Congenital megacolon obser-vation by Frederick Ruysch – 1691. *J. Pediat. Surg., 5*, febr., 1–3.

1498 BAZZI, Franco (1955). Un maestro della tecnica anatomica Federico Ruysch(1638–1731). *Riv. Storia Sci Med. Natur., XLVI*, 255–73, portrs., ill.

1499 GRONDONA, Felica (1965). La struttura dei reni da F. Ruysch a W. Bowman. *Physis, 7*, 281–316, 20 fig.

1500   HALLEMA, A. (1951). De benoeming van Frederik Ruysch tot gerech-
       telijk geneeskundige van de stad Amsterdam (F.R.'s appointment as
       coroner of Amsterdam). *NTG, 95*, II, 1380–3; *BGG, XXXI*, 22–5.

1501   BISSELING, G. H. (1921). Uit de "Amsterdamse Courant", 1695, no
       84; 1720, no 36 (From the "Amsterdam Newspaper".) *NTG, 65*, I,
       3113; *BGG, I*, 280.
       – two advertisements of Fred. Ruysch on public anatomies.

1502   MANN, Gunther (1961). Anatomische Sammlung Frederik Ruysch
       (1638–1731). *SA, 45*, 176–8, 4 ill.
       – On the Ruysch collection at Leningrad.

1503   — (1964). Museums: The Anatomical Collection of Frederik Ruysch
       at Leningrad. *Bull. Cleveland and med. Library, 11*, 10–3, ill.

1504   LINDEBOOM, G. A. (1962). Frederik Ruysch' anatomische preparaten-
       verzameling te Leningrad (The collection of anatomical preparations
       of — at L.). *NTG, 106*, I, 32–3; *BGG, XLII*, 5–6, 2 ill.

1505   FRANKE, H. (1971). Peter der Grosse und die anatomo-pathologische
       Präparatesammlung von F. Ruysch. *Münch. med. Wschr., 11*, 488–91.

1505ᵃ RAPTSCHINSKY, Boris (1935). Frederik Ruysch en Peter de Groote.
       Amstelodamum, 22, 77–9.

1506   ACKERKNECHT, Erwin H. (1971). Gemaniëreerde anatomie: Frederik
       Ruysch en zijn verzameling (Mannered anatomy: F.R. and his collec-
       tion). *Image*, no 43, 27–32, 11 ill.
       – original title: Ruysch und seine Sammlung.

1507   LUYENDIJK-ELSHOUT, A. M. and J. Dankmeijer (1970). De allegorische
       betekenis van de praeparatenverzamelingen van Frederik Ruysch
       (1638–1731) (The allegorical sense of the collections of preparations
       of — —). *NTG, 114*, 1679–80.

1507ᵃ WOLTERSON, Bertha (1939). Frederik Ruysch als romanheld (— — as a
       hero in a novel). *Amstelodamum, 26*, 28–33.

1508   HAZEN, A. T. (1939). Johnson's life of Frederic Ruysch. *Bull. Inst.
       Hist. Med., VII*, I, 324–34.

1509   LUYENDIJK-ELSHOUT, A. M. (1964). *Frederik Ruysch. Dilucidatio
       valvularum in vasis lymphaticis et lacteis 1665.* Facsimile of the first

edition with an introduction by — —. Dutch Classics on History of Science, 49 + 94 pp., ill. B. de Graaf, Nieuwkoop.

– Reviewed by: M. M. Ravitch: *BHM, XL* (1966), 90.

See also: 2921, 3581

1509ª GEYL, A. (1911). Mr Valentijn Ruysworm. *NTG, 55*, I, 1689–95.

– R., a 16th century physician at Leyden and a Paracelsist. The article contains some notarial minutes concerning R.

S

1510 DRAAK, A. M. E. (ed.) (1967). *Het boek Sajet. Opstellen over Aspecten der Sociale Geneeskunde door Vrienden aangeboden aan Dr. B. H. Sajet ter gelegenheid van zijn tachtigste verjaardag.* (The book Sajet. Essays on aspects of Social Medicine presented by friends to Dr. B. H. Sajet on the occasion of his 80th anniversary). 191 pp., portr. Holland-Breumelhof, Amsterdam.

– Dr. B. H. Sajet, born 17 March 1887, an Amsterdam physician was very active in the field of Social Medicine.

1511 LEMOS, Maximiano (1911). Ribeiro Sanches à Leyde (1730–1731). *Janus, XVI*, 237–53.

– Rib. Sanches (1699–1783) came to Leyden in order to hear Boerhaave, who recommended him to the Russian Czarina as court-physician.

1512 WILLEMSE, David (1966). *António Nunes Ribeiro Sanches – élève de Boerhaave – et son importance pour la Russie.* Thesis Amsterdam (Supervisor: J. A. van Praag), XIII + 188 pp. With photostatic reprint of *Catalogue des Livres de feu M. Ant. Nunes Ribeiro Sanches*, Paris 1783. E. J. Brill, Leiden.

– Reviewed by Lester S. King: *BHM, XLI* (1967), 377–8.

See also 1698

EDUARD SANDIFORT

1513 PUTTO, J. A. (1964). Eduard Sandifort (14 nov. 1742 – 12 febr. 1814) *GG, 42*, 103.

1514 GUTIERREZ, J. E. (1961). The "Rarissimo cordis vitio" of Sandifort [Eduard]. *Marquette med. Rev., 26*, 92–4.

1515 PIERRO, F. (1971). Due lettere di Leopoldo M. A. Caldani (1725–1813) all'anatomico leidense Edoardo Sandifort (1742–1814). *Med. Secoli, 7* (4), 19–40, facsims.

1516 [Editorial] (1953). Steensen – Sandifort – Fallot. *NTG*, *97*, II, 1415.
– An editorial note.

See also 4151

SAMUEL SARPHATI

1517 BARUCH, J. Z. (1963). Dr. Samuel Sarphati, medicus, hygiënist, stede-
bouwer (1813–1866). (S.S., physician, hygienist and townbuilder).
NTG, *107*, II, 1932–6; *BGG*, *XLIII*, 20–4.
Also in: *De Opbouw*, orgaan *Port. Isr. Gemeente Amsterdam*, *17*,
(1963), nr. 2, 66–9.

1518 — (1967). Dr. Samuel Sarphati, medicus en planoloog (1813–1866)
(Dr. S.S., physician and planologist). *Sci. Hist.*, *9*, 75–83.
– Also in: *Socialisme en Democratie*, *23* (1966), nr. 6, 453–62.

1519 HARTKAMP, A. Th. (1913). Dr. Samuel Sarphati 1813 – 31 Januari –
1913. *Eigen Haard*, *XXXIX*, 35.

1520 DUBIEZ, F. J. (1966). Dr. Samuel Sarphati, een groot Amsterdammer
(Dr. S.S., a great inhabitant of Amsterdam). *Ons Amsterdam*, *18*,
162–9, ill.

1521 KRUIZINGA, J. H. (1966). Dr. Samuel Sarphati (1813–1866): wegbe-
reider voor het nieuwe Amsterdam (S.: forerunner of the new Amsterdam). *Cobouw*, 6 mei, 13.

1522 SCHELTEMA, B. E. (1917). *Herinneringen van een geneesheer* (Memories of a physician). Zutfen, 8°.
– Autobiographical notices.

1523 VUGS, J. G. (1971). In memoriam Gustav Scherz (1895–1971). *AP*, *4*,
28–9.
– G.S., the editor of works of Nic. Steno.

1524 ANDEL, M. A. van (1940). In memoriam Dr. A. F. C. van Schevensteen 19 I 1882 – 22 V 1940. *NTG*, *84*, IV, 3890; *BGG*, *XX*, 147.

1525 FEYFER, F. M. G. de (1941). A la mémoire du docteur A. F. C. van
Schevensteen. 19 janvier 1882 – 22 juillet 1940. *Janus*, *XLV*, 57–8,
portr.
– Van Schevensteen, a Belgian ophthalmologist living at Antwerp (where he was
"chef de service" of an ophthalmic hospital) contributed to the history of medicine
in several periodicals. (f.e. *Janus*).

1526 WILLINGE PRINS, J. A. (1930). Carl Ludwig Schleich. *NTG*, 74, I, 1099; *BGG*, X, 88.

1527 KUIJJER, P. J. (1957). In Memoriam Dr. Th. H. Schlichting. 14 Januari 1894 – 14 September 1957. *Janus, XLVI*, 281–2. also in: *NTG*, *101*, (1957), 1853–4.

1528 LINDEBOOM, G. A. (1959). In Memoriam Dr. Th. H. Schlichting. *Yperman, VI*, 9–10.

1529 DOOREN, L. (1938). Octrooi aanvraag van Bernardus Schotanus (Application for a patent by —). *GG, XVI*, 333.

1530 SCHLICHTING, Th. H. (1954). De betekenis van Dr. Dirk Schoute voor de beoefening der historia medica in Nederland (The significance of — for the study of the historia medica in the Netherlands). *NTG*, *98*, I, 27–9; *BGG, XXXIV*, 1–3.

1530ª SCHIERBEEK, A. (1953–1955). Dirk Schoute (Deventer, 12 Januari 1873 – Soest, 6 December 1953). *Jbk. Mij Ned. Letterk.*, 78–82.

1531 SNELDERS, H. A. M. (1971). Hendrik Willem Schroeder van der Kolk (1836–1867) en de fysische chemie (— and physical chemistry). *Sci. Hist.*, *13*, 185–97.

1532 ESCH, P. van der (1954). *Jacobus Ludovicus Conradus Schroeder van der Kolk, 1797–1862, leven en werken* (—, life and works). Thesis Amsterdam (Supervisor: A. Querido), 196 pp., no. pl.

1533 KLEIJ, J. J. van der (1929). Schroeder van der Kolk's boek over krankzinnigheid, als voorbeeld van een eenvoudige degelijke Nederlandsche wetenschap (S's book on lunacy, as a model of a simple thorough Dutch science). *VIᵐᵉ Congrès Int. d'Hist. de la Méd. Leyde-Amsterdam 1927*, 286–8, Anvers.

1534 DOESSCHATE, G. ten (1961). *J. L. C. Schroeder van der Kolk als physioloog* (— as a physiologist)., 253 pp. Utrechts Universitair Museum, Utrecht.
– Latin text with Dutch translation of the lecture-notes on physiology of Schroeder van der Kolk (1797–1862), professor of physiology at Utrecht since 1827.

1535 HANEVELD, G. T. (1970). The Schroeder van der Kolk Collection – a rediscovered link between Utrecht and Oxford. *J. Path.*, *101*, Aug., Proc. XX.

1536 ORLOVSKAIA, D. D. (1972). J. L. C. Schroeder van der Kolk. *Zh. Ne-vropat. Psikhiat*, 72, 1088–90 (Russian).
– on the 175th anniversary of his birth.

1537 SCHROEDER VAN DER KOLK, J. L. C. (1835) (1932). *Over het verschil tusschen doode natuurkrachten, levenskrachten en ziel* (On the difference between dead natural forces, vital strengths and soul). With German translation. *Opusc., XI*, 282–359.

1538 – (1838, 1927). *Redevoering over de verwaarlozing der vereischte zorg ter leniging van het (ongelukkig) lot der krankzinnigen en ter genezing derzelve in ons vaderland* (An Address on the neglect of the care required for the assuagement of the Fate of the Insane, and for the cure of same in our country). With English translation. *Opusc., VI*, 294–352.

                                                    See also 942, 5463a

1539 HANEVELD, G. T. (1968). Toers Diesbergen Schubaert 1805–1853. *GeWiNa*, 24, 13–5.

1540 LINDEBOOM, G. A. (1972). Florentius Schuyl und seine Bedeutung für die Verbreitung des Cartesianismus in den Niederlanden. *Janus, LIX*, 25–37, 2 ill.

1540ᵃ — (1974). *Florentius Schuyl (1619–1669) en zijn betekenis voor het Cartesianisme in de geneeskunde* (F.S.; and his significance for Cartesianism in medicine). 158 pp., port. ill. M. Nijhoff, Den Haag.

1541 HOEVEN, J. van der (1921). Letters of Thomas Schwencke on the inoculation of smallpox. *Janus, XXV*, 325–9.
– misnumbered: 225–9.

1542 [   ] (1937). The date of birth and death of Johannes Scultetus. *Isis*, 27, 63.
– Note.

I. SEMMELWEIS

1543 SCHRÖDER, R. G. C. (1923). Portret van Semmelweis (Portrait of —). *NTG*, 67, I, 517.

1544 VERAART, B. A. G. (1929). Welche Bedeutung haben Semmelweis und Lister für den Fortschritt der Medizin? *Janus, XXXIII*, 360–9.

1545   — (1930). Semmelweis en Lister. *NTG*, *74*, I, 1762–75; *BGG*, *X*, 89–
       102.

1546   THOMPSON, Morton (1950). *Pionier van het leven. De tragische strijd
       van dr. Ignaz Semmelweis* (Pioneer of life. The tragic fight of —), 525
       pp., Elsevier Amsterdam-Brussel.
       – Dutch translation of the English original by A. P. Prins.

MICHAËL SERVET

1547   SMIT KLEINE, F. (1909). Michel Servet. *Tijdspiegel*, *I*, 35.

1548   LINDEBOOM, G. A. (1954). Michaël Servet. *G&W*, *52*, 49–60, I ill.

1549   — (1954). Michaël Servet (1511–1553) en de ontdekking van de kleine
       bloedsomloop (and the discovery of the lesser circulation of the blood).
       NTG, *98*, I, 696–708; *BGG*, *XXXIV*, 17–29, 4 ill., portr.

1550   — (1965). Michaël Servet en de geneeskunde (M.S. and medicine
       Soteria, *X*, 135–8, ill.

1551   WYNANDTS FRANCKEN, C. J. C. (1937). *Michael Servet en zijn martel-
       dood* (M.S. and his martyrdom). Tjeenk Willink & Zn., Haarlem.
       – Calvin, Servet, Castellion. A page from the history of the reformation.

1552   BIJLEVELD, W. J. J. C. (1932). *Von Siebold. Bijdrage tot zijn levens-
       beschrijving* (A contribution to his biography), ill., portr., Leiden.
       – The German physician Philipp Franz von Siebold (1796–1866), a famous con-
       noisseur of Japan spent his last years in the neighbourhood of Leiden.

1553   SIEBOLD, F. K. von (1941). Jonkheer Dr. med. Ph., F. von Siebold
       zu seinem 75. Todestag am 18.10.1941. *Janus*, *XLV*, 208–18, ill.

1554   WILDE, P. A. de (1937). In Memoriam Dr. A. Sikkel Azn. *NTG*, *81*,
       5648–50.
       – Abraham Sikkel (1866–1937), a specialist in otorhinology, has been president of
       the Dutch Association of Physicians; he founded in 1923 the periodical "Genees-
       kundige Gids".

1555   KOUWER, B. J. (1912). Professor A. E. Simon Thomas. *Leidsch
       Jbk.*, *IX*, 1.

1556   KLEIBERG, J. (1962). Dr. Albert Simons: The doctor and the man
       [Hebrew] *Koroth*, *2*, 165–72.

1557 SCHIERBEEK, A. (1962). In Memoriam Charles Singer. *NTG, 106*, I, 1201; *BGG, XLII*, 28.
– Charles Singer (1876–1960), the famous English medico-historian.

1557ª VERKROOST, C. M. (1973). De dichter Slauerhoff als medicus (The poet — as a physician) *AP*, no 12, 57–65.
– J. J. Slauerhoff (1898–1937) Dutch poet and physician.

1558 PUTTO, J. A. (1964). William Smellie (1697–1763). *GG, 42*, 136.

1559 [   ] (1970). The dietary surveys of Dr. Edward Smith, 1862–73. *Voeding, 31*, 618.

1559ª POPPER, H. (1973). Isidore Snapper, M. D. (1889–1973). *Mt. Sinai J. Med. N. Y., 40*, 716–9.

1559ᵇ On H. Snellen: see ophthalmology (3661–3).

See also 5399

CORNELIS SOLINGEN

1560 ANDEL, M. A. van (1936). De chirurgijn Cornelis Solingen en zijn instrumentarium (The surgeon Cornelis Solingen and his instruments). *NTG, 80*, I, 47–55; *BGG, XVI*, 10–8; see also: *NTG, 79* (1935), IV, 5165; *BGG, XV*, 228.

1561 BESSERT, HERBERT (1935). *Zahnärztliches bei Cornelis Solingen*, Inaugural Dissertation, 26 pp. Leipzig.

1562 KRUL, R. (1883). Argumentatio fustis. Bijdrage tot het leven van de broeders Stalpert van der Wiel en van Cornelis Solingen. (Argumentatio fustis. Contribution to the life of the brothers S. van W. and C.S.). *NTG, 19*, 871–4.
– Altercation between Solingen and Johan Stalpert van der Wiel.

1563 FEYFER, F. M. G. de (1907). Solingen's nalatenschap (S.'s inheritance). *Cat. Geschiedk. Tent. Nat. en Geneesk. te Leiden 1907*, 176.

1564 SOLINGEN, C. (1684, 1943). *Manuale operatiën der chirurgie* (Manual operations of surgery). – With English translation *Opusc., XVII*, 130–75.

See also 5448n

1565 BROEK, A. J. P. van der (1959). Een en ander uit het leven van de anatoom S. Th. von Sömmering (1755–1830) (Something from the life of the anatomist —). *GeWiNa*, no. 5, 13.

1566 JONG, F. de (1963). Marie Johanna Spaarnaay, 19 januari 1856 – 6 april 1923. *Tegen Tuberculose, 59*, 32–8, ill.

1567 CAPPARONI, P. (1930). Cinque lettere inedite de Adriaan van den Spieghel (Adrianus Spigelius), Professore nel'ateneo Padovano. *Boll. Ist. ital. Arte. san., 10*, 248–53, 1 ill.
– The five letters contain interesting data from the life of A.v.d.S. (1578–1625), professor of anatomy and surgery at Padua.

1567ᵃ ZEN BENETTI, F. and L. ROSETTI (1972). Nuove ricerche sull' anatomico fiammingo Adriaan van den Spieghel (1578–1625). *Quad. Storia Univ. Padova, 5*, 45–89.

1568 NUYENS, B. W. Th. (1927). Een autograaf van Mr. Adr. van den Spiegel (An autograph of —). *NTG, 71*, II, 87–94; *BGG, VII*, 491–8.
– the document is from A.v.d.Sp.Sr., surgeon of the Prince of Orange, father of the Padua professor.

BARUCH DE SPINOZA

1569 SARTON, G. (1928). Spinoza, 1632–1677–1927. *Isis, 10*, 11–5, 4 ill.

1570 DUBIEZ, F. J. (1969). Baruch de Spinoza 1632–1677. *Ons Amsterdam, 21*, 2–12, ill.

1571 COHEN, M. H. (1920). *Spinoza en de Geneeskunde* (S. and medicine). Thesis University of Amsterdam (Supervisor: I. Snapper), 74 pp., De Bussy, Amsterdam.
– Reviewed by F. M. G. de Feyfer in: *NTG, 65*, I, 1274–6; *BGG, I*, 125–7.

1572 COERT, H. J. (1938). *Spinoza's betrekking tot de geneeskunde en hare beoefenaren* (S.'s relation to medicine and its practicers. Meded. Spinozahuis, IV, 18 pp., Brill, Leiden.

1573 ARON, W. (1962). Baruch Spinoza and medicine [Hebrew]. *Harofé Haivri, 35*, 150–77, portr.

1574 — (1963). Baruch Spinoza and medicine [Hebrew and English] *Harofé Haivri, 36*, 105–28, 232–55, portr.

1574ᵃ — (1965). Baruch Spinoza et la médecine. *Revue d'Hist. Méd. hébraïque, 18*, 61–78, 113–21.

1575 HÜHNERFIELD, J. (1939). Die Stellung Spinozas und Hobbes zur Medizin, insbesondere zur Physiologie ihrer Zeit. *SA, 23*, 113–34.

1576 MEERLOO, J. A. M. (1965). Spinoza: coup d'oeil sur ses conceptions psychologiques. *Méd. et Hyg.* (Genève), no. 678, 255–6, ill. and in: *Am. J. Psychiatr.*, *121*, 890–4 [English].

1577 — (1965). Spinoza; a look at his psychological concepts. *Am. J. Psych. 121*, 890–4.

1577ᵃ VYGOTSKII, L. S. (1972). Spinoza's theory of the emotions in light of comtemporary psycho-neurology. *Soviet. Stud. Philos.*, *10*, 362–82.

1578 WUNDERLI, J, (1968). Ueber Spinozas Beitrag zur Leib-Seele-Problematik unter Berücksichtigung der Relation zur modernen Psychosomatik. *Gesnerus*, *25*, 101–11.

1579 ARON, W. (1964). Freud und Spinoza. *Heb. med. J.*, *1*, 265–84. also in *Harofé Haivri*, *37* (1), 119–28 [Hebrew]; 284–65 [Engl.] and: *37* (2) 36–46 [Hebrew]; 260.

1580 — (1967). Freud et Spinoza. *Revue hist. Méd. hébraique*, *20*, 149–60.

1581 BERNARD, W. (1972). Spinoza's influence on the rise of scientific psychology: A neglected chapter in the history of psychology. *J. Hist. behav. Sci.*, *8*, 208–15. *See also:* 3709.

1582 NIERENSTEIN, M. (1932). Helvetius, Spinoza, and transmutation. *Isis*, *17*, 408–11.

1583 FISCHER, J. (1921). De geneesheeren onder Spinoza's vrienden (Physicians among S.'s friends). *NTG*, *65*, I, 1856–75; *BGG*, *I*, 145–64.

1584 MEININGER, J. V. (1972, 1973). Medici in de vriendenkring van Spinoza (I, II en III Physicians in the circle of friends of S.) *AP*, no. 8, 44–51; *ibid.*, no. 10 (1973), 1–10; *ibid.*, no. 12, 45–56.

See also 592, 2088–9

1584ᵃ JOSSELIN DE JONG, R. de (1932). In Memoriam C. H. H. Spronck 18 Februari 1858 – 3 December 1932. *NTG*, *76*, IV, 5726–9 port.
– C.H.H.S., founder of serology and serotherapy in the Netherlands.

1585 BAUMANN, E. D. (1921). Cornelis Stalpart van der Wiel. *NTG*, *65*, II, 1689–1712; *BGG*, *I*, 373–96. *See also* 1562.

NICOLAAS STENO

1586 FEYFER, F. M. G. (1911). De vader van den ductus Stenonianus (The father of the ductus stenonianus). *NTG*, *55*, I, 2168.

1587 PEYER, B. (1954). Nicolaus Steno. *Gesnerus*, *11*, 55–61.

1588 VUGS, J. G. (1968). *Leven en werk van Niels Stensen (1638–1686), on-derzoeker van het zenuwgestel* (Life and Work of Niels Stensen (1638–1686), investigator of the nervous system). Thesis Leiden (Supervisor: J. Dankmeijer), 312 pp., ports., ill. 8°. Universitaire Pers Leiden.

1589 SCHERZ, Gustav (1960). Niels Stensen's first dissertation. *J. Hist. Med.*, *15*, 247–64, pl., facsims.
– Fascimile edition of Stensen's *Disputatio Physica de Thermis*, held under Arnold Senguerd (1610–67) at the Amsterdam Athenaeum, July 8, 1660.

1590 VUGS, J. G. (1970). Het paleontologisch-geologisch werk van Steno (The paleontologic-geological work of Steno). *Sci. Hist.*, *12*, 192–205, also in: *GeWiNa*, *26* (1970), 5–8.

1591 LINDEBOOM, G. A. (1969). Libido Sciendi en Amor Dei. *G&W*, *67*, 201–6.
– on Pascal, Swammerdam and Steno.

1592 VUGS, J. G. (1970). Steno in Amsterdam. *Janus*, *LVII*, 163–73. also in: *Acta Sexti Conventus Hist. Sci. medic. Math. Nat. Excolendae* 163–73, Brill, Leiden (1971).

1593 — (1971). Niels Stensen in Holland (N.S. in Holland). *Aere Perennius*, no. 5, 44–57.

1594 GEURTS, P. A. M. (1960). Niels Stensen en Albert Burgh. *Arch. Gesch. Kath. Kerk in Nederland*, *2*, 139–52.

1595 MAY, M. T. (1950). On the passage of yolk into the intestines of the chick. Nicolaus Steno. *J. Hist. Med.*, *V*, 119–43.
– on Steno. with a translation of his letters to Paulus Barbette on the passage of yolk.
See also 1523, 1630

1596 AERNOUTS, R. and E. Trison (1965). Wetenschappelijk leven te Ant-werpen in de 17de eeuw, de vriendenkring van Frans van Sterbeeck in Zuid- en Noord-Nederland (Scientific life at Antwerp in the 17th century, the cercle of friends of Frans van Sterbeeck in South- and North-Netherland). *Sci. Hist.*, *7*, 5–15.
– see on v.St.: *NBW* (België) (1966), 2, col. 814–9.

B. J. STOKVIS

1597   [   ] (1899). Ter herinnering aan het 25-jarig ambtsjubileum van Prof. Dr. B. J. Stokvis als hoogleeraar (In memory of the 25th anniversary of – as a professor). *NTG, 35,* 2de reeks, I, 1017–8, portr.

1598   PEL, P. K. (1902). In memoriam Prof. Dr. B. J. Stokvis. *DMW, 42.*

1599   [   ] (1902). Nécrologie Barend Joseph Stokvis. *Janus, VII,* 559–60, portr.

WILLEM STORM VAN LEEUWEN

1600   RACKEMANN, F. M. (1958). Professor Willem Storm van Leeuwen and the asthma problem. *Acta allerg., 12,* 407–26.

1601   BEUMER, H. M. (1968). *Willem Storm van Leeuwen und seine Bedeutung für die Asthmaforschung.* 66 pp., Michael Triltsch Verlag, Düsseldorf. Heft 31 der Düsseldorfer Arbeiten zur Gesch. der Medizin. (H. Schadewalt, Ed.).

1602   — (1968). Willem Storm van Leeuwen in Utrecht (W.S. van S. at U.). *Oud-Utrecht, 41,* 85–6.

1603   — (1969). Storm van Leeuwen en de klinische farmakologie (— and clinical pharmacology). *NTG, 113,* 1515.

1604   — (1971). Allergie- und Asthmaforschung von Willem Storm van Leeuwen (1882–1933). *Med. Welt, 22,* 1530–6, portr., 6 ill.

1605   VAREKAMP, H. (1966). Enige herinneringen aan Professor Dr. W. Storm van Leeuwen 1883–1933 (Recollections of —). *NTG, 110,* 2014–6.

     – In 1966 Dr. Varekamp received the "Storm van Leeuwen medal" for his work in the field of allergology and social medicine. *NTG, 110* (1966), 206.

1606   LOUIS, Armand (1966). S t o r m s (Sturmius). *Nat. Biogr. Woordenboek* Brussels, *2,* Col. 831–4.

     – Roland Storms (17th century), born at Louvain, studied in Italy and settled as a practising physician at Delft.

1607   BAUMANN, E. D. (no d.). *Een lijfarts der Oranjes in de XVIIde eeuw* (A court-physician of the Oranges in the 17th century)., 48 pp., ill., portr., Keming en Zoon, Utrecht.

     – On Willem van der S t r a a t e n (1593–1681), professor in the University at Utrecht.

1608 OELE, Walla (1966). "Koppige Piet" ("Obstinate Peter"). *MC, 20,*
243–5, ill.
– On Pieter Stuyvesant (1610–1672).

1609 SURINGAR, P. H. (1874). Bijzonderheden betreffende het leven van Dr.
G. C. B. Suringar (Details from the life of —). *NTG, 2,* 66.
– G. C. B. Suringar (1802–74), professor at Amsterdam and afterwards at Leiden,
commemorated by his brother. *See also* 4136–53.

1610 DANIËLS, C. E. (1887). Pieter Hendrik Suringar 3 januari 1813 –
13 januari 1887. *NTG,* 2de reeks, *23,* I, 81.

JAN SWAMMERDAM

1611 SINIA, R. (1878). *Jan Swammerdam in de lijst van zijn tijd* (J.S. and his
time). Thesis Leiden 178 pp. P. Geerts, Hoorn.

1612 SCHIERBEEK, A. (1920). Jan Swammerdam. *Levende Natuur, XXIV,*
(March 1), 323.

1613 — (1937). Jan Swammerdam. 12 Febr. 1637 – 17 Febr. 1680 – *NTG,
81,* I, 1025–50; *BGG, XVII,* 41–66.

1614 — (1946). *Jan Swammerdam (12 Februari 1637 – 17 Februari 1680)
Zijn leven en Werken* (His Life and Works), 280 pp., ill. De Tijdstroom,
Loghem.
– with a chapter on the geneaology of Swammerdam and some further archivalia,
by H. Engel.

1615 — (1969). *Jan Swammerdam (1637–1680). His life and works.* VI +
202 pp. Swets & Zeitlinger, Amsterdam.
– Reviewed by H. Querner: *SA, 54* (1970), 335–6; by W. Coleman: *BHM, XLIV,*
391–2. English of the previous item.

1616 — (1948). Jan Swammerdam 1637–1680. *Arch. int. d'Hist. des Sci.,
XXVIII,* 246–7.

1617 PÖHLMANN, O. (1944). *Jan Swammerdam, natuuronderzoeker en medicus*
(J.S., naturalist and physician), 208 pp., 8 pl., portr. Amsterdam.
– Translated into Dutch by H. Schaap.

1618 SCHULTHEISZ, Emil (1967). Jan Swammerdam [Hungarian]. *Orvosi
Hetilap, 108,* 1086–9.

1619 SMIT, P. (1972). Jan Swammerdam, ein holländischer Naturforscher
des 17. Jahrhunderts. *Biol. i/d Schule, 21,* 509–14.

1620 FEYFER, F. M. G. de (1923). Een ondergeschoven portret (A sup-
      posititious portrait). *NTG*, *67*, I, 57; *BGG*, *III*, 24.
      – Letter to the editor. Arguing that there does not exist a portrait of Swammerdam.
      Jan Stolk (1724–86) adapted one of the figures of Rembrant's Anatomy, passing it
      off as a portrait of Swammerdam.

1621 COLE, F. J. (1937). Swammerdam's House. *Ann. of Sci.*, *II*, 236, ill.
      – Note.

1622 — (1937). *The birthplace of Jan Swammerdam 1637–1680*. ill. 8°.
      Bruges.
      – Reprint of *Isis*, *XXVII* (3), 75.

1623 ENGEL, H. (1950–51). Records on Jan Swammerdam in the Amster-
      dam archives. *Centaurus*, *I*, 143–55, 3 ill.

1624 NORDSTRÖM, Johan (ed.) (1954–55). Swammerdamiana. Excerpts from
      the Travel Journal of Olaus Borrichius and two letters from Swammer-
      dam to Thévenot. Appendix: The History of Swammerdam's Demon-
      stration of the valves in the Lymphatic Vessels. *Lychnos*, *XV*, 21–65.

1624ª BOUQUET, H. (1912). Le mysticisme d'un anatomiste du XVII⁰ siècle.
      Jean Swammerdam et Antoinette Bourignon. *Aesculape*, 171–6, 2 ill.,
      2 ports.

1625 PAPP, D. (1962). Une expérience galvanique de Swammerdam. *Congr.*
      Hist. Sci., *1962*. also in: *Bull. signal. Hist. Sci. Techn.*, *17* (1), No 7820.
      Abstr. *Actes dixième Congrès int. d'Hist. Sciences*, Ithaca, 1962, II,
      921–3, ill. Hermann, Paris.

1626 FRANCESCINI, Pietro (1964). Il secolo de Galileo e il problema della
      generazione. *Physis*, *6*, 141–204, 18 fig.
      – Discusses also the views of Steno, Swammerdam, De Graaf and Leeuwenhoek.

1627 ENGEL, H. (1952). Jan Swammerdam as an Entomologist. *Trans.*
      Nineth. Int. Congress Entomol., *I*, 11–9, Amsterdam

1628 BRUGGENCATE, H. A. ten (1943). Johannes Swammerdam's specula-
      tiën over het haft of oeveraas (Johannes Swammerdam's speculations
      on the may-fly or ephemeron). *Nieuw Theol. T.*, *32*, 131–43.

1629 LOCY, W. A. (1901). Malpighi, Swammerdam and Leeuwenhoek. *The*
      Popular Science Monthly, *LVIII*, Nov. 1900 – April 1901, 561–84.

1630 SCHULTE, B. P. M. (1968). Swammerdam and Steno. In: G. Scherz (ed.)
      The Historical Aspects of Brain Research in the 17th Century, 35–41.
      (Analecta Medico-Historica, 3). Pergamon Press, Oxford.

1631 BELLONI, L. (1968). Swammerdams Zeichnungen des Seidenspinners, die Malpighi 1675 durch Vermittlung Stensens erhielt. In: G. Scherz (ed.). *The Historical Aspects of Brain Research in the seventeenth century*, 171–80 (= Analecta Medico-Historica, 3). Pergamon-Press, Oxford-London.

1632 STOKVIS, B. J. (1880). *Herdenking van Jan Swammerdams 200-jarigen sterfdag op 17 Februari 1880* (Commemoration of the 200th anniversary of the dying-day of S. on February, 17, 1880.

1633 POLLIN, Fr. W. (1936). *Gedenktage im Jahre 1937*, 68 pp., 8°. Welchert, Ascherleben.
    – a.o. on Swammerdam.

1634 SWAMMERDAM, J. (1667, 1927). *Tractatus physico-anatomico-medicus de Respiratione usuque pulmonum* – with Dutch translation. *Opusc.*, *VI*, 46–181.

1635 — (1737–38, 1907). *Proefnemingen van de particuliere bewegingen der spieren van den kikvorsch* (Experiments of the particular motions of the muscles of the frog). *Opusc.*, *I*, 69–97.
    – From Swammerdam's *Bijbel der Nature* (*Biblia Naturae*, 1737-38), p. 835-61.

GERARD VAN SWIETEN

1636 MÜLLER, Willibald (1883). *Gerhard van Swieten. Biographischer Beitrag zur Geschichte der Aufklärung in Österreich.* 11 + 175 pp. 8°, Wien.

1637 MUNDY, Jaromir von (1883). *Van Swieten und seine Zeit..* Wien.

1638 PETERSEN, J. J. (1901). Gerhard van Swieten. *Ugeskrift for Laeger, 8*, 25–33 and 49–57.

1639 FISCHER, C. L. (1906). Gerhard van Swieten. *Ärztl. Vierteljahresrundschau, 2*, 3–5.

1640 GERSTER, A. G. (1909). The life and times of G. van Swieten. Born 1700, at Leyden. *Bull. John Hopkins Hosp., 20*, 161–8.

1641 SWIETEN, D. L. van (1919). Gerard van Swieten, de lijfarts van Maria Theresia, en zijn geslacht (Gerard van Swieten, courtphysician of Maria Theresia, and his family). *Ned. Leeuw, XXXVII*, 5–11.

1642   — (1929?). *Dr. Gerard van Swieten und seine Vorfahren*, 15 pp., no. d., no. pl., 8°.

1642ᵃ LINDEBOOM, G. A. (1974). Zur Genealogie von Gerard van Swieten. *Clio Med.*, *9*, 45–9.

1643   LIMBURG, Rob [no d.] Gerard van Swieten. In: *Nederlanders in den vreemde*, 148–76, port. Servire, Den Haag.

1644   PROBST, G. (1931). Gerhart van Swieten. *Wien. med. Wschr.*, *81*, 487–90.

1645   SCHÖNBAUER, L. (1944). Van Swieten und seine Zeit. *Völkischer Beobachter*, 23. Jänner.

1646   ATZROTT, E. H. G. (1937). Gerhard van Swieten. "Docet et sanat". Ein Zeitbild. *Med. Welt*, *11*, 737–9.

1647   HEUVELN, H. Th. van (1942). *Gerard van Swieten. Leben, Werk und Kampf.* Thesis Groningen (Supervisor: Prof. Jhr. Dr. G. A. Kreuzwendedich von dem Borne), 64 pp. G. Keizer, Veendam.

1648   BITTNER, Chr. (1953). Le docteur Gérard van Swieten. *Trib. Med.*, Nov.

1649   JONAS, [   ] (1957). Gerard van Swieten 1700–1772. *Ars medici* (Gand), *12*, 311–4.

1650   SCHULTHEISZ, Emil (1962). Gerhard van Swieten. [Hungarian]. *Orvosi Hetilap*, *103*, 1277–80, 1 portr., 3 ill.

1651   ZAUNICK, R. (1964). Schrifttum zu Leben und Werk von Gerhard Freiherrn van Swieten. In: Glaser, H. Gerhard Freiherr van Swieten. *Sudhoffs Klassiker der Mediz. u. Naturw.*, *38*, 74–85, Leipzig.

1652   [Anonym] (1966). Gerhard van Swieten (1700–1772) Boerhaave's Boswell. *JAMA*, *198*, 1028–9.

1653   BRECHKA, Frank T. (1970). *Gerard van Swieten and his world 1700–1772.* 171 pp., 7 ill. Martinus Nijhoff, The Hague.
       – Review by E. Lesky: *Med. Hist.*, *XVII* (1973), 322–4.

1654   DUKA, N. (1972). Gerard van Swieten. [Hungarian]. *Orv. Hetil.*, *113*, 455–7, portr.

1655   KREUZINGER, V. (1922). Zum 150. Todestag Gerard van Swietens. *Janus*, *XXVI*, 177–89.

1656 SCHRÖDER, H. (1922). Gerard van Swieten. Zu seinem 150. Todestage. *Fortschr. Med.*, *50*, 421–6.

1657 BERGHOF, Emanuel (1950). Gerhard van Swieten. Gedenkworte zum 250. Geburtstage. *Wien. med. Wschr.*, *100*, 549–50.

1658 LEJEUNE, Fritz (1951). Gerhard van Swieten zum Gedächtnis. *Der Landarzt*, *27*, 238–9.

1659 ZIMMERMANN, G. (1972). Gerard van Swieten und seine Zeit. Zum 200. Todestag am 18. Juni 1972. *Dtsch. Apoth. Ztg.*, *112*, nr. 24, 929–31; also in: *Österr. Apoth. Ztg.*, *26* (1972), 359–62, ill.

1660 LESKY, E. (1972). Van Swieten, Begründer des österreichischen Gesundheitswesens. Zur 200. Wiederkehr seines Todestages am 18. Juni 1972. *Mitt. Österr. Sanitätsverw.*, *73*, Heft 7–8. 7 pp., portr., 3 ill.

1661 — und A. WANDRUSZKA (ed.) (1973). *Gerard van Swieten und seine Zeit*. Internationales Symposium ... Wien 8–10. Mai 1972. 194 pp., ill. Verlag Hermann Böhlaus Nachf. Wien-Köln-Graz.
– With contributions of E. Lesky, G. A. Lindeboom, Chr. Probst, G. Klingenstein, B. Zanobio, E. H. Ackerknecht, L. Belloni (Morgagni), G. Ricuperati (Nicolò Garelli), H. Balâzs, K. Benda, E. Wangermann; with an extensive bibliography of Van S.

1662 KLINGENSTEIN, G. (1973). Gerard van Swieten and his Time. A symposium held at the University of Vienna, 8–10 May 1972. *Med. Hist.*, *XVII*, 68–9.

1663 DEKKER, C. (1973). Gerard van Swieten und seine Zeit. Internationaal symposium gehouden te Wenen van 8 tot en met 10 mei 1972. (G. van Swieten and his time. International symposium, held at Vienna, 8–10 May 1972). *NTG*, *117*, 113–6.

1664 JUNGE, A. (1901). Gerhard van Swieten als Stenograph. *Arch. Stenogr.*, *53*, 13–22.

1665 MENTZ, A. (1903). Zu "Gerhard van Swieten als Stenograph". *Arch. Stenogr.*, *55*, 52–3.

1666 LEERSUM, E. C. van (1919). Boerhaave's dictaten, inzonderheid zijner klinische lessen. Met een beschrijving van Gerard van Swieten's stenografische nalatenschap (B.'s lectures, particularly his clinical lessons. With a description of the stenographic inheritance). *NTG*, *63*, I, 50–76.

See also 132, 228, 233

1667   LINDEBOOM, G. A. (1973). De Hollandse tijd van Gerard van Swieten (The Dutch period of —). *NTG*, *117*, 1037–42, portr.

1668   — (1972). Het consult van Gerard van Swieten voor Aartshertogin Marianne van Oostenrijk, de zuster van Maria Theresia (Brussel, 1744) (The consult of G.v.S. to Archduchess Marianne of Austria, sister of Maria Theresia (Brussels, 1744). *Sci. Hist.*, *14*, 97–111, portr.

1669   LEERSUM. E. C. van (1919). Hoe van Swieten zijn zaken regelde voor zijn vertrek naar Weenen (How Van Swieten arranged his affairs before his departure to Vienna). *NTG*, *63*, I, 2058–9.

1670   GILBERT, A. and P. CORNET (1922). L'impératrice Maria Theresia d'Autriche et son médecin Van Swieten. *Paris méd.* (annexe), *44*, 3–9.

1670ᵃ GYSEL, C. (1973). Gerard van Swieten, son oeuvre et la Belgique. *Rev. Belg. Méd. Dent.*, *28*, 451–8.

1670ᵇ GLASER, H. (1935). *Österreichs grosze Ärzte.* 71 pp., 1 ill. Bücher der Heimat, Steyerermühl-Verl., Wien. 8°.
       – also on G. van Swieten.

1671   HECKER, J. F. C. (1839). *Geschichte der neueren Heilkunde*, 614 pp. Erstes Buch: Die Volkskrankheiten von 1770. Zweites Buch: Die Wiener Schule, I, Gründung. Van Swieten, 353–97. Verlag Enslin, Berlin.

1671ᵃ LESKY, E. (1974). Van Swieten und die Chirurgie. In *Circa Tiliam*, 140–9. Brill, Leiden.

1672   KREUZINGER, V. (1924). *Gerhard van Swieten und die Reform der Wiener Universität unter Maria Theresia bis zur Errichtung der Studien-Hof-Commission.* Thesis phil., Wien.

1673   JANTSCH, Marlene (1949). Van Swieten als Begründer der Schulmedizin in Wien. *Österr. Gemeindezeitung*, *15*, Sonderheft Spitalstadt Wien, nr. 8 vom 15. April, S. 8.

1674   HOFFMANN, K. F. (1960). Gerhard van Swieten (1700–1772), der Begründer der älteren Wiener Medizinschule im 18. Jahrhundert. *Med. Monatschr.*, *14*, 535–7.

1675   MISSITS, Gheorghe (1933). *Gerhard van Swieten, primă scoală medicală vieneză si Ardealul medical din epoca tereziana-josefină.* Thesis. Cluj.

1776   LINDEBOOM, G. A. (1950). Gerard van Swieten als hervormer der Weense medische faculteit (Gerard van Swieten as reformer of the medical faculty at Vienna). *NTG, 94*, II, 1277–85; *BGG, XXX*, 12–20.

1677 LESKY, E. (1971). Wiener Krankenbettunterricht, Van Swieten und die Begründung der Medizinischen Fakultät Tyrnau. *Orvostort. Közl.*, nos. 57–59, 29–39.

1678 LEERSUM, E. C. van (1910). Een tweetal brieven van G. van Swieten over den liquor Swietenii en de kinderpokinenting (Two letters of Van Swieten on the "liquor Swietenii" and on the inoculation of smallpox). *NTG, 54*, I, 1708–25.

1679 — (1910). A couple of letters of Gerard van Swieten on the "liquor Swietenii", and on the inoculation of smallpox. *Janus, XV*, 345–71, facs.

1680 BILANCIONI, Guglielmo (1917). Le prime esperienze cliniche col Liquore de van Swieten. *Riv. Stor. crit. Sci. Med. Nat., 5*, 300–7.

1681 LECLERC, Henri (1972). La liqueur de van Swieten. *Presse méd., 30*, 1950–1.

1682 LESKY, E. (1959). Van Swietens Syphilistherapie und die Schule von Montpellier. *Bull. Soc. int. Hist. Med.*, special no. *Compt. rend., 16ᵉ Congr. int. Hist. Méd.*, vol. I, 59–62.

1683 KLEIJ, J. J. van der (1921). G. van Swieten's *Constitutiones epidemicae et morbi potissimum Lugduni-Batavorum observati. NTG, 65*, II, 33–9; *BGG, I*, 286–92.

1684 IDELER, H. (1902). *Die Pharmakodynamik van Swietens. Auf Grund seines Commentars zu H. Boerhaaves Aphorismen zusammengestellt.* Thesis. Greifswald.

1685 FRITZ, Joseph (1928). Zu G. van Swietens Kommentaren von Boerhaaves Institutionen. In: *Internationale Beiträge zur Geschichte der Medizin, Max Neuburger zur Feier seines 60. Geburtstages am 8.XII. 1928 gewidmet.*, 115–9, Wien.

1686 SEIDE, J. (1933). Die Geschwülste in den "Commentaria" des Gerardus van Swieten. *SA, 26*, 76–82.

1687 LESKY, E. (1972). Neue Dokumente zum Streit Haller-Van Swieten. *Clio Medica, 7*, 120–7.

1688 GLASER, Hugo (1948). Van Swietens Rat an die Alten. In: Festschrift zum 80. Geburtstag Max Neuburgers, 190–2. (= *Wiener Beiträge zur Geschichte der Medizin 2*). Wien.

1689   — (1964). Gerhard Freiherr van Swieten – Rede über die Erhaltung der Gesundheit der Greise (Wien 1778). *Sudhoffs Klassiker der Medizin und der Naturwissenschaften*, 38. Leipzig.

1689[a] SCHOUTEN, J. (1974). Gerard van Swieten, a Pioneer in the Field of Geriatrics. *Geront. clin.*, *16*, 231–5.

1690   LESKY, Erna (1972). Van Swieten über Kriterien des Todes. *Wien. Klin. Wschr.*, *84*, 244–5.

1691   HERSCHE, Peter (1972). Gerard van Swieten's Stellung zum Jansenismus. *Int. Kirchl. Ztschr.*, *61*, 33–5.

1692   LESKY, Erna (1973). Van Swietens Hypochondrie. Zur Berufskrankheit der Gelehrten und zur Musiktherapie. *Clio Medica*, *8*, 171–90, 1 ill.

1692[a] GYSEL, C. (1973). Gerard van Swieten, son oeuvre et la médecine dentaire. *Rev. Belg. Méd. Dent.*, *28*, 429–50.

1693   LEERSUM, E. C. van (1906). Gerard van Swieten en qualité de censeur. *Janus, XI*, 381–98; 446–69; 501–22; 588–606., ill. Reprint: 81 pp.

1694   PINKHOF, H. (1923). Een advies van Gerard van Swieten (An advice of Gerard van Swieten); *NTG*, *67*; II, 478–9; *BGG, III*, 189–90.
        – On Van Swieten's advice on Jewish physicians, midwives, etc. Review.

1695   LESKY, E. (1968). Van Swietens Vorschlag für Herman Kaau Boerhaaves Nachfolge am Zarenhof (1755). *Clio Medica*, *3*, 273–7.

1696   BONNE, H. la (1908). Voltaire et van Swieten. *Médecin*, *15*, 219.

1697   SIMILI, A. (1965). Carteggio inedito di Gerardo van Swieten con Giovanni Bianchi (Iano Planco). *Accad. Stor. Arte sanit.*, S. II, *31*, 82–91, portrs., facsims. Also in: *Rass. Clin. Ter.*, *64*, suppl. 83–91.

1698   WILLEMSE, David (1972). Gerard van Swieten in zijn brieven aan Antonio Nunes Ribeiro Sanches (1739–1754) (G.v.S. in his letters to A. Nunes Ribeiro Sanches (1739–1754)). *Sci. Hist.*, *14*, 113–43.

1699   LINDEBOOM, G. A. (1973). Acht brieven van Gerard van Swieten uit zijn Hollandse jaren (1730–1754) (Eight letters of — from his Dutch years (1730–44)). *Sci. Hist.*, *15*, 73–89, portr.

1700   — (1972). Gerard van Swieten, Herr und Landstand von Tirol. *Adler*, *9*. (XXIII.), Heft 8, 187–8.

1701   — (1973). Gerard van Swietens erster Lebensabschnitt. In: E. Lesky und A. Wandruszka (ed.) *Gerard van Swieten und seine Zeit.* 63–79. Verlag H. Böhlaus, Wien-Köln-Graz.

1702   TIETZE-CONRAT, E. (1921). Ein unbekanntes Bildnis des Gerard van Swieten. *Oud-Holland, 39,* 49–51.
       See also 2009, 4842, 5411

1703   BAKER, Frank (1909). Two Sylviuses. *Bull. Johns Hopkins Hosp., XX,* 329–39.
       – on Jac. Sylvius (1478–1555) and Franc. dele Boë Sylvius (1614–72).

1704   O'MALLEY, C. D. (1962). Jacobus Sylvius. Regimen for poor scholars. *J. Hist. Med., 17,* 141–51.

FRANÇOIS DELE BOË SYLVIUS

1705   DANA, Ch. L. (1917). Franciscus Dela Boë Sylvius. *Ann. Med. Hist.,* s. 1, *I,* 422–3.

1706   BAUMANN, E. D. (1949). *François dele Boe Sylvius.* 242 pp., portr., E. J. Brill, Leiden.

1707   BOCHALLI, R. (1954). Franz de le Boë Sylvius. *Med. Mschr., 8,* 39–40.

1708   DIENST, G. J. C. van (1960). Over leven en werken van Franciscus Deleboe Sylvius (On life and works of Franciscus Deleboe Sylvius) *Tegen Tuberculose, 56,* 4–8, portr.

1709   DANN, G. E. (1965). Beitrag zur Biographie und Familiengeschichte des Leidener Professors François de la Boë Sylvius. *Veröffent. int. Gesell. Gesch. Pharm., 26,* 29–46, ill.

1710   KING, Lester S. (1970). *The road to Medical Enlightenment 1650–1695,* 224 pp., MacDonald, London and American Elsevier Inc., New York.
       – on Franciscus dele Boë Sylvius, 93–112.

1711   BOË SYLVIUS, F. dele (1658, 1927). *Oratio inauguralis de Hominis Cognitione* – with Dutch translation. *Opusc., VI,* 1–45.

1712   KELLETT, C. E. (1961). Sylvius and the reform of anatomy. *Med. Hist., 5,* 101–6.

1713   UNDERWOOD E. ASHWORTH, (1972). Franciscus Sylvius and his Iatrochemical School. *Endeavour, XXXI,* no. 113, 73–6.
       – on the occasion of the tercentenary of the death of Franciscus Sylvius (François dele Boë Sylvius) (1615–72).

1714 SEIFFERT, O. (1907). Franciscus de le Boë Sylvius, de *Phthisi*. Neu herausgegeben und zum ersten Mal in das Deutsche übersetzt von —, Berlin.

1715 GUBSER, Alfred (1966). The Positiones variae medicae of Franciscus Sylvius. *BHM, 40,* 72–80, facs.

1716 REY, Albert (1930). *De Sylvius à Régnier de Graaf. Quelques considérations sur les idées médicales au XVIIᵉ siècle.* 86 pp. Thèse doctorat en médecine, 1929–1930, no. 126. Université Bordeaux, Bordeaux.

See also 2789, 4142

THOMAS SYDENHAM

1717 FEYFER, F. M. G. de (1924). Thomas Sydenham (1624–1924). *NTG, 68,* II, 1747–53; *BGG, IV,* 255–61, portr.

1718 WEYDE, A. J. van der (1924). Nog iets over Thomas Sydenham (Something more on —). *NTG, 68,* II, 2240–1; *BGG, IV,* 277–8.

1719 SCHLICHTING, Th. H. (1952). De wetenschappelijke methodologie van Sydenham (The scientific methodology of —). *NTG, 96,* II, 827–8; *BGG, XXXII,* 12–3.
– review of an article by R. M. Yost Jr. (1950) in: *Osiris, 19,* 84.

1720 KLEIJ, J. J. van der (1930). Thomas Sydenham en zijn verhandelingen over de hysterie (T.S. and his treatises on hysteria). *NTG, 74,* II, 4911–8; *BGG, X,* 271–8.

T

1721 (1924). Nicolaas Philip Tende loo. In: Grote, L.R. (ed.) *Die Medizin der Gegenwart in Selbstdarstellungen,* deel III, 245–79, portr. Felix Meiner, Leipzig.
– Autobiography of N. P. Tendeloo (1864–1945), professor of pathology and pathological anatomy at Leyden.

1722 THOMASSEN À THUESSINK VAN DER HOOP, E.J. (1930). *Het geslacht Thomassen à Thuessink van der Hoop.* (Genealogy of the family —).
– With data on Evert Jan Thomassen â Thuessink (1762–1832), from 1794 professor of medicine at Groningen. Reviewed by M. A. van Andel: *NTG, 75* (1931), IV, 5017–8; *BGG, XI,* 280–1.

1723 DEELMAN, H. T. (1920). De geneeskunst voor honderd jaar, ontleend aan het dagboekreisjournaal van C. B. Tilanus (Medicine hundred years ago, quoted from the diary of the journeys of —). *NTG, 64,* I, 1-79; with an introduction by C. C. Delprat.

– Christiaan Bernard Tilanus (1796-1883), father of J. W. R. Tilanus, was professor of surgery and obstetrics at Amsterdam.

1724 TILANUS, C. B. (1974). *Surgery 150 years ago* [Diary of a 19th century surgeon]. EP Publ. Ltd., Wakefield, Yorkshire.

– Reprint of no. 3406; *See also* 4232n

1725 WAL, de (1893). Prof. J. W. R. Tilanus. *NTG, 29,* [2de reeks, 37], I, 689-92.

– In commemoration of the 70th birthday of — (1823-1914), professor of surgery at Amsterdam since 1867.

ABRAHAM TITSINGH AND ISAÄC TITSINGH

1726 KRUL, R. (1891). Abraham Titsingh. Harrewarrerijen en schermutselingen tusschen Amstels Doctoren en chirurgen, in verband met het gildewezen (Squabbles and skirmishes between the Amsterdam doctors and surgeons, in connection with the guilds). *NTG, 27,* II, 429-48.

– With appendices: 1. fracture of the collum femoris. 2. m.orbicularis uteri (Ruysch). 3. professional secret. 4. title of F. Ruysch. A. Titsingh (1684-1776).

1727 GEYL, A. (1912). *Abraham Titsingh, de deken der Amsterdamsche chirurgijns* (the dean of the Amsterdam surgeons). 44 pp., *Gen. Bl. 16*de reeks, 1-44.

1728 VLES, A. B. van der (1917). Iets over Abraham Titsingh en zijne familie (Something on — and his family). *Wapenheraut, 21,* 170 and 233.

1729 CALKOEN, L. (1917). Titsingh. *Wapenheraut, 21,* 232.

1730 LIMBURG, Rob (no d.) Isaäc Titsingh. In: *Nederlanders in den vreemde,* 177-98, Servire, Den Haag.

– I. Titsingh (1744/5-1812), was trained for a surgeon, but became later a government official; as such he visited Japan twice.

1730ᵃ VINHUIZEN, J. (1916). De Brillenslijper Willem Trapman (The optician — —). *Groningen, I,* 13-7.

HECTOR TREUB

1731 KOUWER, B. J. (1904). *Prof. Hector Treub en het Nieuw Malthusianisme* (H.T. and New-Malthusianism), 16 pp., 2nd ed. Kampen.

1732 NIEUWENHUIS, A. W. (1912). Professor Dr. H. Treub. Zu seinem fünf-
undzwanzigjährigen Jubiläum am 26en Januar 1912. *Janus, XVII,* 1–2,
portr.

1733 KOUWER, B. J. (1920). In memoriam Hector Treub. *NTG, 64,* I, 1317.

1734 PEKELHARING, G. A. (1921). In memoriam Hector Treub. *Janus, XXV,*
51–3, portr.

1735 NIJHOF, G. C. (1922). In memoriam Hector Treub. geb. Voorschoten
1 Aug. 1856, overleden Utrecht 7 April 1920. *N.T. Verl. Gyn., XXVIII,*
81.

1736 DONGEN, J. A. van (1956). Rede bij de eeuwherdenking van de geboorte van Hector Treub (Oration at the 100th anniversary of the birthday of —). *N.T. Verl. Gyn., 56,* 408–21.

1737 — (1956). *Hector Treub. 1 augustus 1856 – 7 april 1920. Zijn persoon
en zijn arbeid* (personality and work). 117 pp., portr., ill., Scheltema &
Holkema, Amsterdam.

1738 BURGER, H. (1912). Hector Treub. *NTG, 56,* I, 197–9. Also in: H.
Burger (1930). *Uitgezochte opstellen en toespraken,* 525–7.

1739 [   ] (1912). *Feestbundel door vrienden en vereerders opgedragen aan
Hector Treub bij de feestelijke herdenking van zijn vijf en twintig jarig
professoraat 1887 – Leiden-Amsterdam – 1912* (Memorial volume dedicated by friends and admirers to H.T. at the commemoration of the
25th anniversary of his professorship). 705 pp., 4°, portr. S. C. van
Doesburgh, Leiden.

1739ᵃ TREUB, H. (1892). *Patient en geneesheer* (Patient and physician). 24
pp. S. C. van Doesburgh, Leiden.
– refers a.o. to the then well-known quack Sequah.

THÉODORE TRONCHIN

1740 GEYL, A. (1907). Dr. Théodore Tronchin. Een karakterteekening
(Th.T. A character sketch). *Gen. Crt., 61,* 16 and 23 March.
– rev. by C. E. Daniëls: *Janus, XII,* 358–9.

1741 — (1908). Dr. Theodor Tronchin. *SA, I,* 81–101, 289–309.

1742 LINDEBOOM, G. A. (1956). Theodore Tronchin (1709–1781). *NTG, 100,*
III, 1999–2006; *BGG, XXXVI,* 49–56, 1 ill., portr.

1743 — (1958). Tronchin and Boerhaave. *Gesnerus*, *15*, 141–50.

1744 LINT, J. G. de (1926). Une lettre de Tronchin et la méthode de l'inoculation. *Ve Congrès Int. d'Hist. Méd. (Genève 1925)*, 38–42, Genève 1926.

1745 EEGHEN, I. H. van (1957). De papieren uit de zolderbalken of Dr. Theodorus Tronchin en Jacob van Ghesel (The papers from the ceiling-beams or Theodorus Tronchin and Jacob van Ghesel). *Jbk. Amsteldamum*, *49*, 96–109, portr.

– Reviewed by A. A. G. Ham in: *AP*, no. 6 (1972), 12–4; on copies of letters, found in the house O.Z.Voorburgwal 316 at Amsterdam, from Jacob van Ghesel to his brother-in-law Th. Tronchin on the liquidation of his affairs after his departure to Switzerland (1754).

1746 LINDEBOOM, G. A. (1957). Vrouwe Trotula van Salerno (Lady Trotula of Salerno). in: *Liber amicorum van Bouwdijk Bastiaanse*, 167–71. Bohn, Haarlem.

NICOLAAS TULP

1747 THIJSSEN, Eduard Hendrik Marie (1881). *Nicolaas Tulp als geneeskundige geschetst. Een bijdrage tot de geschiedenis der geneeskunde in de XVIIde eeuw* (N.T. sketched as a physician. A contribution to the history of XVIIth century medicine). Thesis University of Amsterdam (Supervisor: A. H. Israëls), 146 pp., Schröder, Amsterdam, 4°.

1748 SCOLTEN, Adrian [translator] (1929). Nicolaas Tulp. A contribution to the History of the medical Science of the seventeenth century by Eduard Hendrik Marie Thijssen. Translated from the Dutch by —. *Med. Life*, *36*, 394–442, ill.; *39*, 297–330, portr., ill.

1749 GOLDWYN, Robert M. (1961). Nicolaas Tulp (1593–1674). *Med. Hist.*, *5*, 270–6, 2 pl.

1750 MULLER, H. A. L. (1967). Nicolaas Tulp – 11 october 1593 – 15 september 1674. *Voeding*, *28*, 361–2, portr.

1751 QUERIDO, A. (1970). Nicolaas Tulp en zijn manuscript (N.T. and his manuscript). *Spiegel Historiael*, *5*, 304–11, 12 ill.

1752 BALBIAN VERSTER, J. L. F. de (1932, 1970). Nicolaes Tulp 1593–1674. In: *Burgemeesters van Amsterdam in de 17e en 18e eeuw*, 51–7, W. J. Thieme & Cie., Zutfen (1932) "Vrienden van het Amsterdamboek", Amsterdam (1970).

See also 5242–46 (Anatomy lesson).

1753   deleted

U and V

1754   WITTOP KONING, D. A. (1960). In memoriam Georg Urdang. *Bull. Pharm.*, *XXII*, Umschlag.

1755   HAMERS, N. A. (1965). Een Katholiek lector aan de Nijmeegse Academie (A Catholic lector in Nijmegen Academy). *Numaga*, *12*, 37–40.
– Dr. Jacob Uwens taught anatomy and chemistry at the Quarterly Academy at Nijmegen, 1656–'59.

ANDREAS VESALIUS

General background

1756   NUYENS, B. W. Th. (1915). Kerk en wetenschap in Vesalius' dagen (Church and Science in Vesalius' days). *NTG*, *61*, I, 364.

1757   KNAPPERT, L. (1914). L'Eglise et la science au temps de Vésale. *Janus*, *XIX*, 420–34.

1758   — (1915). Kerk en wetenschap in Vesalius' dagen (Church and science in the time of Vesalius). *NTG*, *59*, I, 17–30 and 461.

1759   BALEN, A. van (1915). Kerk en wetenschap in Vesalius' dagen (Church and science in the time of Vesalius). *NTG*, *59*, I, 340.

1760   LUYENDIJK-ELSHOUT, A. M. (1972). De duisternis rondom Vesalius. Het veranderend patroon der geneeskunde in de Lage Landen in de zestiende eeuw (The darkness around Vesal. The changing face of medicine in the Low Countries in the 16th century). *T. Gesch.*, *83*, 390–409, ill.

Biographica

1761   DANIËLS, C. E. (1905). Andreas Vesalius. *Onze Kunst*, *II*, 16–21, portr.

1762   LEERSUM, E. C. van (1914). André Vésale. *Janus*, *XIX*, 397–409.

1763   — (1915). Andreas Vesalius. *NTG*, *59*, I, 4–15.
– Address.

1764   HOFFMAN, A. C. A. (1915). Vesalius. *NTG*, *59*, I, 265.

1765 KLEY, J. J. van der (1914). Von wo stammen die Vorfahren von Vesalius her? *Janus, XIX,* 523.

1766 — (1915). Vanwaar stammen de voorvaderen van Vesalius? (From where do the forefathers of Vesalius originate), *NTG, 59,* I, 264.

1767 RIJNBERK, G. van (1915). Andreas Vesalius, *NTG, 59,* I, 2–3.

1768 — (1915). Vesalius als proefondervindelijk physioloog (V. as an experimental physiologist), *NTG, 59,* I, 113–30.

1769 — (1917). Vésale comme physiologiste expérimentateur. *Arch. néerl. Physiol. de l'homme et des animaux,* I, 129.

1770 VETH, Jan (1915). *Andreas Vesalius en de kunst* (A.V. and Art). *Gids,* (febr.), *I,* 264–75.
      – Address delivered on the occasion of the Vesalius-commemoration 4 january 1915.

1771 SUDHOFF, K. (1920) Andreas Vesalius zu Ehren. *Verhandl. der Gesch. dt. Naturf. u. Ärzte,* 162–90, Leipzig. Also in: *SA, 21,* 131–55.

1772 ZILBOORG, G. (1943). Psychological sidelights on Andreas Vesalius. *BHM, XIV,* 562–75.

1773 EDELSTEIN, L. (1943). Andreas Vesalius, the Humanist. *BHM, XIV,* 547–61.

1774 SINGER, C. (1945). Some Vesalian problems. *BHM, XVII,* 425–37, 1 ill.

1775 LEROY, F. (1960). *Andreas Vesalius,* 214 pp., Oosterbaan & Le Cointre, Goes.
      – A "vie romancée" of Vesalius, according to Bocksteale (*Sci. Hist. 4* (1962), 106), historically not justified.

1778 SCHIERBEEK, A. (1919–20). Andreas Vesalius. *Levende Natuur, XXIV,* (1 Dec.), 225.

1779 SONDERVORST, M. F. (1964). Influence of Vesalius on the development of medical sciences in the 16th century. *Scalpel, 117,* 917–28. [French].

1780 [Anonym] (1964). Andreas Vesalius (1514–1564). *Organorama, I,* no. 3, 23–5, ill.

1780ᵃ DRIESSCHE, A. van (1954). Vesaliana. *Wetensch. Tijdingen, 14,* col. 217–8.

1781 LINDEBOOM, G. A. (1964). *Andreas Vesalius 1514–1564*. Een schets van zijn leven en werken (A sketch of his life and works). 193 pp., ill., Bohn, Haarlem, f°.

– Reviewed by M. W. Woerdeman: *NTG, 109* (1965), I, 40; *BGG, XLV*, 13.

1782 BARUCH, J. Z. (1964). Andreas Vesalius. Zijn leven en werken in historisch perspectief (His life and works in historical perspective). *GG, 42,* 253–62.

1783 — (1964). *Het leven en werken van Andreas Vesalius in het kader van zijn tijd* (Life and works of — in the framework of his time). 104 pp., ill. Pantheon Reeks, Kruseman, Den Haag.

1784 ROTH, M. (1965). *Andreas Vesalius Bruxellensis*. 500 pp., Asher & Co., Amsterdam.

– Photostatic reprint of the 1892 edition, with a preface by G. A. Lindeboom.

1785 O'MALLEY, C. D. (1965). *Andreas Vesalius of Brussels 1514–1564*. 480 pp., ill., portr. University of California Press, Berkeley and Los Angeles.

1786 FEYFER, F. M. G. de (1914). Die Schriften des Andreas Vesalius. Eine Bibliographie mit einer iconographischen Tafel und 8 Abbildungen. *Janus, XIX,* 435–507.

1787 — (1915). Lijst der geschriften van Andreas Vesalius (List of the writings of —). *NTG, 59,* I, 86–113.

1788 DONGEN, J. A. van (1965). De Incunabelen en Postincunabelen in de Bibliotheek van de Maatschappij XV. Andreas Wesalius Paraphrasis in nonum librum Rhazae... (The Incunabula and Post-incunabula in the Library of the "Maatschappij" XV.))port. *MC, 20,* 1023–4.

1789 DANKMEIJER, J. (1964). Herdenking van Andreas Vesalius (Commemoration of —). *Leids Universiteitsblad, 30,* 4.

1790 — (1964). Vesalius' betekenis voor de hedendaagse wetenschap (V.'s significance for present-day science). *Commémoration solennelle du quatrième Centenaire de la mort d'André Vésale, 10,* 19–24. Also in: *Acad. Royale de Méd. de Belgique,* 43–52, (Bruxelles).

Anatomy

1791 BOEKE, J. (1914). André Vésale comme réformateur de l'anatomie. *Janus, XIX,* 508–22.

1792 — (1915). Andreas Vesalius als hervormer der ontleedkunde (A.V. as a reformer of anatomy). *NTG*, *59*, I, 31–45.

– Address (delivered at the 400th anniversary of Vesalius), also as a reprint, Bohn, Haarlem.

1793 BROEK, A. J. P. van den (1915). Iets over de verhouding van de ontleedkunde van Vesalius tot die van Leonardo da Vinci (Something on the relation of the anatomy of — to that of —). *NTG*, *59*, I, 74–85.

1794 BALL, James Moores (1910). *Andreas Vesalius the Reformer of Anatomy*. 149 pp., Saint Louis, 4°.

1795 VERMEULEN, H. A. (1915). Andreas Vesalius, de grondlegger van de hedendaagsche ontleedkunde 1 Jan. 1515 – 1 Ian. 1915 (A.V., the founder of modern anatomy). *T. Veearts*, *XLII*, 195.

1796 BRUNN, W. von (1940). Andreas Vesalius aus Brüssel. Der Schöpfer der modernen Anatomie und sein Werk. *Brüsseler Ztg*, nr. 94, 2 oct. 1940, 1 ill.

1797 SCHMUTZER, R. (1941). Anatomische Beobachtungen bei Tisch aus Andreas Vesals "Fabrica" (1543). *SA*, *34*, 162–8.

1798 KLEIJ, J. J. van der (1943). De indirecte invloed van Vesalius op de ontleedkunde (The indirect influence of — on anatomy). *GG*, *21*, 235–9.

1799 CODELLAS, P. S. (1943). Vesalius – Valverde – Patousas: The unpublished manuscript of the first Modern Anatomy in the Greek language. *BHM*, *XIV*, 688–702, 5 ill.

1800 SCHULTE, B. P. M. (1966). Vesalius on the Anatomy of the Brain. *Janus*, *LIII*, 40–9, ill.

1801 — (1967). Vesalius on the anatomy of the brain. *Acta quarti conventus historiae scientiae medicinae, matheseos naturaliumque excolenda*, Lovanii 1964, 45–54, Brill, Leiden.

Fabrica and Epitome

1802 RIJNBERK, G. van (1915). De ontleedkundige afbeelding voor en in den tijd van Vesalius (The anatomical picture before and after —). *NTG*, *59*, I, 45–62.

1803 — (1916). Le dessin anatomique avant Vésale et de son temps. *Arch. néerl. scienc. exact. et nat.* Série III B, Tome III, 176.

1804   BOEKE, J. (1917). De platen van de Fabrica van Vesalius (The plates of the Fabrica of —). *NTG*, *61*, I, 946–7.

1805   ROZENKRANZ, K. (1937). Die Initialen in Vesals Anatomie. *SA*, *30*, 35–46, 30 ill.

1806   SCHMUTZER, R. (1938). Die Initialen in Vesals Anatomie. *SA*, *31*, 328–30.

1807   BENJAMIN, J. A. (1943). A discussion of the twenty-first illustration of the fifth book of *De Humani corporis fabrica* (1543). *BHM, XIV*, 634–51, 6 ill.

1808   BROEK, A. J. P. van den (1943). Andreas Vesalius, *De humani corporis fabrica libri VII* (1543), *NTG*, *87*, I, 28–34; *BGG, XXIII*, 1–7.

1809   IVINS, Jr, W. M. (1943). A propos of the *Fabrica* of Vesalius. *BHM*, *XIV*, 576–93.

1810   NUYENS, B. W. Th. (1944). Het oordeel van tijdgenoten en nageslacht over Vesalius en zijn *Fabrica* (The judgement of contemporaries and posterity on V. and his *Fabrica*). *NTG*, *88*, I, 27–30; *BGG, XXIV*, 1–4.

1811   LINDEBOOM, G. A. (1955). De tweede druk van Vesalius' Fabrica (1555) (The second edition of —). *NTG*, *99*, III, 2213–27; *BGG, XXXV*, 56–70, 7 ill., 3 portrs.

1812   ELAUT, L. (1964). De derde en vierde druk van Vesalius' *Fabrica*: 1568, 1604 (The third and fourth edition of — —). *Sci. Hist. 6*, 124–34.

1813   — (1965). De Franse vertaling van Vesalius' Fabrica door J. Verschaffelt (The French translation of — — by —). *Sci. Hist.*, *7*, 156–62
     – See on Verschaffelt: *Nat. Biogr. Wdbk* (Brussels), *2*, col: 903–6.

1814   SCHMUTZER, R. (1934). Vesals Darstellung des Baues der Niere. *SA*, *27*, 187–8.
     – Ein Nachtrag zur gleichnamigen Arbeit Holls im: *Arch. Gesch. Mediz. VI* (1913), 129–48.

1815   SIGERIST, H. E. (1943). Albanus Torinus and the German edition of the *Epitome* of Vesalius. *BHM, XIV*, 652–66.

1816   ELAUT, L. (1961). Nog meer bibliographische kanttekeningen bij het enig bekende Nederlandse eksemplaar van A. Vesalius' "*Epitome*"

(Some more bibliographical notes to the only known Dutch copy of
— —). *De Gulden Passer, 9*, 125–38, ill.

1817   [   ] (1569, 1947). *Dat Epitome ofte Cort Begrip der Anatomien
And. Vesalii*, uit het Latijn in het Nederduitsch naer den oprechten
zinne over-ghestellt, door Jan Wouters ... te Brugge 1569. (The Epitome or abridged edition of the Anatomy of A.V., from the Latin into
Dutch by — at Bruges). Facsimile *MKVAW*, Verhandelingen IX, no.
1, Brussel.
  – Reviewed by A. Schierbeek: *NTG, 92* (1958), IV, 3207; *BGG, XXVIII*, 10.

Dentistry

1818   GYSEL, C. (1966). Over de betekenis van Andreas Vesalius voor de
tandheelkunde (On the significance of — for dentistry). *Ned. T. Tandheelk., 73*, 68–76.

1819   — (1966, 67). Vesalius en de zestiende-eeuwse tandheelkunde. (V.
and 16th century dentistry). *Ned. T. Tandh. 73*, 399–404; 566–74;
643–50. II. Bij de vierhonderdste verjaardag van Vesalius' dood (At the
400th anniversary of — death). *Ned. T. Tandh. 73*, 729–37. III. De
culturele betekenis van de "Fabrica" (The cultural significance of the
"Fabrica"). *Ned. T. Tandh. 74* (1967), 63–8. IV. Rondom Vesalius'
brief aan Rolandus (Around – letter to —). *Ned. T. Tandh. 74*, 136–47.

1820   — (1968). André Vésale et les historiens de la médecine dentaire.
Med. et Hygiène (Genève), *26*, 590–1.

Letters

1821   RIJNBERK, G. van (1915). Vesalius' brief over het afkooksel van de
chynawortel (A Vesalian letter on the decoction of the Chyna root)
NTG, 59, I, 717.

1822   SCHULLIAN, D. H. (1953). A Vesalian letter. *J. Hist. Med., VIII*, 448,
ill.
  – Note on a letter by Vesalius to the Prince of Orange, Count of Nassau.

1823   BOEYNAEMS, P. (1964). De brief van Vesalius aan Johannes Gast (1546)
(The letter of — to —). *Sci. Hist., 6*, 164–8.
  – Johannes Gast was deacon of St. Martin's Church in Basel. Translated into Dutch.

1824   LINDEBOOM, G. A. (1963). A Vesalian letter. *Janus, L* (1961–3), 258–63.

1825   — (1964). De brief van Vesalius aan Oporinus (Letter of — to O.).
       NTG, 108, I, 28–31; *BGG, XLIV*, 10–4. Also in *TMA* 19, 144–50.

See also 1909

1826   — (1964). Twee brieven van Vesalius (Two letters of —). *NTG*, 108,
       I, 32–6; *BGG, XLIV*, 14–8.

1827   VESALIUS, A. (1539, 1929). *Epistola docens venam axillarem dextri
       cubiti in dolore laterali secandam* – with Dutch translation. *Opusc.*,
       VIII, 1–75.

1828   — Andreas (1546, 1915). Brief, behelzende de aanwending van het de-
       coct van Chynawortel (Letter, concerning the use of the decoction of
       Chyna-root), 214 pp., *Opusc.*, *III*.

1829   — (1564, 1935). *Vesalii Consilium ad Petrus Forestum* (ante annum
       1564). (With Dutch translation). *Opusc.*, *XIII*, 9–16.

Iconography

1830   GEYL, A. (1905). De echtheid van den Andreas Vesalius uit het me-
       disch-pharmaceutisch museum ontkend (The authenticity of the por-
       trait of A.V. in the medico-pharmaceutical museum denied). *Geneesk.
       Crt.*, *59*, no. 46, 371.

1831   ARKEL, G. van (1915). Een portret van Andreas Vesalius? (A portrait
       of —?). *Eigen Haard*, *XLI*, 73.

1832   VETH, J. (1923). Een portret van Vesalius door Titiaan? (A portrait of
       — by —?). *Gids*, *I*, 478.

1833   LINT, J. G. de (1914). Les portraits de Vésale. *Janus*, *XIX*, 410–9, ill.

1834   — (1915). Iets over de portretten van Vesalius (Something on the por-
       traits of —). *NTG*, *59*, I, 62.

1835   — (1925). *The Iconography of Andreas Vesalius*, with notes, critical,
       literary and bibliographical (London 1925). *NTG*, *69*, II, 2566–73;
       BGG, *V*, 307–14, ill.
       – An extensive review of M. H. Spielman's book (same title).

1836   FEYFER, F. M. G. de (1926). Een onbekend portret van Andreas Vesa-
       lius (An unknown portrait of —). *Meded. Ned. Hist. Inst. te Rome*, *VI*,
       123–32, ill. Nijhoff, 's-Gravenhage.

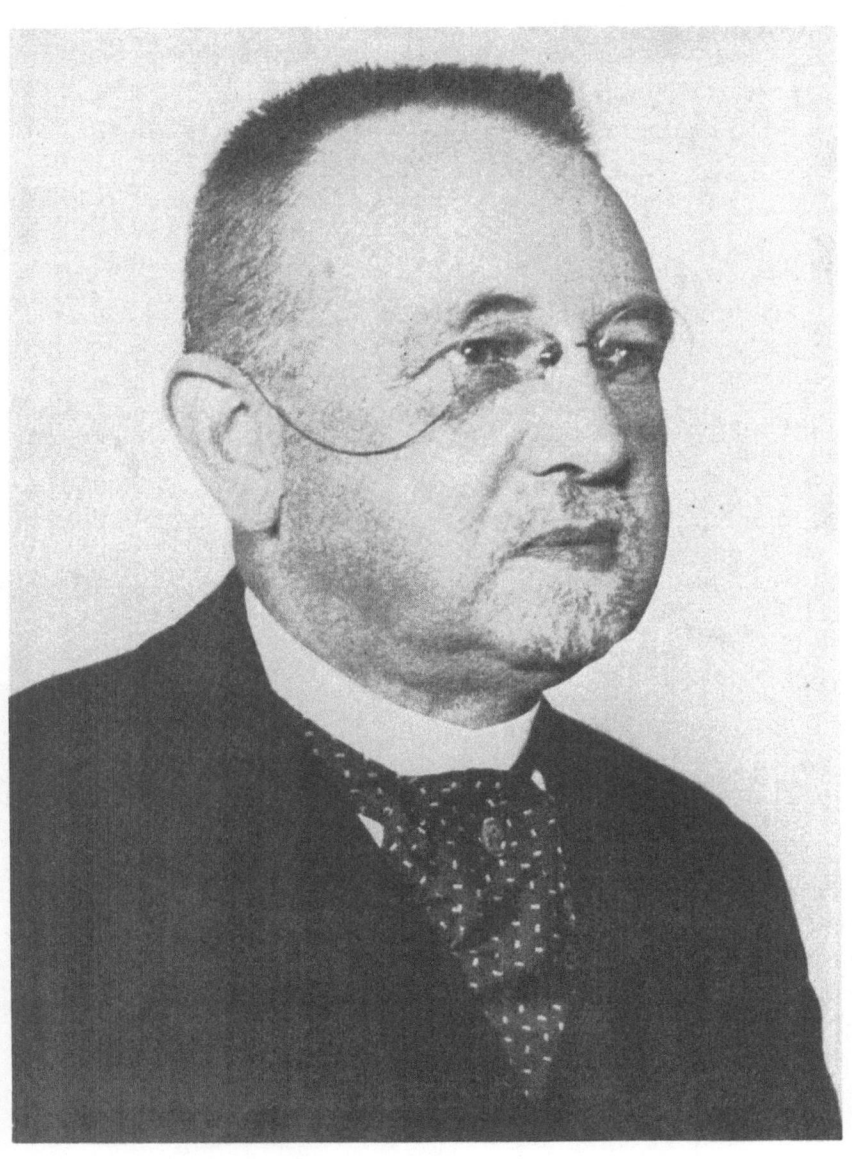

F. M. G. de Feyfer (1873–1950)

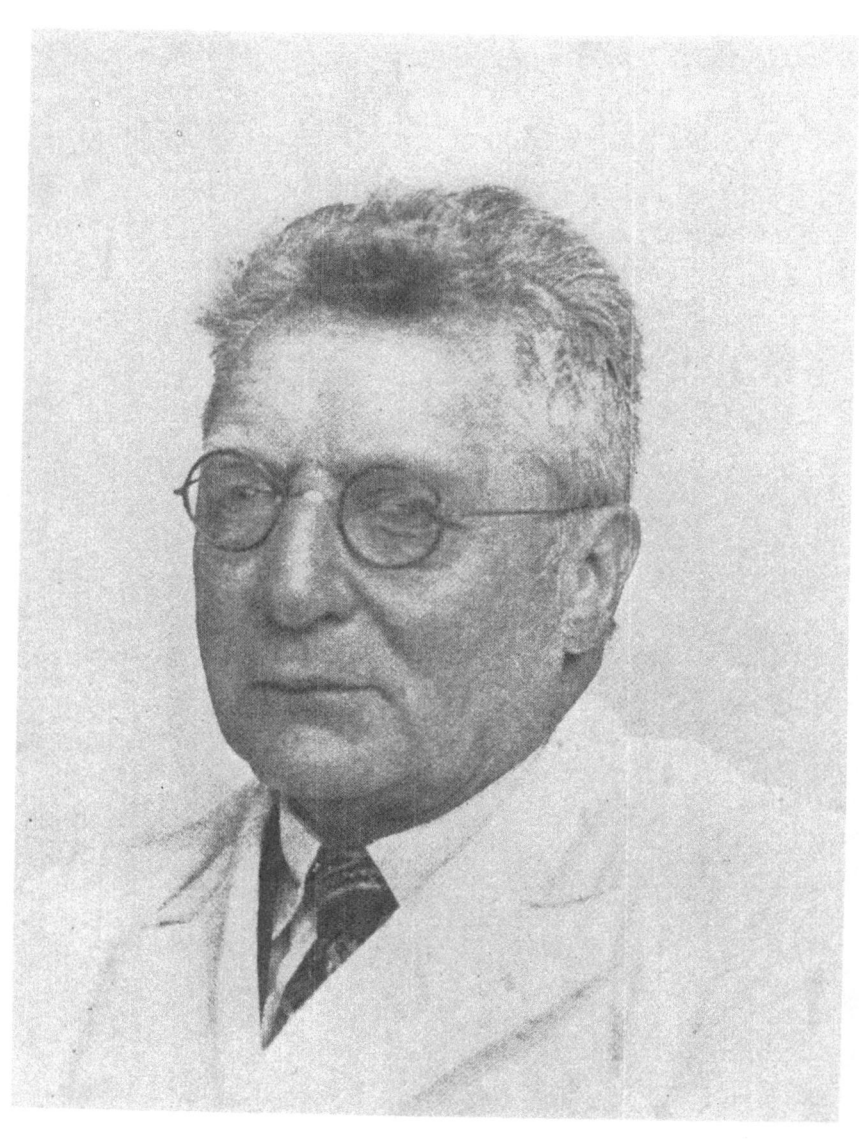

E. C. van Leersum (1862–1938)

1837 — (1926). Het nieuwe portret van Vesalius (The new portrait of —).
NTG, 70, II, 2580; *BGG, VI*, 339.
- Letter to the editor.

1838 — (1932). Een portret van Andreas Vesalius (A portrait of —). *NTG,
76*, I, 60–73; *BGG, XII*, 1–14.

Various subjects

1839 STRAUSS, Jr. W. L. and O. Temkin (1943). Vesalius and the problem of
variability. *BHM, XIV*, 609–32, 12 ill.

1840 ETZIONY, M. (1946). The Hebrew-aramaic element in Vesalius. A critical
Analysis. *BHM, XX*, 36–57.

1841 LINDEBOOM, G. A. (1963). Vesalius on Manardus. *Atti Convegno Internationale per la Celebrazione del V Centenario della nascita di Giovanni Manardo (1462–1536)*. Università degli studi di Ferrara, 182–5.
See also 5495

LEONARDO DA VINCI

1842 NIEUWENBURG, C. J. van (1914). Over de natuurkennis van Leonardo
da Vinci (On the natural science of —). *Vrag. Dag., XXIX*, 284.

1843 BROEK, A. J. P. van den (1917). Iets over de *Quaderni d'Anatomia* van
Leonardo da Vinci (Something on the *Quaderni d'Anatomia* of —).
Haarlem. *NTG, 61*, II, 277–83.

1844 — (1919). Iets over het natuurwetenschappelijk werk van Leonardo da
Vinci (Something on the scientifical work of —). *NTG, 63*, I, 1555–63.

1845 — (1919). Einiges über Harn- und Geschlechtsorgane, im besonderen
über das Koitusbild, in der Anatomie des Leonardo da Vinci. *Janus,
XXIV*, 85–100, 3 ill.

1846 DANKMEIJER, J. (1959). *Leonardo's beeld van de natuurmens* (L.'s image
of natural man), 14 pp., and 12 facsimileplates, Kon. Ned. Gist- en
Spiritusfabriek, Delft.
See also 1793, 2996, 5230, 5231

1847 KRUIZINGA, J. H. (1964). Dr. J. J. Viotta 1814–1859, geneesheer,
componist, orgelist en pianist (Physician, composer, organist and pianist). *Op de Uitkijk*, januari, 192–5.

VIRCHOW

1848   VERAART, B. A. G. (1959). Virchow en de geschiedenis (V. and history).
       NTG, 103, I, 1265; *BGG, XXXIX*, 6.

1849   STOKVIS, B. J. (1901). Virchow und die niederländische Medizin.
       Berl. Klin. Wschr., (no. 41), 1038.
       – review ed. by Pergens: *Janus, VI* (1901), 612–4.

1850   LINDEBOOM, G. A. (1958). Virchow en zijn cellulaire pathologie (V.
       and his cellular pathology). *NTG, 102*, II, 2166–70; *BGG, XXXVIII*,
       27–31, (portr.).

1851   — (1959). Virchow en de geschiedenis der geneeskunde (V. and the
       history of medicine). *NTG, 103*, I, 567–70, 2 ill.; *BGG, XXXIX*, 1–4,
       2 ill.

1852   — (1959). Virchow en de geneeskunde (V. and medicine). *NTG, 103*, I,
       567–70; *BGG, XXXIX*, 1–4.

1853   VERAART, B. A. G. (1959). Virchow en de geneeskunde (V. and medi-
       cine). *NTG, 103*, I, 1265; *BGG, XXXIX*, 6.

1854   LINDEBOOM, G. A. (1959). Virchows miskenning van Semmelweis,
       naschrift (Virchows misjudgment of Semmelweis, postscript). *NTG,
       103*, I, 1265; *BGG, XXXIX*, 6.

1855   SCHULTE, J. E. (1959). Virchow, Semmelweis en Pasteur. *NTG, 103*,
       II, 1811; *BGG, XXXIX*, 13.

1856   ELAUT, L. (1963). Een Nederlandse vertaling van Virchow's Cellu-
       larpathologie (A Dutch translation of Virchow's Cellularpathologie).
       Sci. Hist., *5*, 62–7.

1857   POSTMUS, S. (1954). Adolphe Guillaume V o r d e r m a n. 1844–1902.
       Voeding, *15*, 185–7, portr.

1857ª VERKROOST, C. M. (1972). Een vroeg negentiende-eeuws hoogleraar
       in de medische encyclopaedie, Jacob V o s m a e r (An early 19th century
       professor of medical encyclopaedia, — —) *AP*, no. 7, 29–31.

1858   VEER, P. H. de (1969). *Leven en werk van Hugo de Vries* (Life and
       work of —) Thesis R.C. University Nijmegen. VIII + 252 pp., Wol-
       ters-Noordhoff, Groningen.

See also 2836

1859 BIERENS DE HAAN, J. A. (1940). Hoe W. Vrolijk een butskop ontleed-
de (How W. Vrolijk did anatomise an Atlantic right whale). *NTG*, *84*, ,I
34–41; *BGG*, *XX*, 1–8.

1860 KRUIZINGA, J. H. (1963). Willem Vrolik. *Ons Amsterdam*, *15*, 354–9.
See also 1382a

W

JOHANNES WALAEUS

1861 STEPHENS, G. Arbour (1922). Les découvertes de Walaeus sur la circulation du sang. *Bull. Soc. Fr. Hist. Méd.*, *XVI*, 406–8.

1862 [   ] (1942). *Jan de Wale. Zwei Briefe über die Bewegung des Chylus
und Blutes an Thomas Bartholinus, Sohn des Caspar, 1640*. Übersetzt
u. erläutert von Bernward Josef Gottlieb (Klassiker der Medizin,
Bd. 33), 87 pp., 3 ill., 8°, J. A. Barth, Leipzig.

1863 SCHOUTEN, J. (1972). *Johannes Walaeus. Zijn betekenis voor de verbreiding van de leer van de bloedsomloop* (His significance for the spread of
the theory of the circulation of the blood). Thesis Free University Amsterdam (Supervisor: G. A. Lindeboom). 260 pp., 18 ill. Van Gorcum,
Assen.
– Also as a monograph. Reviewed by J. R. Prakken: *NTG*, *117* (1973), 1060; and
by W. Pagel: *Med. Hist.*, *18* (1974), 377–9.

1863[a] — (1974). Johannes Walaeus (1604–1649) and his Experiments on the
Circulation of the Blood. *J. Hist. Med.*, *XXIX*, 259–79.

1864 WALE, J. de (1650, 1922). *Epistolae duae de motu chyli et sanguinis* –
with Dutch translation. *Opusc.*, *IV*, 36–159.
See also: 2987n.

1865 KANNEGIETER, J. Z. (1964). Dr. Nicolaas Jansz. van Wassenaar
1571/2–1629. *Jbk. Amstelodamum*, *56*, 71–99.
See also 5357, 5358

1865[a] ANDEL, M. A. van (1936). Sir Henry Wellcome (1854–1936). *NTG*,
80, IV, 5447–8; *BGG*, *XVI*, 220–1.
– short commemorative note on the founder of the Wellcome Historical Medical
Museum at London.

KAREL FREDERIK WENCKEBACH

1866 HITZENBERGER, Karl (1940). Ein Wohltäter der Menschheit ist tot. [K. F. Wenckebach]. *Neues Wiener Tageblatt*, Thursday, 14 November.

1867 A. A. HIJMANS VAN DEN BERGH (1940/41). Levensbericht van Karel Frederik Wenckebach (Biographical notice of —). Jbk. *NAW*, 258–65.

1868 FALTA, W. (1940). Wenckebach zum Gedenken. *Wiener Klin. Wschr.*, 53, 1067–73.

1869 OOSTERHUIS, R. A. B. (1941). Professor Dr. K. F. Wenckebach. De geneesheer en philantroop herdacht (The physician and philantropist commemorated). *Stemmen des Tijds*, 30, 122–33.

1870 KEITH, Sir (1941). Prof. K. F. Wenckebach. *Lancet*, I, 299.

1871 HIJMANS VAN DEN BERGH, A. A. (1940). In Memoriam K. F. Wenckebach. *NTG*, 84, 4498–9, port.

1872 [Obituary] (1941). Prof. K. F. Wenckebach. *Brit. med. J.*, I, 219.
      – with some notes of Sir Thomas Lewis.

1873 RITCHIE, W. T. (1941). Karel Frederik Wenckebach. *Brit. Heart J.*, III, 141–4.

1874 WILLIUS, Frederik A. and Thomas J. Dry (1948). Karel Frederik Wenckebach (1864–1940). in: *A History of the Heart and the Circulation*, 341–6, portr., Saunders, Philadelphia & London.

1875 [   ] (1964). *Karel Frederik Wenckebach*. Franckensche Buchdruckerei, Berlin, pr. pr.

1876 [Anonymous] (1964). Karel Frederik Wenckebach 1864–1940. *Triangle*, 6, 207.

1877 [Anonymous] (1964). Prof. Dr. Karel Frederik Wenckebach (1864–1940). *Organorama*, I, no. 4, 19–21, ill.

1878 [Anonymous] (1964). Karl Friedrich Wenckebach 1864–1940. *Triangle*, 6, 207.

1879 WINCKELMANN, J. (1964). Karel Frederik Wenckebach. Zur 100. Wiederkehr seines Geburtstages am 24. März 1964. *Med. Welt.*, 641–7, portr.

1880 — (1964). Zur Erinnerung an Karel Frederik Wenckebach. *Berliner Medizin, 15,* Sonderheft 6/7, 142–4.

1881 LINDEBOOM, G. A. (1965). *Karel Frederik Wenckebach (1964–1940); Een korte schets van zijn leven en werken* (A short sketch of his life and works). 127 pp., portr., ill., letters, Bohn, Haarlem, 8°.

1882 — (1965). Karel Frederik Wenckebach. Nederlands arts van Europees formaat (Karel Frederik Wenckebach. A Dutch physician of European stature). *Elseviers Wbl.,* 16 october.

1883 — (1967). Two letters from Sir James Mackenzie to Karel Frederik Wenckebach, *Clio Medica, II,* 128–33.

1883ª — (1974). Karel Frederik Wenckebach (1864–1941) und Österreich. In: E. Lesky (ed.) (1974). *Wien und die Weltmedizin,* 214–8, port. Hermann Böhlau, Wien-Köln-Graz.

1884 LANGEN, C. D. de (1966). Karel Frederik Wenckebach (24 mai 1864 – 11 novembre 1940). *Angiologie, 18,* 5–8.

1885 KENÉZ, J. (1966). Karel Frederik Wenckebach [Hungarian]. *Orv. Hetil., 107,* 134–6.

1886 WYKLICKY, H. (1968). Vom Landarzt zum klinischen Lehrer. *Österreich. Ärztezeitung,* 25 July, front page, portr.
– on Karel Frederik Wenckebach.

1887 SCHERF, D. (1968). A cardiologist remembers. *Perspect. in Biol. Med., 11,* 615–30.
– on Karel Frederik Wenckebach.

1888 KEYS, F. E. and F. A. Willius (1942). Cardiac Clinics XCV. The achievements of Karel Frederik Wenckebach. *Proc. Staff Meeting Mayo Clinic, 17,* 330–2.

1889 PICK, E. P. (1955). Karl Friedrich Wenckebach und seine Bedeutung für die Wiener medizinische Schule. *Wiener Klin. Wschr., 67,* 636–7.

1890 SCHÖNBAUER, L. (1955). Wenckebachs Verdienste um das Institut für Geschichte der Medizin. *Wiener Klin. Wschr., 67,* 640–1.

1891 BEVERWIJK, Agatha L. van (1962). In Memoriam Prof. Dr. Johanna Westerdijk 1883–1961. *Antoni van Leeuwenhoek J. Microbiol., 28,* 1–4, portr.

1892 [   ] (1958). Bibliography of scientific publications of Prof. Dr. H. J. M. Weve. *Ophthalmology (Basel)*, *13*, 237–45.

1893 DOESSCHATE, G. ten (1962). In Memoriam H. J. M. Weve 1888–1962 (Commemoration H. J. M. Weve 1888–1962). *Bull. Soc. belge d'Ophthalm.* 303–5, portr.

1894 DOESSCHATE, J. ten (1962). To the Memory of Hendricus Jacobus Marie Weve. *Ophthalmologica*, 143, 1–3.

JOHANNES WIER (WEYER)

1895 BINZ, Karl (1896). *Doctor Johann Weyer, ein rheinischer Arzt, der erste Bekaempfer des Hexenwahns.* Ein Beitrag zur Geschichte der Aufklaerung und der Heilkunde. VII + 189 pp., portr., 1st ed. 1885 (Bonn), 2nd ed., Hirschwald, Berlin, 8°, 3rd. ed. 1972 or 1973.

1896 LEERSUM, E. C. van (1916). Joh. Wier, de bestrijder der heksenvervolgingen (— —, the fighter against witch-persecutions). *NTG, 60*, II, 963–9.

1897 KLEINE, A. O. (1931). Der Hexendoktor (Zur Erinnerung an Dr. Johann Weyer). *DMW, 57*, 1296–7.

1898 VOGEL, M. (1938). Johann Weyer. Zur 350. Wiederkehr seines Todestages am 24. Februar 1938. Zugleich ein Beitrag zur Geschichte des Skorbuts. *Hippokrates*, 270–5, 3 ill.

1899 KRONHEIMER, H. (1938). In memoriam Johannes Wier 1588–1938. *NTG, 82*, IV, 5776–7; *BGG, XVIII*, 324–5, portr.

1900 DOOREN, L. (1940). *Doctor Johannes Wier. Leven en Werken* (Life and Works). Thesis Utrecht (Supervisor: H. C. Rümke), 156 pp., De Graafschap, Aalten.

1901 — (1958). Een tot heden niet gepubliceerde brief van Johannes Wier aan Coiter (An up to the present unpublished letter of Johannes Wier to Coiter). *NTG, 102*, II, 2162–6; *BGG, XXXVIII*, 23–7, 2 ill.

1902 MORA, G. (1963). On the 400th anniversary of Johann Weyer's "De praestigiis daemonum" – its significance for today's psychiatry. *Amer. J. Psychiatry, 120*, 417–28.

1903 COBBEN, J. J. (1960). *De opvattingen van Johannes Wier over bezetenheid, hekserij en magie* (The ideas of — on demonic possession, witch-

craft and magic). Thesis Free University Amsterdam (Supervisor: G. A. Lindeboom), 193 pp., portr., Van Gorcum, Assen.
– also as a monograph.

1904 — (1966). Jan Wier 1515–1588. *GeWiNa*, *19*, 12–3.

1905 — [   ]. Johannes Wier. *Actuele onderwerpen*, no. *859*. 5–16. Stichting IVIO, Amsterdam.

1906 EHRLICH, G. E. (1960). Johann Weyer and the witches. *New Engl. J. Med.*, *263*, 245–6.

1907 PUESCHEL, E. (1958). Die "Varen" in der medizinischen Literatur seit Johann Weyer (1515–1588). In: *Medicinae et Artibus. Festschrift f. Wilhelm Katner*, Michaël Trilsch, 110–20.

1908 HABERLING, W. (1926). Rede zur Einweihung der Johann Weyer-Gedächtnistafel am Hause des Vereins der Ärzte in Düsseldorf. *Rhein. Ärzteblatt*, *XXIV*, no. 19, 2 oct.

1909 GEYL, A. (1911). Der Oporinusbrief an Johann Weyer. *Arch. f. Gesch. Mediz.*, *IV*, 425–30. See also 1825.

1910 SCHIERBEEK, A. and L. Dooren (1962). Drie tot heden niet gepubliceerde brieven van Caspar Bauhin aan Galenus Wier, zoon van Johannes, en een aan Johannes Wier zelf gerichte brief (Three letters of — to Galenus Wier (the son of Johannes) and one to Joh. W. himself, unpublished up to the present). *Jbk. Dodonaea*, *30*, 527–43, 2 facs.

1911 WIER, J. (1582, 1583, 1935). *Three letters on the state of the Countess of Berg* – English translation from the German. *Opusc.*, *XIII*, 95–106.

1912 — (1586, 1970?). *De praestigiis daemonum.* Reprint of the 1586 edition (Frankfurt) J. G. Bläschke, Darmstadt.

1913 SNELLEN, Sr. H. (1900). De operatiën van G. J. van Wij, van H. Küchler en van Wenzel (The operations of G.J.v.W., of H.K. and of W.) *Ned. Oogheelk. Bijdrage.*, no. 9, 18.
– on the instrument of Van Wij for lens extraction. G. J. van Wij (1748–1819); see also: *Bio-Lex 5*, 1010, *sub voce* Van Wij.

1914 JONGKEES, L. B. W. (1962). Sir William Wilde, zoals hij beschreven wordt door T. G. Wilson in zijn boek *A Victorian doctor* (Sir — as described by T.G.W. in his book *A Victorian doctor*). *NTG*, *106*, I, 1202–5; *BGG*, *XLII*, 29–32.
– Sir William was the father of the famous Oscar Wilde.

1915 KRUYTZER, E. M. (1962). In memoriam dokter C. Willemse, Oud-voorzitter van het Natuurhistorisch Genootschap in Limburg, lid van verdienste (Commemoration of doctor —, past-president of the Society of Science in Limburg, member of merit). *Natuurhist. Mbl.*, *51*, 59–93, portr.

1916 NUYENS, B. W. Th. (1943). Paulus de Wind, 1714–1771 als verloskun-dige (as an obstetric surgeon). *NTG*, *87*, II, 1084–9; *BGG*, *XXIII*, 47–53.

1917 ELAUT, L. (1962). "Der eingeklemmte Kopf gerettet". Das Geburts-hilfliche Instrument Paul de Winds. *SA*, *46*, 183–91.

CORNELIS WINKLER

1918 STENVERS, Sr. H. W. (1955). Winkler als neuroloog, Rede, gehouden bij de 100ste verjaardag van prof. dr. C. Winkler, op vrijdag 25 fe-bruari 1955 (W. as a neurologist. Address held at the 100th anniversary of —). *NTG*, *99*, I, 632–42; *BGG*, *XXXV*, 1–11.

1919 VALKENBURG, C. T. van (1955). Winkler als psychiater (W. as a psychiatrist). *NTG*, *99*, I, 643–7; *BGG*, *XXXV*, 12–6.

1920 WINKLER, Cornelis (1947). *Herinneringen van Cornelis Winkler 1855–1941* (Memories of —), 173 pp., portr., ill. Van Loghum Slaterus, Arnhem.
      – An autobiography. Rev. by B. Brouwer in: *Psych. en Neurol. Bladen*, *50* (1947), no. 6.

1921 NAPJUS, J. W. (1936). De hoogleeraren aan de Hoogeschool en het Athenaeum te Franeker (1585–1843): Menelaus Winsemius (The professors of medicine at Franeker Academy and Athenaeum). *NTG*, *80*, III, 3559–62; *BGG*, *XVI*, 119–22.

1922 — (1937). Een portret van Winsemius (A portrait of —). *NTG*, *81*, II, 1955; *BGG*, *XVII*, 85.

1923 — (1941). De hoogleeraren aan de Hoogeschool en het Athenaeum te Franeker (1585–1843): XX en XXI: Frederik Winter (The professors of medicine at Franeker Academy and Atheneum). *NTG*, *85*, I, 73–9; *NTG*, *85*, II, 1907–11; *BGG*, *XXI*, 1–7: *BGG*, *XXI*, 61–5, portr.
      See also 4148

1924 GROEN, J. J. and C. de Wit (1964). Martine Wittop Koning en Jeanette Polak-Kiek, twee pioniersters van de diëtistenopleiding in Nederland (M.W.K. and J.P.-K., two pioneers of the training for dietetics in the Netherlands). *Voeding*, 25, 244–7, 2 portrs.

1925 GRESHOFF, M. (1909). Nicolaas Witsen als Maecenas (N.W. as a Maecenas). *Alb. Nat.*, 125.

1926 MIJSBERG, W. A. et al. (ed.) (1950). *Prof. Dr. M. W. Woerdeman, hoogleraar in de anatomie en de embryologie aan de Universiteit van Amsterdam.* Schets van zijn wetenschappelijk werk uitgegeven ter gelegenheid van zijn 25–jarig hoogleraarschap op 18 Mei 1950 (Professor of anatomy and embryology, University of Amsterdam. A sketch of his scientific work, published on the occasion of his 25–years professorship), 132 pp., portr., No. pl.
– W., born April 10, 1892.

1927 SCHIERBEEK, A. (1921). Caspar Friedrich Wolff. *Levende Natuur*, *XXVI* (1 Nov.), 161.

1928 EMMERIE, A. (1953). Prof. L. K. Wolff (1879–1938). *Voeding*, *14*, 397–9, portr.

1929 TILANUS, J. W. R. (1905). *Herinneringswoord over wijlen prof. C. L. Wurfbain* (Commemoration —), Amsterdam.

1930 [editorial] (1970). Dr. W. A. H. van Wylick. *Gamma*, 20, 289.

Y

JOHAN YPERMAN

1931 LEERSUM, E. C. van (1912). Meester Jan Yperman, Vlaamsch chirurg uit de 14de eeuw (Master —, a Flemish surgeon from the 14th century). *NTG*, *66*, II, 1712.

1932 — (1913). Notes concerning the life of Jan Yperman. *Janus*, *XVIII*, 1–15, 1 ill.

1933 — (1914). Note concernant l'année de la mort de Jan Yperman. *Janus*, *XIX*, 33–4.

1934 — (1909). Est-ce en 1310 que Jan Yperman est mort? *Janus*, *XIV*, 393–8.

1935 — (1905). Bemerkungen über Broeckx' Ausgabe der Chirurgie des Jan Yperman. *Janus*, *X*, 544–9, ill.

1936 — (1912). De "Cyrurgie" van Meester Jan Yperman. Naar de hand-
schriften van Brussel, Cambridge, Gent en Londen uitgegeven door —
(The "Cyrurgie" of Master —. After the manuscripts of Brussels,
Cambridge, Gand and London edited by —). Bibliotheek Middel-Ned.
Letterk., 285 pp., 6 ill., 8°. Sijthoff, Leiden. (no. d.).
– Reviewed by E. Pergens: *Janus, XVIII* (1913), 86–8.

1937 — (1913). Master Jan Yperman's Cyrurgia. *Janus, XVIII*, 197–209.

1938 TABANELLI, Mario (1969). *Jehan Yperman, padre della chirurgia fia-
minga*. Bibl. Revista Storia Scienze Mediche, 360 pp., 17 pl., Leo S.
Olschki, Firenza.
– Reviewed by D. de Moulin: *Epistème, III* (1969), 277–8.

1939 ELAUT, L. (1972). *De Medicina van Johan Yperman* (The Medicina
of Johan Yperman), 151 pp., 1 facs. Naar het middelnederlands HS.
15624–41 (14e eeuw) uit de Koninklijke Bibliotheek te Brussel.) (After
the Middle Dutch manuscripts 15624–41 (14th century) from the Royal
Library at Brussels). E. Story-Scientia P.V.B.A., Gent.
– Reviewed by W. Braekman: *Sci. Hist.*, *14* (1972), 61–3.

1940 — (1972). Etymologie en betekenis van enige leen- en bastaardwoorden
in de vaktaal van Johan Ypermans *Medicina* (Etymology and significance of some loan-words in the professional language of — — —).
Leuvense Bijdr., *61*, 13–28.

1941 HOMBLÉ, A. G. (1972). De Phlebotomie en de invloed van de maan-
gestalten in de "Cyrurgie van Jehan Yperman" (1260–1333?) naar de
handschriften van Brussel, Londen, Gent en Cambridge (Phlebotomy
and the influence of the phases of the moon in the "Cyrurgie of —
after the manuscripts of Brussels, London, Ghent and Cambridge).
Oostvlaamse Zanten, XLVII, no. 1, 1–18, ill.

1942 METZ, A. de (1939). *Jehan Yperman* – La chirurgie, Livre I and II,
Paris.

1943 LAFAUT, J. (1869). Jan Yperman – vader der heelkunde in Vlaanderen
(Jan Yperman – father of surgery in Flanders). *Soc. d'Hist. de la ville
d'Ypres, IV*, 34.

1944 DEWACHTER, P. J. (1863). De la chirurgie de maître Jehan Yperman. *Ann. Soc. Médec.*, Anvers, 521.

See also 1972

Z

1945 DANIËLS, C. E. (1903). *Levensbericht van T. Zaayer* (Biographical notice of T. Zaayer). Leiden, 8°.

1946 KASTLER, Alfred (1966). Notice nécrologique sur Frits Zernike. *Compt. Rend. hebd. Séances acad. Sciences.*, *263*, 7–9.
– Zernike, physicist, was the inventor of the "phase-contrast" microscope. (Nobel-prize 1953).

1947 GROENEWOLD, H. J. (1966). In memoriam Prof. Dr. F. Zernike. *Ned. T. Natuurk.*, *32*, 77–9, portr.

1948 KAMPEN, N. G. (1966). Frits Zernike, *Nature*, *211*, 465.

1949 TOLANSKY, S. (1967). Frits Zernike: 1888–1966. *Biogr. Mem. Fellows Roy. Soc.*, *13*, 393–402.

1950 KLAY, D. (1951). Hertog Karel neemt Hendrik van Zitterd aan tot zijnen medicijnmeester, 15 augustus 1500 (Duke Karel engages H. van Z. as his physician, August 15, 1500). *NTG*, *95*, 2202; *BGG*, *XXXI*, 41.

1951 BURGER, H. (1922). Zilveren ambtsfeest van Professor Zwaardemaker (Silver professional feast of —). In: H. Burger (1930). *Uitgezochte opstellen en toespraken*, 311–9.
– Address delivered on October 10, 1922 in the Physiological Laboratory at Utrecht.

1952 KOOPMAN, J. (1938). Een collega en musicoloog uit de 15e eeuw Hendrik Arnaut van Zwolle (A colleague and musicologist from the 15th century — of Z.). *GG*, *16*, 485–6.

C. Surgeons

1953 [   ] (1550, 1935). *Master Arent and Master Albert, barbers. Visum repertum. Opusc.*, *XIII*, 1–8.

1954 BROUWERS, J. (1969). Guillaume Berckenbosch – chirurgijn te Smeermaas (1740). (— —, surgeon at S.). *Limburg*, *48*, 132–5.

1955 DONKERSLOOT, H. (1933). *Willem Donkersloot, stads-chirurgijn, operateur en heelmeester te Rotterdam, 1758–1824. Een levensschets.* (— —, town-surgeon, operating surgeon, and surgeon at R. A sketch of his life). [Rotterdam].

1955ᵃ Zɪᴊʟ, H. van (1974). met schuldige eerbiedigheit... Durgerdam en de chirurgijns in 1738 (with due respect... D. and the surgeons in —). *Ons Amsterdam, 26*, 216–7, 2 ill.

1955ᵇ Rɪɴɢoɪʀ, D. J. B. (1974). Een Durgerdamse chirurgijn in de 18de eeuw (A Durgerdam surgeon in the 18th century). *Herv. Durgerdam, 27* no 6, 6–9.
    – on Anthonie Egberts.

1956   Andel M. A. van (1919–20). J. H. Francken, een reizende meester in de 18de eeuw (— —, a travelling master in the 18th century). *Med. Wbl., 26*, 349, 361 and 373.

1957   Oᴜᴅsᴄʜᴀɴs Dᴇɴᴛᴢ, F. (1931) Van slaaf tot geneesheer (From slave to physician). *De West-Indische Gids*, July-August.
    – on Adolf Frederik Gravenbergh (1811–1906), from 1855 city surgeon in Surinam. Reviewed by F. M. G. de Feyfer: *NTG, 75* (1931), IV, 5506–7; *BGG, XI*, 301– 2.

1958   Hᴀᴀs, J. H. (1893). Gerard ten Haaff. *NTG, 29*, I, 906–9.
    – G. ten Haaff (1720–91), surgeon, lithotomist at Delft.

1959   Pɪᴊᴘᴇʀ, C. and H. Zwarenstein (1922). The "Account-book" of Jan Haszing. *Janus, XXVI*, 317–33.
    – Jan Haszing was a Dutch-speaking surgeon who practiced at Capetown in the middle of the 18th century.

1959ᵃ Dᴜᴅok ᴠᴀɴ Hᴇᴇʟ, S. A. C. (1970). Rembrandt in de verzameling van de chirurgijn Jacob Fransz. Hercules (— in the collection of the surgeon — —). *Amstelodamum, 57*, 45.

1960   Bʀoᴜᴡᴇʀs, J. (1966). Een vermaard chirurgijn: Meester Matthijs Hollenders uit Hoepertingen (17e eeuw) (A famous surgeon: Master — — from H. (17th century)). *Limburg, 45*, 222–4.

1961   Wɪᴇʀsᴜᴍ, E. van (1918). Een receptenboek van Barent Hovius, chirurgijn te Rotterdam (A prescription-book of — —, surgeon at R.) *NTG, 62*, II, 1300–7.
    – with reference to this article a letter to the editor by J. Ph. Elias (same title), relating some prescriptions of Thomas Willis (1621–75): *NTG, 63* (1919), I, 408; and another letter by W. J. F. Nuyens, entitled Een aphorisme van Barent Hovius (An aphorism of — —). *NTG, 63*, I, 479.

1962   Hᴜʟsᴍᴀɴ, G. (1966). Frederik Willem Krieger, heelmeester (F.W.K., surgeon). *NTG, 110*, 18–20.

1963   Zᴜɪᴅᴇɴ, D. S. van (1919). Een overeenkomst tussen [de chirurgijn)

Corn. Sasbout en G. van Dulcken (An agreement between [the surgeon] C.S. and G. van D.). *NTG, 58*, II, 2047;

See also 4625

1964 BAUMANN, E. D. (1919). *Een Haarlemsche Chirurgijn uit de XVIIde eeuw* [Wouter Schouten] (A Haarlem surgeon from the 17th century) no. pl., 36 pp., 8°.

1965 BEYERMAN, J. J. (1936). Mr. Nicolaes Servaessen chirurgijn en Janneken Joosten vroedvrouw, getuigen... (Mr. N.S., surgeon and J.J., midwife, testify...) *NTG, 80*, III, 3172; *BGG, XVI*, 116.
– certificate of the absence of small-pox.

1966 HOEVEN, J. van der (1936). Arnoldus Soek (1760–1795), "beroemd heel- en vroedmeester te Leiden" ("famous surgeon and accoucheur at Leiden"). *NTG, 80*, IV, 5027–33; *BGG, XVI*, 177–83.

1967 ROEKEL, G. van (1940). De Jisper ledenzetter (The limb-setter of Jisp). *NTG, 84*, III, 2562–3; *BGG, XX*, 118–9.
– On Willem Thomasz (d. 1613) a famous setter of the small Noord-Holland village Jisp, where also other setters have been active.

1968 KATE, W. ten (1937). Verzoekschrift van Hendrik van Ulhoorn operateur (Uit de notulen van de Staten van Overijsel, 9 april 1731) (Petition of —, surgeon. (From the minutes of the States of Overijsel, April 9, 1731)). *NTG, 81*, II, 965–6; *BGG, XVII*, 95–6.

1969 BISSELING, G. H. (1922). Uit "De aanmerkingen van Hendrik Ulhoorn" (From "the considerations of —"). *NTG, 66*, II, 2608–20; *BGG, II*, 352–64.

1970 SCHEER, Hermann (1925). *Meister Peter Volck aus Holstein; Wunderarzt zu Delft. Vorrede zu seiner Uebersetzung des ersten Buches des grossen Wundarznei des Theophrast von Hohenheim.* Inaugural Dissertation, 27 pp., Leipzig.
– On the Preface of the Dutch translation of Paracelsus' *Grosze Wundarznei* (Antwerp, 1555) by Peter Volck (d. 1572).

1971 WAAL, H. van der (1959). Albertus Welcker (Alkmaar, 11 januari 1884 – Amsterdam. 11 juli 1957). *Jbk. Mij Ned. Letterk. Leiden, 1958–1959*, 109–14, Brill Leiden.
– Welcker was an Amsterdam surgeon.

See also 1931–44 (J. Yperman), 3443, 3460–93.

D. Military physicians

1972 HANEVELD, G. T. (1964). De eerste met name genoemde legerartsen van Nederlandse afkomst (The first Army physicians of Dutch origin called by name). *Ned. MGT, 17,* 407–9.

– Jan Yperman and Volcher Coiter.

1973 SONDERMEYER, F. A. J. (1959). Dr. Johan Christaan Basting. *Ned. MGT, 12,* 153–8, portr.

– Dr. Basting (1817–70), military physician, translated the book of Henry Dunant *Un souvenir de Solférino* into Dutch, and played a role in the foundation of the Red Cross, in Geneva as well as in the Netherlands.

1974 BEERSTECHER, H. J. P. (1964). Petrus Lambertus Beckers, inspecteur van de geneeskundige dienst der landmacht van 5 maart 1841 tot 8 november 1950 (Inspector of the medical corps of the land-forces). *Ned. MGT, 17,* 57–8, portr.

1975 — (1964). Josephus Chrysostomus Bernardus Bernard, inspecteur-generaal van de geneeskundige dienst van land- en zeemacht van 15 September 1824 tot 5 Maart 1841 (General inspector of the medical corps of the army and navy). *Ned. MGT, 17,* 55–6, portr.

– J. C. B. Bernard (1774–1852), professor of medicine at Leyden (1817–24).

1976 — (1964). Jan Binnendijk (1842–1924). Inspecteur van de Geneeskundige Dienst der Landmacht van 11 juli 1902 tot 1 november 1905 (Inspector of the medical Corps of the Army). *Ned. MGT, 17,* 176–7.

1977 VEERSEMA, H. J. (1957). S. J. Brugman (1763–1819). *Ned. MGT, 5.*

1978 — (1954). *Sebald Justinus Brugman.* (1763–1819).

– Edition of the Nederlandsche Roode Kruis.

1979 — (1964). Sebald Justinus Brugman. *Ned. MGT., 17,* 1–6 portr.

– S. J. Brugmans (1763–1819), son of a Franeker professor of philosophy. As professor at Leyden (1786–1813), he taught several disciplines (botany, physics, natural history, chemistry). General Inspector of the medical corps of the Army in the North and South Netherlands, 1814, he deserved well after the battle at Waterloo.

1980 Esso Bzn., I. van (1940). Gevatte antwoorden (Clever answers). *NTG, 84,* III, 3516; *BGG, XX,* 143.

– Two answers of S. J. Brugman (1763–1819).

1981 BEERSTECHER, H. J. P. (1964). Carel Joan van der Burcht van Lichtenbergh, inspecteur van de geneeskundige dienst der landmacht van 2 Mei 1892 tot 1 Juli 1898 (Inspector of the medical corps of the Army). *Ned. MGT.*, *17*, 96–7, portr.

1982 — (1964). Hermanus Franciscus Ambrosius Giesbers, inspecteur van de geneeskundige dienst der landmacht van 23 October 1905 – 28 April 1908 (Inspector of the medical corps of the Army). *Ned. MGT.*, *17*, 177–8, portr.
– H. F. A. Giesbers (1843–1923).

1983 — (1964). Franz Joseph Harbaur, inspecteur-generaal van de geneeskundige dienst van land- en zeemacht van 22 Augustus 1819 tot 26 Maart 1824 (General-inspector of the medical corps of the Army and Navy). *Ned. MGT.*, *17*, 21–2, portr.
– F. J. Harbaur (1776–1824), Rector of the University of Louvain, 1817–19.

1984 — (1964). Alexander Willem Michiel van Hasselt, inspecteur van de geneeskundige dienst der landmacht van 23 Maart 1873 tot 26 Augustus 1880 (Inspector of the medical corps of the Army). *Ned. MGT.*, *17*, 91–2, portr.
– A. W. M. van Hasselt (1814–1902).

1985 — (1964). Cornelis Johannes van Hees, inspecteur van de geneeskundige dienst der landmacht van 26 Augustus 1880 tot 4 Mei 1886 (Inspector of the medical corps of the Army). *Ned. MGT.*, *17*, 93–5, portr.
– C. J. van Hees (1814–94).

1986 — (1964). Klaas Hennes, inspecteur van de geneeskundige dienst der landmacht van 28 April 1908 tot 15 April 1910 (Inspector of the medical corps of the Army). *Ned. MGT*, *17*, 178–9, portr.

1987 STOPPELAAR, P. de (1958). Cornelis de Mooy (1834–1926)., *Het Reddingswezen*, *47*, 7–10, ill.
– de Mooy was a pioneer of first aid, who made some apparatus for transport and nursing of sick and wounded people.

1988 SYPKENS SMIT, J. H. (1958). Cornelis de Mooy 1834–1926. *GeWiNa*, no *3*, 21–2.

1988ª — (1974). Cornelis de Mooy, Arzt und Erfinder (1834–1926). In: *Proc. XXIII Int. Congr. Hist. Med., London 2–9 Sept. 1972*, Vol. I., 483–7. Wellcome Institute of the History of Medicine, London.

1989 BEERSTECHER, H. J. P. (1964). Wilhelmus Theodorus Philipsen in-

specteur van de geneeskundige dienst der landmacht van 28 Juni 1898
16 Juli 1902 (Inspector of the medical corps of the Army from — till
—). *Ned. MGT.*, *17*, 175.

1990 — (1964). Jacob Johannis Sas, inspecteur van de geneeskundige dienst
der landmacht van 26 October 1865 tot 23 Maart 1873 (Inspector of
the medical corps of the Army from — till —). *Ned. MGT.*, *17*, 61–2,
portr.
– J. J. Sas (1808–74).

1991 — (1964). Louis Philip Jacob Snabilié, inspecteur van de geneeskun-
dige dienst der landmacht van 31 januari 1851 tot 5 October 1865
(Inspector of the medical corps of the Army) *Ned. MGT.*, *17*, 59–60.
– L. Ph. J. Snabilié (1797–1865).

1992 HANEVELD, G. T. (1969). Officieren-arts – Natuuronderzoekers (Medical officers-investigators of nature). *Ned. MGT.*, *22*, 183–5.

See also 1052–54 (Larrey), 1239–55 (A. Mathijsen).

E. Naval surgeons

General

1993 HANEVELD, G. T. (1961). De vroegste zeevarende artsen, tot 1500 na
Christus (The earliest seafaring physicians, till 1500 A.D.) *NTG*, *105*,
I, 37–9; *BGG*, *XLI*, 5–7.

1994 SCHOUTE, D. (1923). Gescheurde beelden (Torn pictures). *NTG*, *67*,
II, 1603–4; *BGG*, *III*, 257–8.
– A reflection on the picture we have, for example, of the former ship's surgeons.

1994[a] KOPUIT, R. (1974). Scheepsarts in dienst van de compagnie (Naval
physician in the service of the Company). *Organorama*, *11*, no 3, 16–22.

Biographical

1995 BIJL, A. (1966). Simon Bake, 1724–1772. Een Rotterdamse marine-
dokter die de Deij van Algiers met kaneelwater kureerde (A Rotterdam naval surgeon, who healed the Dey of Algeria with water of cin-
namon). *Rott. Jbk.*, 7de reeks, *4*, 238–48.

1996 SCHOUTE, D. (1948). Scheepschirurgijns-journaal van een slavenschip
der Middelburgse Commercie Compagnie (log-book of a ship's-sur-

geon of a slave-ship of the Middelburg Commercial Company). *NTG*, *92*, IV, 3645–62; *BGG*, *XXVIII*, 19–36.

– on the journal (1761–63) of Petrus Couperus, naval surgeon, of his voyage on "De Eenigheyt".

1997 STAPEL, F. W. (1927). *Pieter van Dam's beschryvinge van de Oostindi-sche Compagnie. Eerste boek, Dl I* (P.v.D.'s description of the East-Indian Company. First Book. Vol. I). 772 pp., Rijksgeschiedkundige publicatiën, Martinus Nijhoff, The Hague.

– with some particulars on the medical service; reviewed by A. J. van der Weyde: *NTG*, *73* (1939); *BGG*, *XIX*, 335–6.

1998 FONTAINE VERWEY, H. de la (1972). De scheepschirurgijn Exqueme-lin en zijn boek over de flibustiers (The naval surgeon — and his book on the buccaneers). *Jbk. Amstelodamum*, *64*, 94–116, 7 ill.

1998ᵃ MOULIN, D. de (1974). Uit 't leven van een Hollandse scheepschirur-gijn uit de zeventiende eeuw (From the life of a Dutch naval surgeon from the 17th century). In: *Circa Tiliam*, 211–29. Brill, Leiden.

– on Nicolaus de Graaff (ca 1620 – ca 1701).

1999 SCHOUTE, D. (1953). Het scheepsjournaal van Robertus Padtbrugge, 1670–1671 (The log-book of —). *NTG*, *97*, II, 1135–41; *BGG*, *XXXIII*, 17–23.

2000 BOERMA, N. J. A. F. (1942). Van een opper-barbier die een deugniet was (From a chief-barber, who was a rascal). *NTG*, *86*, I, 33; *BGG*, *XXII*, 12.

– Jacob Veeger, naval surgeon at the ship Mauricio.

2001 JENSEN, J. N. J. (1916). Van een Duitschen arbeider op Hollandsche schepen in de 18e eeuw (On a German labourer on board Dutch ships in the 18th century). *Nederl. Zeewezen*, no. 20 (15 oct.); no. 22 (15 nov.).

– On Adrian Gottlieb Volckart.

F. Quacks

2002 HAGELAND, A. van (1962). Dokter of kwakzalver? Martin van But-chell *b.* 1735 (Physician or quack?). *Periodiek 17*, 70–2.

2003 WIELEN, P. van der (1915). Beroemde kwakzalvers (de Graaf de St. Germain) (Famous quacks (the Count of —). *Mndbl. v. Bestrijd. Kwakz.*, *35*, no 5 (mei).

2003^a LANGEVELD, L. A. (1930). *Der Graf von Saint Germain.* Den Haag.

2003^b RIJNBERK, G. van (1939). *Saint Germain in de brieven van zijn tijdgenoot
den Prins Karel van Hessen Cassel* (St. G. in letters of his contemporary,
Prince Charles of H.C.). 29 pp. Servire, Den Haag.
- Reprint from *Uitzicht1*, 241–50; 273–87; Saint Germain (?–1784), a quack who
also founded a factory for dyeing cotton at Moscow.

2004 HEUPERS, E. (1964). Jan Muus, de laatste medicijnman van Soest
(The last medicine-man from Soest). *Neerlands Volksleven, 14,* 281–6.
- Jan Muus (1846–1922).

2005 VERZIJL, Jan (1959). Pater Joannes Neijt, minderbroeder (Father —,
Minorite). *Bijdr. Gesch. Prov. Minderbroeders in de Nederl., 11,* 196–7.
- The Franciscan friar of a monastery near Maastricht gave medicines for further-
ing fertility to the town-midwives. A difference arose (1770).

2006 DANIËLS, C. E. (1907). Giovanni Francesco Pivati. Un charlatan de
bonne foi? *Janus, XII,* 129–39.

2007 ZUIDEN, D. S. van (1916). Niets nieuws onder de zon (Nothing new
under the sun). *NTG, 60,* II, 506–7; 1042–4.
- On a quack Jacques Raynaud (*ca* 1778) who pretended to be able to cure cancer
of the mouth without operations (The Hague).

2008 BITTER, H. (1912, 1913). Claes of (or) Nicolaas Tilly als uitvinder van de
Haarlemmerolie (As an inventor of the Haarlem oil). *Maandbl. t.
Kwakzalv.*, no. 11 and 12; 1913: no. 4.

                                    See also 4564–82 (Quackery)

G. Pathographies

Scientists, Artists and Statesmen

2009 SIMON, Carl W. and M. T. Arco (1959). Das Ende Adrians VI (2. März
1459 – 14. September 1523). Ein medizinisch-historischer Versuch.
Med. Monatschr., 13, 303–6.
- Adrianus VI, the only Dutch Pope, would have died from general infection by
staphylococci.

2010 SOLETO, R. (1968). La maladie des yeux de Charles Bonnet dans sa
correspondance avec van Swieten. In: *Verhandlungen des XX. Inter-*

nationalen Kongresses für Geschichte der Medizin Berlin, 22. – 27. August 1966, 848–9. G. Olms, Hildesheim.
– Ch. Bonnet (1720–93), Swiss naturalist.

2011 HEMPHILL, R. E. (1965). The personality and problem of Hieronymus Bosch. *Proc. Roy. Soc. Med.*, *58*, 137–44.

2012 PLOKKER, J. H. (1972). Jérome Bosch et sa vision du monde. *55*, no. 8, 3–65, ill.

2013 ANDEL, M. A. van (1925). De Zeeuwsche koorts van Jacob Cats (The Zealand fever of Jacob Cats), *NTG*, *69*, I, 1127–32; *BGG*, *V*, 60–5.

2014 AARDWEG, G. J. van den (1965). De neurose van Couperus (The neurosis of —). *Ned. T. Psychol.*, *20*, 293–307.

2015 DOESSCHATE, G. ten (1946). Leed Dürer aan strabismus? (Did D. suffer from strabismus?). *NTG*, *90*, IV, 1969–72; *BGG*, *XXVI*, 50–3.

Erasmus

2016 O'MALLEY, C. D. (1970). Some incidents in the medical history of Desiderius Erasmus. *Essays in biohistory ... presented ... to Frans Verdoorn*, 153–62.

2017 MEURON-LANDOLT, M. de (1967). Erasme insolite. *Hist. de la Méd.*, *17*, no. 1, 2–40, 25 ill., 1 portr.
– on the skeleton and the cranium of E.

2018 BAUMANN, E. D. [n.d.]. *Medisch-Historische Studiën over Des. Erasmus*, 82 pp., portr., Arnhem.

2019 DEELMAN, H. T. (1948). Het skelet van Erasmus (The skeleton of Erasmus). *NTG*, *92*, IV, 3663–7; *BGG*, *XXVII*, 37–41.

2020 FEIS, O. (1921). Die Pesterkrankung des Erasmus von Rotterdam. *Dtsch. Arch. klin. Med.* B5, Heft 5.

2021 SCHENK, V. W. D. (1947). *Erasmus'* karakter en ziekten (Erasmus' character and diseases). *NTG*, *91*, I, 702–8; *BGG*, *XXVII*, 1–7.

2022 WERTHEMANN, A. (1930). *Schädel und Gebeine des Erasmus von Rotterdam*. 80 pp. 13 ill. Birkhäuser u. Cie, Basel.

2023 — (1965). Grabstätte, Schädel und Gebeine des Erasmus von Rotterdam. *Mediz. Monatsspiegel*, 27–33, ill.

2024 VELTHEER, W. (1970). Een historische botafwijking (bij Erasmus van Rotterdam) (An historic case of bone disease (Erasmus of Rotterdam)). *NTG*, *114*, 1313–4.

2025 GYSEL, C. (1969). Craniofacial morphology of Erasmus of Rotterdam [French]. *Europ. orthodont. Soc. Rep. Congr.*, 465–8.

See also 734–62

Vincent van Gogh

2026 SHIKIBA, R. (1932). *Vincent van Gogh, His life and Psychosis.* 2 vols., Tokyo.

2027 BETT, W. R. (1954). Vincent van Gogh (1853–90), artist and addict. *Brit. J. Addict.*, *51*, 7–14, bibliogr.
      – Followed by discussion.

2028 VALLERY-RADOT, P. (1955). La vie tourmentée de Vincent van Gogh (1853–90): les dernières années (1888–1890), d'après les lettres à son frère Theo. *Presse méd.*, *63*, 279–80, portr.

2029 MIREK, R. (1965). Personality of Vincent van Gogh. *Przegl. lek.*, *21*, 467–70. [Polish].

2030 PEERY, I. H. (1947). Vincent van Gogh's Illness. A Case Record. *BHM, XXI*, 146–72.

2031 RIESE, W. (1927). Vinzent van Gogh in der Irrenanstalt. Krankheiten und Kunstwerk. *D. mediz. Welt*, nr. 36, 1381.

2032 ROELANDT, L. (1954). Les maladies de Vincent van Gogh. *Aesculape*, *35*, 73–8, ill.

2033 GASTAUT, H. (1956). La maladie de Vincent van Gogh envisagée à la lumière des conceptions nouvelles sur l'épilepsie psychomotrice. *Ann. méd. psychol.*, *114*, 196–238.

2034 TRALBAUT, E. (1957). Vincent van Gogh chez "Aesculape". Quelques apports nouveaux à la connaissance de la santé, la maladie et la mort du grand peintre. *Aesculape*, *40*, Déc., 2–62, portrs., ill.

2035 KOOPMAN, J. (1930). Aan welke ziekte leed Vincent van Gogh? (What illnes did — suffer from?). *GG*, *8*, 985–97.

2036 BOLTEN, G. C. (1930). De ziekte van Vincent van Gogh (The illness of —). *GG*, *8*, 1058–62.
      – letter to the editor.

2037 NAVIATIL, L. (1959). Woran litt Vincent? Zur Beurteilung der Krankheit von Goghs auf Grund seines Werkes. *Ciba Symp.*, 7, 210–6, ill.

2038 HEMPHILL, R. E. (1961). The illness of Vincent van Gogh. *Prov. roy. Soc. Med.*, 54, 1083–8, 16 refs.

2039 RIESE, W. (1926). *Vincent van Gogh in der Krankheit.* In: *Grenzfragen des Nerven- und Seelenlebens.* München.

2040 EVENSEN, H. (1926). Die Geisteskrankheit Vincent van Goghs. *Allg. Ztschr. f. Psychiatrie u. Psychische gerichtliche Medizin, F. 15*, 84–133.

2041 COCHRANE, A. [   ]. Van Gogh's Madness. *Art Digest, X*, April 15.

2042 STAMM, J. L. (1971). Vincent van Gogh, identity crisis and creavity. *Amer. Imago, 28*, 363–72.

2043 GRANT, V. W. [1968]. *Great abnormals: the pathological genius of Kafka, Van Gogh, Strindberg, and Poe.* 248 pp., Hawthorn Books New York.

2044 LEONHARD, K. (1968). Schizophrene mit typischen Defektzuständen nach ihren eigenen Schriftstücken (Mit Bemerkungen über die Briefe und die Psychose Van Goghs). *Arch. Psychiatr. Nervenkr., 211*, 7–22.

2045 DOITEAU, V. (1926). La folie de Vincent van Gogh. *Progrès méd., XCI*, suppl., 17–20, ill.

2046 — and E. Leroy (1930). *La folie de Vincent van Gogh.*, ill., Coll. "sous le signe de Saturne", Editeur Aesculape, Paris.
– Préface de P. Gachet.

2047 — (1930). *Vincent van Goghs Leidensweg.* Neue Dokumente-Klärung Übertrag. v. H. J. Ken-Flory. 204 pp., 12 ill, 8°. Urban-Verl., Freiburg i. Br.

2048 BEER, J, (1935). Essai sur les rapports de l'art et de la folie chez Vincent van Gogh. *Le Médecin d'Alsace et de Lorraine*, pp. 40, 322, 345 and 369.

2049 PERRUCHOT, H. (1955). La folie de van Gogh. *Progr. méd.* (Paris), 83, 276.
– abstract from "Revue de Paris", March, 1955.

2050 HOLSTIJN, A. J. Westerman (1957). The psychological development of Vincent van Gogh. *J. ment. Sci., 103*, 1–17.

2051 [Anonym] (1970). Litt Van Gogh an psychomotorischer Epilepsie? *Unteilbare Neurologie* (Documenta Geigy), Basel, 6–7, ill.

2052 MUELLER, K. K. (1960). Vincent van Gogh betegsége ès pszichiàtria újabb szempontjai. *Orv. Hétil, 22,* 781–4, portrs.

2053 FAIRBAIRN, R. H. (1966). Vincent van Gogh – his psychopathology as reflected in his oil paintings. *Canad. psychiat. Ass. J., 11,* 443–4.

2054 [Anonym] (1971). Vincent van Gogh and glaucoma. *JAMA, 218,* 595–6.

2055 MAIRE, F. W. (1971). Van Gogh's suicide. *JAMA, 217,* 938–9.

2056 FINKELSTEIN, E. A. (1971). Van Gogh's suicide. *JAMA, 218,* 1832.

2057 DESTAING, F. (1972). Le soleil et l'orage ou la maladie de Van Gogh. *Nouv. Presse méd., I,* 3141–3.

2058 DOITEAU, V. (1957). Deux "copains" de van Gogh, inconnus, les frères Gaston et René Secrétan, Vincent, tel qu'ils l'ont vu. *Aesculape, 40,* mars, 39–58, portrs., ill.

2059 ZIEGLER, E. (1961). Vincent van Gogh und seine Ärzte. *Schweiz. med. Wschr., 91,* 949–53.
   – German and English summaries.

2060 GAUCHET, P. (1957). Les médecins de Théodore et de Vincent van Gogh *Aesculape, 40,* Mars, 4–37, portrs., ill.

2061 FRIESE, H. (1959). Doktor Gachet und die Maler von Anvers ([Vincent van Gogh]. *Neue Z. ärzt. Fortbild. 12,* 1027–9, portrs. ill.

2062 RIESE, W. (1925). Über den Stilwandel bei Vincent van Gogh. *Z. f. die ges. Neurologie und Psychiatrie, 98,* 1–16.

2063 PAREJO MORENO, M. (1958). "Fouroux". Notas acerca de Vicente v. Gogh. *Acta méd. Tenerife, 9,* 215–31.

2064 VICTORIA, M. (1967). Psicografia de Van Gogh. *Rev. Neuro-psiquiat. 30,* 219–46.

2065 DAHLGREN, K. G. (1968). Psykiatrin och van Gogh. *Sydsvenska medhist Sällsk. Arsskr., 5,* 31–45, ill.

2066 [Anonym] (1964). Van Gogh seen by a psychoanalyst. *Rassegna* (Milano), *41,* 17–24, ill.

2067 [Anonym]. (1964). Van Gogh visto da uno psicanalista. *Rass. med. cult.*, *41*, 35–42, ill.

2068 MILLER, P. W. (1965–66). Provenience of the death symbolism in Van Gogh's cornscapes. *Psychoanal. Rev.*, *52*, 60–6.

2069 LEROY, E. (1926). Le séjour de Van Gogh à l'asile de St. Remy de Provence. *Ausculape*, *7*, 16, 137, 154, 180.

2070 ALVES GARCIA, J. (1959). A influência da esquizofrenia sôbre a vida e a obra artistica de Van Gogh e de Paul Gauguin. *Rev. bras. Med.*, *16*, 125–31.

2071 PONCE, R. (1960). El caso y la obra de Van Gogh. *Rev. Neuropsychiat.*, *23*, 460–72.

2072 URSI, C. G. and J. L. Molinari (1963). La enfermedad de Van Gogh (Nuevos aportaciones). *Rev. Asoc. med. Argent.*, *77*, 197–204, ill.

See also 799

2073 RIJKENS, R. G. (1901). De ziekte en lijdensgeschiedenis van Heinrich Heine (The illness and suffering of Heinrich Heine). *Vrag. Dag. XVI*, 609.

2074 GILS, J. B. F. van (1925). John Hunter's ziekte en dood (J.H.'s illness and death.) *NTG*, *69*, I, 1138; *BGG*, *V*, 71.
– A short note.

2075 OOSTERHUIS, R. A. B. (1961). De homeopatische behandeling van de ziekte van Dr. A. Kuyper in het jaar 1894 (The homoeopathic treatment of the illness of —). *De Natuurgeneeswijze*, *13*, 34–8, portr.
– A. Kuyper (1837-1920), theologian, politician, statesman, founder of the Free University of Amsterdam.

2076 KRUL, R. (1901). De laatste dagen van Mirabeau (The last days of —). *Tijdspiegel*, *I*, 196.

2077 SCHLICHTING, Th. H. (1954). De lijkopening van St. Philip Neri (The autopsy of —). *NTG*, *98*, II, 1372–8; *BGG*, *XXXIV*, 34–40.
– Neri was the founder of the order of the Oratorium.

2078 SCHOLTENS, M. (1958). *Études medico-psychologiques sur Pascal.* Thesis Utrecht (Supervisor: H. C. Rümke), 199 pp., portrs., ill., Joh. Enschedé, Haarlem.

2079 FEYFER, F. M. G. de (1926). De hand van Paul (The hand of Paul). *NTG*, *70*, I, 1813; *BGG*, *VI*, 116.
 – Short note on the bronze hand of the surgeon F. T. Paul, being in the possession of the Liverpool Medical Institution (In Pavia the head, an index and a thumb of Ant. Scarpa are preserved).

Rembrandt van Rijn

2080 LENNEP, J. van (1957). Les maladies et la mort de Rembrandt van Rijn. *Le Scalpel*, *110*, 635–41.

2081 DIEKMEIER, L. (1958). Rembrandts Alterwandlung im Spiegel seiner Selbstbildnisse. Beitrag zur Biomorphose der Physiognomie. *Z. Altensforsch.*, *11*, 301–9, portr.

2082 ROSSEEUW, Karel (1958). Was Rembrandt een dronkaard? (Was Rembrandt a drunk?). *Wetensch. Tijdingen*, *18*, 53–6.

2083 [   ] (1970). Famous TB's in history. Saskia wife of Rembrandt van Rijn. *Santa News*, *9* (12), 6–7, ill.

See also 5296–5303 (Art)

2084 VERBEEK, Ernst (1957). *Arthur Rimbaud. Een pathografie.* (Arthur Rimbaud. A pathography). Thesis Utrecht (Supervisor: H. C. Rümke), 607 pp., Swets & Zeitlinger, Amsterdam.

2085 BOEYNAEMS, P. (1959). Anna Roemers Visschers en de Antwerpse arts L. Nonnius (Anna Roemers Visschers and the Antwerp physician L. Nonnius), *Periodiek*, *14*, 77–82, portr.

2086 BOLK, L. (1912). De schedel van Schiller (The skull of Schiller). *NTG*, *56*, I, 1669.

2087 [   ] (1969). Benedictus de Spinoza (1632–77). Famous men and their poor health. *Minn. Med.*, *52*, 1818.

2088 SCHULTZIK, R. (1933). Die Krankheit Spinozas (Ein Beitrag zur Geschichte der Glasschleifer-krankheiten). *SA*, *26*, 84–8.

2089 [   ] (1969), Famous T.B.'s Tuberculosis in history. Baruch Spinoza ... the gentle philosopher. *Santa News*, *8* (9), 6 portrs.

2090 HANEVELD, G. T. (1972). "Het wonder Lit van Jan de Witt (onderzoek van de tong van Jan de Witt ("The famous limb of —; examination of the tongue of —). *NTG, 116,* 626–7.

– Included in a report of the 92th Meeting of the Dutch Association of pathologists-anatomists, held on February 22, 1969. On the murder of the brothers De Witt (20–8–1672). The corpses were mutilated, and parts of the corpses, as the tongue, the fingers, ears etc., were removed. So the tongue of Jan de Witt and a toe of Cornelis de Witt are preserved (in the Hague Municipal Museum, no 368).

Royalties

2091 DOOREN, L. (1939). Reinoud II, Hertog van Gelderland (1326–1343) van het graveel genezen (Reinoud II, Earl of Guelderland, cured of the stone). *NTG, 83,* III, 4328; *BGG, XIX,* 210.

2092 HOCKE HOOGENBOOM, J. (1941). Enkele mededelingen omtrent Carel Gustaaf, graaf van Waldeck en Culemborg (Some information concerning Carel Gustaaf, count of — and —). *NTG, 85,* IV, 3932–3; *BGG, XXI,* 140–1.

– died 1675.

2093 SCHILFGAARDE, A. P. van (1928). Een ziektegeschiedenis uit 1656, met naschrift van M. A. van Andel (Case history from 1656, with a postscript by —). *NTG, 72,* II, 3302–8; *BGG, VIII,* 172–8.

– A case history by Dr. A. W. Peelen (1601–67) at Boxmeer concerning the illness and death of Albert, Count van den Berg (1607–1656).

2094 ANDEL, M. A. van (1933). Willem van Oranje als patient (W. of O. as a patient). *NTG, 77,* II, 2041–5; *BGG, XIII,* 105–9.

2095 FRUIN, R. (1886). Over eenige ziekten van Prins Willem I (uit de aanteekeningen van zijn lijfarts Pieter van Foreest). (On some illnesses of Prince William I – from the notes of his physician-in-ordinary —). *Bijdr. voor Vaderl. Gesch. en Oudheidk.,* 3de reeks, 3de deel, 1. (Verspreide geschriften III, 40; *Historische opstellen,* vol. III).

2096 BLANKENHORN, M. A. (1957). The medical history of William the Silent. *Bull. Cleveland med. Libr.,* 4, (3), 39–44, portr.

2097 HALLEMA, A. (1956). Ziekte en overlijden van Filips Willem, Prins van Oranje, 19 en 20 februari 1618. Een bijdrage tot de geschiedenis van zijn doodsoorzaak blijkens berichten van tijdgenoten (Illness and death of —, Prince of Orange, 19 and 20 February 1618. A contribution to the history of his cause of death according to notices of contemporaries.) *NTG, 100,* II, 1321–5; *BGG, XXXVI,* 39–43.

2098   VREEDE, G. W. [*ca* 1840]. De laatste ziekte van Prins Maurits (The
       last illness of —). In: *Nijhoff's Bijdragen voor Vaderlandsche geschie-
       denis en Oudheidkunde*, 1ste reeks, Vol. III, 77.

2099   ESSO Bzn., I. van (1965). *Het consult van Dr. Jozef Bueno aan het ziek-
       bed van Prins Maurits van Oranje* (The consultation of Dr. J.B. at the
       sick-bed of Prince Maurits of Orange). 64 pp., portrs. M. Hertzber-
       ger, Amsterdam.

2100   HALLEMA, A. (1935). Een medisch rapport in brieven over de verwon-
       ding en het overlijden van den Frieschen stadhouder Willem Frede-
       rik, prins van Nassau, anno 1664 (A medical report in letters on the
       injuries and the death of the Frisian Stadtholder William Frederick,
       prince of Nassau, A.D. 1664). *NTG*, *79*, IV, 5150; *BGG*, *XV*, 213–20.

2101   BIDLOO, G. (1702). *Verhaal der laatste ziekte en het overlijden van
       Willem IIIde ... Koning van Groot Britanje, enz.* (The Story of the last
       illness and the death of — ... King of Great Britain, etc.). 2nd ed.
       Leide, 8°.

2102   VERAART, B. A. G. (1934). G. Bidloo's verhaal van de laatste ziekte en
       het overlijden van Willem III, koning van Engeland (G.B.'s story of
       the last illness and the death of —, king of England). *NTG*, *78*, IV,
       5057–64; *BGG*, *XIV*, 203–10.

2103   DITMAR, J. van (1937). Dood (ziekte) van den stadhouder Willem III
       (Death (illness) of the stadtholder —). *NTG*, *81*, III, 4273–4; *BGG*, *XVII*,
       165–6.
       – with some quotations from letters to the Grand Pensionary Heinsius.

2104   HALLEMA, A. (1935). Geneeskundige bulletins betreffende den ziekte-
       toestand van Z.K.H. den prins-veldmaarschalk (later koning Willem
       II) in Januari 1835 (Medical bulletins concerning the illness of H.R.H.
       prince-marshall (the later king William II) in January 1835). *NTG*, *79*,
       II, 1605–10; *BGG*, *XV*, 92–7.

                                                              See also 1607

2105   MENDES DE LEON, D. E. (1964). Historische aspecten van jicht bij en-
       kele illustere monarchen (historical aspects of gout in some illustrious
       monarchs). *NTG*, *108*, 2204–4.

2106   WALSEM, G. C. van (1912). De krankzinnigheid (?) van Karel den
       Stouten (The madness (?) of Charles the Bold). *Navorscher*, *LXI*, 17.

2107   BRIL, P. van den (1959, 1960). Psycho-somatische studie van Keizer

Karel (Psycho-somatic study of Emperor Charles). *Annales Collegii Medici Antverpiensis*, 13, 239–41, 255–8, 273–5, 307–10; *14*, 51, 97, 111 and 147.

2108 O'MALLEY, C. D. (1958). Some Episodes in the Medical History of Emperor Charles V. *J. Hist. Med.*, *XIII*, 469–82.

2109 KROON, J. E. (1912). Ziekte en dood van Koning Karel II (Illness and death of King Charles II). *NTG*, *56*, II, 142.

2110 SCHULTEN, C. M. (1970). Lodewijk XIV prenataal (Louis XIV prenatal). *Spiegel Historiael*, *5*, May, 268–73, 7 ill.

2111 STUYT, J. C. L. M. (1956). Examen médical de Naundorff. *Hist. de la Méd.*, (Paris), *6*, no. 7, 31–43.
– on Naundorff who pretended to be Louis XVII.

2112 — (1956). *Examen médical de Naundorff*. 61 pp., ill., A. Sijthoff, Den Haag.
– Thesis for the grade of *docteur ès lettres* (Paris). Naundorff pretended to be Louis XVII. Reviewed by: Th. H. Schlichting: *NTG*, *100*, III, 2007; *BGG*, *XXXVI*, 57.

2113 DITMAR, T. van (1939). Dood van een vorstelijk kindje (Death of a royal child). *NTG*, *83*, II, 2633–4; *BGG*, *XIX*, 167–8.
– On the daughter of Leopold I and Empress Margaretha Theresia, who died February 23, 1672, after having lived for 14 days.

2114 RIJKENS, R. G. (1903). Napoleon Bonaparte. Van psychologisch en medisch standpunt beschouwd (Considered from a psychological and medical point of view). *Vrag. Dag*, *XVIII*, 34.

2115 SCHELTEMA, M. W. (1928). Het lijden van Napoleon op St. Helena en de geneesheeren die hem aldaar behandelden (The suffering of — on —, and the physicians, who treated him there). *NTG*, *72*, I, 2670–8; *BGG*, *VIII*, 154–62.

2116 VERBEEK, A. D. J. M. (1958). Autopsie-preparaat van Napoleon I (Autopsy-preparation of —). *NTG*, *102*, II, 2386; *BGG*, *XXXVIII*, 41.

2117 LINDEBOOM, G. A. (1957). Waaraan stierf Napoleon? (What was the cause of death of —?). *G&W*, *55*, 203–4.

2118 GROEN, J. J. (1961–3). La dernière maladie et la cause de mort du Napoléon. Étude psychologique historique et médicale. *Janus*, *L* (1961–3), 88–157.
– also as a monograph: Brill, Leiden 1962. 70 pp. Reviewed by P. Huard in: *Arch. Int. Hist. des Sci.*, *18* (1965), 147–51.

2119 NATER, J. P. (1972). Napoleon's ziekte en dood: een nieuwe theorie (N.'s illness and death: a new theory). *Arts en Wereld*, *5*, no. 12, 11–3, 1 ill.

2120 QUERIDO, A. (1973). Napoleon's ziekte en dood (Napoleon's illness and death). *Arts en Wereld*, *6*, no. 1, 12–3.

2121 NIEUWENHUIJZEN, H. J. W. A. (1942). De ziekte van Koning Lode, wijk Napoleon, onzen "lamme" Koning (The illness of King — our "paralysed" King). *NTG*, *86*, I, 27–32; *BGG*, *XXII*, 6–11.

2122 BURGER, H. (1912). De oorsprong van het gelaatstype der Habsburgers (The origin of the form of the face of the —). *NTG*, *66*, II, 946.

2123 RIJKENS, R. G. (1904). Frederik de Groote als patient (Frederick the Great as a patient). *Vrag. Dag, XIX*, 28.

2124 JONG, H. de (1928). De ziektegeschiedenis van Keizer Friedrich III (The case-history of Emperor —). *NTG*, *72*, I, 53; *BGG*, *VIII*, 16.

2125 WENTGES, R. Th. R. (1973). De ziekte van Keizer Frederik III van Duitsland (The disease of Emperor — of Germany). *Organorama*, *10*, no. 5, 12–8, ill, 5 portrs.

2126 GERLINGS, P. G. (1966). Enkele beschouwingen over het larynxcarcinoom naar aanleiding van de ziekte van Keizer Friedrich III (Reflections on laryngeal carcinoma in relation to the illness of Emperor Friedrich III). *NTG*, *100*, II, 1977–80. cf. *ibid.*, 2274 and *NTG*, *111* (1967), 145.

(See also 792–3)

2127 BEYER, T. (1967). Victoria's legacy: haemophilia in royal houses. *Organorama*, *4*, 9–14.

2128 PORTIGLIOTTI, G. (1926). La morte di Margherita de Brabante. *Illust. med. Ital. VII*, 140–5.

Chapter II

History and Historiography of Medicine

History of medicine is quite another science than medicine itself; it is not a natural science, it has another scope, uses other methods and other resources. Medical thinking in the past and present is governed by special systems, ideas and concepts of disease. It has had narrow connections with philosophy, religion, culture and society. Fundamental contributions to these different aspects made by Dutch scholars have been relatively rare.

As may be seen from the Table of Contents of the present volume a variety of sections has found a place here. General surveys of the history of medicine and of Dutch medicine or of some periods of it in particular have been included, as well as sections with entries on libraries, catalogues, bibliographies, archives, medical-historical institutes and so on.

A. Philosophy and Ideas

2129 SIGERIST, H. E. (1933). *Geneeskunde. Encyclopaedisch overzicht.* (Medicine. Encyclopaedic survey). 360 pp., Leiden-Amsterdam.
– Translated and edited by J. G. de Lint. Introduction by J. A. J. Barge.

2130 LINDEBOOM, G. A. (1954). Geneeskunde en wijsbegeerte. (Medicine and philosophy). *Alg. Ned. T. Wijsb. Psych.*, 47, 44–7.

2131 — (1965). *Natuur en Geest in de Geneeskunde.* (Nature and mind in medicine). 32 pp., Bohn, Haarlem.
– Oration held on the occasion of the 85th Dies Natalis of the Free University at Amsterdam, October 20, 1965, in the presence of H. M. Queen Juliana and the Royal Family.

2132 — (1956). *Begrippen in de geneeskunde.* (Concepts in medicine). 65 pp., Bohn, Haarlem. 2nd ed.: 1967, 76 pp., Bohn, Haarlem.

2133   — (1957). Begripsvorming in de pathologie. (Forming of concepts in pathology). In: *De vorming van wetenschappelijke begrippen*, 20–39. Kok, Kampen.

– Interfaculty addresses delivered in 1953 at the Free University at Amsterdam.

2134   — (1957). From the history of the concept of specificity. *Janus, XLVI*, 12–24. Also in Dutch: *NTG, 101*, I, 357–62; *BGG, XXXVII*, 1–6.

2135   — (1933). Teleologie en Natuurwetenschap. (Teleology and Natural Science). *Org. Chr. Ver. Nat. – en Geneesk.*, no 1, 42 pp.,

2136   — (1948). Doeloorzakelijkheid en doelmatigheid in het verstaan der natuur. (Teleology and purposeness in understanding of the nature). *G&W, 46*, 9.

2136ª   MEININGER, J. V. (1973). De begrippen orgaan en organisch in de geschiedenis der geneeskunde (The concepts "organ and organic" in the history of medicine). I: *AP*, no 11, 25–35; II: *AP*, no 15 (1974), 31–43.

2137   SNELDERS, H. A. M. (1970). De ontvangst van Kant bij enige Nederlandse wetenschapsbeoefenaars omstreeks 1800 (The reception of — in the work of a number of Dutch natural scientists about 1800). *Sci. Hist., 12*, 23–38.

See also 1027

2138   BUMA, J. T. (1950). *De Huisarts en zijn patient. Grondslagen van het medisch denken en handelen* (The family doctor and his patient. Bases of medical thinking and acting). 264 pp., portrs. Allert de Lange, Amsterdam.

2138ª   ROCHAT, G. F. (1937). Beschouwingen over de "crisis" in de geneeskunde (Observations on the "crisis" in medicine). In: *Jbk. R.U. Groningen*, 9–32.

2138ᵇ   DROGENDIJK, A. C. (1952). Geneeskunst en Existentialisme. (Medicine and Existentialism). *Gen. Bl.*, 45ste reeks, V, 143–86.

2139   LINDEBOOM, G. A. (1932). De anatomische gedachte in de geneeskunde. (The anatomical thought in medicine). *Reformatie*, 23 and 30 September.

2140   — (1936). De functionele gedachte in de moderne Geneeskunde. (The functional thought in modern medicine). *Org. Chr. Ver. Nat. en Geneesk.*, november, 139–62.

2141 — (1941). Ontwikkelingslijnen in de moderne Geneeskunst. (Lines of development in modern medicine). *Org. Chr. Ver. Nat. en Geneesk.*, no 3, 93–108.

2142 — (1955). The changing face of medicine. *Free Univ. Quart.*, IV, 66.

2143 DROGENDIJK, A. C. (1961). Aus der Geschichte der Kybernetik. *Münch. med. Wschr.*, *103*, 1517–20.

2143ᵃ KRUYVER, G. P. M. (1974). Metabletica van de obstetrie-gynaecologie ("Metabletics" of obstetrics and gynecology). *GG, 5*, no 8, 33–8.
– general reflections with a short historical introduction.

2144 WEIJDE, A. J. van der (1925). De cirkelgang der menschheid. (The circular course of mankind). *NTG, 69*, I, 1120–6; *BGG, V*, 53–9.

2145 VOS, T. A. (1973). Geschiedkundige bijdragen. V. Meditatie over het Denken. (Historical contributions. V. Meditation on thinking). *Arts en Wereld, 6*, no 9, 23–32, 12 ill.

2146 LINDEBOOM, G. A. (1954). De mens in de geneeskunde (Man in medicine). *G&W, 52*, 101–17

2146ᵃ METZ, W. (1964). *Het verschijnsel pijn. Methode en mensbeeld der geneeskunde* (The phenomenon pain. Method and view on men in medicine). 171 pp., F. Bohn, Haarlem.
– with a chapter on the history of the scientific view on men.

2147 TOURNIER, P. (⁶1957) *Bijbel en geneeskunde* (Bible and medicine). 239 pp. W. ten Have, Amsterdam.
– Reviewed by G. A. Lindeboom: *Horizon* (1955), 18–19 maart, 80.

2148 LOON, L. van (1949). Geloof en Geneeskunde (Faith and medicine). *G&W, 47*, 1–15.

2149 SCHULTE, J. E. (1961). Geneeskunde en godsdienstig geloof – bij een recente publicatie (Medicine and religion – at a recent publication). *Kath. Artsenblad, 40*, 190–4.
– on an article by P. H. Futcher. "William Osler's Religion" in: *Arch. int. Med.*, april 1961.

2150 VERMEULEN, H. (1943). De katholieke kerk en de geneeskunde in vroeger tijd (The Roman-catholic Church and medicine in former times). *NTG, 87*, III, 1495–8; *BGG, XXIII*, 71–4.

2151 ROGGE, C. W. L. (1967). Sanguis et Ecclesia. *Ned. T. Med. Stud.*, febr., 7 pp.

2152 LEE, S. van der (1951). *Clerus en Medicijnen in de geschiedenis van het Kerkelijk Recht* (Clergy and Medicine in the history of Ecclesiastical Law). 142 pp. Dekker & Van de Vegt, Utrecht-Nijmegen.

2153 LINDEBOOM, G. A. (1951). The significance of a Medical Faculty in a Christian University. *Free Univ. Quarterly, I,* 107.

See also 2586, 2587, 3052–65 (Concepts of diseases).

B. History of Medicine as a Science

2154 PEYPERS, H. F. A. (1901). L'avancement de l'historie de la médecine. *Janus, VI,* 490–2.

2155 HOFFMAN, A. C. A. (1919). De historische eenheid der geneeskunde en haar tweevoudig karakter van steeds voortschrijdende wetenschap en overgeleverde kunst. (The historical unity of medicine and its two-fold character of ever progressing science and traditional art). *NTG, 63,* I, 1603.
      – included in a report of the 17th Congress of the Dutch physicists and physicians, held on April 24–26, 1919.

2156 RIJNBERK, G. van (1921). De beteekenis van de geschiedenis der geneeskunde. (Significance of the history of medicine). *NTG, 65,* I, 51–3; *BGG, I,* 1–3.

2157 ANDEL, M. A. van (1918). Tweeërlei opvatting over de geschiedenis der geneeskunde. (Two conceptions on the history of medicine). *NTG, 62,* I, 1520–2.

2158 — (1922). Apologie der historia medica. (Apology of the —). *NTG, 66,* I, 339–40.

2159 LINT, J. G. de (1924). *De herleving van de geschiedenis der geneeskunde.* (The revival of the history of medicine). 29 pp., Noorduyn & Zn., Gorinchem.
      – Public lecture, March 12, 1924.

2160 NUYENS, B. W. Th. (1933). Het nut van de geschiedenis der geneeskunde. (The benefit of the history of medicine). *NTG, 77,* II, 1427–9; *BGG, XIII,* 102–4.

2161 BAUMANN, E. D. (1952). De betekenis der Historia Medicinae voor

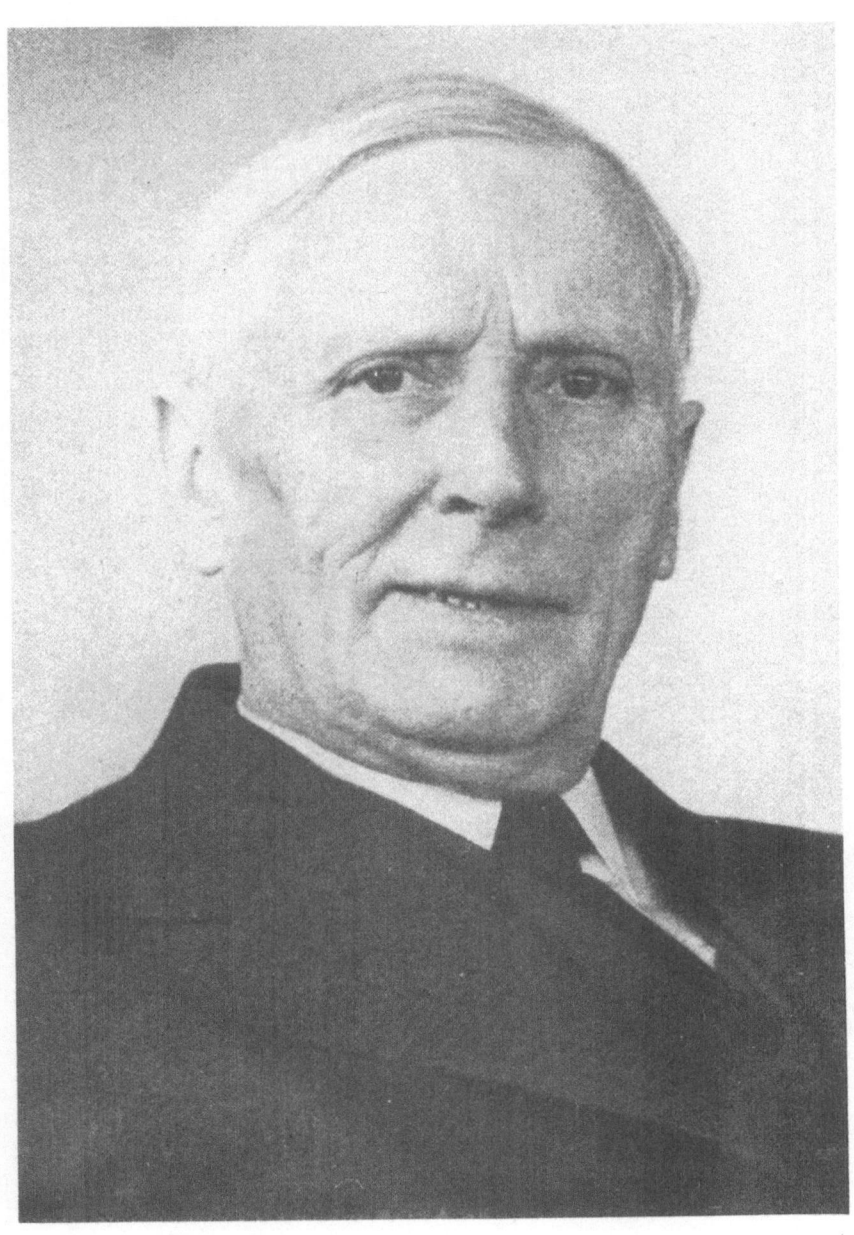

D. Schoute (1873–1953)

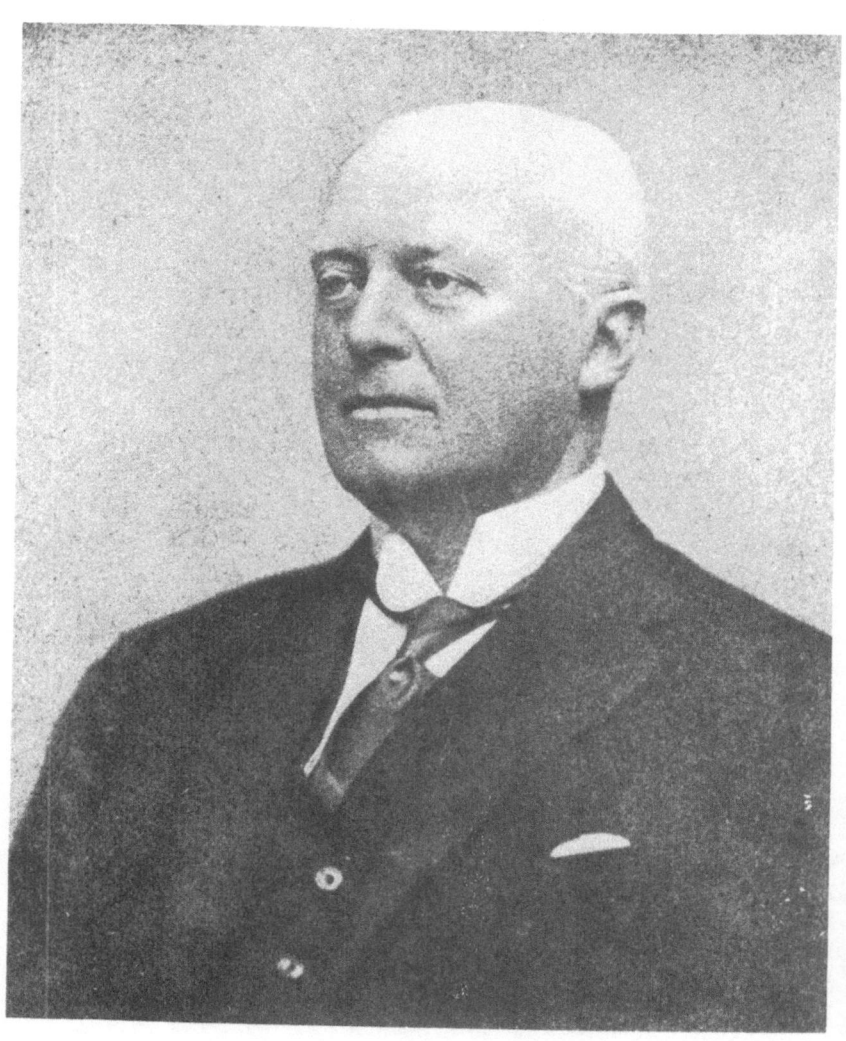

B. W. Th. Nuyens (1865–1945)

onzen tijd. (The significance of the — for our time). *Jbk. Verbond Med. Studentenfac. Ned.*, 16–25.

2162 VELDE, A. J. J. van de (1955). L'histoire des sciences et la division de l'histoire de l'humanité. *Rev. d'Hist. Sci.*, *VII*, 97–102.

2163 ELAUT, L. (1962). Geschiedenis van de geneeskunde. Waarom en waarheen? (History of medicine. Why and where to?). *Sci. Hist.*, *4*, 1–11.

2164 LEERSUM, E. C. van (1904). *De arts en de geschiedenis zijner wetenschap.* (The physician and the history of his science). 36 pp., E. J. Brill, Leiden, 4°.
– Inaugural address, December 7, 1904 (Leiden). Reviewed by V.d.B.: *Janus*, *X* (1905), 157–8.

2165 SYPKENS SMIT, J. H. (1955). De geschiedenis der geneeskunde. (History of medicine). *Ned. T. Med. Stud.*, *1*, 108–12.

See also Congresses (4700–22).

C. Methods

2166 LENNEP, J. van (1954). Obituaries as contemporary medical history. *WMJ*, *1*, 201–2.

2167 LUYENDIJK-ELSHOUT, A. M. (1973). De gedaanten van Proteus. Nieuwe mogelijkheden voor de geschiedeniswetenschap der geneeskunde. (The shapes of Proteus. New possibilities for the science of the history of medicine). *Metamedica*, *52*, no. 1, 319–24.

2168 VERBRUGH, H. S. (1973). De actualiteit van de geschiedenis der geneeskunde in het medisch onderwijs. (The actuality of the history of medicine in the teaching of medicine). *GeWiNa*, no 31, 11–4.

2168ª JAPPE ALBERTS W. and A. G. van der STEUR (1968). *Handleiding voor de beoefening van lokale en regionale geschiedenis* (Manual to the study of local and regional history). 142 pp., 40 ill. Fibula – Van Dishoeck, Bussum (no 32).

See also 1020, 5420

D. Surveys

2169 FEYFER, F. M. G. de (1907). Geschiedenis der geneeskunde. Inleiding I en II. (History of medicine. Introduction I and II). *Med. Revue, VII*, 114 and 301.

2170 — (1915). *De geneeskunde*. (Medicine). Uit onzen Bloeitijd, Serie III, no 10, Baarn, 8°.

2171 — (1917). Geschiedenis der Geneeskunde. (History of medicine). In: *Geschiedenis der Wetenschappen*, 187–220. Hollandia Drukkerij.

2172 BAUMANN, E. D. (1918). *Geschiedenis der Geneeskunde*. (History of Medicine). Amsterdam.

2173 HAGGARD, Howard H. (1931). *Van medicijnman tot geneesheer*. Vijftig eeuwen strijd voor zieke en kraamvrouw. (From medicineman to physician. Fifty years of fight for the sick and the woman in childbed). 287 pp., ill. G. J. A. Ruys, Amsterdam.
 – Translated from the English by W. Schuurmans Stekhoven. Reviewed by D. Schoute: *NTG, 96* (1942), II, 829; *BGG, XXXII*, 14.

2174 HÜHNERFELD, Paul 1957. *Korte Geschiedenis van de geneeskunde*. (Short history of medicine). Translated from the German by Hans Jacobs. With introduction by J. J. C. Marlet, 214 pp., Prisma books, no 269. Het Spectrum, Utrecht-Antwerpen.

2175 STAROBINSKI, Jean (1965). *Geschiedenis van de geneeskunst*. (History of medicine). 104 pp., 167 ill. (some col. pl.), Scheltema & Holkema, Amsterdam.
 – Dutch translation by J. G. M. Wellen and P. G. M. Wellen-Leeuwenberg.

2176 LINDEBOOM, G. A. (1961). *Inleiding tot de geschiedenis der geneeskunde*. (Introduction to the history of medicine). 342 pp., ill., ports. Bohn, Haarlem. 2nd ed.: 1971, 346 pp., ill., ports., Bohn, Haarlem.

2177 PROOSDIJ, C. van (1952/53). De Geschiedenis der Geneeskunde. (History of Medicine). *TMA, 7* (1952), Part I: 30–1; II: 42–5; III: 58–60; IV: 68–71; V: 82–3; VI: 96–9; VII: 109–11; VIII: 116–8; IX; 131–4; *ibid., 8* (1953), X: 4–5; XI: 23–5; XII: 41–2; XIII: 61–3; XIV: 74–6; XV: 112–4.

E. History of Dutch Medicine

2178 ISRAËLS, A. H. (1873). Bijdragen tot de geschiedenis der geneeskunde in Nederland. (Contributions to the history of medicine in the Netherlands). *NTG, 9*, II, 1.

2179 ALI COHEN, L. (1887). Kleine bijdragen tot de geschiedenis der geneeskunde. (Small contributions to the history of medicine). *NTG*, n.r. *23 [32]*, I, 481.

2180 GODEFROI, M. J. (1894). Oud en nieuw uit de geschiedenis der geneeskunde. (Old and new from the history of medicine). *NTG, 30, [48]*, II, 1006.

2181 FEYFER, F. M. G. de (1918). Over de geschiedenis der geneeskunde in Nederland. (On the history of medicine in the Netherlands). *NTG, 62*, I, 1297–8; 1591.

2182 SCHOUTE, D. (1918). Over de geschiedenis der geneeskunde in Nederland. (On the history of medicine in the Netherlands). *NTG, 62*, I, 945–52; 1141.

2183 — (1936). Eer en vergetelheid in onze vaderlandsche geneeskunde. (Honour and oblivion in our national medicine). *NTG, 80*, III, 4312–7; *BGG, XVI*, 158–63.

2184 MÜLLER, L. R. (1935). Medizinische Eindrücke in Holland. *Münch. med. Wschr., 82*, 1365–70, 13 ill.
  – Also on Boerhaave and Sylvius.

2185 BAUMANN, E. D. (no d.) [1950]. *Uit drie eeuwen Nederlandse geneeskunde*. (From three centuries of Dutch medicine). 320 pp., ill., ports. Meulenhoff, Amsterdam.

2186 CALKOEN, Jhr G. Th. A. (1973). Grepen uit de geschiedenis der geneeskunde (Analecta from the history of medicine). *Arts en Auto, 39*, 2171–83, 12 ill., 6 ports.

2186ᵃ — (1974). Medische geschiedschrijving in opmars? (Medical history in progress?) *Arts en Auto, 40*, 897–905, 8 ill., 4 ports.
  II. Historia Medicinae in Nederland. Leidens groei tot grote bloei (1575–1700). (Leiden's growth to great prosperity). *Ibid.*, 2073–82, 6 ill., 5 ports. [To be continued].

2187 LINDEBOOM, G. A. (1972). *De geschiedenis van de medische wetenschap in Nederland.* (History of medical science in the Netherlands). 198 pp., 63 ill., Fibula-Van Dishoeck, Bussum (Grote Fibula Serie, 2).

- Reviewed by J. R. Prakken: *NTG, 117* (1973), 1060; by D. de Moulin: *Janus, LX* (1973), 309.

2188 LEERSUM. E. C. van (1923). De beoefening der geschiedenis der geneeskunde in Nederland. (The study of the history of medicine in the Netherlands). *NTG, 77,* II, 1597–1602; *BGG, III,* 251–6.

- Address delivered on October 21, 1923 at Gorinchem, on the occasion of the 10th anniversary of the "Vereeniging voor de geschiedenis der Geneeskunde", etc.

2189 SIGERIST, H. E. (1928). Hollands Bedeutung in der Entwicklung der Medizin. *Deutsche Med. Wschr.,* 1489–92

See also 1446–50 (V. Rijnberk).

F. Periods and Progress

2190 KLEIJ, J. J. van der (1918). Ziektebeschrijving in kronieken uit de vijftiende eeuw. (Case-history in chronicles from the 15th century). *NTG, 62,* I, 100.

2191 SCHULTETUS AENEAE, B. W. (1905). *De Renaissance der medische wetenschappen.* Met een terugblik op Hippocrates. (The Renaissance of medical sciences. With a retrospective view on H.) 198 pp., Martinus Nijhoff, 's-Gravenhage.

2192 GEYL, A. (1905). De renaissance der medische wetenschappen. (The — of medical sciences). *Ned. Spectator,* no 39 and 40.

2193 LEJEUNE, F. (1928). De geest der geneeskunde in de 16de eeuw. (The spirit of medicine in the 16th century). *NTG, 72,* I, 1104–7; *BGG, VIII,* 71–4.

2194 LUYENDIJK-ELSHOUT, A. M. (1973). The situation in Medicine in the Low Countries of the sixteenth century. *Materia Med. Polona, 5,* fasc. 1, 95–6.

2195 ACKERKNECHT, Erwin H. (1971). Holland im 17. Jahrhundert: medizinisch und kulturell. *Gesnerus, 28,* 1–6.

2196 GREVENSTUK, J. G. Th. (1923). Geneeskundige hulp op het platteland in de 17e en 18e eeuw. (Medical care in the country in the 17th and 18th century). *Jbk. Oudhk. Gen. Niftarlake, 11,* 1–5.

2197 KING, Lester S. (1962). A glimpse into eighteenth century medicine. *Quart. Bull. Northw. Univ. med. Sch.*, *36*, 160–6.
– Also on Boerhaave.

2198 PUTTO, J. A. (1936). De geneeskunst onder de Bataafsche republiek. (Medicine during the Batavian Republic). *GG*, *14*, 18–9.

2199 GUYE, A. A. G. (1901). De geneeskunde van de negentiende eeuw. (Nineteenth century medicine). *NTG*, *37*, *45*, I, 803–8.
– Opening address of the medical section of the 8th Congress of science and medicine. [Rotterdam]

2200 — (1901). La médecine du dix-neuvième siècle. Discours d'ouverture de la section de médecine du huitième Congrès Néerlandais des Sciences et de la médecine, Rotterdam 11 avril 1901, *Janus*, *VI*, 274–8.

2201 TILANUS, C. B. (1920). *De Geneeskunde voor honderd jaren*. (Medicine a hundred years ago). Bohn, Haarlem.

2202 WEIJDE, A. J. van der (1924). De toestand der geneeskunde omstreeks 1860. (Medical situation about 1860). *NTG*, *68*, I, 38; *BGG*, *IV*, 1–2.

2203 ROTGANS, J. (1899). Eenige bladzijden uit de geschiedenis der chirurgie dezer eeuw. (Some pages from the history of surgery of this century) *NTG*, *35*, I, 573–93.

2204 NIERSTRASZ, J. J. (1968). Ziek zijn en beter worden 150 jaar geleden (Being ill and recovering 150 years ago). *Sci. Hist.*, *10*, 87–93.

2205 SCHULTE, B. P. M. (ed.) (1963). *Vijftig jaren beoefening van de geschiedenis der geneeskunde, wiskunde en natuurwetenschappen*. (Fifty years of studying history of medicine, mathematics and natural sciences). 118 pp., 2 pl. Publ. by the "Genootschap voor Geschiedenis der geneeskunde, wiskunde en natuurwetenschappen". no pl.
– With a preface by D. A. Wittop Koning.

2206 LINDEBOOM, G. A. (1963). De beoefening van de geschiedenis der geneeskunde. In: Schulte, B. P. M. (ed.). *Vijftig jaren beoefening van de geschiedenis der geneeskunde*, ..., 9–23.
– with an extensive bibliography (19–23).

2207 — (1946). Oorlogswinst der Geneeskunde. (War-gain of medicine). *Voortgang*, no 1, september.
– of this periodical only three issues have appeared.

2208 LOGHEM, J. J. van (1951). Het aandeel van Nederland in de vooruitgang der geneeskundige wetenschap van 1900 tot 1950. Gezondheidsleer. (The share of the Netherlands in the progress of medical science from 1900 till 1950. Hygiene). *NTG*, *95*, I, 4–8.

– This is the first article in a series of Dutch medicine (1900–1950), in which also the following six items have appeared:

2209 GISPEN, R. (1951). Microbiologie en Immunologie (Microbiology and Immunology). *NTG*, *95*, I, 830–9; 961–8.

2210 ARIËNS KAPPERS, J. (1951). De bouw van het zenuwstelsel. (The structure of the nervous system). *NTG*, *95*, II, 1406–12.

2211 RUYS, A. C. (1951). Epidemiologie (Epidemiology). *NTG*, *95*, II, 1666–74.

2212 JONGH, C. L. de (1951). Inwendige geneeskunde. (Internal medicine. *NTG*, *95*, III, 2762–8, *See also* 3306

2213 KOUWENAAR, W. (1951). Tropische geneeskunde. (Tropical medicine). *NTG*, *95*, IV, 3814–22.

2214 WAARDENBURG, P. J. (1953). Erfelijkheidspathologie. (Hereditary pathology). *NTG*, *97*, I, 650–6; II, 905.

2215 HEES, C. A. van (1952). De ontwikkeling van de geneeskunde in de laatste 75 jaren. (The development of medicine in the last 75 years). *Landbouwk. T.*, *64*, 451–60.

2216 DONGEN, J. A. van (ed.). (1966). *De vooruitgang van de geneeskunde in onze eeuw.* (Progress of medicine in our century). 288 pp., ill., ports, De Bussy, Amsterdam.

– Published on the occasion of the 60th anniversary of the "Amsterdamsche Specialisten Vereeniging" (Amsterdam Association of specialists); with surveys of the 20th century development of 33 branches of medicine.

2216ª MEIJNE, N. G. (1974). Vijfentwintig jaar spiegel van de Nederlandse chirurgie (25 years reflection of Dutch surgery). *NTG*, *118*, 1822.

– on the occasion of the 25th anniversary of the periodical *Archivum chirurgicum neerlandicum.*

See also 4282a

G. Linguistics

2217 KLUYVER, A. (1923). Over termen met -geen als tweede lid. (On terms with -gen as suffix). *NTG*, *67*, II, 1616–7; *BGG*, *III*, 270–1.

2218 BROEK, A. J. P. van der (1932). Over het ontstaan van spraak en schrift. (On the genesis of language and script). *Gen. Bl.*, *32*, 289–315.

2219 ESSO Bzn, I. van (1936). De etymologie der woorden "kinkhoest, mazelen, roode hond, bof, quinte de toux, en coqueluche". (Etymology of the words — — —). *NTG*, *80*, III, 3565–6; *BGG*, *XVI*, 125–6.

2220 LINDEBOOM, G. A. (1972). Moeilijkheden met oude en nieuwe spelling in 1701. (Troubles with old and new spelling). *NTG*, *116*, 1145.
– a small note on change of spelling.

2221 [Anonymous] (1971). Uit de vaktaal van medicus en chirurgijn; Hondschoote 1643. (From the professional language of physician and surgeon; —). *Biekorf*, *72*, 120–1.

See also 1136–7 (Leeuwenhoek)

H. Chronology and Calendars

2222 WIJK, W. E. van (1920). De Juliaansche en Gregoriaansche kalenders vergeleken. (Comparison of the Julian and the Gregorian calendar). *Natuur*, *XL*, 177.

2223 HENINGER Jr., S. K. (1961). Some Renaissance versions of the Pythagorean telrad. *Stud. Renaiss.*, *8*, 7–35.

2224 deleted

2225 WINTER, J. J. (1964). A shepherd's time-stick, Nagari inscribed. *Physis*, *6*, 377–84.

2226 BRAEKMAN, Willy and M. Gysseling (1967). Het Utrechts Kalendarium met de Noordlimburgse gezondheidsregels (The Utrecht Calendarium with the Northern Limburg health rules) *MKVAB*, 575–635, 11 ill.

I. Teaching of History of Medicine

2227 MUNTENDAM, P. (1921). Leergang over geschiedenis der geneeskunde. (Course on the history of medicine). *NTG*, *65*, II, 1204; *BGG*, *I*, 371.
– Announcement of a course on the history of medicine, to be given by M. A. van Andel at Gorinchem.

2228 SCHOUTE, D. (1937). Universitair onderwijs in de geschiedenis der geneeskunde. (University education of the history of medicine). *NTG, 81*, IV, 5815–6; *BGG, XVII*, 201–2.

2229 — (1943). Enkele vragen inzake het geneeskundig onderwijs. 13. Onderwijs in de geschiedenis der geneeskunde. (Some questions concerning medical education. 13. Teaching of the history of medicine). *NTG, 87*, I, 53–4.

2230 FORBES, R. J. (1947). The teaching of the history of Science. In postwar Holland. *Isis, 38*, 98–9.

2231 KOUWENAAR, W. (1953). Het onderwijs in de geschiedenis der geneeskunde. (Teaching of the history of medicine). *NTG, 97*, I, 586–7;

2232 LINDEBOOM, G. A. (1953). De betekenis van het onderwijs in de geschiedenis der geneeskunde. (The significance of the teaching of the history of medicine). *NTG, 97*, II, 1149; *BGG, XXXIII*, 30–1.
      – Included in the report of the meeting of the "Genootschap" November 15–16, 1952.

2233 — (1953). De betekenis van het onderwijs in de geschiedenis der geneeskunde. (The significance of the teaching of the history of medicine). *Gen. Bl.*, 45ste reeks, *XI*, 345–64.

2234 HOEVEN, J. van der (1933). L'enseignement de l'histoire des sciences. IV. The teaching of the History of Medicine at the Dutch Universities. *Archeion, XV*, 81–2.

2235 BARUCH, J. Z. (1964). Medisch Universitair Onderwijs. Onderricht in de geschiedenis van de geneeskunde. (University Medical Education. Teaching of the history of medicine). *MC, 19*, 551–3.

2236 MOULIN, D. de (1972). De geschiedenis der Geneeskunde, wiskunde, natuurwetenschappen en techniek aan de Nederlandse Universiteiten en Hogescholen van 1968–1971. (The history of Medicine, Mathematics, Natural Sciences and Technics at the Dutch Universities and Academies from 1968–1971). *GeWiNa*, nr 29, 4–16.

2237 ANDEL, M. A. van (1939). Lessen in de geschiedenis der geneeskunde voor aspirant-reserve-officieren van gezondheid. (Lessons in the history of medicine for candidate reserve-medical officers). *NTG, 83*, III, 4048 and 4329; *BGG, XIX*, 220.

2238 MOULIN, D. de (1967). Medical History in the United States of America. *Janus, LIV*, 252–5.

2239 LINDEBOOM, G. A. (1971). De evolutieleer versus de Historia Medicinae in de medische opleiding. (The theory of evolution versus the — in medical education). *G&W, 69,* 168.
— a short note.

See also 1857a

J. History of Medical Ethics

2240 ALETRINO, A. (1889). *Eenige beschouwingen over den beroepseed der artsen.* (Some observations on the professional oath of physicians). Thesis Amsterdam (Supervisor: C. H. Kuhn), 89 pp., F. S. van Staden, Amsterdam.

2241 STASSEN, M. J. W. (1947). *Medische ethiek in grijze oudheid.* (Medical ethics in antiquity). Thesis Utrecht (Supervisor: A. J. P. van den Broek). 151 pp., port. (of Hippocrates). Ernest van Aelst, Maastricht.

2242 LINDEBOOM, G. A. (1932). Euthanasie. (Euthanasia). *Predikant en Dokter,* 205–29.

2243 — (1944). Grondslag en beginselen der medische ethiek. (Foundation and principles of Medical Ethics). *Stemmen des Tijds,* June–July, 281–96; Aug.–Sept., 358–78.

2244 — (1960). *Opstellen over Medische Ethiek* (Essays on Medical Ethics)., 176 pp., ill. Kok, Kampen.

2245 — (1964). Origin and Foundation of Medical Ethics. In: *The service of the Christian doctor in a modern* society, [= *Ministerium medici,* no 4], 51–63, Van Gorcum, Assen.

2246 — (1969). Medical Ethics in Medical Education. In: J. B. Natvig and N. J. Lavik (ed.). *The Responsibility of the Christian Physician in the Modern World,* 26–31. Oslo.

2247 — (1970). Medisch-ethische bezinning in Protestantse kring. (Medical-ethical reflection in Protestant circle). *Metamedica, 49,* 411–5.

2248 LAER, P. H. van (1973). Paus Innocentius XI en abortus provocatus. (Pope Innocentius XI and abortion). *Metamedica, 52,* 523–4.

See also 3488

K. Bibliographies and Catalogues

2249 [   ] (1931). *Geneeskundige Bibliograghie.* (Medical Bibliography). Scheltema & Holkema Amsterdam
– Original Dutch works published in the years 1921–30.

2250 [   ] (1957). Bibliographie (Bibliography). *NTG, 101*, II, 1270; *BGG, XXXVII*, 21.

2251 [   ] (1958). Bibliographie van een eeuw geleden. (Bibliography from a century ago). *NTG, 102*, I, 27; *BGG, XXXVIII*, 6.

2252 [   ] (1958). Bibliographie. (Bibliography). *NTG, 102*, I, 1160; *BGG, XXXVIII*, 12.

2253 RHIJN, Jr. W. P. (1918–19). Bibliotheecq librorum medici, anatomici et botanici. *Med. Wbl., XXV,* 396.

2254 KRUMBHAAR, E. B. (1926). Seventeenth century medical literature as exemplified in the Elzevier presses. *Ve Congrs Int. d'Hist. de la Méd., Genève 1925,* 109–13. Genève.

2255 NUYENS, B. W. Th. (1930, 1949) *Bibliotheca Medica Neerlandica. Catalogus librorum quos collegit societas Neerlandica ad promovendam Artem Medicam ab anno MDCCCXLIX ad annum MCMXXX.* 659 pp., De Bussy, Amsterdam, 4°.
Vol. II (E. J. van der Linden): MCMXXXI–MCMIL, 286 pp., Ibid.
Vol. III. (J. A. van Dongen): 1949–1954, 88 pp., J. v. Campen, Amsterdam.
Vol. IV. (J. A. van Dongen): 1954–1960, 118 pp., *ibid.*

2256 DIBON, P. (1957). *Le Fonds néerlandais de la bibliothèque académique de Herborn,* 165 pp., MKNAW, afd. Letterkunde, Nieuwe Reeks, deel 20, no 14. Noord-Holl. Uitg. Mij, Amsterdam.
– The "Alte Bibliothek" of the "Hohe Schule" at Herborn contains several small 17th century Dutch medical works (e.g. of Regius) not present in the Netherlands.

2257 [   ] (1893, 1961). *Bibliotheca Erasmiana. Répertoire des oeuvres d'Erasme.,* 3 vols: 186, 68 and 65 pp., Gand. Reprint 1961, De Graaf, Nieuwkoop.

2258 BOEYNAEMS, P. [no d.]. *Nederlandsche bibliographie van de Vlaamsche geneesheeren 1919–1934.* (Dutch bibliography of Flemish physicians 1919–1934). Antwerpen.

2258ᵃ SMIT, P. (1974). *History of the Life Sciences: an annotated Bibliography.* XIII + 1071 pp. A. Asher & Co, Amsterdam.

2259 BOCKSTAELE, Paul (1959–1968). Bibliografie van de geschiedenis der wetenschappen in de Nederlanden (Bibliography of the history of sciences in the Netherlands). *Sci Hist., 1,* 31–52; 107–16; 162–75; 219–28. *Ibid., 2,* 30–45; 86–100, 39–51 (= 143–55); 203–21. *Ibid., 3,* 50–6; 102–13; 209–26. *Ibid., 4,* 91–112; 212–25. *Ibid., 5,* 82–94; 178–94. *Ibid., 6,* 97–107; 222–35. *Ibid., 7,* 127–36; 229–40. *Ibid., 8,* 114–24. *Ibid., 9,* 48–60; 91–105; *Ibid., 10,* 42–55; 234–45. *Ibid., 11,* 190–208.

2260 KROON, J. E. (1923). *Catalogus van werken en artikelen van Nederlanders op historisch genees-, schei-, wis-, natuurkundig en natuurwetenschappelijk gebied. 1 Januari 1900 to 30 September 1923.* (Catalogue of works and articles of Dutchmen on the history of medicine, mathematics, chemistry, physics and natural sciences. 1 January 1900 till 30 September 1923). Leiden.
– Published by "GeWiNa" on the occasion of its 10th anniversary.

2261 [   ] [no d.] *Catalogus van de Bibliotheek van de Christelijke Vereeniging van Natuur- en Geneeskundigen in Nederland.* (Catalogue of the library of the Christian Society of natural and medical scientists in the Netherlands). 12 pp., 212 nrs. K. Kleywegt, Loosduinen.

2262 [   ] (1899). *Catalogus van de Bibliotheek van het Bataafsch Genootschap der Proefondervindelijke wijsbegeerte.* (Catalogue of the Library of the Batavian Society of Experimental Philosophy). 215 pp., Rotterdam.

2263 [   ] (1830). *Katalogus der Bibliotheek van de Maatschappij Felix-Meritis.* (Catalogue of the library of the Society —). 144 pp., no pl.
– Catalogue of a disappeared library. F. M. was established at Amsterdam.

2264 MULLER, Fred. (ed.) (1856, 1868). *Catalogus van de Bibliotheek van de Vereeniging ter Bevordering van de belangen des Boekhandels.* (with Supplement: 1868). (Catalogue of the library of the Association for the furtherance of the interests of booksellers). 2 vols. XIV + 144 pp., 91 pp., Amsterdam.
– In 1885 appeared again a Catalogue of the Ass.: 265 pp.

2265 VRIES, A. G. C. de, and E. DRONCKERS (ed.) (1920–65). *Catalogus der bibliotheek van de Vereeniging ter bevordering van de belangen des boek-*

handels. (Catalogue of the Library of the Association for the furtherance of the interests of the booksellers). 7 vols, 's-Gravenhage.

– With supplement catalogues: 1920–26; 1927–1939; 1940–49 and 1949–64; system-
atical catalogue of the rich possessions of the Dutch Booksellers Association.

2266 [no d.] *Catalogue of books printed in the XVth century in the British
Museum*. Fasc. I. Holland; Fasc. II. Belgium) XXXIV + 123 pp.,
XXXV–LXI, 125–222; Facs: 3 pp., 10 photo's, Trustees of the British
Museum, London.

2267 WITTOP KONING, D. A. (1956). Farmaceutisch-Historische Bibliografie van Nederland .(Pharmaceutical-historical Bibliography of the
Netherlands). *Ph. W.*, *91*, 705–20; *Bull. Pharm.*, *XIII*, 1–16.

2268 GUISLAIN, A. (1960). Bibliografie van de geschiedenis der farmacie in
België. (Bibliography of the history of pharmacy in —). *Ph. T. Belg.*,
37, 1–16.

See also 366–368, 508, 1150

L. Libraries and Collections

2269 BRUMMEL, L. (1972). De Bibliotheken (Libraries). *Spiegel Historiael*, *7*,
165–71, 9 ill.
– a.o. on the Leiden University Library.

2270 MOLHUYSEN, P. C. (1905). *Geschiedenis der Universiteits-bibliotheek te
Leiden*. (History of the Leiden University library). 80 pp., 1 port.,
ill., Leiden.

2271 SOMEREN, J. F. van (1909). *De Utrechtsche Universiteitsbibliotheek.
Haar geschiedenis en kunstschatten vóór 1880*. (The Utrecht University
Library. Its history and art-treasures before 1880). VI + 160 pp., ports,
Utrecht, 4°.

2272 MOLL, W. (1920). Een vrijwel onbekende geneeskundige boekerij.
(An almost unknown medical library). *NTG*, *64*, I, 157–60. Also in:
Med. Dienst Kunst en Wetensch. Den Haag (1919–20), 29.
– On the libraries of Dr. J. de Cocq (1639–1721) and of the Collegium Pharmaceut-
icum.

2273 KROON, J. E. (1921). De grootste geneeskundige bibliotheek. (The
largest medical library). *NTG*, *65*, I, 1898–9; *BGG*, *I*, 189–90.
– on the library of the Surgeon-General's office at Washington, possessing many
Dutch medical books, some of which are no longer present in the Netherlands.

2274 HOUTZAGER, H. L. (1972). Medische boeken uit de bibliotheek van Daniel van der Meulen. (Medical books from the library of —). *Spiegel Historiael*, 7, 422–8.
– The auction-catalogue of the library of —, a 16th century merchant, includes about 1200 items, a number of which refer to important medical works.

2275 [   ] (1892). *Catalogus der Boekerij*, geschonken door Dr J. N. Ramaer, aan de Nederlandsche Vereeniging voor Psychiatrie en geplaatst in het Rijkskrankzinnigengesticht te Medemblik (Catalogue of the Library, given by — — to the Association of Psychiatry and placed in the State Mental Asylum at M.) 97 pp. (1388 items). F. van Rossen, Amsterdam.

2276 KROON, J. E. (1931). Aanvulling der bilbiotheek van het "Instituut voor Geschiedenis der Genees-, natuur- en wiskunde". (Supplement to the library of the —). *NTG*, 75, IV, 5912; *BGG*, XI, 332.

2277 SCHLICHTING, Th. H. (1954). De boekerij van het *Tijdschrift*. (The library of —). *NTG*, 98, III, 2335. (not in: *BGG*).
– "Tijdschrift" is the same as *NTG*.; This library, containing some 4600 books, has a mainly historical character.

2278 LINDEBOOM, G. A. (1968). De Bibliotheek der Maatschappij in het heden, en in de toekomst. (The Library of the [Dutch Society for the promotion of Medicine], at present and in the future. *MC*, 23, 933–5.

2279 BURKE, M. N. (Compiler), (1946). The Miller collection in the library of the Richmont Academy of medicine. *BHM*, *XIX*, 200–25; 319–44.
– Mentioned are a.o. works of B. S. Albinus, E. D. Baumann, H. Boerhaave, Joh. van Beverwijck, J. Bontius, R. Descartes, Ch. Drélincourt, Galenus, A. Geyl, R. de Graaf (*Opera omnia*), J. Palfijn, C. Stalpert van der Wiel, a.o.

2280 [   ] (1960). *Livres anciens des Pays Bas. La collection Lessing J. Rosewald provenant de la Bibliothèque d'Arenberg*. Exposition. La Hay, 29 août – 9 octobre 1960; Bruxelles. 21 octobre – 31 décembre 1960., 148 pp., ill. Bibliothèque Royale de Belgique, Bruxelles.

2281 ROOSEBOOM, M. (1964). De Collectie De Lint. (Collection De Lint). *GeWiNa*, *16*, 11–2
– The collection of J. G. de Lint (1867–1936), external university lecturer is in the "Rijksmuseum vor Geschiedenis der Natuurwetenschappen" at Leiden. It comprises 3500 portraits (also of giants and dwarfs; and caricatures) and other pictures, and *ca* 1700 books and theses.

2282 [   ] (1877). *Catalogus der boekerij van het provinciaal geneeskundig gesticht voor krankzinnigen "Meerenberg" bij Bloemendaal* (Catalogue of the library of the provincial lunatic asylum − near −). 277 pp. no pl. *See also* 4420.

See also 1153, 1310, 1450, 2603

M. Medical-historical Institutes

2283 VERDOORN, Frans (1971). History of Science institutions and their universities. *Janus, LVIII*, 277–88.

2284 SMIT, P. (1968). Das Biohistorische Institut der Reichsuniversität Utrecht. Ein Institut für die Grenz- und Übergangsgebiete zwischen den organischen Naturwissenschaften und den Geisteswissenschaften. *Mediz. Hist. J.*, *3*, 195–205.

2285 VERDOORN, F. (1970). A bird's-eye view of the Utrecht Biohistorical Institute. *Utrecht biohist. Bull.*, Summer, Suppl. no 1, 4 pp.

2286 VISSER, R. P. W. (1970). "Miquel Huis" and its Residents. *Essays in Biohistory and other Contributions, presented to Frans Verdoorn, on the occasion of his 60th birthday*, 401–4. Ed. by P. Smit and R. J. Ch. V. ter Laage.

2286ª LINDEBOOM, G. A. (1970). Korte geschiedenis van het Instituut (Short history of the Institute). *AP*, no 1, 6–15.

– Medical-encyclopaedic Institute of the Free University, Amsterdam.

See also 1270-1

N. Archives

2287 GOUW, J. L. van der (1955). *Inleiding tot de archivistiek.* (Introduction to archivistics). *Archivistica* no 1, Tjeenk Willink, Zwolle.

2288 — H, HARDENBERG, W. J. van HOBOKEN and G. W. A. PANHUYSEN (1962). Nederlandse archiefterminologie. (Dutch terminology of archivistics). *Archivistica*, no 2, Tjeenk Willink, Zwolle.

2289 GRASWINCKEL, Jhr D. P. M. (1930). *De archieven der gasthuizen en fundatiën, gilden, schutterijen en vendels.* (The archives of hospitals and foundations, guilds, citizen soldieries and companies 413 pp. Alg. Landsdrukkerij, 's-Gravenhage.

– From the Old Archive of Arnhem.

2290 WEE, H. van der (1966). Les archives hospitalières et l'étude de la pauvreté aus Pays-Bas du XVe au XVIIIe siècle. *Rev. Nord, 48,* 5–16.

2291 VEDER, W. R. (1908). *Het Archief van de Gasthuizen te Amsterdam
(tot 1875).* (The Archives of the hospitals at A.). 304 + CII pp.
Stadsdrukkerij, Amsterdam.
  – reviewed by J. F. M. Sterck: *Jbk Amstelodamum, 8* (1910), 181–7.

2292 EEGHEN, I. H. van (1946). *Inventarissen van archieven betreffende de
Latijnsche School, het Athenaeum en gezelschappen van studenten aan
het Athenaeum te Amsterdam.* (Inventories of the archives concerning
the Latin School, the Athenaeum and Associations of students at the
— at —). Historische Commissie der Univ. Amsterdam.

2293 BAART de la FAILLE, R. D. (1920). Inventaris der Archieven van het
Geneeskundig Staatstoezicht in Noord-Holland, 1801–1865 (Inventory of the Archives of the Medical State Supervision in —). *Versl.
'sRijks Oude Archieven, XLIII,* deel 2, 139–56.

2293^a FORMSMA, W. J. (1967). *Gids voor de Nederlandse archieven* (Guide for
the Netherlands Archives). 112 pp., 35 ill. Fibula-Van Dishoeck,
Bussum (no 21).

2293^b GOUW, J. L. van der (1963). *Oud Schrift* (Old Script). 256 pp. Tjeenk
Willink. Zwolle.
  – introduction into old (medieval – 17th century) script with many examples.
                              See also 4512, 4633–7, 4996, (Medical profession).

O. Incunabula, Postincunabula and rare books

2294 DONGEN, J. A. van (1964–70). Incunabelen en Postincunabelen in de
Bibliotheek der Maatschappij (Incunabula and Postincunabula in the
Library of the Dutch Society for the promotion of medicine).
  – a series of short notes of one column or one page.

2295   I. Des. Erasmus: *Encomium artis medicae,* Basileae apud
              Joan. Frobenium, 1518. *MC, 19,* (1964), 870–1.

2296   II. *Der Vrouwen Natuere ende Complexie.* Jan van Does-
              borch, Utrecht [1540]. *MC, 19,* 908–9.

2297   III. *Chirurgie meester Lanfrancks van Meylanen.* Antwerpen,
              1529. *MC, 20* (1965), 68–9.

2298   IV. Guido de Cauliaco. *Die Cyrurgie van meester Guido de Cauliaca...* Antwerpen, 1507. *MC, 20,* 112–4.

2299   V. *Den Roseghaart van den bevruchten vrouwen.* [Antwerpen], 1528, *MC, 20,* 146–8.

2300   VI. Jasonis à Pratis Zyricaei. *De pariente et partu, liber obstetricibus, puerperis nutricibusque utilissimus.* S.I. 1527. *MC, 20,* 206–7.

2301   VII. Bartholomeus de Glanvilla Engelsman, *Van den proprieteyten der dinghen,* Haerlem 1485. *MC, 20,* 289–90.

2302   VIII. *Fasciculus medicine ...,* 1512. *MC, 20,* 448–50.

2303   IX. *Dat Licht der Apothekers ...,* 1529. *MC, 20,* 565–8.

2304   X. Jeronimus Bruynswijck. *Dits dat hantwerck der cirigien ende leert alle wonden...,* Utrecht 1535. *MC, 20,* 616–9.

2204ᵃ   XI. Albertus Magnus. *Liber aggregationis ...,* Adelardus Bathoniensis. *Questiones naturales perdifficiles – Questiones naturales philosophorum.,* Antwerpen, tussen 1485–91. *MC, 20,* 666–8.

2305   XII. Petrus Sylvius. *Tfundament der Medicinen ende Chyrurgien...,* Antwerpen 1530. *MC, 20,* 731–3.

2306   XIII. *Dat chyrurgylick werk D. Johanis de Vigo Genuensis* Antwerpen, 1533. *MC, 20,* 852–5.

2307   XIV. Petrus Yspanus. *Summa experimentorum sive Thesaurus pauperum.* Antwerpen, 1497. *MC, 20,* 922–4.

2308   XV. *Paraphrasis in nonum Rhazae Medici Arabis Clarissimi ad Regem Almansorem, de affectuum singularum corporis partium curatione, Andrea Wesalio Bruxellensi auctore.* Basel, 1537. *MC, 20,* 1022–4.

2309   XVI. *Ioachimi Ringelbergii Antverpiani Liber de Homine.* Antwerpen, 1529. *MC, 20,* 1126–7.

2310   XVII. Annotatiunculae aliquot Cornelii Petri Leydensis Physici, in quatuor libros Dioscoridis Anazarbei. *Experimenta et Antidota contra varios morbos. De rebus occultis in natura mirandis ...,* Antwerpen, 1533. *MC, 21* (1966), 84–5.

2311   XVIII. Aurelii Cornelii Celsi *de sanitate tuenda liber plurimis in locis antea nemini suspectis...*, Antwerpen, 1539. *MC, 21*, 204–5.

2312   XIX. Andreae Wesalii Bruxellensis, ... *Espistola, docens venam axillarem dextri cubiti in dolore laterali secandam: et melancholicum succum ex venae portae ramis ad sedem pertinentibus, purgari.* Basel, 1539. *MC, 21*, 296–9.

2313   XX en

2314   XXI. *Dit is der bien boeck* (door Thomas Cantipratensis), Swolle 1488.
Hier beghint der bijen boeck ende is tracterende van den prelaten ende den ondersaten (door Thomas Cantipratensis). Leyden 1515. *MC, 21*, 407–10.

2315   XXII. *Libri duo de uteris* Jasonis à Pratis Zyricei ... Antwerpen, 1523. *MC, 21*, 728–30.

2316   XXIII. *Den Tresoor van den Preservatyve remedien ende cure.....* Ghemaect bij Meester Jan Thibault Medecijn ende Astrologijn ..., Antwerpen, 1531. *MC, 21*, 871–3.

2317   XXIV. *Den Herbarius in dyetsche.* Antwerpen, 1511. *MC, 21*, 947–9.

2318   XXV. *Epitome medices summam totius medicinae complectens,* autore Otthone Brunsfelsio, ... Antwerpen, 1540. *MC, 21*, 990–1.

2319   XXVI. *Instructie voer die Barbyers Jonghers ende den ghemeynen simpelen man.* Kampen, ca 1540. *MC, 21*, 1056–7.

2320   XXVII. *Die fleubothomia dat is dat bloet te laten* van meester Avicenna ..., Antwerpen, 1529. *MC, 21*, 1119–21.

2321   XXVIII. *Alberti cognomento Magni Libellus, qui inscribitur de Formatione hominis in utero Materno,* ... 1538. *MC, 21*, 1166–8.

2322   XXIX. *Dije Anathomia magistri Gwidonis*, Antwerpen, 1529. *MC, 22* (1967), 100–1.

2323   XXX. D. Iasonis Pratensis Medici *De tuenda sanitate Libri quatuor.* Antwerpen, 1538. *MC, 22*, 171–3.

2324   XXXI. *Spiegel der Artznij* des geleichen vormals nie von keinen Doctor in tütsch uszgangen .... Laurentio Phryesen von Colmar..., Straszburg, 1518. *MC, 22,* 271–4.

2325   XXXII. Joachimi Fortii Ringelbergii Antverpiani *Institutiones Astronomicae...,* Antwerpen 1530. *MC, 22,* 483–5.

2326   XXXIII. *De usu pharmaceutices in consarcinandis medicamentis, Isagoge...* Autore Theobaldo Lepleignio Vindocinensi., 1539. *MC, 22,* 574–6.

2327   XXXIV. *Hieremiae Thriveri Brachelii in primum Aphorismorum Hippocratis librum Commentarius, ... MC, 22,* 785–8.

2328   XXXV. Henrici Cornelii Agrippae ab Nettesheym, *Splendidissimae noblitatis Viri, et armatae militiae* Equitis aurati, ac. LL. Doctoris, ... *de Incertitudine et Vanitate Scientiarum et Artium, ...* Antwerpen 1531. *MC, 22,* 1007–10.

2329   XXXVI. Jacobi Castrici Hasebrocani ... *de sudore Epidemiali quem Anglicum vocant,* ad Medicos Gandenseis (!) Epistola. Antwerpen, 1529. *MC, 22,* 1177–8.

2330   XXXVII. *Liber de arcenda sterilitate et progignendis liberis,* D. Jasonis Pratensis Zyricei. Antwerpen, 1531. *MC, 22,* 1257–8.

2331   XXXVIII. Hieremias Thriverus Brachelius ... *de temporibus morborum et opportunitate auxiliorum.* Adiectus est ... L. Fuchsii nuper *emissae de missione sanguinis in pleuritide.* Leuven, 1535. *MC, 23,* (1968). 297–9.

2332   XXXIX. *Epitome opusculi de curandis pusculis, ulceribus et* doloribus morbi Gallici ... autore Laurentio Phrisio, Basel 1532. *MC, 23,* 941–2.

2333   XL. Hieremiae Thriveri Brachelii... *de missione sanguinis in pleuritide, ac aliis phlegmonis tam externis quam internis omnibus* ... Eiusdem commentarius de victu ab arthiticis morbis vindicante, ubi quam male diris illis ... Leuven, 1532. *MC, 23,* 1195–7.

2334   XLI, XLII,
        XLIII en
        XLIV. *Den Rosenghaert van de bevruchte vrouwen.* Antwerpen 1529. *MC, 23,* 1383–5.

2335 XLV. Aurelii Cornelii Celsi, *De Re Medica*; *libri octo eruditissimi*. Haganoae, 1528. *MC, 24* (1969), 94–6.

2336 XLVI. *Galeni de curandi ratione per sanguinis missionem*, Liber... Theodorico Gaudano interprete. Parijs, 1529. *MC, 24*, 266–8.

2337 XLVII. Claudii Galeni Pergameni, *medicorum omnium fere principis opera*... Basel, 1529. *MC, 24*, 681–4.

2338 XLVIII. Claudii Galeni Pergameni *de sanitate tuenda libri sex*, Thoma Linacro Anglo interprete... Parijs, 1530. *MC, 24*, 1010–1.

2339 IL. *Hippocratis Aphorismi*, cum Galeni commentariis, Nicolao Leoniceno Vicentino interprete. Item eiusdem Hippocratis *Praedictiones*, cum Galeni etiam commentariis, Laurentio Laurentiano interprete. Parijs, 1532. *MC, 24*, 1188–90.

2340 L. Huberti Barlandi ... qua docetur non paucis abuti nos vulgo medicaminibus simplicibus ... Antwerpen, 1532. *MC, 24*, 1405–6.

2341 LI. Pauli Aeginetae *Salubria de tuenda valetudine praecepta*, Guilielmo Copo Basileiensi interprete. Neurenberg, 1525. *MC, 25* (1970), 261–2.

2342 LII. [Epistola] Andreae Thurini Pisciensis, ... ad Matthaeum Curtium Ticinen *de vena in curatione pleuritidos incidenda*. Secunda impressio. [Bologna,] 1533. *MC, 25*, 359–61.

2343 NUYENS, B. W. Th. (1925). Een zeldzaam geneeskundige incunabel. (A rare medical incunabulum). *NTG, 69*, I, 2021–39; *BGG, V*, 89–107.

– Albertus Magnus' *De virtutibus herbarum, lapidum, animalium et mirabilibus mundi*, M. van der Goes, Antwerpen, *ca* 1485, together bound up with: *Questiones naturales perdifficiles Adelardi Bathoniensis* and *Questiones naturales philosophorum*. Present in the Library of the University of Amsterdam.

P. Manuscripts

2344 ZUIDEN, D. S. van (1919). Een merkwaardig boekje. (A remarkable booklet). *NTG, 63*, I, 278.

– note on two little manuscript books with notes on all the deliveries attended by Dr Samual Elias Stein (1778–1851), a Jew, born at The Hague, graduated at Leyden in 1799 (*de hydrope*). In 1814 he became a member in some important committees.

2345 ANDEL, M. A. van (1924). Een geneeskundig handschrift uit de 18de eeuw. (An 18th century medical manuscript). *NTG, 68*, II, 2242; *BGG, IV*, 279.

– The ms contains an anatomical part by the priest Carolus Antonius Bodonus, written in 1749–98, "chemiae institutiones" and a botanical atlas.

2346 SCHMITT, Charles B. (1970). A survey of some of the manuscripts of the Biblioteca Lancisiana in Rome. *Med. Hist., 14*, 289–94.

– The library's mss possessions are mainly from the 16th–18th centuries and include some correspondence between William Harvey and Marco Aurelius Severino, as well as materials by Marcello Malpighi and Herman Boerhaave.

2347 BJÖRCK, Gudmund (1938). Remarques sur trois documents médicaux de la bibliothèque universitaire de Leyde. *Mnemosyne*, 3th series, *VI*, 139–50.

2348 KROON, J. E. (1928). Zoekgeraakte werkjes. (Books that got lost). *NTG, 72*, I, 1711; *BGG, VIII*, 112.

– Letter to the editor.

2349 SCHMITZ-CLIEVER, E. (1966). Ein seltener medizinischer Einblattdruck aus der ersten Hälfte des 16. Jahrhunderts. In: *Medizingeschichte im Spektrum. Festschrift Johannes Steudel*, 178–86. F. Steiner, Wiesbaden.

Q. Theses

2350 KROON, J. E. (1920). Leidsche geneeskundige proefschriften. (Leyden medical theses). *NTG, 64*, I, 446.

2351 — (1923). Enkele mededeelingen omtrent de Leidsche geneeskundige proefschriften der 16de, 17de en 18de eeuw (Some communications concerning Leyden medical theses of the 16th, 17th and 18th century). *NTG, 67*, II, 37–48; *BGG, III*, 145–56, 11 ill.

2352 — (1928). De Leidsche geneeskundige proefschriften der 16e, 17e en 18e eeuw. (The Leyden medical theses from the 16th, 17th and 18th century). *NTG, 72*, I, 568; *BGG, VIII*, 44.

– Letter to the editor.

2353 WOUDE, S. van der (1963). De oudste Nederlandse dissertaties. (The oldest Dutch theses). *Bibliotheekleven, 48*, 1–14, ill.

2354 ELAUT, L. (1954). Al snuffelend in oude proefschriften van medici uit het Noorden. (Looking into old theses of physicians from the north). *Ann. Noorden, 2*, 1–7.

2354ᵃ MULDER, R. D. (1950). De oudste medische dissertatie over Drenthe en haar verband met de "Tegenwoordige Staat" (The oldest medical thesis on D. and its relation with the "Present Situation"). *NweDrentsche Volksalm., 68*, 61–8, 1 ill.

R. Periodicals

2355 SARTON, George (1913). Le but d'"Isis". *Isis, 1*, 193–6.

2356 GARRISON, F. H. (1934). The medical and scientific periodicals of the 17th and 18th centuries. *Bull. Inst. Hist. Med., II*, 285–343.
– With a revised Catalogue and Checklist; contains also Dutch periodicals.

2357 KOUWER, B. J. (ed.) (1932). *Nederlandsch Tijdschrift voor Verloskunde en Gynaecologie. Inhoudsopgave over de jaren 1887 tot 1931, met een geschiedkundig overzicht.* (Dutch Journal for Obstetrics and Gynaecology. Table of contents on the years 1887 till 1931, with a historical survey). 174 pp., Bohn, Haarlem.
– Edited on the occasion of the 45th anniversary of the periodical and of the Dutch Gynaecological Association.

2358 DELPRAT, C. C. (1927). De geschiedenis der Nederlandsche Geneeskundige tijdschriften van 1680 tot 1857 (History of the Dutch medical periodicals from 1680 till 1857). *NTG, 71*, I, 3–116; I, 1711–1824; II, 13–86; *BGG, VII*, 1–114; 201–314; 417–90.

2359 — (1932). *De Geschiedenis van de eerste 50 jaren van het Nederlandsch Tijdschrift voor Geneeskunde 1857–1907* (History of the first 50 years of — ("Dutch Journal of Medicine")). XI + 413 pp., ill., many ports. Bohn, Haarlem.

2359ᵃ LINDEBOOM, G. A. (1974). Janus. *AP*, no 14, 17–8.
– on the history of the periodical *Janus*.

See also 1554, 2216a, 4988–9

Chapter III

Prehistoric, Primitive and Folkmedicine; Magic.

Studies on prehistoric medicine in the Netherlands or elsewhere made by Dutch scholars are relatively rare. Contributions on primitive medicine as observed in the Far East and elsewhere are more numerous. Especially in the ages in which medical care was rare in the country, but also long afterwards, folk medicine was necessarily applied extensively in the Netherlands, and it is still practised on a smaller scale.

Though there may have been some knowledge of effective medicinal herbs or procedures, most of folk medicine rested on popular belief and superstition. Exorcizing and the use of materials that go against the grain with us have been practised for a long time. Indeed, folk medicine has much in common with magic and sometimes with witchcraft. All this accounts for the contents of this chapter.

Some formerly well-known quacks are referred to in Chapter I, quackery is dealt with in Chapter XVIII (Medical Profession).

A. Prehistoric Medicine

2360 KLEIWEG de ZWAAN, J. P. (1914-15). Over prae- en protohistorische geneeskunde. (On prae- and protohistorical medicine). *Med. Wbl.*, *21*, 9, 61, 73, 85, 97 and 110.

2361 LINDEBOOM, G. A. (1955). Praehistorische geneeskunde. (Prehistoric medicine). *Trouw*, 17 december.

2362 BROEK, A. J. P. van de (1934). Over recente vondsten van menschelijke fossielen en hunne beteekenis. (On recent discoveries of human fossils and their significance). *Gen. Bl.*, *31*, 249–77, 4 ill.

2363 [Anonym] (1966). De mens at in het voorhistorisch tijdperk onkruid-zaden. (Man ate seeds of weeds in the prehistoric area). *Voeding*, *27*, 434.

2364   PUTTO, J. A. (1938). Tandcaries in het steenen tijdperk. (Tooth decay in the Stone Age). *GG*, *16*, 698.

See also 3410

Trepanation

2365   ANDEL, M. A. van (1923). Getrepaneerde praehistorische schedels. (Trephined prehistoric skulls). *NTG*, *67*, II, 63–4; *BGG*, *III*, 171–2.
– Review of T. Wilson Parry's article: The prehistoric trephined skulls of Great Britain, etc. (*Proc. Roy. Soc. Med. Hist. Section, XIV*, August, 192).

2366   MUSKENS, L. J. J. (1929). Praehistorische trepanatie. (Prehistoric trepanation). *NTG*, *73*, II, 4636–43; *BGG*, *IX*, 237–44, ill.

2367   LUYENDIJK, W. (1959). *De trepanatie in de loop der tijden*. (Trepanation in the course of times). Public lecture June 9, 1959. 26 pp., no pl.

2368   BOELES, P. C. J. A. (1943). Schedelnapjes uit terpen te Stiens en Marrum (Skull cups from terps at — and —). *De Vrije Fries*, *37*, 81–3, ill.

2369   SYPKENS SMIT, J. H. (1943). Een te Winsum (Fr.) gevonden, getrepaneerde schedel. (A trepanned skull, found at —). *De Vrije Fries*, *37*, 66–80, ill.

2370   BRONGERS, J. A. (1965–66). Evidence for Trepanning Practice in the Netherlands during Pre- and Protohistoric Times. Ultraviolet Fluorescence Photography of a soil Silhouette of an Interred Corpse. *Ber. ROB.*, *15–16*, 221–8, 24 ill.

2371   — (1967). Pre- en protohistorisch trepanaties toegelicht aan Nederlandse vondsten. (Pre- and protohistoric trepanations illustrated by Dutch finds). *Sci. Hist.*, *9*, 106–7.
– Report of a lecture.

2372   — (1967.) Protohistoric worked human skull bone in the Netherlands. *Ber. ROB*, *17*, 29–34, 18 ill.

2373   — (1968). Een trepanatiecentrum uit het begin van de jaartelling in het Noord Nederlands kustgebied. (A trepanning-centre from the beginning of the era in the Northern-Netherland coastal area). *GeWiNa*, *24*, 7–8.

2374   — (1968). Another Rondelle from the Netherlands: Garnwerd, Groningen. *Ber. ROB*, *18*, 263–5, ill.

2375   — (1969). Schedeltrepanaties. (Skull-trepanations). *Spiegel Historiael*, *4*, 41–6, 12 ill.

2376   — (1969). Ancient Old-World Trepanning Instruments. *Ber. ROB, 19,* 7–16, ill.

- also in: *Acta Sexti Conventus Historiae Scientiae medicinae Mathesos naturaliumque Excolendae Luxemburg 1970,* 131–3 (extract). E. J. Brill, Leiden.

See also 5034

2377   HENGEN, Otto P. (1973). Palaeogeneeskunde in Europa tijdens Oudheid en begin van de Middeleeuwen. (Palaeomedicine in — during Antiquity and the beginning of the Middle Ages). *Image, 12,* nr 51, 31–40, 23 ill.

B. Primitive Medicine

General

2378   BURG, C. L. van der (1904). Contribution à l'étude de la pathologie des races humaines. *Janus, IX,* 43–53.

2379   NYÈSSEN, D. J. H. (1927). De Nederlandsche arts als anthropoloog (The Dutch physician as an anthropologist). *NTG, 71,* II, 1028–39; *BGG, VII,* 602–13.

2380   BEUKERING, J. A. and H. W. A. Voorhoeve (1972). De westerse arts en de inheemse medicijnman. (The western physician and the native medicine-man). *Arts en Wereld, 5,* no 8, 20–3.

2381   OEFELE, F. Freiherr von (1899). *Over het gebruik van kruiden en dranken ter voorkoming van zwangerschap. Een ethnografisch historische studie.* (On the use of herbs and draughts in order to prevent pregnancy. An ethnografical-historical study). 127 pp. W. J. van Hengel, Rotterdam.

2382   NIEUWENHUIS, A. W. (1928). Die ursprünglichsten Ansichten über das Geschlechtsleben des Menschen. *Janus, XXXII,* 289–314.

2383   KLEIWEG de ZWAAN, J. P. (1916). Kleidung und Krankheiten. Ethnologische und historische Betrachtungen. *Janus, XXI,* 63–110.

2384   NIEUWENHUIS, A. W. (1924–25). Die Anfänge der Medizin unter den niedrigst entwickelten Völkern und ihre psychologische Bedeutung. 1. *Janus, XXVIII,* 42–60; 2. *ibid.,* 92–109; 3. *ibid.* 174–91; 4. *ibid, XXIX* (1925), 33–51; 5. *ibid.* 98–111; 6. *ibid.* 198–209; 7. *ibid.* 290–301.

2385 RENSELAAR, H. C. van (1965). Ziekte en maskers. (Disease and masks). *Organorama*, 2, nr 2, 19–24, 5 ill.

2386 NIEUWENHUIS, A. W. (1929). Meinungen der primitiven Völker über das Geschlechtsleben der Menschen. *VIme Congrès Int. d'Hist. Méd. Leyde-Amsterdam 1927*, 24–31, Anvers.

Indian Archipel

2387 KLEIWEG de ZWAAN, J. P. (1913). Die Heilkunde der Niasser. *Janus*, *XVIII*, 454–61.

2388 — (1914). *Denkbeelden der Inlanders van onzen Indischen Archipel omtrent het ontstaan van ziekten.* (Ideas of the natives of our Indian Archipel concerning the cause of diseases). Serie: Onze Koloniën, I, no 7, Baarn, 8°.

2389 — (1915). De hond in het volksgeloof der inlanders van den Indischen Archipel. (The dog in popular belief of the natives of the Indian Archipel). *Ind. Gids*, *XXXVII*, I, 173.

2390 — (1915). De aap in het volksgeloof der inlander van den Indischen Archipel. The monkey in popular belief of the natives of the —). *T. Kon. Ned. Aardrk. Gen.*, 2de serie, *XXXII*, 35.

2391 — (1930). L'île de Nias et ses habitants. *Rev. anthropol.*, *40*, 116–35.

2392 OSSENBRUGGEN, F. D. E. [1915]. *Het primitieve denken zooals dit zich uit voornamelijk in pokkengebruiken op Java en elders. Bijdrage tot de prae-animistische theorie.* (Primitive thinking, as it manifests itself mainly in smallpox-usages on Java and elsewhere. Contribution to the pre-animistic theory). 369 pp. [The Hague].

2393 KREEMER, Jr. J. (1915). Volksheilkunde im Malaiischen Archipel. *Janus*, *XX*, 46–71; 113–42; 202–31 and 365–408.

2394 NIEUWENHUIS, A. W. (1906). Die medicinischen Verhältnisse unter den Bahau- und Kenja-Dajak auf Borneo. *Janus*, *XI*, 108–18; 145–63.

2395 ELSHOUT, Jac. Mar. (1923). *Over de geneeskunde der Kênja-Dajak in Centraal Borneo, in verband met hun godsdienst.* (On the medicine of the — in Central-Borneo, in relation to their religion). Thesis Amsterdam (Supervisor: J. P. Kleiweg de Zwaan), 218 pp. Joh. Muller, Amsterdam.

2396   ROMER, D. (1907). Die Heilkunde der Batak auf Sumatra. *Janus, XII,* 382–92; 466–74; 511–24; 572–89 and 630–48, ill.

2397   NIEUWENHUIS, A. W. (1925). Der Fetischismus im Indischen Archipel und seine psychologische Bedeutung. *Arch. f. Religionswissensch., XXIII,* 265–78.

2398   KEERS, W. (1939). Over de verschillende vormen van het bijzetten der dooden bij de Sa'dan-Toradja. (On the different fashions of interring the dead with the —). *T. Kon. Ned. Aardrk. Gen.,* 2 (56), 207–13, 12 ill.

2399   EERDE, J. C. van (1911). Vingermutilatie in Centraal Nieuw-Guinea. (Finger mutilation in Central New Guinea). *T. Kon. Ned. Aardrk. Gen.,* 2de serie, *XXVIII,* 49.

2400   HANEVELD, G. T. (1971). On the early history of tattooing. *Acta Sexti conventus Hist. Sci. medic. math. nat. excolendae,* 150–5. E. J. Brill, Leiden. Also in *Janus, LVII* (1970), 150–5, 5 ill.

Africa

2401   PIJPER, C. (1919). *De volksgeneeskunst in Transvaal* (Folkmedicine in the Transvaal). Thesis Leiden (Supervisor: E. C. van Leersum). 71 pp., ill. Groen & Zn., Leiden, 8°.

2402   MBITI, J. (1967). Afrikaanse begrippen van tijd, geschiedenis en de dood (African ideas of time, history and death). *Afrika, 21,* 68–75, 4 ill. Den Haag.

2403   ZURING, J. (1970). *Leven, ziekte en dood in Afrika.* Gedachten over de niet-westerse geneeskunst (Life, disease and death in Africa. Thoughts on non-western medicine). 75 pp., ill. Gist-Brocades NV, Delft.

2404   JANSEN, G. (1973). *The doctor-patient relationship in an African tribal society.* Thesis Free University Amsterdam (Supervisor: G. A. Lindeboom). 224 pp., ill. Van Gorcum, Assen.
        – Also as a monograph with an introduction by H. G. Schulte Nordholt, (co-supervisor, professor of cultural anthropology).

C. Folkmedicine

General

2405 SCHRIJNEN, D. (1902). Volksgeneeskundige aanteekeningen (Notes on folk-medicine). *Ph. W.*, *39*, 1004–06.

2406 LEERSUM, E. C. van (1914). Over de waardeering van oude en volksgeneesmiddelen (On the appreciation of old and popular remedies). *NTG*, *58*, I, 1952–60.

2407 COHEN, M. H. (1921). Over enkele volksgeneeskundige gebruiken (On some folk-medical customs). *NTG*, *65*, II, 2795–2805; *BGG, I*, 427–37.

2408 GEWIN, Everard (1925). *Nederlandsch volksgeloof* (Dutch popular belief). 94 pp., Neerlandia, Arnhem.

2409 LINT, J. G. de (1919). Volkstümliche Bilder auf dem Gebiete der Medizin in den Niederlanden. *Janus, XXIV*, 253–315, 11 ill.

2410 BAUMANN, E. D. (1934). *Drie opstellen over volksgeneeskunde* (Three essays on folk-medicine). Primitieve opvattingen over lijf en leven. De bok en de geit in de volksgeneeskunde. De dood door den bliksem in volksgeloof en wetenschap. (Primitive views on body and life. He- and she-goat in folk-medicine. Death by lightning in popular belief and in science). 47 pp. "Eigen Volk", Scheveningen.

2411 WAAL, M. de (1934). *Nederlandsche land- en tuinbouwgewassen in de Volksgeneeskunst* (Dutch agricultural en horticultural plants in Folk-medicine). 125 pp., Veeneman, Wageningen.

2412 ROECK, Remy de (1959). Over geschiedenis der volks- en andere geneeskunde (On the history of folk- and other medicine). *De Brabantse folklore*, no. 141, 35–9.
   – Some general considerations with reference to E. D. Baumann's *Geschiedenis der Geneeskunde* (1918) (see 2172).

2413 HOMBLÉ, A. G. (1971). Bijdrage tot het geschied- en volkskundige aspekt van de geneeskunde (Contribution to the historical and folkloristic aspect of medicine). *Oostvl. Zanten, 46*, 82–8; 126–32; 166–73, ill.

2414 COCK, Alphonse de [1921]. *Spreekwoorden, gezegden en uitdrukkingen op volksgeloof berustend* (Proverbs, sayings and expressions based on popular belief). Vol. I. 240 pp., Vol. II, 116 pp. "De Sikkel", Antwerpen.

– Reviewed by M. A. van Andel. Vol. I: *NTG, 65* (1921), I, 1887–8; *BGG, I,* 178–9; Vol. II: *NTG, 67* (1923), II, 482–3; *BGG, III,* 193–4.

2415   HOMBLÉ, A. G. (1972). Geneeskundige volksboeken (Medical popular books). *Oostvl. Zanten, 47,* 122–38.

2416   SIMONS, R. D. G. Ph. (1959). Volksgeloof in de geneeskunde, in het bijzonder betreffende de lepra in de Atlantische negerzones met de overeenkomst tussen Zuid-Amerika en West-Afrika (Popular belief in medicine, particularly regarding leprosy in the Atlantic negro-zones with the resemblance between South-America and Western Africa). *NTG, 103,* 2288.

2417   ANDEL, M. A. van (1909). *Volksgeneeskunst in Nederland* (Folkmedicine in the Netherlands). Thesis Leiden (Supervisor: E. C. van Leersum). J. van Boekhoven, Utrecht. 8°.

2418   — (1910). Dutch Folk-medicine. I. no sub-title: *Janus, XV,* 452–61; II. Diseases of the nervous system and of the organ of sense. *Ibid.,* 609–21; III. Children's diseases. *Ibid.,* 698–711; IV. Diseases of the respiratory organs. *Ibid.,* 730–51; V. Infectious diseases. *Ibid.,* 858–72, ill. VI. Chirurgical diseases. *Janus, XVI* (1911), 254–70; VII. Inflammations and suppurations. *Ibid.,* 351–9; VIII. Diseases of the urogenital organs *Ibid.,* 719–31.

2419   — (1929). Volksgeneeskundige motieven in sprookjes, sagen en legenden (Folk-medical themes in folk-tales, myths and legends). *NTG, 73,* I, 2163–72; *BGG, IX,* 113–22.

2420   — (1929). Folk-medical themes in myths, legends and folk-tales. *VIme Congrès Int. d'Hist. de la Méd. Leyde-Amsterdam 1927,* 19–23. Anvers.

2421   — (1941). Volksgeneeskunst en haar betekenis voor de Nederlandse volkskunde (Folk-medicine and its significance for Dutch folk-lore). *NTG, 85,* II, 2697–2705; *BGG,* XXI, 68–76.

See also 532, 644–47, 4902a, 4903, 5073a

Customs and remedies

2422   — (1923). Das Sympathie-pulver und Verwandtes in der niederländischen Volksmedizin. *Janus, XXVII,* 54–5.

– Report of a paper read at the 15th meeting of the "Deutsche Gesellschaft für die Geschichte der Medizin und der Naturwissenschaften Leipzig, 19–22 September)

2423   — (1920). Over het gebruik van bloed in de volksgeneeskunst (On the use of blood in folk-medicine). *NTG*, *64*, I, 425–30.

2424   — (1923). De tanden in het volksgeloof en volksgebruik (The teeth in popular belief and customs) *T. Tandhk.*, *XXX*, 105.

2425   Voo, B. P. van der (1911). Volksmiddelen tegen kiespijn (Popular remedies against toothache). *Vrag. Dag*, *XXVI*, 498.

2426   Bakker, C. (1926). Volksgeneeskundige aanteekeningen omtrent de hik (Folk-medical notes concerning hiccough). *NTG*, *70*, I, 975–8; *BGG*, *VI*, 55–8.

2427   Leersum, E. C. van (1913). Polygonum aviculare als volksmiddel tegen diabetes mellitus (— as a popular remedy against diabetes mellitus). *NTG*, *57*, II, 173–80.

2428   Stapelkamp. Chr. (1941). Agrimonia Eupatoria in de volksgeneeskunde (— in folk-medicine). *Org. Chr. Ver. Nat. Geneesk.*, *39*, 34–62.

2429   Waal, M. de (1924). Steen en aarde in de Nederlandsche volksgeneeskunst (Stone and earth in Dutch folk-medicine). *NTG*, *68*, I, 1544; *BGG*, *IV*, 96. Also in: *Ph. W.*, *61* (1924), 1046–9, 1053, 1055. Literature 1056–7.

2430   Enckels, Raym (1966). Volksgeneesmiddelen uit de XVIIIde eeuw (1765). (Popular remedies from the 18th century). *Limburg*, *45*, 229–30.

2431   Feyfer, F. M. G. de (1922). De omhulling in de volksgeneeskunst ("Enveloping" in folk-medicine). *NTG*, 66, *I*, 48–58; *BGG*, *II*, 13–23.

2432   Grolman, H. C. A. (1923). Volksgebruiken bij sterven en begraven in Nederland (Popular customs at dying and burying in the Netherlands). *T. Kon. Ned. Aardr. Gen.*, 2de serie, vol. 40.

2432ᵃ   Kok, H. L. (1970). *De geschiedenis van de laatste eer in Nederland* (History of the funeral honours in the Netherlands) 326 pp., ill. De Tijdstroom, Lochem.

See also 3612

Animals

2433   Waal, M. de [after 1936]. *Dieren in de volksgeneeskunst* (Animals in folk-medicine). 122 pp., ill. "De Vlijt", Antwerpen.

2434 KALSBEEK, G. (1915). De dieren als boden van den dood (Animals as messengers of death). *Vrag. Dag, XXX,* 636.

2435 CORNELISSEN, J. (1920, 1921). De muizen en ratten in het volksgeloof (Mices and rats in popular belief). *Vrag. Dag, XXXV,* 350; *XXXVI* (1921), 367.

2436 HARTOG, C. den (1958). Haring in de volksgeneeskunde (The herring in folk-medicine). *Voeding, 19,* 267–70.
      – Addition and correction: *Voeding, 19,* 545.

2437 [C.] (1935). De rol van den hond in oude geneeswijzen (The role of the dog in old modes of treatment). *De Drogist,* no 25.

                                                        See also 2389–90

      Local and regional

2438 BAKKER, C. (1925). Enuresis nocturna in de volksgeneeskunst in en om Broek in Waterland (Enuresis nocturna in folk-medicine in and around —). *NTG, 69,* II, 1123–31; *BGG, V,* 210–8.
      – The author was a family doctor at Broek in Waterland, a small village in Noord-Holland, about 20 KM to the north of Amsterdam.

2439 — (1925). Aanteekeningen van volksgeneeskunst in en om Broek in Waterland (Notices of folk-medicine in and around —). *NTG, 69,* I, 1603–8; *BGG, V,* 77–82.

2440 — (1927). Volksgeneeskundige aanteekeningen in en om Broek in Waterland verzameld (Folk-medical notices collected in and around —). *NTG, 71,* I, 2506–19; *BGG, VII,* 356–69.

2441 — (1928). *Volksgeneeskunde in Waterland. Een vergelijkende studie met de geneeskunde der Grieken en Romeinen* (Folk-medicine in Waterland. A comparative study with the Greek and Roman medicine). 631 pp. H. J. Paris, Amsterdam. 4°.

2442 — (1928). Volksgeneeskundige aanteekeningen in en om Broek in Waterland verzameld (Folk-medical notices collected in and around —). *NTG, 72,* I, 1078–94; *BGG, VIII,* 45–61.

2443 KOOI, D. van der (1933). Folkloristische en volksgeneeskundige sprokkelingen in de Friesche wouden (Folkloristic and folk-medical gleanings in the Frisian woods). *NTG, 77,* I, 50–66; *BGG, XIII,* 1–17.

2444 WIT, J. de (1924). Volksgeneeskunde in West-Friesland (Folk-medicine in —). I. *NTG, 68*, II, 1252–7; *BGG, IV*, 215–20. II. *NTG, 69* (1925), I, 588–96; *BGG, V*, 29–37.

2445 VADER, J. (1964). Walcherse Volksgeneesmiddelen (Walcheren folk remedies). *Neerlands Volksleven, 14*, 163–6.

2446 SCHEVENSTEEN, A. F. C. van (1921). Over Folklore der bedevaarten voor ooglijders in België (On Folk-lore of the pilgrimages for eye-patients in Belgium). *NTG, 65*, I, 62–7; *BGG, I*, 12–7.
– Lecture delivered to the Dutch Association for the History of medicine at Gorinchem.

2446ᵃ COCK, A. de (1891) *Volksgeneeskunde in Vlaanderen* (Folk-medicine in Flanders). Gent.

2446ᵇ HEESTERS, Wiro (1968). Resten van volksgeneeskunde in ons heem (Rests of folk-medicine in our country). *Heemschild* (St. Oedenrode), *2*, 27–32; 58–60.

See also 2458, 5316, 5317

D. Magic

2447 DEUTMANN, L. (1914). De opleiding van den arts en de occulte wetenschappen (The education of the physician and the occult sciences). *Vrag. Dag, XXIX*, 1.

2448 DIETHELM, O. (1970). The medical teaching of demonology in the 17th and 18th centuries. *J. Hist. Behav. Sci., 6*, 3–15.
– Also on Anton de Haen (1704–76).

2449 ANDEL, M. A. van (1910). Magische geneeskunde (Magic medicine). *NTG, 64*, II, 393–401.

2450 JONGKEES, L. B. W. (1960). Magie en geneeskunde (Magic and medicine). *NTG, 104*, I, 529–34.

2451 JONG, K. H. E. (1938). *De zwarte magie* (Black magic). 290 pp. Parapsychol. Bibl., Vol. III. Leopold's Uitg. Mij., Den Haag.

2452 ZUIDEN, D. S. van (1916). Verstandige inmenging der Middelburgsche vierschaar in een geval van tooverij, anno 1629 (A wise interference of the Middelburg tribunal in a case of witchcraft, A.D. 1629). *NTG, 60*, II, 1818–9.

2453 BRAEKMAN, W. (1966). Magische experimenten en toverpraktijken uit een Middelnederlands handschrift (Magic experiments and witchcraft practises from a Middle-Dutch manuscript). *MKVAW*, afd. Taal en Letterk., 53–118, facs. afl. 1–4.

2454 LINDEBOOM, G. A. (1969). De magie van het dieet (Magic of the diet). *NTG*, 113, I, 362–4. Also in: *T. Ned. Ver Diëtisten*, 24 (1969), no 6, 3–11 and in *Soteria*, 13, 1969. 57–60.
– cf. *Soteria*, 13, 60–1 (remarks by D. J. Hoens).

2455 HAVERMANS, F. M. (1938). *De magie in het denken van schizophrenen en natuurvolken* (Magic in the thinking of schizophrenics and primitive nations). Thesis Leiden (Supervisor: E. A. D. E. Carp). 144 pp. J. J. Romen, Roermond-Maaseik.

2456 KLEIWEG de ZWAAN, J. P. (1906). De astrologie in de geneeskunst (Astrology in medicine). *Geneesk. Crt.*, 28 April.

2457 BAUMANN, E. D. (1938). Magische Identificatie (Magic Identification). *Mensch en Maatschappij*, 14, nr 5, 334–47.
See also 885, 2513, 2514, 2559, 2646, 2707

Witchcraft and exorcism

2458 ANDEL, M. A. van (1934). De heks en de volksgeneeskunst (The witch and folk-medicine). *NTG*, 78, III, 3140–61; *BGG*, *XIV*, 123–44.

2459 MEYERE, Victor de (1929). De tooverij in Vlaanderen. Toovenaars, tooverheksen, aflezers en stuiters. Hunne practijken en geheimen (Witchcraft in Flanders. Magicians, witches, readers and big marbles. Their practises and secrets). *Ned. T. Volksk.*, nr 4, 5 and 6.
– Reviewed by M. A. van Andel: *NTG*, 74 (1930), II, 5397; *BGG*, *X*, 297.

2460 MEERLOO, A. M. (1960). Unwitching the witches. A trip to two towns in Holland. *Int. Rec. Med.*, 173, 770–3, facs.

2461 — (1963). Four hundred years of "witchcraft", "protection" and "Delusion". *Amer. J. Psychiat.*, 120 (1), 83–6, port.

2462 PEIPER, A. (1966). Verhexte Kinder. *Pädiat. Pädol.*, 2, 361–6.
– Also on Anton de Haen (1704–76).

2462ª WEYDE, A. J. van der (1927). Iets over toovenaars en heksen (Something on magicians and witches). *Jbk. Oud-Utrecht*, 155–69.

2463 BAKKER, C. (1903). Iets over kollen en belezen (Something on witches and exorcizing). *NTG, 47,* I, 679–97.

2464 — (1921). Iets over belezen (Something on exorcizing). *NTG, 65,* II, 52–5; *BGG, I,* 305–8.

2465 — (1922). Geesten- en heksengeloof in Noord-Holland boven het Y (Belief in spirits and witches in — beyond the Y). *Gids, II,* 84; 267.

2466 — (1931). De kerksleutel en de magische gordel in de volksgeneeskunde en signatura rerum (The church key and the magic girdle in folk-medicine and —). *Mensch & Maatschappij, 7,* 360–73.

2467 PENNING, C. P. J. (1932). Iets over vampyrs (Something on —). *NTG, 76,* III, 3861–5; *BGG, XII,* 149–53.

2468 DOOREN, L. (1938). Veroordeeling van een chirurgijn in den tijd der heksenprocessen (Conviction of a surgeon in the time of the witch-trials). *GG, 16,* 333.

2469 GEYL, A. (1908). Beschouwingen en opmerkingen naar aanleiding van de waterproef bij heksenprocessen (Reflections and remarks with reference to the water-ordeal in witch-trials). *Geneesk. Crt.,* 4 Apr. 31 pp.

2470 BASCHWITZ, Kurt (1948). *De strijd met den duivel. De heksenprocessen in het licht der massapsychologie* (The fight with the devil. The witch-trials in the light of mass-psychology). Amsterdam.

2471 TIMMER, M. (1971). Een epidemie van vrouwenhaat (An epidemic of misogyny). *Soteria, 15,* 153–63, 8 ill.
– On persecutions of witches.

2471ᵃ EMSTEDE, E. J. Th. A. M. van (²1971). *Heks en seks in Nederland.* Een geschiedenis der heksen en heksenprocessen in de Nederlanden met De Peel als middelpunt (The witch and sex in the Netherlands. A History of the witches and witch-trials in the Netherlands with the region "De Peel" as central point). 358 pp., ill. Deurne.

2472 OLBRACHTS, Frans M. (1931). Een oud Mechelsch Bezweringsformulier. (An old Mechlin incantation). *MKVAW,* 202 pp., ill., Gent.
– Reviewed by M. A. van Andel: *NTG, 75,* IV, 5905–6; *BGG, XI,* 325–6.

2473 BIJLSMA, R. (1915). Het "Boos" oog (The "evil" eye). *Natuur, XXXV,* 322.

2474 TEIXEIRA de MATTOS, E. (1928). Een geval van "het booze oog" met duivelbanning, Ao. 1598 te Antwerpen, bij een gehuwde dame met typisch hysterische aanvallen (A case of "the evil eye" with exorcism Ao 1598 at—, in a married woman with typical fits of hysteria). *NTG*, *72*, I, 1095–1103; *BGG*, *VIII*, 62–70.

2475   HAVER, J. van (1968). Bezweringen, recepten en z.g. liefdetover uit een 17e-eeuws handschrift (Exorcism, prescriptions and the so-called love magic from a 17th century manuscript). *Volkskunde*, *69*, 189–202.

2476   PANHUYS, Jhr L. C. van (1924). About the "trafe" superstition in the colony of Surinam. *Janus*, *XXVIII*, 357–68.

2477   NATER, J. P. (1972). De heks en de dermatologie (The witch and derma-tology). *Arts en Wereld*, *5*, nr 4, 26–7.

2478   MUNTENDAM, P. (1925). De breukebomen in Drenthe (The hernia-trees in —). *NTG*, *69*, II, 2123; *BGG*, *V*, 292.
       – A short note on so-called hernia-trees, wherein the sufferer from hernia should hit a nail in order to get rid of his hernia.

2479   KNIPPENBERG, W. (1956). Het spijkeroffer in de Magdalenakapel op Esdonk bij Gemert en enige hiermee verwante gevallen (The nail sacrifice in the Magdalena-chapel at — near — and some related cases). *Brabants Heem*, *8*, 106–15.

2480   VISSER, C. (= pseudon. for K. Baschwitz) (no d.). *Van de Heksenwaag te Oudewater en andere te weinig bekende zaken* (On the Witch Weigh-house at — and other not well-known things). Lochem.

2481   VRIES, Thom. J. de (1956). *Speculum Superstitionis*, 35 pp., 10 ill. Tjeenk Willink, Zwolle.

See also 1895–1912 (Joh. Wier), 5505–06

Chapter IV

Antiquity

In this chapter the few items referring to the ancient medicine of Babylon, India, Egypt and Israël precede those dealing with medicine and medical writers of the Greeks and the Romans whose ideas prevailed untill the end of the seventeenth century.

Whereas, in the eighteenth century, Boerhaave published a new edition of the works of Aretaeus of Cappadocia provided with a critical apparatus, and, in the nineteenth century, F. Z. Ermerins published a new edition of the Corpus Hippocraticum, in this country little or no philological work has been done in our age on the writings of classical medical authors. Nevertheless, a.o. Van Andel, Lulofs and Schlichting wrote some essays in the field of Graeco-roman medicine, and Baumann who was not only a medical historian but also a cultural philosopher wrote many articles on various diseases and topics related to medicine in antiquity.

A. Babylonian and Assyrian Medicine

2482 BAKKER, C. (1932). De geneeskunst der oude Arische volken (Medicine of the ancient Aryan peoples). *NTG, 76*, I, 564–81; *BGG, XII*, 21–38.

2483 PROOSDIJ, B. A. van (1954). De jongste literatuur over de Assyrische geneeskunde (Recent literature on Assyrian medicine). *NTG, 98, III,* 1863–7; *BGG, XXXIV*, 61–5.

2484 DIJK, J. van (1964). Le motif cosmique dans la pensée sumérienne. *Acta orient. Copenhagen, 28,* 1–60.

2485 SCHLICHTING, Th. H. (1957). Het oudste medische geschrift (The oldest medical writing). *NTG, 101*, I, 362; *BGG, XXXVII*, 6.
– Review of an article from the *Illustrated London News,* 26 Febr. 1956, on an old Sumerian clay tablet with description of chemical, vegetable, and animal medicines.

2486 BARUCH, J. Z. (1967). Opvattingen over ziekte in het oude Babylon en

Egypte (Ideas on disease in ancient Babylon and Egypt). *NTG, 111*,
1214; cf: *NTG, 112* (1968), 45.

2487 JONG, H. W. M. de (1959). *Demonische ziekten in Babylon en Bijbel*
(Demonic diseases in Babylon and the Bible). Thesis University of
Amsterdam (Supervisor: P. van der Meer). XVI + 132 pp. E. J. Brill,
Leiden.
– Reviewed by J. J. Versluys in: *Janus, XLVIII* (1959), 279–81.

2488 — (1959). Medical Prognostication in Babylon. *Janus, XLVIII*, 252–7.

2489 ELZAS, M. (1973). La Boulimie, d'après le Talmud Babylonien. *Rev.
d'Hist. Méd. hébraique*, 26, no 105, 145–9.

See also 2696

B. Indian Medicine

2490 HALBERTSMA, K. T. A. (1941). Iets over de oogheelkunde der oude
Indiërs, in het bijzonder van Susrata (Something on the ophthalmology of the ancient Indians, particularly of Susrata). *NTG, 85*, 1899–
1906; *BGG, XXI*, 53–60.

2491 KLAIJ, D. (1952). Indiaanse badkuur (Indian bathing-cure). *NTG, 96*,
II, 1545–6; *BGG, XXXII*, 31–2.

2492 SUBBA REDDY, D. V. (1972). A Dutch traveller of the 16th century on
"Social conditions, drugs, diseases, physicians and hospitals in India".
BHM Hyderabad, 1, 31–43, 135–40.

2492ᵃ MEULENBELD, G. J. (1974). *The Mādhavanidāna and its chief commentary. Chapters 1–10. Introduction, Translation and notes*. Thesis University Utrecht (Faculty of Arts, Supervisor: J. Gonda). 709 pp. E. J.
Brill, Leiden.

C. Egyptian Medicine

2493 LINT, J. G. de (1923). De Edwin Smith Papyrus (The papyrus —). *NTG,
67*, II, 474–8; *BGG, III*, 185–9.
– Extensive review of an article by James Henry Breasted (*Bull. Soc. Med. Hist.*,
Chicago, 1923).

2494 — (1924). De papyri Ebers en Smith (The papyri — and —). *NTG*, 68, I, 940–3; *BGG, IV*, 63–6.
– Report.

2495 — (1935). De achterzijde van den papyrus Edwin Smith (The reverse of the papyrus —). *NTG, 79*, I, 880–9; *BGG, XV*, 42–51.

2496 — (1931). De papyrus Edwin Smith (I). (The papyrus —). *NTG, 75*, III, 3563–81; *BGG, XI*, 193–211.

2497 — (1931). Chirurgische tekst van den papyrus Edwin Smith (II) (Surgical text of the papyrus —). *NTG, 75*, III, 3581–3602; *BGG, XI*, 211–32.

2498 GISPEN, J. G. W. (1968). A remark on the "Heart-treatise" in the Ebers papyrus. *Atti XXI Congr. Storia Med. Siena 22–28 Settembre 1968*, 956–8.

2499 LINT, J. G. de (1923). Egypte en de geneeskunde (Egypt and medicine). *NRC*, 5 maart.

2500 — (1925). Oud-Egypte en de geneeskunst (Ancient Egypt and medicine). *NTG, 69*, I, 610–1; *BGG, V*, 51–2.
– Report of a lecture, drawn up by P. Muntendan.

2501 ANDEL, M. A. van (1931). Oud-Egyptische geneeskunde. Lezing van prof. H. Ranke op 18 maart 1931 te Utrecht (Ancient egyptian medicine. Lecture by prof. H. Ranke on —). *NTG, 75*, II, 2390–2; *BGG, XI*, 166–8.

2502 STOUTENBEEK, W. C. P. (1970). Over de Oud-Egyptische geneeskunde en haar invloed op de Oud-Griekse (On the influence of ancient Egyptian on ancient Greek medicine). *Soteria, 10*, 131–48.

2503 LINT, J. G. de (1915). Oudste bronnen van onze anatomische kennis (Oldest sources of our anatomical knowledge). *NTG, 59*, II, 2423–8.
– On some old Assyrian and Egyptian data.

2504 DUTILH, J. M. (1922). Iets over leven en dood in het oude Egypte (Something on life and death in ancient Egypt). *Vrag. Dag, XXXVII*, 305.

2505 MACKENZIE-van der NOORDA, M. C. (1964). Een medisch aspect van de verwantschap tussen Akhnaton, Smenkha Re en Toetankamon (A medical aspect of the relationship between —, —, and —). *Organorama, I*, no 4, 23-6.

2506 LINT, J. G. de (1923). Champollion and Egypt. *Med. Life, XXX*, 115.

2507 BER, Artur (1973). Was de god Bes een hypothyreoïde dwerg? (Was the god Bes a hypothyroid dwarf?) *Organorama, 10*, nr 4, 27-30, 8 ill.

2508 WAGENAAR, M. (1937). Kennis der artsenijen uit het oude Egypte (Knowledge of the drugs from ancient Egypt). *NTG, 81*, II, 1967-8; *BGG, XVII*, 97-8.
– included in a report of a meeting of the "Genootschap".

2509 STOUTENBEEK, W. C. P. (1962). De arts in het oude Egypte (The physician in ancient Egypt). *Soteria, 6*, 172-81.

2510 LINT, J. G. de (1934). Egyptische specialisten (Egyptian specialists). *NTG, 78*, I, 1023-7; *BGG, XIV*, 48-52.

2511 — (1918). Afbeeldingen van geneesheren uit Oud-Egypte (Pictures of physicians from ancient Egypt). *NTG, 62*, II, 372-9.

2512 SYPKENS SMIT, J. H. (1947). F. Jonckheere. *Une Maladie Egyptienne. L'Hématurie parasitaire*, Brussels, 1944. *Bibl. Orient., 4*, no 2.
– Review of J.'s book. The disease discussed is considered as Bilharziosis.

2513 LINT, J. G. de (1928). Die Beschwörung in der Medizin des alten Aegyptens. *Janus, XXXII*, 119-51.

2514 — (1928). De bezwering in de geneeskunde van het oude Egypte Conjuration in the medicine of ancient Egypt). *NTG, 72*, I, 541-52; *BGG, VIII*, 17-28.

2515 — (1934). De "BNW-T"-ziekte der Egyptenaren (The "BNW-T" disease of the Egyptians). *NTG, 78*, I, 1020-2; *BGG, XIV*, 45-7.

2516 — (1935). Massage in het oude Egypte (Massage in ancient Egypt). *NTG, 79*, III, 3744-7; *BGG, XV*, 168-71.

2517 GISPEN, J. G. W. (1967). "Measuring" the patient in ancient Egyptian medical Texts. *Janus, LIV*, 224-7.

2518 MEERLOO, J. A. M. (1972). De geneeskunde en het helende oog van Horus (Medicine and the healing eye of —). *Arts en Wereld, 5*, nr 3, 3-7.

2519 ROOYEN, P. H. van (1948). Het balsemen van lijken (Embalming of corpses) *GG*, *26*, 311–4.
  – With translation of the passage on embalming with the Egyptians of Herodotus.

2520 LINT, J. G. de (1922). Notice sur la nomenclature anatomique des Egyptiens au temps des anciens pharaons. *Compt. rend. 2e Congr. Int. Hist. Méd., Paris, 1–7 July 1921.*

2521 — (1925). *Die Aegyptischen Krankheitsnamen*, von B. Ebbell *(Ztschr. ägyptische Sprache und Altertumskunde, 59*, Zweiter Heft, 55–9 and 144–9), reviewed by —. *Janus, XXIX*, 306–9.

2522 — (1932). Beitrag zur Kenntnis der anatomischen Namen im alten Ägypten. *SA, 25*, 382–90.

2523 GISPEN, J. G. W. (1968). Is the Origin of our Concept "Inflammation" to be found in the Ancient Egyptian Medical Texts? *Verh. XX. Int. Kongress Gesch. Mediz. Berlin, 22–27 August 1966*, 228–30. Olms, Hildesheim.

2524 FORBES, R. J. (1940). Problemen om een koning (Problems about a king). *NTG, 84*, III, 2949–57; *BGG, XX*, 128–36.
  – On the Pharao Achnaton.

2525 GRAY, P. H. (1966). Radiological aspects of the mummies of ancient Egyptians in the Rijksmuseum van Oudheden, Leiden. *Oudheidk. Med. Rijksmus. Oudh., 47*, 1–30.

                                       See also 1265

2525ᵃ WAGENAAR, M. (1930). Over het mummificatieproces der aegyptenaren (On the proces of mummification of the Egyptians). *Chem. Wbl., 27*, no. 23, 348–55.

D. Israël

2526 TEUNISSEN, J. V. (1972). Het boek Ecclesiasticus (The book —) *Arts en Wereld, 5*, nr II, 55–9.

2527 STRUYS, Th. (1968). *Ziekte en genezing in het Oude Testament* (Illness and cure in the Old Testament). Thesis Free University Amsterdam (Supervisor: N. H. Ridderbos). 466 pp., J. H. Kok, Kampen.

2528 BRONGERS, H. A. (1951–52). Enkele opmerkingen over het verband tus-

sen zonde en ziekte enerzijds en vergeving en genezing anderzijds in
het Oude Testament (Some remarks on the relation between sin and
disease on the one side, and remission and healing on the other side,
in the Old Testament). *Ned. Theol. T.*, *6*, 129–42.

2529 BARUCH, J. Z. (1960). De betekenis van ziekte en ziekzijn in de Bijbel
(The sense of illness and being ill in the Bible). *De Opbouw*, *14*, 2–6.

2530 — (1964). The Relation between Sin and Disease in the Old Testament.
Janus, *LI*, 295–302.

2531 — (1969). Het verband tussen zonde en ziekte in het Oude Testament
(The relation between sin and disease in the Old —). *NTG*, *113*, 30–2.

2532 — (1973). Le Rapport entre le péché et la maladie dans l'ancien Testament. *Rev. hist. Méd. hébraique*, *26*, (1), 5–9.

2533 ESSO, Izaak van (1954). L'angine de poitrine est-elle mentionnée dans
la Bible et le Talmud? *Rev. hist. Méd. hébraique*, *7*, no 3, 173-8.

2533ª LIEBURG, M. J. van (1974). Ziekten in de Bijbel (Diseases in the Bible).
Daniel, *XXVIII*, 16, 304–7.

2534 PINKHOF, H. (1925). Geneesheer of Balsemer? (Physician or Embal-
mer?) *NTG*, *69*, I, 1139; *BGG*, *V*, 72.
 – on the translation of the word "rofé" in Genesis 50:2. Letter to the editor.

2535 ELZAS, M. (1950). Numeri XI, 31–33 in het licht van de moderne wetenschap en van middeleeuwse commentaren (Numeri XI, 31–33 in
the light of modern science and of medieval commentaries). *NTG*, *94*,
IV, 2982–5; *BGG*, *XXX*, 42–5.
 – letter to the editor by A. G. J. Hermans (1950). Vergifitiging na het nuttigen van
kwartels (Poisoning after eating quails): *NTG*, *94*, IV, 3135.

See 2553

2536 KULSDOM, M. E. (1957). Naar aanleiding van Salomo's rechtspraak
(Concerning S.'s jurisdiction). *NTG*, *101*, II, 1264–9; *BGG*, *XXXVII*,
15–20.
 – 1st Book of the Kings 3:16–28. On the depiction of this event and the occurrence
of it in the 17th and 18th century.

2537 [Editorial] (1961). Een voedingsexperiment in de bijbel (A nutrition
experiment in the Bible). *Voeding*, *22*, 319–20.
 – On Daniël 1:5.

2538 DROGENDIJK, A. C. (1938). Is de melaatschheid van den bijbel een zui-

ver religieus begrip? (Is the leprosy of the Bible a pure religious conception?). *GG*, *16*, 824–34 and 850–5.

2539   TAS, J. (1953). On the leprosy in the Bible. *Actes du Septième Congrès
Int. d'Hist. Sci., Jérusalem, Août 1953*, 583–7.

2540   GRAMBERG, K. P. C. A. (1957/58). Lepra en Bijbel (Leprosy and Bible).
Soteria, *2*, no 5, 4–11.

2541   GISPEN, W. H. (1945). *De Levietische wet op de melaatsheid* (The Leviti-
cal leprosy law). Kok, Kampen.

2542   WIERSMA, J. H. (1959). Over melaatsheid van huizen i.v.m. Leviticus
14:33–53 (On leprosy of houses in relation to —). *Lucerna*, *1*, 70–7.

2543   LEIBOWITZ, J. O. (1968). A Caslari's (14th century) Hebrew manuscript
Pestilential fevers edited by H. Pinkhof. *Koroth*, *4*, 517–20 [Hebrew].

2544   SIMONS, R. D. G. Ph. (1959). Wie was Lazarus en aan welke ziekte leed
hij? (Who was — and what disease did he suffer from?) *NTG*, *103*, I,
688–90, 2 ill.

2545   BARUCH, J. Z. (1971). Gebedsgenezing (Faith healing). *Arts en Auto*,
37, nr 17, 1585.
   – on the prayer of Moses for Mirjam's leprosy (Exodus XV:26).

2546   ESSO Bzn, I. van (1949). Kende het Oude Testament het ziektebeeld
van angina pectoris? (Did the Old Testament know the syndrome of
—?). *NTG*, *93*, II, 1878–84; *BGG, XXIX*, 31–7.

2547   — (1956). Medica sacra experimentalia. Certains notions médicales
bibliques confirmées par des expériences pharmacologiques modernes.
Rev. hist. Méd. hébraique, *9*, nr 30, 5–16.

2548   WAAL, M. de (1922). *Medicijn en Drogerij in den bijbel* (Medicine and
drugs in the Bible). Amsterdam, 8°.
   – with register.

2549   SCHULTE, J. E. (1952). Was de evangelist Lucas geneesheer? (Was
Luke the Evangelist a physician?) *NTG, 96*, IV, 3211; *BGG, XXXII*, 48.
   – included in a report of a meeting of the "Genootschap" on 17 and 18 may 1952.

2550   LINDEBOOM, G. A. (1965). Luke the Evangelist and the ancient Greek
writers on medicine. *Janus, LII*, 143–8.

2551   — (1965). *Dokter Lukas* (Doctor Luke)., 175 pp., ill. Carillon-reeks
no 48, W. ten Have, Amsterdam.

2552 BARTSTRA, S. (1912). Persoonsnamen – Diernamen in den bijbel en bij het Friesche volk (Personal names – names of animals in the Bible and with the Frisian people). *Vrag. Dag, XXVII*, 130.

2553 LINDEBOOM, G. A. (1949). Vergiftige kwartels in Algerië (Poisonous quails in —). *G&W, 47*, no 4, 127–8.

See also 2535

2554 PINKHOF, H. (1921). De eenhoorn in den bijbel (The unicorn in the bible). *NTG, 65*, II, 2592.

2555 BALEN BLANKEN, G. C. van (1917–18). Erotisch-sexueele symboliek in het Oude Testament (Erotic-sexual symbolism in the Old Testament). *Med. Wbl., 24*, 609.

2556 BARUCH, J. Z. (1960). Joodse opvattingen over het verband tussen zonde en ziekte (Jewish views on the relationship between sin and disease) *G&W, 58*, 59–73.

2557 — (1961). De arts in het Joodse spreekwoord (The physician in the Jewish proverb). *GG, 39*, 315–7.

2558 — (1961). *Geneeskunde in het oude Israël* (Medicine in ancient Israël). 168 pp. Joachimsthal, Amsterdam.

2559 — (1962). Magie in de Israëlitische geneeskunde (Magic in Israelian medicine). *G&W, 60*, 241–51.

2560 — (1962). De sociale positie van de arts in het klassieke Israël (The social position of the physician in classical —). *T. Soc. Geneesk., 40*, 1–5.

2561 — (1963). De praktische therapie in het oude Israël (Practical therapy in ancient —). *Soteria, 7*, 172–5.

2562 — (1963). De juridische verantwoordelijkheid van de arts in het oude Israël (The juridical responsibility of the physician in ancient —). *Sci Hist., 5*, 147–54.

2563 — (1964). The social position of the physician in ancient Israël. *Janus, LI*, 161–8.

2564 HES, J. P. and S. WOLLSTEIN (1964). The attitude of the ancient Jewish sources to mental patients. *Israel Ann. Psychiat., 2*, 103–16.

2565 LINT, J. G. de (1917–18). De besnijdenis bij de volken der oudheid (Circumcision with ancient nations). *Med. Wbl.*, *24*, 641.

2566 [Editorial] (1973). Verbod varkensvlees te eten (Prohibition of eating pork). *Voeding*, *34*, 273.
– A review of the book: Simoons. *Food avoidances in the old world.* University of Wisconsin Press, Madison 1961. Discusses the prohibition of eating pork in Eastern Countries (Israel, etc.).

2567 KOOPMAN, J. (1930). Aan welke ziekte stierf Koning Herodes de Groote? (Of what disease died King Herodes the Great?) *NTG*, *74*, II, 5951–3; *BGG*, *X*, 330–2.

See also 1213–18 (Maimonides)

2568–81 transposed.

E. Ancient Western Medicine

General

2582 SIRKS-JOUSTRA, A. A. (1916). Oude Geneeskunde (Ancient medicine). *Vrag. Dag, XXXI*, 453.

2583 POLLAK, K. (1970). *Oude Geneeskunst* (Ancient medicine). 347 pp. ill. Stafleu, Leiden.
– *Wissen und Weisheit der alten Ärzte* translated into Dutch by Ir J. A. Maas Geesteranus.. Reviewed by W. P. C. Stoutenbeek in: *Soteria*, *15* (1971), 150–2.

2584 LINT, J. G. de (1917–18). Het verband tusschen de geneeskunde der oudheid en die der Grieken (The connection between ancient and Greek medicine). *Med. Wbl.*, *24*, 481 and 497.

2585 ELAUT, L. (1960). *Antieke Geneeskunde.* In teksten van Griekse en Latijnse auteurs vanaf Homerus tot het begin van de Middeleeuwen (Ancient medicine. In texts of Greek and Latin writers from Homer till the beginning of the Middle Ages). 439 pp. Standaard Boekhandel, Antwerpen-Amsterdam.

2586 WESTERINK, L. G. (1964). Philosophy and Medicine in late Antiquity. *Janus, LI*, 169–77.

2587 MANSFELD, J. (1973). *Theorie en Empirie. Filosofie en geneeskunst in*

de voorsokratische periode (Theory and Empiricism. Philosophy and medicine in the pre-socratic period). 38 pp., Van Gorcum, Assen.
– Inaugural address delivered february 12, 1973 Utrecht University.

GREEK MEDICINE

General

2588 WAGENINGEN, J. van (1924). De iatromathematici (The iatromathematicians). *NTG, 68,* I, 46–7; *BGG, IV,* 12.
– on the Greek physicians relating medicine to mathesis (i.e. astrology).

2589 KERSBERGEN, L. C. (1936). De geneeskunde in de Grieksche oudheid (Medicine in Greek antiquity). *NTG, 80,* III, 3305–21.

See also 150–1; medical profession

Various topics

2590 EYKEL Jr, N. M. (1955). Voeding bij de Grieken en Romeinen (Nutrition with the Greeks and Romans). *Voeding, 16,* 799–802, 2 ill.

2591 BROEKSMIT, P. L. (1905). Over spijzen en dranken in ouden tijd (On food and drinks in ancient times). *Vrag. Dag, XX,* 16 and 215.

2592 BAUMANN, E. D. (1923). Een probleem uit de antieke physiologie (A problem from ancient physiology). *NTG, 67,* II, 468–74; *BGG, III,* 179–85,
– The Ancients thought that fluids went from the mouth to the lungs.

2593 — (1931). An Antique Physiological Problem. *Ann. Med. Hist.,* n.s. *III,* 21–6.

2594 STRICKER, B. H. (1964). De nederdaling van het slijm (The descent of the phlegm). *Oudheidk. Med. Rijksmuseum van Oudheden te Leiden, XLV,* 15–24.

2595 LULOFS, H. J. (1929). Antieke beschouwingen over de menschelijke stem (Antique observations on the human voice). *NTG, 73,* II, 5730–43; *BGG, IX,* 314–27.

2596 LAIN-ENTRALGO, P. (1969). De geneeskracht van het woord in de Oudheid (The curative power of the word in Antiquity). *Doc. Geigy,* issue "Het woord en de geneeskunst".

2597 ZWAN, Jr, A. van der (1962). Antiek Hermafroditisme (Antique her-
mafroditism). *G&W*, *60*, 219–35, 10 ill.

2598 BAUMANN, E. D. (1940). Antike Betrachtungen über Nutzen und Schade des Koïtus. *Janus*, *XLIV*, 123–38.

2599 VOS, T. A. (1962). De moderne en de antieke medicus (The modern
and the ancient physician). *Hermèneus*, *33*, 172–4.

2600 ESSER, A. A. M. (1932). Gefährliche Augenärzte der Antike. *Klin.
Mbl. Augenheilk.*, *89*, 243–6.

2601 LINT, J. G. de (1920). Afbeeldingen van geneesheeren uit de oudheid
(Pictures of physicians from antiquity). *NTG*, *66*, I, 447.
– included in a report of a meeting of the "Genootschap" by M. A. van Andel.

2602 — (1921). Afbeeldingen van enkele geneesheeren uit de oudheid
(Pictures of some physicians from antiquity). *NTG*, *67*, I, 1262–71;
BGG, *I*, 113–22.

2603 SCHLICHTING, Th. H. (1955). De bibliotheek van Alexandrië (The
Alexandrian library). *NTG*, *99*, I, 973; *BGG*, *XXXV*, 35.
– Letter to the editor, with an answer of J. Ariëns Kappers.

Aesculapius

2604 SCHELTEMA, M. W. (1931). Aesculapius. *NTG*, *75*, II, 1807–10; *BGG*,
XI, 130–3.

2605 WELCKER, A. (1951). Aesculapius en Hygieia. *NTG*, *95*, II, 1373–6;
BGG, *XXXI*, 15–8, 2 ill.

2606 VOS, T. A. (1963). Asklepios en zijn heiligdommen (— and his sanctu-
aries). *Hermèneus*, *34*, 222–38.

See also Emblems (5326–36)

Homer

2607 KLEIWEG de ZWAAN, J. P. (1913). De geneeskunde ten tijde van Homerus (Medicine in the time of Homer). *NTG*, *57*, II, 352–8.

2608 VÜRTHEIM, J. J. G. (1917). Homerus' gulden keten (The golden chain
of Homer). *Gids*, *IV*, 466.

2609 STASSEN, M. J. W. (1943). Homerus en de geneeskunde (Homer and
medicine). *NTG*, *87*, I, 275–6; *BGG*, *XXIII*, 13–4.

2610   KERKHOFF, A. H. M. (1973). De artsen in Ilias en Odyssee (Physicians in Iliad and Odyssey). *NTG*, *117*, 1055–9, 1 ill.

Hippocrates

2611   LINDEBOOM, G. A. (1948). *Hippocrates*. 72 pp., 7 ill. "Het Kompas", Antwerpen – L. J. Veen, Amsterdam.

2612   SCHLICHTING, Th. H. (1936). De grondgedachten van Hippocrates (The basic ideas of —). *NTG*, *80*, III, 4023–30; *BGG*, *XVI*, 133–40.

2613   KLEIWEG de ZWAAN, J. P. (1914–15). Aanteekeningen omtrent de geneeskunde der Hippocratici (Notes concerning the medicine of the Hippocratics). *Med. Wbl.*, *21*, 314.

2614   BAUMANN. E. D. (1934). Du médecin philosophe d'Hippocrate. *Janus*, *XXXVIII*, 25–32.

2615   HOEVEN, J. A. van der (1963). *Hippokrates. Arts en ethiek.* (Hippocrates. Physician and ethics). 169 pp. Stafleu, Leiden.
         – Anthology.

                                                      See also 5218–5220

2616   LULOFS, H. J. (1920). Hippocrates' de Arte. *NTG*, *64*, I, 445–6.

2617   — (1923). Hippocrates over de kunst (— on Art). *NTG*, *67*, II, 49–58; *BGG*, *III*, 157–66.

2618   — (1926). Over het begrip "Natuur" bij Hippocrates. Poging tot analyse (On the conception "Nature" in —. Attempt at analysis). *NTG*, *70*, II, 1535–40; *BGG*, *VI*, 272–7.

2619   LINT, J. G. de (1921). Hippocrate en vers. *Bull. Soc. franç. hist. méd.*, *XV*, 314.

2620   SCHLICHTING, Th. H. (1937). De hippocratische behandeling van inwendige ziekten (The hippocratic treatment of internal diseases). *NTG*, *81*, II, 1452–60; *BGG*, *XVII*, 73–81.

2621   VOS, T. A. (1941). De oogheelkunde van Hippocrates (Ophthalmology of —). *NTG*, *85*, IV, 4023–4.

2622   — (1970). Ophthalmologie in de hippocratische geschriften (Ophthalmology in hippocratic writings). *Hermèneus*, *41*, 213–5.

2623   BAUMANN, E. D. (1960). Hippocrates over voeding (— on nutrition). *Voeding*, *21*, 89–95, ill.

2624 DOBROVICI, Antoine (1949). Hippocrates, les origines de la biologie.
      NTG, *93*, I, 47; *BGG*, *XXIX*, 14.
      – included in a report of a meeting of the "Genootschap" by D. Burger.

2625 LULOFS, H. J. (1919). Ethiek en practijk uit de school van Hippocrates
      (Ethics and practise from the hippocratic school). *Vrag. Dag*, *XXXIV*,
      581.

Hippocratic oath

2626 COHEN, M. H. (1919). Over den eed van Hippocrates (On the oath of
      —). *NTG*, *63*, II, 1390.

2627 LINT, J. G. de (1921). De eed van Hippocrates (The oath of —). *NTG*,
      65, II, 2322–3; *BGG*, I, 425–6.

2628 LINDEBOOM, G. A. (1946). *De eed van Hippocrates* (The oath of —).
      19 pp.
      – Address delivered at the Congress of the Medical Faculty Association at Amster-
      dam, on the occasion of the 10th lustrum (mid-November). [Reprint].

2629 DROSSAART LULOFS, H. J. (1965). De eed van Hippocrates (The oath
      of —). *Voordrachtenreeks Ned. Ver. psychiaters in dienstverband*, *VII*,
      no 24, 105–35.

2630 — (1965). De eed van Hippocrates (The oath of —). *MC. 20*, 1075–80;
      1104–9.

2630ᵃ DAEMS, W. F. (1973). Ärztliche Ethik in der Antike. Der Sogenannte
      Eid des Hippokrates und die Abtreibungsproblematik. *Drei* (Stutt-
      gart), no 9, 429–32, 40–1.

Hippocratic writings

2631 LULOFS, H. J. (1916). Hippocrates' geschriften: "Over lucht, water
      en bodem", en zijn historisch-geographische beteekenis (Hippocratic
      writings: "On air, water and soil" and its historical-geographical signi-
      ficance). *T. Kon. Ned. Aardrk. Gen.*, *XXXIII*, 2de serie, 206–35 and
      518–38.

2632 — (1921). Hippocrates' geschrift: παραγγελίαι, Praecepta. Hippo-
      cratic writing: —, Praecepta). *NTG*, *65*, I, 650–60; *BGG*, *I*, 64–74.

2633 — (1924). Hippocrates' geschrift περὶ ἀρχαίης ἰητρικῆς – de prisca
      medicina: over de oude geneeskunst. (Hippocrates' writing — — — —

de prisca medicina: on ancient medicine). *NTG, 68*, II, 2253–4; *BGG, IV*, 290–1.
– Report.

2634 BAUMANN, E. D. (1926). *Studiën over Hippocratici* (Studies on the Hippocratics). 112 pp. Naeff, Den Haag.

On the *Corpus Hippocraticum*, the oath, the physician and his art, on Hippocrates' relation to the philosophy of his time, on his books *Air, Water and Soil* and *On Dreams*, as well as on his prognostics.

2635 — (1938). Die pseudohippokratische Schrift Peri Maniès. *Janus, XLII*, 129–44.

2636 VOS, T. A. (1970). Decorum en Diversen (Decorum and sundries). *Hermèneus, 41*, 246–9.

2637 UNGER, Fred. Car. (ed.). (1923). *Hippocrates.* περι καρδιης. Spec. litt. inaug. [Rheno Traject]. Lugd. Bat., 8°.

2638 — (1927). De groote Hippocrates-uitgevers en de geschiedenis der geneeskunde (The great Hippocrates-publishers and the history of medicine). *NTG, 71*, I, 2493–2505; *BGG, VII*, 343–55.

2639 — (1943). Het Hippocratisch geschrift περὶ ἀρχαίης ἰητρίκῆς over de oude geneeskunde (The Hippocratic writing — on ancient medicine) *NTG, 87*, IV, 1705–9; *BGG, XXIII*, 88–92.

2640 PINKHOF, H. (1932). Hippocrates in "Onze Tuinen". (— in "Our Gardens"). *NTG, 76*, II, 2238; *BGG, XII*, 104.

– Short note on a quotation from H. on vinegar in: ΠΕΡΙ ΔΙΑΙΤΗΣ Lat. ed. Foes, II, Tome I, 359.

2641 DROSSAART LULOFS, H. J. (1954). Kanttekeningen bij Hippocrates' "Over heilige ziekte" (Marginal notes on H. "on sacred disease"). *NTG, 98*, III, 1852–63; *BGG, XXXIV*, 50–61.

2641ᵃ JONG, H. W. M. de (1973). Hippocrates en de heilige ziekte (— and the sacred disease). *GeWiNa*, no 32, 8–9.

2642 VOS, T. A. (1970). De betekenis van de hippocratische geschriften (The significance of the Hippocratic writings). *Hermèneus, 41*, 213–5.

Aristotle

2643 WASSENAAR, Th. (1916). Het tastzinbedrog van Aristoteles (A.'s deception of the sense of touch). *NTG, 60*, II, 1208–13.

2644 LULOFS, H. J. (1927). Aristoteles over eugenese (A. on eugenics). *NTG*, *71*, II, 2363–70; *BGG*, *VII*, 694–701.

2645 — (1930). Aristoteles over uiterlijk en innerlijk (A. on outward and inward). *NTG*, *74*, II, 4904–10; *BGG*, *X*, 261–70.

2646 BAKKER, C. (1930). Iets over den invloed van Empedocles en Aristoteles op de geneeskunde en de magie bij de oude Grieken en Romeinen (Something on the influence of E. and A. on medicine and magics with the ancient Greeks and Romans). *NTG*, *74*, I, 507–22; *BGG*, *X*, 29–44.

2647 SCHILFGAARDE, P. van (1938). *De zielkunde van Aristoteles* (Psychology of A.) Thesis Amsterdam (Supervisor: H. J. Pos). Leiden.

2648 SCHIERBEEK, A. (1943). Aristoteles' beschouwingen over bevruchting en erfelijkheid (A's views on conception and heredity). *NTG*, *87*, I, 270–4; *BGG*, *XXIII*, 8–12.

2649 KRAAK, W. K. (1960). Voeding bij Aristoteles (Nutrition in A.) *Voeding*, *21*, 301–7, port.

See also 2844, 2847, 2848

Galen

2650 LEERSUM, E. C. van (1913). Galen and the pulse. *Janus*, *XVIII*, 327–31, 1 ill.

2651 LULOFS, H. J. (1922). Galenus over sport (G. on sports). *NTG*, *66*, I, 486–504; *BGG*, *II*, 43–52.

2652 — (1923). Galenus' klacht: "Dokter word weer filosoof"! (G.'s complaint: Doctor, be philosopher again"!). *NTG*, *67*, II, 1634–6; *BGG*, *III*, 288–90.

2653 — (1928). Galenus over gewoonte (G. on custom). *NTG*, *72*, II, 4968–77; *BGG*, *VIII*, 305–14.

2654 BAUMANN, E. D. (1960). Galenus over "Gezonde voeding" (G. on "Healthy nutrition"). *Voeding*, *21*, 497–503, ill.

2655 ELAUT, L. (1964). Le traité galénique des clystères et de la colique traduit en latin par François de Ravelengien. *Janus*, *LI*, 136–51.

See also 751, 927, 928, 933 (Van Helmont).

Various Greek authors

2656   BALEN, J. C. F. van (1921). Basiliskos en Cockatrice. *De Natuur, XXXI,* 203.

2657   NAPJUS, J. W. (1941). De "Codex Constantinopolitanus" van Dioscorides (The — of D.). *NTG, 85,* IV, 3916–23; *BGG, XXI,* 124–31.

2658   SCHIERBEEK, A. (1919). Theophrastus, Dioscorides, Plinius, Galenus. *Levende Natuur, XXIV* (1 sept.), 135.

2659   — (1940). Theophrastus van Eresos, de vader der plantkunde (Th. of Eresos, father of botany). *Jbk Dodonaea,* 7, afl. 1.

2660   GILS, J. B. F. van (1937). Epignathus. *NTG, 81,* IV, 5838; *BGG, XVII,* 224, ill.
- On Minerva born from the head of Jupiter.; letter to the editor.

2661   BAKKER, C. (1930). Enkele fragmenten uit de werken van Oribasius, waaruit de waardeloosheid der signatuurleer blijkt (Some fragments from the works of —, showing the worthlessness of the theory of signature). *NTG, 74,* II, 5385–93; *BGG, X,* 285–93.

2662   LULOFS, H. J. (1931). Degeneratie der Galaten. Een anthropologisch moment bij Livius (Degeneration of the Galatians. An anthropological moment in L.). *NTG, 75,* II, 2371–6; *BGG, XI,* 147–52.

2663   — (1925). De eubiotiek van Plutarchus (The eubiotics of P.). *NTG, 69,* II, 1557–67; *BGG, V,* 237–47.

2664   BAUMANN, E. D. (1937). Praxagoras von Kos. *Janus, XLI,* 167–85.

2665   LINDEBOOM, G. A. (1931). Een verdediging der Geneeskunst (A defence of medicine). *Hermèneus, 3,* 73–8.
- on a small writing of a sophist.

2666   LULOFS, H. J. (1931). Seneca als medisch censor (S. as a medical censor) *NTG, 75,* IV, 5911; *BGG, XI,* 331.
- included in a report of a meeting of the "Genootschap", October 17 and 18, by M. A. van Andel.

2667   — (1932). Seneca als censor van zijn tijd (S. as a censor of his time). *NTG, 76,* III, 3293–3304; *BGG, XII,* 125–36.

2668   KREVELEN, D. A. van (1964). Quintus Smyrnaeus und die Medizin. *Janus, LI,* 178–83.

2669 VRIES, J. de (1930). Le jet de la dent. *Rev. Anthropol.*, *40*, 87–9.
– o.a. on the myth of Deukalion and Pyrrha.

2670 SNEIRO, B. (1930). A propos du jet de la dent. *Rev. Anthropol.*, *40*, 400.
– Observations from Portugal, with reference to the article of De Vries.

Roman medicine

2671 BECK, J. W. (1914). Iets over artsen en de uitoefening der geneeskunde in de Romeinse wereld (Something on physicians and the practice of medicine in the Roman world). *NTG*, *58*, I, 1902–6.

2672 SCHULTE, J. E. (1967). Keizer Hadrianus en zijn artsen (Emperor H. and his physicians). *NTG*, *III*, 1220.

2673 HAVERMANS, F. M. (1942). Krankzinnigenrecht bij de Romeinen (Lunatics law with the Romans). *NTG*, *86*, IV, 2484–5; *BGG*, *XXII*, 138–9.

2674 JONKERS, E. J. (1946). Plinius en het begin van de geneeskunde (P. and the beginning of medicine). *NTG*, *90*, III, 784–7; *BGG*, *XXVI*, 26–9.

2675 BAUMANN, E. D. (1961). De voeding in Nederland in de Romeinse tijd voornamelijk ontleend aan Plinius Major (Nutrition in the Netherlands in the Roman time mainly borrowed from —). *Voeding*, *22*, 401–8, ill.

2676 ANDEL, M. A. van (1921). Cosmetica in de Romeinsche oudheid (Cosmetics in Roman antiquity). *NTG*, *65*, II, 2164–76.

2677 HABETS, J. [1884]. Over heelkundige instrumenten uit den Romeinsche tijd, onlangs te Maastricht en omstreken gevonden (On surgical instruments from the Roman time, recently found at M. and its environs). *MKNAW*, afd. Letterk., 3de reeks, 1ste deel.

See also 503a

Diseases in Antiquity

2678 BAUMANN, E. D. (1923). *De heilige ziekte. Een bijdrage tot de geschiedenis der geneeskunde in de Oudheid* (The sacred disease. A contribution to the history of medicine in Antiquity). 323 pp. Nijgh & Van Ditmar, Rotterdam.

2679 — (1925). Die heilige Krankheit. *Janus*, *XXIX*, 7–32.
– Review of the previous item by the author himself.

2680   — (1927). Die heilige Krankheit der Skythen. *Janus, XXXI*, 447–63.

2681   — (1929). Ueber den rätselhaften Morbus Cardiacus der Antiken. *Janus, XXXIII*, 371–99.

2682   MOULIN, D. de (1961). Aneurysm in Antiquity. *Arch. Chir. néerl., XIII*, 49–63.

2683   BAUMANN, E. D. (1930). De phtisi antiqua. *Janus, XXXIV*, 209–25 and 253–72.

2684   — (1934). De asthmate antiquo. *Janus, XXXVIII*, 139–62.

2685   — (1928). Über die Erkrankungen des Blutes und der Milz im klassischen Altertum. *Janus, XXXII*, 321–37.

2686   — (1931). Ueber die Erkrankungen der Leber im klassischen Altertum. *Janus, XXXV*, 153–68 and 185–206.

2687   — (1934). Ueber die Magenkrankheiten im klassischen Altertum. *Janus, XXXVIII*, 241–65.

2688   — (1924). Over de dysenterie in de oudheid (On dysentery in antiquity). *NTG*, 68, II, 2878–98; *BGG, IV*, 307–27.

2689   — (1933). Ueber Erkrankungen der Nieren und Harnblase im klassischen Altertum. *Janus, XXXVII*, 33–47, 65–83, 116–21 and 145–52.

2690   — (1933). De Diabete antiquo. *Janus, XXXVII*, 257–70.

2691   — (1924). Over hondsdolheid in de oudheid (On rabies canina in Antiquity). *NTG*, 68, I, 458–81; *BGG, IV*, 25–48.

2692   — (1928). Ueber die Hundswut im Altertume. *Janus, XXXII*, 137–69.

2693   — (1927). *Psyché's lijden*. Studiën over de ziekten der ziel in de oudheid (The suffering of P. Studies on mental diseases in antiquity). 241 pp., Van Ditmar, Rotterdam.

2694   — (1932). Der Wahnsinn der IO. *SA*, 25, 307–14.

2695   — (1932). *De goddelijke waanzin*. Vier studiën over de ekstase. (The divine madness. Four studies on ecstasy). 113 pp., Van Gorcum, Assen.

2696   — (1935). Ueber den Boulimos und die fames canina. *Janus, XXXIX*, 165–74.

See also: 2489

2697   — (1936). Der Spasmos Kunikos der Antiken. *Janus, XL*, 34–42.

2698 JONG, H. W. M. de (1961). Demonic diseases in Sophronios' *Thaumata*. *Janus, L,* 1–8.

2699 BAUMANN, E. D. (1922). Over de kennis aangaande jicht in de oudheid (On the knowledge regarding gout in Antiquity). *Ned. Mndschr. Geneesk., XI* (N.R. III), 145.

2700 LULOFS, H. J. (1924). Antieke melancholie (Melancholy in Antiquity). *NTG, 68,* I, 944–6; 1521–33; *BGG, IV,* 67–9; 73–85.

2701 — (1925). Plato over psychisch lijden (P. on mental diseases). *NTG, 69,* II, 2552–8; *BGG, V,* 293–9.

2702 BAUMANN, E. D. (1938). Die Katalepsie der Antiken. *Janus, XLII,* 7–24,

2703 — (1939). Die Krankheit der Jungfrauen. *Janus, XLIII,* 189–94.

2704 HERMANS, A. G. J. (1963). Zelfmoord in de oudheid (Suicide in Antiquity). *NTG, 107,* I, 966–7; *BGG, XLIII,* 8–9.

2705 BAUMANN, E. D. (1923). De ziekte van Titus Pomponius Atticus. (The disease of —). *NTG, 67,* II, 1614–5; *BGG, III,* 268–9.

2706 LINT, J. G. de (1927). The Treatment of the Wounds of the Abdomen in Ancient Times. *Ann. Med. Hist.,* s. 1. *IX,* 403–7, ill.

Various topics

2707 OEFELE, F. Freiherr von (1897–98). Variétés. *Janus, II,* 634–5.
– on the double names of drugs in a Greek papyrus (on magic), Leyden Museum 7384.

2708 WAGENINGEN, J. van (1918). Die Namen der vier Temperamente. *Janus, XXIII,* 48–55.

2709 SCHLICHTING, Th. H. (1935). *De Temperamenten.* Een historisch-kritische studie (The temperaments. A historical-critical study). 220 pp. Dekker & Van de Vegt, Utrecht-Nijmegen.

2710 VOS, T. A. (1956). Epidaurus. *Hermèneus, 27,* 109–14.

2711 ESVELD, W. H. C. van (1908). *De balneis lavationibusque Graecorum.* Spec. litt. inaug. Rheno-Traject. Amersfortiae, 8°.

2712 KRAAK, W. K. (1973). Vechtende zwanen, witte pontische muizen: de oud-griekse biologie op zijn best en zijn zwakst (Fighting swans, white pontic mouses: ancient Greek biology at its best and its weakest). *GeWiNa*, no 31, 10.

2713   LULOFS, H. J. (1923). De Ouden over afstamming en erfelijkheid (The Ancients on descent and heredity). *NTG*, *67*, I, 878–84; *BGG*, *III*, 53–69.

2714   GEURTS, P. M. M. (1941). *De erfelijkheid in de oudere Grieksche wetenschap* (Heredity in ancient Greek science). Thesis Nijmegen (Supervisor: F. L. R. Sassen).

2715   HERMANS, A. G. J. (1966). Oogheelkundigen in de Griekse anthologie (Ophthalmologists in Greek anthology). *NTG*, *110*, 698–9.

2716   BAUMANN, E. D. (1938). Over het Daimonion Semeion van Socrates (On the — of S.) *Alg. Ned. T. Wijsbeg. & Psych.*, *31*, 256–65.

2717   — (1934). Tychè. *Alg. Ned. T. Wijsbeg. & Psych.*, *27*, 12–20.

2718   HOLWERDA, J. H. (1902). Een Grieksch Lourdes (A Greek L.). *Onze Eeuw*, *IV*, 665.

2719   SCHENK, V. W. D. (1955). Het mes in de wijn (The knife in the wine). *NTG*, *99*, III, 2232–3, *BGG*, *XXXV*, 75–6.
       – On the legend of childless Iphiklos. cf: A. G. J. Hermans *NTG*, *98* (1954), 359.

2720   KLEIWEG de ZWAAN, J. P. (1913). Over de heilgoden der klassieke oudheid (On the healing Gods in Antiquity). *NTG*, *57*, I, 1572–81.

2721   BAUMANN, E. D. [1936]. *Varia antiqua*, inhoudende: Over raadselachtige volken, Apolloon en de muis, Zeus de Wolfgod, Dierennamen als ziektenamen. Vespacianus als wondarts. Het bloed van den zwaardvechter (Varia antiqua, containing: On enigmatical people, A. and the mouse, Zeus and wolf-god. Names of animals as names for diseases. V. as wound physician. The blood of the gladiator). 89 pp. No pl., no d.

2722   — [no d.]. *Varia Antiqua*, IIde reeks, inhoudende: De mythe van den manken God. Asklepios en de dood. Het giftige bloed van den stier. De magische kracht van de maan (Varia Antiqua, 2nd series, containing: The myth of the lame God. The poisonous blood of the bull. The magic power of the moon. A. and death). 90 pp. Misset, Arnhem.

2723   — (1938). *Antieke Wetenschap en Folklore, Melissa*, een studie over de Bij in het Volksgeloof. Over de z.g. Ontwikkelingsideeën bij de Antieken (Ancient Science and Folk-lore. Melissa, a study on the Bee in popular belief. On ideas of generation with the Ancients). 68 pp. Misset, Arnhem.

2724 DRIESSEN, L. A. (1948). Het antieke slakkenpurper (The antique murex purple). *NTG*, *92*, I, 45; *BGG*, *XXVIII*, 3–4.
       – short note included in the report of a meeting of the "Genootschap".

2725 BAKKER, C. (1929). De aanwending van het kruid echium in de oude geneeskunde (The use of the herb – in ancient medicine). *NTG*, *73*, I, 2634–6; *BGG*, *IX*, 149–51.

2726 HANEVELD, G. T. [1966]. Cleopatra, de eeuwige minnares (C., the eternal lover). *Organorama*, *III*, no 4, 13–6, ill.

Military and naval medicine in Antiquity

2727 BOEKELMAN, W. A. (1954). De geneeskunde tijdens het beleg van Troje (Medicine during the siege of —). *NMGT*, *7*, 200–2.

2728 KERKHOFF, A. (1972). Militaire geneeskunde in de wereld van Homerus (Military medicine in the world of Homer). *NMGT*, *25*, 273–83, I ill.

2729 GOELL, Herm. (1870). *Hoe hebben de oude Grieken en Romeinen in den oorlog hunne zieken en gekwetsten verpleegd?* (How did the ancient Greeks and Romans nurse their sick and wounded persons in time of war?). Translated from German into Dutch by —. Arnhem, 8°.

2730 FEYFER, F. M. G. de (1916). Militair geneeskundige dienst bij de Romeinen (The Military medical corps with the Romans). *NTG*, *60*, I, 58–9.

2731 HANEVELD, G. T. (1965). De geneeskundige dienst bij de Romeinse vloot (The Medical corps in the Roman Navy). *NMGT*, *18*, 288–90.

2732 FEYFER, F. M. G. de (1909). Review of: Die Militärlazarette im alten Rom, vom Stabsarzt Dr Haberling (*Dtsch. Militärärztl. Ztschr.*, 1909, Heft II). *Janus*, *XIV*, 844–5.

Chapter V

Medieval Medicine

Medieval medicine occupies an intermediate place between ancient and modern medicine. Some knowledge of ancient medicine was preserved in various books of classical medical writers, copied in monasteries, and by another route transmitted bij the Arabs who had a strong sense for science; in the late Middle Ages Arab medicine had a distinct influence upon Western European medicine. However, medieval medicine was for the greater part merely empirical; theoretically it rested upon some poorly understood notions of old Greco-Roman and Arab medicine.

From this period date some herbals and antidotaries derived from the Salernitan Antidotarium Nicolai. Two books on surgery, written by two Flemish practitioners: Yperman and Scellinck, show a fresh approach to the practice of surgery. On the whole our knowledge of Dutch medicine in theory and practice in medieval times is still highly fragmentary.

The literature on some infectious diseases that prevailed in the late Middle Ages is incorporated in the chapter on Pathology (VII).

A. General

2733 DOESSCHATE, G. ten (1948). *Rolduc als middeleeuwse voorpost der wis-, natuur- en geneeskunde in de Nederlanden* (Rolduc as a medieval outpost of mathematics, natural sciences and medicine in the Netherlands) 154 pp. Lochem.

2734 BOEYNAEMS, P. (1955). De invloed van Salerno op de Nederlanden voor de Stichting der Leuvense Universiteit (The influence of Salerno on the Netherlands before the foundation of Leuven University). *Belg. T. Geneesk.*, *11*, 988-98.

2735 VERMEULEN, H. (1944). Iets over de beoefening der geneeskunde in de Benedictijner kloosters (Something on the practice of medicine in the Benedictine monasteries). *NTG*, *88*, II, 494-5; *BGG*, *XXIV*, 9-10.

2736 BARUCH, J. Z. (1967). Geneeskunde van middeleeuwen tot renaissance (Medicine from the Middle Ages till the Renaissance). *GG, 45*, 286–91.

2737 SYPKENS SMIT, J. H. (1942). Pathologie en chirurgie in de Middeleeuwen (Pathology and surgery in the Middle Ages). *NTG, 86*, III, 2236–8; *BGG, XXII*, 124–6.

2738 MOULIN, D. de (1964). *De heelkunde in de vroege Middeleeuwen.* (Early medieval surgery). Thesis Nijmegen (Supervisor: E. J. Moeys). 166 pp., 23 ill. (of which 7 col.). E. J. Brill, Leiden.
– Also as a monograph. Reviewed by E[laut] in *Sci. Hist., 6* (1964), 213–4 and by C. H. Talbot in: *Med. Hist., IX* (1965), 96–7.

2739 — (1966). Chirurgische Illustrationen aus dem frühen Mittelalter. *Curr. Problems in Hist. Med.*, 284–5. S. Karger, Basel-New-York.

2739ª BERENTS, D. A. (1974). Middeleeuwse heelmeesters. *Spiegel Historiael, 9*, 194–7, 5 ill.

2740 LINT, J. G. de (1926). Afbeeldingen uit de handschriften van Guy de Chauliac (Pictures from the manuscripts of —). *NTG, 70*, I, 530–41; *BGG, VI*, 25–36, 5 ill.

2741 [   ] (1928). Het *"Boeck van surgiën"* van Meester Thomas Scellinck van Thienen (The "Book of Surgeries" of Master — from —). *Opusc., VII*, 334 pp.
– with English translation.

2742 SUDHOFF, Karl (1919). Eine niederländische Übersetzung des frühmittelalterlichen Leitfadens für die Kinderpraxis. *Janus, XXIV*, 218–21.

2743 ANDEL, M. A. van (1913). Public hygiene in a medieval Dutch town. *Janus, XVIII*, 626–31.
– The town is Gorinchem.

2744 GEYL, A. (1909). Der Gerichtsarzt des Mittelalters. *Janus, XIV*, 81–93.

2745 — (1909). Un traité de médecine du quatorzième siècle. *Janus, XIV*, 354–89.
– see also: J. Verdam. Quelques observations littéraires sur le manuscrit, publié par le Dr Geyl. *Janus, XIV*, 390–2.

2746 WIELEN, P. van der (1900). Pharmacie in Nederland gedurende de middeleeuwen (Pharmacy in the Netherlands during the Middle Ages). *Ph. W., XXXVII*, nr 26 (27 Oct.) and nr 27 (3 Nov.).

2747   DIJK, Th. G. van (1971). Een merkwaardige schedel uit de St. Pieterskerk te Utrecht (A remarkable skull from St. Peter's Church at —).
Westerheem, *XX*, no 4 (August), 211–3, ill.

      – on a skull with a stigma in the form of a cross.

2748   CATE, C. L. ten (1971). De schedel uit de St. Pieterskerk te Utrecht
(The skull from the St. Peter's Church at —). *Westerheem*, *XX*, no 4,
213–23, 5 ill.

      – see previous item; cf: review by D. de Hoop in: *AP* (1974), no 16–17, 103–4.

2749   — (1972). Une étrange découverte: un crane du moyen-âge marqué au
fer chaud. *Archeologia*, no 49 (August), 68–71, 7 ill.

         See also 30, 1931–44 (Yperman), 3041a, 3336a, 3473,
4102–04 (Universities), 5034.

B. Manuscripts

2750   MUNK, J. (1917). *Een Vlaamsche leringe van Orinen uit de veertiende
eeuw* (A Flemish teaching of "Urine" from the fourteenth century).
Thesis Leyden. 96 pp. Leiden.

      – Ms 15624/41 Royal Library, Brussels. Reviewed by F. M. G. de Feyfer: *Janus*,
XXII (1917), 415–6.

2751   KOOI, D. van der (1924). Een oud "Meysterboek" (An old "Master-
book"). *NTG*, *68*, I, 51–2; *BGG*, *IV*, 17–8.

      – Report. A written copy of an old writing on uroscopy with a collection of
prescriptions.   *See also* 3305.

2752   BRAEKMAN, W. L. (1968). Een onbekend Mnl-handschrift uit de veertiende eeuw (An unknown Middle Dutch manuscript from the 14th
century). *MKVAW*, afd. Taal en Letterk., Nieuwe reeks, 99–131, ill.

2753   MEYIER, K. A. de (1961). Un manuscrit de Leyde contenant le "Régime du corps" d'Aldebrandin de Sienne. *Scriptorium* (Brux.), *5*,
112–4.

2754   VANDEWIELE, L. J. (1970). Some notes about the Dutch incunabulum
"Van de eygenschappen der dingen" (1485) of Bartolomeus Engelsman
XIIIth. c.) In: P. Smit and R. J. ter Laage. *Essays in biohistory*, 389–
93. Utrecht.

2755   BOEYNAEMS, P. (1964). Mechtild von Hackeborn's waarneming van de
3de en 4de harttoon (M.v.H.'s observation of the third and fourth
cardiac sounds). *Sci. Hist.*, *6*, 25–9.

2756 BRAEKMAN, W. L. and A. DEVOLVER (1969). Het Boec van .XIJ. goeden wateren. Een alchemistisch traktaatje uit de veertiende eeuw (The
Book of .XIJ. good waters. An alchemistic treatise from the 14th
century). *Sci. Hist., 11*, 65–81.

2756ᵃ ELAUT, L. (ed.). (1974). *Der Vrouwen Heimlicheid. Een middeleeuws
leerdicht over gynekologie en verloskunde.* (Women's secrets. A medieval didactic poem on gynecology and obstetrics). XLIV + 62 pp., ill.
E. Story-Scientia P.V.B.A., Gent-Leuven-Antwerpen-Brussel.
– Composed in modern Dutch by L. Elaut.

2757 DAEMS, W. F. (1966). Die MNL Macerglossen im MS 6838 A der Nationalen Bibliothek zu Paris. *Janus, LIII*, 17–29.

2758 VANDEWIELE, L. J. (1964). Dit zijn. 24. tekene der doot die Ypocras
met hem dede graven (On 24 signs of death, according to Hippocrates).
Jbk Dodonaea, 32, 393–401, facs.

2759 — (1964). Een middelnederlands tractaat over fysiognomiek (A Middle
Dutch treatise on physiognomy). *Sci Hist., 6*, 49–65.

2760 — (1966). Een Middelnederlands tractaat over chiromantie (A Middle
Dutch treatise on chiromancy). *Sci Hist., 8*, 181–202, fig.

2761 ELAUT, L. (1956). *Van Smeinscen lede. Een Middelnederlands geneeskundig geschrift.* (A Middle Dutch medical writing). Thesis for the
grade of "Geaggregeerde" to the academic teaching of the history of
medicine, Ghent). 167 pp., ill. Scheerders-Van Kerckhove, Sint-
Niklaas. 8°.

2762 — (1963). De Nederlandse bewerking (1514 en 1554) van Maguinus'
Regimen Sanitatis (The Dutch adaptation of —). *Het Boek, 36*, 80–8,
facs.

2763 BRAEKMAN, W. L. (1967). Een gecommentarieerd Antidotarium en de
Circa Instans van Platearius in een Oostmiddelnederlandse bewerking
(A commented Antidotarium and the *Circa Instans* of P. in an East
Middle Dutch version). *Sci. Hist., 9*, 182–210.

2764 DAEMS, W. F. (1961). De Middelnederlandse vertalingen van het Antidotarium Nicolai (The Middle Dutch translations of the —). *Sci.
Hist., 3*, 1–20.

2765 BOEYNAEMS, P. (1963). Een onbekende middelnederlandse vertaling
van het Antidotarium Nicolai (An unknown Middle Dutch translation
of the —). *Sci. Hist., 5*, 118–9.

2766 DAEMS, W. F. (1967). *Boec van Medicinen in Dietsche.* Een Middelnederlandse compilatie van medisch-farmaceutische literatuur (—. A Middle Dutch compilation of medical-pharmaceutical literature). *Janus*, Suppléments, VII. VI + 361 pp., 6 pl. E. J. Brill, Leiden.
  – Reviewed by D. de Moulin: *BHM, XLIII* (1969), 191–2; also by G. Rosen: *J. Hist. Med., 25* (1970), 362 and by G. Keil: *Niederdtsch. Mitt., 24* (1968), 141–8.

2767 — (1968). Die Clareit- und Ypocrasrezepte in Thomas van der Noots' "Notabel Boecxken van Cokeryen" (um 1510). In: *Fachliteratur des Mittelalters. Festschrift für Gerhard Eis*, 205–24. Metzlersche Verlagsbuchh., Stuttgart. *See also* 3040.

See also 4811–3, 4843–4, 4884, 5361a

2768 VANDEWIELE, L. J. and W. L. BRAEKMAN (1968). Een Latijns-Mnl. plantenglossarium uit het midden van de 14e eeuw (A Latin-middle Dutch glossary of plants from the middle of the 14th century). *Sci. Hist., 10,* 115–44.

2769 BRAEKMAN, W. L. (1965). De Middelnederlandse recepten in W. de Vreeses uitgave. Bestemming botanisch glossarium (The Middle Dutch prescriptions in — edition. Destination of the botanical glossary). *MKVAW*, afd. Taal en Letterk., 65–110.

2770 — (1966). Middelnederlandse recepten uit handschriften in Engeland (Middle Dutch prescriptions from manuscripts in England). *Volkskunde, 67,* 65–78.

2771 — (1971). Twee Middelnederlandse prozatraktaten en enkele recepten tegen de pest (Two Middle Dutch prose-treatises and some prescriptions against the plague). *Sci. Hist., 13,* 65–91.

2772 — and G. DOGAER (1972). Laatmiddelnederlandse pestvoorschriften (Late Middle Dutch plague regulations). *MKVAW*, afd. Taal en Letterk., no 1, 98–122.

2773 SUDHOFF, K. (1915). Die Fragmenta Emmeranensia des Pseudo-Apuleius in München und der Leidener Sammelkodex (cod. voss. lat. Q. 9). *Arch. Gesch. Mediz., VIII,* 446–9.

2774 BRAEKMAN, W. L. (1968). A middle Dutch version of Arnold de Villanova's *Liber de Vinis. Janus, LV,* 96–133.

2775 — (1968). "Van der Hulpen des Ghebrecs des Wiins". Een onbekend wijntractaat uit de vijftiende eeuw (An unknown winetreatise from the 15th century). In: *Fachliteratur des Mittelalters. Festschrift für Gerhard Eis*, 177–204, ill. Metzlersche Verlagsbuchh., Stuttgart.
  – Ms 517 Wellcome Historical Medical Library. A medieval treatise on wine.

2776 DAEMS, W. F. (1958). Ein mittelniederländisches Fragment des Liber de Vinis des Arnoldus de Villanova. *Janus, XLVII*, 87–100.

2777 DOORMAN, G. (1955). *De Middeleeuwse Brouwerij en de Gruit* (The brewery in the Middle Ages and the "gruit" [a herb later replaced by hop]. 105 pp., M. Nijhoff, Den Haag. 8°.

See also 2828, 2864–8 (herbals), 2872, 3113a, 3136, 3392–3, 3748

C. Arab Medicine

2778 KONING, P. de (1896). *Traité sur le calcul dans les reins et dans la vessie par Abu Bekr Muhammed Ibn Zakariya al-Razi*. Traduction accompagnée du texte par —. VI + 285 pp. E. J. Brill, Leiden.

2779 — (1903). *Trois traité's d'anatomie arabes par Muhammed ibn Zakariya al-Rāzi, Ali ibn Abbas et Ali ibn Sina*. Texte inédit de deux traités. Traduction par —. Leyden. 8°.

2780 BAUMANN, E. D. (1916). Razes over de pokken en mazelen (R. on smallpox and measles). *NTG, 60*, I, 1554–60.

2781 BOER, Tj. de (1920). De "Medicina Mentis van den arts Razi" (The — — of the physician —). *MKNAW*, afd. Letterkunde, *53*, serie A.

2782 GEYL, A. (1909). Zwei lateinische Handschriften aus dem 11. Jahrhundert, respective von Gariopontus und Constantinus Afer. *Janus, XIV*, 161–6.

2783 — (1909). Un traité de Médecine du quartorzième siècle. *Janus, XIV*, 354–89. cf: *ibid.*, 390–2 (remarks by J. Verdam).

2784 HOOG, P. H. van der (1938?). *Ik, Ibn Sina*. 212 pp. Zuid-Holl. Uitg. Mij., Den Haag.

2785 RIET, S. van (1963). La traduction latine du *De Anima* d'Avicenne. Préliminaires à une édition critique. *Rev. phil. Louvain, 61*, 583–626.

See also 361, 362, 2791, 3799

D. Saints

2785ᵃ WIELEN, P. van der (1934). De beschermheiligen van geneeskunst en pharmacie, St. Cosmas en Damianus (The patrons of medicine and

pharmacy, St. Cosmas and Damianus). *NTG*, *78*, III, 3165–6; *BGG*, *XIV*, 148–9.
– included in a report of a meeting of the "Genootschap" by M. A. van Andel.

2785[b] WITTOP KONING, D. A. (1968). Cosmas en Damianus in de Nederlanden (Cosmas and Damianus in the Netherlands). *Sci. Hist.*, *10*, 8–12.

2785[c] ELAUT, L. (1967). Le culte des Saints Côme et Damien dans les pays de Bénélux. *Janus*, *LIV*, 161–7, ill.

2785[d] — (1968). Kosmas en Damiaan in de Beneluxlanden. *Sci. Hist.*, *10*, 13–20.

2785[e] GEYL, A. (1911). Lidewijde van Schiedam en andere ziekten (Lidewijde of Schiedam and other diseases). *NTG*, *55*, I, 2239.

2785[f] HUDDLESTON SLATER. W. B. (1911). Lidewijde van Schiedam. *NTG*, *55*, I, 2396.

2785[g] ELAUT, L. (1960). Het skelet van Liduina van Schiedam (The skeleton of —). *Sci. Hist.*, *2*, 21–2.

2785[h] WEYDE, A. J. van der (1925). Behandeling van zieken door heiligen, priesters en monniken (Treatment of the sick by saints, priests and monks). *NTG*, *69*, II, 1118–22; *BGG*, *V*, 205–9.

2785[i] LAMERS, A. J. M. (1921). Schutspatronen en patronessen der zwangere, barende en zoogende vrouwen (Patrons and patronesses of the pregnant, child-bearing and nursing women). *NTG*, *65*, II, 2829–30; *BGG*, *I*, 461–2.

2785[j] LOGHEM, J. J. van (1932). Montpellier en de heilige Rochus (Montpellier and Saint Rochus). *NTG*, *76*, II, 2816–9; *BGG*, *XII*, 121–4, 2 ill.

2785[k] MÖNNICH, C. W. (1962). *Martinus van Tours. Naar de beschrijving van zijn leven door Sulpicius Severens*. Reidans der heiligen (Martinus of Tours. After the description of his life by Sulpicius Severens. Round dance of the saints). 124 pp., Moussault, Amsterdam.

2785[l] HEERES, P. A. (1970). *Elisabeth van Thüringen*. 68 pp., 1 col. pl., 17 ill., St. Elisabeth's of Groote Gasthuis, Haarlem.

2785[m] SCHOUTEN, J. (1973). De H. Sebastianus, erfgenaam en opvolger van Apollo (St. Sebastian, heir and successor to Apollo). *Antiek*, *8*, nr. 3, 220–8.

2785[n] CATE, C. L. ten (1971). Sankt-Antonius Abt, der Schweinheilige. *Der prakt. Tierarzt*, *52*, 178–82, 5 ill.

Chapter VI

Basic Sciences

With the rise of anatomy in the sixteenth century a new era of medicine dawned. Botany, of which some knowledge was indispensable for the collecting of medicinal herbs, developed to a more mature science. Although in our time it is considered as an auxiliary science of lesser importance, in former ages it was, to a certain extent, the basic science of therapeutics and thus it was taught for centuries in the medical faculty only.

In the seventeenth century physics was developed into a science by such genial physicists as Galilei and by the introduction of mathematics into physics. Chemistry, however, remained essentially alchemistry till the second half of that century, and even then, for a long time it continued to be an auxiliary to pharmacists. It should be remembered that the iatrochemists still based themselves on rather rough chemical notions and that it was Boerhaave who made lifelong efforts to raise chemistry to the rank of a science. It was also Boerhaave who definitively introduced the basic sciences into medical education.

The knowledge of the structure and functioning of the animal and human body was for many centuries based solely on the works of Aristotle and Galen. The appearance of the *Fabrica* of Andreas Vesalius in 1543 is the milestone marking the beginning of the Medical Renaissance and a new and most fruitful approach.

The discovery of the circulation of the blood by William Harvey in 1628 (*De motu cordis*) made the development of a new physiology possible; Dutch scientists should be given considerable credit for the early spreading of this theory initially so vehemently opposed.

In the seventeenth century Dutch research workers, as for example Antoni van Leeuwenhoek, Frederik Ruysch and Jan Swammerdam, made important contributions in the field of anatomy and physiology through the use of the first microscopes, through the new technique of injecting preserving or colouring substances into blood and lymphatic vessels, and through vivisectory physiological experiments.

Also in this chapter a section on nutrition as a basic science for health and wellbeing has been inserted.

A. Chemistry and Physics

Chemistry

2786 HORN van den BOS, H. P. M. (1904). *Matériaux pour l'histoire de la chimie dans les Pays-Bas*. A. Paets van Troostwijk, Haarlem.

2787 ZACHAR, O. (1912). Die Bedeutung der Holländer in der ältesten Geschichte der Chemie. *Janus, XVII*, 535–56.

2788 DEVENTER, Charles M. van (1924). *Grepen uit de historie der Chemie. Voordrachten*. (Analecta from the history of chemistry. Addresses). XVIII + 543 pp. Tjeenk Willink, Haarlem.

2789 PARTINGTON, J. R. (1961). *A History of Chemistry*. Vol. II: Franciscus dele Boë Sylvius, 281–90, Herman Boerhaave, 740–59. MacMillan, London. Reprint 1969.

2790 SMITS, A. (1907). *De chemie in haar oude en nieuwe banen* (Chemistry on its old and new roads). 34 pp. Delft.
– Address

2791 HOOYKAAS, R. (1937). Julius Ruska's werk over de Arabische alchemie (J.R.'s work on Arab alchemistry). *NTG, 81*, IV, 5440–1; *BGG, XVII*, 191–2.
– included in the report of a meeting of the "Genootschap" 23–24 October 1937 on Rhasis and Avicenna.

2792 JONG, H. M. E. de (1965). Michel Maier's Atalanta fugiens, commentary on Emblem XLVIII. *Janus, LII*, 81–112.

2793 — (1969). *Michael Maier's Atalanta Fugiens: Sources of an Alchemical Book of Emblems*. XIV + 461 pp., ill. E. J. Brill, Leiden.
– Reviewed by W. Pagel: *Med. Hist., XVII* (1973), 100–2.

2794 BACKER, H. J. (1918). *Oude chemische werktuigen en laboratoria van Zosimos tot Boerhaave* (Old chemical instruments and laboratories from — till —). Groningen, 8°

2795 TOWNSEND, G. L. (1966). The Alchemist. *J. Hist. Med., 21*, 408–11.
– on an engraving of Pieter Bruegel (1558).

2796 SNELDERS, H. A. M. (1972). De bekeerde alchimist (The converted alchemist). *Spiegel Historiael*, 7, 85–91, 8 ill.

2797 ALPHEN, J. van (1933). *Overzicht van de geschiedenis der organische Chemie voor 1870* (Survey on the history of organic chemistry before —). XII + 139 pp. Leiden-Amsterdam.

2798 HENIGER, J. and J. W. van SPRONSEN (1969). Driehonderd jaar schei-kunde in Leiden (Three hundred years of chemistry at L.) *Chem. Wbl.*, 65, no 32, 17–8, ill.

2799 COHEN, E. (1923). Chemisch-historische aanteekeningen. VII. Pas-teur's échec in het "Institut" (Chemical-historical notes. VII. P's failure in the "Institut"). *NTG*, 67, II, 1621–3; *BGG, III*, 275–8, 2 ports.
   - The first six articles have been published in *Chem. Wbl., 3* (1906), 341; 4 (1907), 787; 6 (1909,) 439; 8 (1911), 87; *11* (1914), 870 and *16* (1919), 168.

2800 WESTENBRINK, H. G. K. (1955–56). Biochemistry in Holland. *Clio Med., 1*, 153–9, ill.
   - a.o. on G. J. Mulder (1802–80), Jac. Moleschott (1822–93) and C. A. Pekelharing (1848–1922).

2801 METZGER, H. (1923). *Les doctrines chimiques en France (17e et 18e siècle)*. 496 pp., Paris.

2802 BACKER, H. J. (1923). De zeven metalen en de zeven planeten (The seven metals and the seven planets). *NTG*, 67, II, 1630–2; *BGG, III*, 284–6.

2803 — (1924). De namen der elementen (The names of the elements). *NTG, 68*, I, 56–7; *BGG, IV*, 22–3.

2804 HOOYKAAS, R. (1939). Die chemische Verbindung bei Paracelsus. *SA, 32*, 166–75.

2805 — (1937). Die Elementenlehre der Iatrochemiker. *Janus, XLI*, 1–28.

2806 BOAS, Marie (1956). Acid and alkali in seventeenth century chemistry. *Arch. Int. d'Hist. Sci., 9* (XXXV), 13–28.
   - also on: Dele Boë Sylvius, R. de Graaf, J. van Helmont a.o.

2807 JORISSEN, W. P. and J. H. WIETEN (1915). Het gebruik van phosphores-ceerend zwavelcalcium bij de bacchantische ritus (The use of phospho-rescent sulfurated calcium in the bacchantic rite). *Chem. Wbl., XII*, 768.

   See also 49–52 (Barchusen), 90, 271–303 (Boerhaave), 926, 1011, 1027, 1029, 1233–4 (v. Marum), 1347, 1372, 1713 4902a.

Physics

2808 COHEN, Ernst (1909). Wer had die Verbrennung einer Uhrfeder in
      Sauerstoffgas zuerst ausgeführt? *Janus, XIV,* 21–32, 2 ports (of Ingen
      Housz).
      – in Dutch: *Chem. Wbl., 2* (1907), 187.

2809 — (1909). Zur Geschichte der Erfindung des Luftballons. *Janus, XIV,*
      304–10.
      – the rôle of Joseph Black.

2810 CROMMELIN, C. A. (1935). Die holländische Physik im 18. Jahrhundert
      mit besonderer Berücksichtigung der Entwicklung der Feinmechanik.
      SA, 28, 129–42.

2811 BRUNET, P. (1926). *Les Physiciens hollandais et la Méthode expéri-
      mentale en France au XVIIIe siècle.* A. Blanchard, Paris.
      – Reviewed by F. M. G. de Feyfer: *NTG, 72* (1928), I, 567–8; *BGG, VIII,* 43–4.

2812 ALEXANDER, M. (1959). Early Acceptance of Lavoisier's theories in
      Holland. *J. Hist. Med., XIV,* 81–4.

2813 NABER, H. A. (1915). De Amsterdamsche proef van 1789 (The Am-
      sterdam test from 1789). *Nieuwe Gids, 30,* I, 66.

2814 ALBURY, W. R. (1971). Halley and the "Traité de la lumière" of Huy-
      gens: new light on Halley's relationship with Newton. *Isis, 62,* 445–68.

2815 KUENEN, J. P. (1919). *Het aandeel van Nederland in de ontwikkeling der
      Natuurkunde gedurende de laatste 150 jaren* (The share of the Nether-
      lands in the development of physics during the last 150 years). 341 pp.,
      ports., fig. Rotterdam. 4°.
      – Memorial volume of the "Bataafsch Genootschap der Proefondervindelijke Wijs-
      begeerte" at Rotterdam, 1769–1919.

2816 HAMBURGER, H. J. (1910). 25 Jahre "Osmotische Druck" in den me-
      dizinischen Wissenschaften. *Janus, XXV,* 787–96.

2817 FEYFER, F. M. G. de (1920). Geschiedenis der osmose (History of
      osmosis). *NTG. 64,* I, 446.
      – included in a report of a meeting of the "Genootschap"

2818 — (1921). Uit de geschiedenis der osmotische verschijnselen (From the
      history of osmotic phenomena). *NTG, 65, II,* 40–6; *BGG, I,* 293–9,
      3 ill.

2819 CROMMELIN, C. A. (1929). Physics and the Art of Instrument-making at Leyden in the 17th and 18th centuries. *VIme Congrès Int. d'hist. de la Méd. Leyde-Amsterdam 1927*, 62–74, Anvers.

See also 1946–49 (Zernike)

B. Biology

General

2820 [   ] (1931). *Die Entwicklung der Naturwissenschaften in den Niederlanden während des letzten halben Jahrhunderts*. 116 pp., ports. Leiden.

2821 JAEGER, F. M. (1919). *Historische studiën. Bijdragen tot de kennis van de geschiedenis der natuurwetenschappen in de Nederlanden gedurende de 16e en 17e eeuw* (Historical studies. Contributions to the knowledge of the history of natural sciences in the Netherlands during the 16th and 17th century). 275 pp., ports and ill. J. B. Wolters, Groningen.

– a.o. on Th. van Hogelande, Boëtius de Boodt, and on 300 years chemical education at Groningen University.

2822 DELAUNAY, P. (1929). L'Evolution philosophique et médicale du biomécanicisme de Descartes à Boerhaave = de Leibniz à Cabanis. *VIme Congrès int. d'hist. Méd. Leyde-Amsterdam 1927*, 133–5, Anvers.

2823 BAUMANN, E. D. (1933). *De Harmonie der Dingen*. Drie studies over Doeloorzaken en Doelmatigheid in de Natuur (The Harmony of things. Three studies on final causes and suitability in Nature). Leiden.

2824 HOOYKAAS, R. (1946). Rede en ervaring in de natuurwetenschap der XVIIIe eeuw (Reason and experience in the natural science of the 18th century). *Org. Chr. V. Nat.- en Geneesk*, 44, 1–61.

2825 SMIT, P. (1973). De situatie in de Nederlandse biologie rond 1875 (The situation in Dutch biology about 1875). *Sci. Hist.*, 15, 39–48.

2826 WAERDEN, B. L. van der (1963). *Science awakening*. 306 pp., ill. Wiley, New York.

– English translation by A. Dresden; with additions by the author. Also published by Oxford Univ. Press 1961.

2827 HOOYKAAS, R. (1959). *Natural law and divine miracle*. A historical-

critical study on the "principle of uniformity" in geology, biology and theology. XIV + 237 pp., E. J. Brill, Leiden.
– Reviewed by P. H. van Laer: *Janus, L* (1961), 72–4.

2828 VIJVER, E. van de (1960). Henricus Bate: *Speculum divinorum et quorundam naturalium*. I. Introductio, littera dedicatoria, tabula capitulorum, Prooemium, Pars I. *Philosophes Médiévaux, IV*, CIX + 261 pp., ill. Publ. Univ. Louvain. Béatrice-Nauwelaerts, Paris.

2829 OYE, P. van (1961). De geschiedenis der Natuurwetenschappen in de Koninklijke Vlaamse Academie voor Wetenschappen, Letteren en Schone Kunsten (History of Natural Sciences in the Royal Flemish Academy for Sciences, Literature and Arts). *Sci. Hist.*, *3*, 25–40.

See also 846, 875, 2624

Doctrine of evolution

2830 SCHIERBEEK, A. (1961). *Opkomst en bloei der evolutieleer* (Origin and flourishing of the doctrine of evolution). Bohn, Haarlem.

2831 LINDEBOOM, G. A. (1971). De evolutieleer versus de historia medicinae in de medische opleiding (The theory of evolution versus the historia medicinae in medical education). *G&W*, *69*, 168.
– a short note.

2832 HEGEMAN, J. G. (1970). Darwin en onze voorouders. Nederlandse reacties op de evolutieleer 1860–1875 (D. and our forefathers. Dutch reactions on the theory of evolution). *Bijdr. Gesch.*, vol. *85*, afl. 3, 261–314. (An abstract in *GeWiNa*, no 31 (1973), 6–9.

2833 SCHIERBEEK, A. (1943). De pangenesis-theorie van Darwin (The pangenesis-theorie of D.). *NTG*, *87*, II, 651–7; *BGG, XXIII*, 29–35.

2834 BOTS, J. (1972). *Tussen Descartes en Darwin. Geloof en natuurwetenschap in de 18e eeuw in Nederland* (Between D. and D. Faith and natural sciences in the 18th century in the Netherlands). 216 pp. Assen.
– with facsimile of the title page of B. Nieuwentyts book: *Regt gebruik der Wereltbeschouwingen* (1714). With a chapter on physico-theological books in the 18th century present in the Republic.

2835 LINDEBOOM, G. A. (1933). Goethe en Darwin. *Wbl. Reformatie*, 27 october.

See also 566, 567, 690

2836 SCHIERBEEK, A. (1943). De pangenesistheorie van Hugo de Vries

(The pangenesis-theorie of — —). *NTG*, *87*, III, 1488–91; *BGG*, *XXIII*, 64–7. *See also* 1858

2837 SIRKS, M. J. (1942). *De ontwikkeling der biologie* (The development of biology). VIII + 183 pp., 24 fig., 13 pl. Noorduyn's Wetenschappelijke reeks, no 2. Gorinchem.

2838 VERDOORN, Frans (1958). *Iter biohistoricum*. M. Nijhoff, Den Haag.
– inaugural address Utrecht.

2839 VERDOORN, Frans (1963). A concise review of Netherlands contributions to biohistory, during the past half century, including works relating to the Malayan Archipelago, Surinam and the Netherland Antilles. *Comm. biohist. Ultraj.*, no 2.
Reprint from: B. P. M. Schulte (ed.) *Vijftig jaren beoefening van de geschiedenis der Geneeskunde, Wiskunde en Natuurwetenschappen in Nederland 1913–1963*, 42–68. Published by the "Genootschap" (GeWiNa), no pl.

2840 ROOSEBOOM, Maria (1960). Ernst Haeckel over bastaardering (E. H. on bastardizing). *Vakbl. Biologen*, *40*, 132.
– Letter of H. to H. M. Bernelot Moens, teacher of biology at Maastricht (1903–05).
See also 875

Zoology

2841 ENGEL, H. (1948). *Over de geschiedenis van de zoölogie* (On the history of zoology). Amsterdam.
– public lecture.

2842 SCHIERBEEK, A. (1961–3). The main trends of zoology in the 17th century. *Janus*, *L*, 159–75.

2843 POSTMA, N. (1965). 50 jaar zoöphysiologie in Nederland (50 years zoophysiology in the Netherlands). *Vakbl. Biologen*, *45*, 189–93, ill.
See also 1114

Various authors on biology

2844 SCHIERBEEK, A. (1919). Aristoteles. *Levende Natuur*, *XXIV*, (1 aug.), 97.

2845 — (1921). Koelreuter en Sprengel. *Levende Natuur*, *XXV*, (1 Maart), 240.

2846   — (1921). Hales, Knight, Dutrochet. *Levende Natuur, XXVI* (1 juni), 33.

2847   — (1919–23). Van Aristoteles tot Pasteur (From A. till P.) *Levende Natuur, XXIV–XXVII*, 18 articles separately listed.

2848   — (1923). *Van Aristoteles tot Pasteur. Leven en werken der groote biologen* (From A. till P. Life and works of the great biologists). ill. Versluys, Amsterdam, 8°.

2849   — (1922). Hedwig, Brown, Ehrenburg, Unger. *Levende Natuur, XXVII* (1 oct.), 161.

Genetics and Heredity

2850   NIJHOFF, G. C. (1924). Praeformatie en epigenesis in verband met historisch belangrijke medische theorieën en systemen (Preformation and epigenesis in view of historical important medical theories and systems). *NTG, 68*, I, 44–5; *BGG, IV*, 10–1.
– Report.

2851   SETERS, W. H. van (1930). Een erfelijkheidsonderzoek in de 18de eeuw (An investigation on heredity in the 18th century). *NTG, 74*, I, 1775–9; *BGG, X*, 102–6.

2852   BARGE, J. A. J. (1938). *Praeformatie èn epigenese* (Preformation and epigenesis). 22 pp., Stenfert Kroese, Leiden.
– Address delivered on the occasion of the 363th dies natalis of the Leyden University on Febr. 8, 1938.

2853   HERMANS, A. G. J. (1953). Dominant erfelijk akyloglosson (Dominant transmissible akyloglosson). *NTG, 97*, II, 1413–4; *BGG, XXXIII*, 47–8.

2854   WAARDENBURG, P. J. (1955). Zur Geschichte der Zwillungsmethode. *SA, 39*, 123–33.

See also 566, 2214, 2713–14

C. Botany

General

2855   STEARN, W. T. (1961). *The influence of Leyden on botany in the seventeenth and eighteenth century*. Lecture delivered at Leyden, November

11, 1960. In: *Early Leyden Botany*. Leidse Voordrachten, *37*. 63 pp. Leiden University Press. Leiden.

– Followed by addresses by C. C. G. J. van Steenis and W. T. Stearn, on the occasion of the awarding of a honorary degree to Dr S. Also read in a meeting of the Brit. Soc. Hist. Science (March 20, 1961), slightly modified and enlarged; published in: *Brit. J. Hist. Sci.*, *I* (1961), 137–58.

2856 SMIT, P. (1971). Über den Einfluss einiger Deutscher Botaniker auf die Entwicklung der niederländischen Botanik im 19. Jahrhundert. *Janus*, *LVIII*, 368–77, 3 ports.

2857 SWAVING, C. (1864). Eene Bijdrage tot de studie der Oost-Indische Geneesmiddelen uit het Plantenrijk (A Contribution to the study of East-Indian remedies from the vegetable kingdom). *NTG*, *1*, 425–60.

2858 BOELMAN, H. A. C. (1936). *Bijdrage tot de geschiedenis der genees-kruidcultuur in Nederlandsch Oost-Indië* (Contribution to the history of the culture of medicinal herbs in the Dutch East Indies). Thesis Utrecht (Supervisor: De Graaff). 114 pp. Van Doesburgh, Leiden.

2859 WIELEN, P. van der (1914). Van de kruiden die genazen (On herbs that healed). *NTG*, *58*, I, 1961–9.

2860 WESTER, D. H. (1915). Over geneeskruiden. Het inzamelen en kweken in Nederland (On medicinal herbs. Collection and cultivation in the Netherlands). *Vrag. Dag, XXX*, 280.

2861 RIJNBERK, G. van (1922). Van de oude kruidkunde (On old botany). *NTG*, *66*, I, 1254–8.

2862 COHEN, H. (1927). *Bijdrage tot de geschiedenis der geneeskruidcultuur in Nederland* (Contribution to the history of the culture of medicinal herbs in the Netherlands). Thesis Utrecht (Supervisor: De Graaff). Rotterdam.

2862ᵃ OPSOMER, J. E. (1972). Cinq cents ans de botanique exotique en Belgique XIIIe – XVIIe siècle. *Bull. Séanc. Acad. roy Sci. Outre-Mer*, 446–79.

2863 VOO, B. P. van der (1910). De leer der teekenen. Een schets uit de geschiedenis der plantaardige geneesmiddelen (The doctrine of signs. A sketch from the history of the vegetable remedies). *Vrag. Dag, XXV*, 869.

See also 304–10 (Boerhaave), 510–31 (Clusius), 832, 968–9 (Hermann), 1154–84 (Linnaeus), 1194, 1270–1, 2659.

Herbals

2864 VANDEWIELE, L. J. (1965). *De "Liber magistri Avicenne" en de "Her-barijs", Middelnederlandse handschriften uit de XIVe eeuw* (Ms 15624–15641 Kon. Bibliotheek te Brussel) (The — and the —, Middle Dutch manuscripts from the 14th century (Ms 15624–15641, Royal Library Brussels). *MKVAW, 27*, no 83, 2 vols, 511 pp.

2865 — (1965). Den Herbarius in Dyetsche en de verwantschap met Her-barius Latinus in Latino cum Figuris (The Herbarius in medieval Dutch and the relationship with — in Latino cum Figuris). *Jbk. Dodonaea, 33*, 419–514, ill; *Bull. Pharm.*, no 35 (nov.), 98 pp, ill.

2866 HUNGER, F. W. T. (1931). Apuleius Platonius. *NTG, 75*, IV, 5910; *BGG, XI*, 330.
      – on the oldest Ms of Apuleius' *De virtutibus herbarum*. Included in a report of a meeting of the "Genootschap" 17 and 18 October.

2867 — (1935). De Herbarius van Pseudo-Apuleius. *NTG, 79*, IV, 5164; *BGG, XV*, 227.
      – included in a report of a meeting of the "Genootschap".

2868 — (1935). *The Herbal of Pseudo-Apuleius*, from the ninth century manuscript in the Abbey of Monte Cassino Codex Casinensis, 97, together with the first printed edition of Joh. Phil. de Lignamine Editio princeps Romae 1481 both in facsimile. Described and annotated by —. L + 172 pp., 2 ports, E. J. Brill, Leiden. f° (43 × 56 cm).
      – Reviewed in *Janus, XXXIX* (1935), 218–20.

2869 BISSELING, G. H. (1922). *Uit een oud kruidboek van 1514* (From an old herbal of 1514). Utrecht.

2870 SCHIERBEEK, A. (1946). Het Wageningse handschrift van een kruid-boek (The Wageningen manuscript of a herbal). *NTG, 90*, IV, 1316–9; *BGG, XXVI*, 35–8.

2871 RIJNBERK, G. van (1921). Van oude kruidboeken (From old herbals). *NTG, 65*, II, 2528–33, 3 ill.; 2656–61, 4 ill.; 2768–76, 8 ill.

2872 DAEMS, W. F. (1966). Die Mnl. Macerglossen in Ms 6838A der natio-nalen Bibliothek zu Paris. *Janus, LIII*, 17–29, 1 pl.
      – Macer Floridus *de viribus herbarum* is a long middle-age didactic poem on herbs.

2873 HUNGER, F. W. T. (1933). Botanische éénblad-drukken uit de 16^e

eeuw (Botanical one-leaved prints from the 16th century). *NTG*, *77*, III, 3058; *BGG*, *XIII*, 173.
– Review of a lecture held for the "Genootschap".
See also 623–53 (Dodonaeus), 1418, 1492, 2768–9, 3751.

Botanical Gardens

2874 STEARN, W. T. (1961). Botanical Gardens and botanical Literature in the eighteenth century. In: *Catalogue of Botanical Books in the Collection of Rachel McMasters Miller Hunt*, vol. II, p. XLIII–CXL. (Also as a separate volume with original pagination). Hunt Foundation, Pittsburgh, Pennsylvania.
– The three first chapters deal with 1). The Amsterdam *hortus medicus*: The Commelins; 2). The Leyden botanic garden: Boerhaave and Linnaeus; 3). The Hartecamp: Clifford and Linnaeus.

2875 METS, A. (1930). Ein Beitrag zur Geschichte der botanischen Gärten in Holland und der Kolonien. *Scalpel*, no 25–32, 8 pp., 2 ill.

2876 LAREN, A. J. van (1915). De Hortus Botanicus te Amsterdam en zijn beteekenis in vroeger en later tijd (The — — at A. and its significance in earlier and later times). *Vrag. Dag*, *XXX*, 228.

2877 SETERS, W. H. van (1954). De voorgeschiedenis der stichting van de Hortus Medicus te Amsterdam (The previous history of the foundation of the — — at A.). *Jbk. Amstelodamum*, *46*, 35–45.

2878 WITTOP KONING, D. A. (1948). De toegangspenningen voor de Hortus Medicus te Amsterdam (The admission badges to the — — at A.). *Jbk. Munt- en Penningk.*, *35*, I, 52–7.

2878ª WIJNANDS, D. O. (1974). De hortus, mensen en planten. (The hortus, men and plants). *Ons Amsterdam*, *26*, 171–3, 5 ill., 4 ports.
– on the Hortus Botanicus of Amsterdam University.

2878ᵇ FRISON, E. et R. AERNOUTS (1973). Le jardin botanique d'Anvers 1797–1926. *Janus*, *LX*, 149–92.

2879 NAPJUS, J. W. (1923). De hortus botanicus van de Franeker hoogeschool (The hortus botanicus of the Franeker Academy). *NTG*, *67*, II, 1658–60; *BGG*, *III*, 312–4.

2880 SERVAAS van ROOYEN, A. J. (1902). De 's-Gravenhaagsche hortus medicus (The hortus medicus at The Hague). *Alb. Nat.*, 24.

2881   ANDREAS, Ch. H. (1953). *Hortus Muntingiorum. Geschiedenis van de*
        Groningse hortus in de zeventiende eeuw (History of the Groningen bo-
        tanical garden in the 17th century). 105 pp., ill. Groningen.

2882   — (1962). Uit de geschiedenis van de Hortus Botanicus te Groningen
        (From the history of the — — at G.). *GeWiNa*, no 11, 12–3.

2883   BITTER, H. (1914). *De "Hortus Medicus" of Stadskruidtuin van het*
        Collegium medico-pharmaceuticum te Haarlem. Een en ander uit de
        notulenboeken van het collegium medicum te Haarlem (The — — or
        the municipal botanical garden at H. Something from the minutes of
        the collegium medicum at H.). Haarlem. 8°.   *See 4555*

2884   VEENDORP, H. and L. G. M BAAS BECKING (1938). *1587–1937. Hortus*
        Academicus Lugduno Batavus. The development of the gardens of Ley-
        den University. by H. Veendorp, hortulanus and L. G. M. Baas Becking,
        praefectus horti. With a preface by Arthur Hill, Director Royal
        Botanic Gardens, Kew. 218 pp.; ill. Enschedé, Haarlem. 4°.
        – History of the Leyden Academic Garden, containing short biographies of its
        supervisors in the foregoing three centuries.

2885   B[OCKSTAELE], P. (1961). De "Hortus Botanicus" en het "Theatrum
        Anatomicum" te Leiden gezien door een Poolse jezuiet (The Leyden
        — — and — —, seen by a Polish Jesuit) *Sci. Hist.*, *3*, 45.
        – on the (Latin) report of Bartholomeus Wasowski (1617–87), who visited Utrecht
        and Leyden during a journey through Europe, (1650–56).

2886   OOMEN, H. C. J. (1960). Een hortus botanicus in Nijmegen (A botani-
        cal garden at N.). *Numaga*, *7*, 201–10, ill., 3 ports.

2887   GROOT Sr, J. de (1931). De hortus botanicus te Rotterdam (The bo-
        tanical garden at R.). *GG*, *9*, 220.

2888   HENIGER, J. (1969). Hortus Academicus Ultrajectinus 1639–1811.
        Reflexen (of Utrecht University), no 99, 6–7.

2888ᵃ   — (1974). De Roos onder de Linden (The Rose under the Limetrees).
        Jbk. Oud-Utrecht, 1–32, 7 ill. Also in: *Comm. Biohist. Ultraj.*, nr 52.
        – Published on the occasion of the 250th anniversary (1723–1973) of the house on
        Nieuwe Gracht 187 at Utrecht as an academical building.
                                                See also 408 (Breda), 972 (Antwerp).

Plants

2889 VERDOORN, F. (ed.) (1935–1957). *Chronica botanica.* Vol. 1–17. Int. Plant Science Publ. Soc., Chronica Botanica House, Waltham 54, Mass., USA.

2890 — (1970–71). De plant in de biohistorie (The plant in biohistory). *Comm. Biohist. Ultraj.*, 19. Also in: *Jbk. Ned. bot. Ver.* (1970) 33–84; 1971: 29–32 (Engl. abstr.).

2891 VOO, B. P. van der (1912). Uit de geschiedenis der voedingsplanten (From the history of food-plants). *Vrag. Dag, XXVII*, 537.

2892 — (1919). Bedwelmende en prikkelende planten (Drugging and stimulating plants). *Vrag. Dag, XXXIV*, 266.

2893 ECK, P. N. van (1911). Iets over planten, voorkomende in de literatuur (Something about plants, figuring in literature). *Natuur, XXXI*, 15, 42 and 68.

2894 — (1916). Eenige der oudste aanwijzingen over het gebruik van planten (Some of the oldest directions for the use of plants). *Natuur, XXVI*, 122, 154 and 183.

2895 DAEMS, W. F. (1962). Bijdrage tot de geschiedenis van Euphrasia (Contribution to the history of —). *Sci. Hist.*, *4*, 53–62.

2896 — (1965). Der Misteltraktat des Wiener Kodex 3811. *SA, 49*, 90–3.

2897 BELLMANN, P. G. and W. F. DAEMS (1965). Ist die Mistel ein altes Krebsheilmittel? *SA, 49*, 355–63.

2898 ROOS, W. H. de (1920). De Alruin of Mandragora (Mandrake). *Eigen Haard, XLVI*, 291.

2899 BOON, B. (1905). De Alruinwortel (Mandragora) (Mandrake). *Natuur, XXV*, 156.

2900 VANDEWIELE, L. J. (1962). Mandragora ook in de Nederlanden (Mandrake also in the Netherlands). *MKVAW, 24*, no 3, 21 pp., 16 ill.

2901 HARMS, H. (1962). Über die Britannica, eine alte friesische Heilpflanze. *Med. Wschr., 16*, 113–7, ill.

2902 VOO, B. P. van der (1912). Tooverplanten (Magic plants). *Tijdspiegel, I*, 122, 234 and 336. *ibid., II*, 18.

2903 — (1915). De brandnetel als tooverplant (The stinging nettle as a magic plant). *Vrag. Dag, XXX*, 321.

2904 VEN, D. J. van der (1911). St Jan en het St-Janskruid (St John and St John's wort). *Eigen Haard, XXXVII*, 431 and 442.

2905 KLEYN, H. (1943). Paddenstoelen en de geneeskunde (Toadstools and medicine). *NTG, 87*, I, 452–7; *BGG, XXIII*, 15–20.

2906 GILS, J. B. F. van (1939). De wijnruit, de basilicus en het wezeltje (The herb of grace, the basilicus and the little weasel). *NTG, 83*, IV, 5656–62; *BGG, XIX*, 254–60.

2907 — (1940). Van wilde polei en wild plagiaat (From pennyroyal and wild plagiarism). *NTG, 84*, III, 2550–4; *BGG, XX*, 106–10.

2908 — (1942). Dolle kervel en volle verstand (Hemlock and sanity). *NTG, 86*, I, 319–25; *BGG, XXII*, 13–9.

See also 1001, 2768, 4932–3, 4960, 5364, 5504

D. Anatomy

General

2909 BOON Czn, A. van der (1851). *Geschiedenis der ontdekkingen in de ontleedkunde van den mensch*, gedaan in de Noordelijke Nederlanden, tot aan het begin der negentiende eeuw (History of discoveries on the anatomy of man, made in the Northern Netherlands till the beginning of the 19th century). 258 pp. C. van der Post Jr. Utrecht.

2910 BOEKE, J. (1925). Geschiedenis der ontleedkunde (History of anatomy). In: A. J. P. van den Broek, J. Boeke and J. A. J. Barge. *Leerboek der beschrijvende ontleedkunde van den mensch*, Vol. I, Chapter I, 13–43, 14 ill., 10 ports. 2nd ed. A. Oosthoek, Utrecht.

2911 VELDE, Jean van de (1959). Grepen uit de geschiedenis der anatomie (Analecta from the history of anatomy). *MKVAW, 21*, no 6, 38 pp., 25 pl.
      – Discussion of 79 "anatomies".

2912 LINT, J. G. de (1925). *Atlas van de geschiedenis der geneeskunde*. I. De ontleedkunde (Atlas of the history of medicine. I. *Anatomy*). 96 pp., 199 ports and ill. S. J. van Looy-Menno Hertzberger, Amsterdam. f°.

– With a foreword by J. A. J. Barge, professor of anatomy at Leyden. Reviewed by P. Muntendam: *NTG, 70* (1926), I, 547–9; *BGG, VI*, 42–4. Also published in English: *Atlas of the history of Medicine*, I. London 1926.

2913 PUTTO, J. A. (1938). Ordonnantie op de Anatomie (Ordinance on Anatomy). *GG, 16*, 920–1.

2914 HERMANS, A. G. J. (1951). Uit de geschiedenis van het onderwijs in de ontleedkunde (From the history of the teaching of anatomy). *NTG, 95*, IV, 3892; *BGG, XXXI*, 101.

2915 DANKMEIJER, J. (1957). *Petite histoire de l'anatomie de Leyde.* 24 pp., 9 ill., ports. Ydo, Leiden.

2916 NUYENS, B. W. Th. (1909). Een en ander over ontleedkundige boeken door Nederlanders geschreven vóór de 2de helft der achttiende eeuw (Something on anatomical books written by Dutchmen before the second half of the 18th century). *NTG, 53*, II, 659–74.

2917 VEEN, S. J. van (1908). Anatomie in de 16e eeuw (Anatomy in the 16th century). *Gelre, XI*, 390.

2918 VOS, T. A. (1973). Geschiedkundige bijdragen. VII. Renaissance der anatomie (Historical contributions. VII. Renaissance of anatomy). *Arts en Wereld, 6*, no 11, 13–26, 10 ill.

2919 LUYENDIJK-ELSHOUT, A. M. (1965). Le système lymphatique au dix-septième siècle. Réalités et Fantaisies. *Janus, LII*, 283–8.

2920 KLAAUW, C. J. van der (1922). Historique de l'osselet ou de cartilage situé dans le tendon du muscle de l'étrier. *Janus, XXVI*, 260–73.
– with an extensive bibliography.

2921 HERRLINGER, R. (1958). Die Milz. *Ciba-Ztschr.*, 8, 2982–3012, ill., port.
– also on Fred. Ruysch.

2922 ARIENS KAPPERS, J. (1954). Opvattingen over de bouw en de functie van het ventrikelsysteem in de hersenen, van de Griekse tijd tot aan het begin van de 19e eeuw (Conceptions on the structure and the function of the ventricle-system in the brains, from the Greeks till the beginning of the 19th century). *NTG, 98*, IV, 3569–87; *BGG, XXIV*, 82–100, 4 ill.

2922ª RINGOIR, D. J. B. (1971). Het begrip Urachus. Een historische inleiding (The concept of Urachus. A historical introduction). *AP*, no 5, 58.

2923 FRANCESCHINI, P. (1961). Epistemologia del concetto di epitelio. *Physis* (Firenze), *3* (1), 49–81.
      – also on F. Ruysch, R. de Graaf a.o.

2924 CATE, C. L. ten (1969). Casings with "Patches of Peyer" ΠΕΡΙ ΑΔΕΝΩΝ. From Sausage to Hippocrates. *Janus, LVI*, 22–45, 14 ill., 4 ports.

2925 HANEVELD, G. T. (1973). Sleutelbeen (Clavicle). *Arts en Wereld, 6*, no 9, 60–3, 4 ill.

2926 COLE, F. J. (Editor). (1938). *Observationes Anatomicae selectiores Amstelodamensium 1667–1673.* University of Reading, England.
      – Reprint of the *Observationes anatomicae selectiores Collegii privati Amstelodamensis.* Amsterdam 1667, and the "pars altera" of 1673. Introduction XI pp. Reviewed by D. McKie: *Ann. Sci., IV* (1939), 109–10.

2927 PRICE, Dorothy [1967]. *A historical review of embryology and intersexuality.* 20 pp., E. J. Brill, Leiden.
      – Address delivered on the occasion of the entering upon the Boerhaave-chair for the year 1967.

2928 MOLL, J. (1962). *De recente geschiedenis van de anatomische wetenschappen* (Recent history of the anatomical sciences). Groningen.
      – Inaugural address.
                    See also 1791–1817 (Vesalius), 2503, 2520, 2522, 2779, 2797, 4991, 5001, 5190a, 5190b.

Plates

2929 LINT, J. G. de (1916). The plates of Jenty. *Janus, XXI*, 129–35, ill.

2930 — (1923). Une planche anatomique inconnue. *Bull. Soc. franç. hist. méd., XVII*, 11–6, ill.

2931 — (1923). Losse anatomische prenten (Single anatomical engravings). *NTG, 67*, 1429–50; *BGG, III*, 77–98, 7 ill.

2932 — (1924). Fugitive anatomical sheets. *Janus, XXVIII*, 78–91, 7 ill.

Anatomical theatres and Collections

2933 BARGE, J. A. J. (1933). De oudste inventaris der oudste Nederlandsche anatomie (The oldest inventory of the oldest Dutch anatomy). *NTG, 77*, III, 3627–8; *BGG, XIII*, 247–50.
      – included in a report of a meeting of the "Genootschap".

2934   — (1944). *Inventaris der anatomische verzameling van de Universiteit te Leiden; De oudste academische anatomie in Nederland* (Inventory of the anatomical collection of Leyden University; the oldest academic anatomy in the Netherlands). Leiden.

2935   — (1923). *De Leidsche Anatomie herdacht* (Leyden Anatomy commemorated). 29 pp., 3 ill. S. C. van Doesburgh. Leiden.
   – Address delivered on the occasion of the opening of the Anatomical Laboratory of the Leyden University, October 2, 1923. Reviewed by P. Muntendam: *NTG, 68* (1924), I, 1977–8; *BGG, IV,* 108–9.

2936   ELSHOUT, A. M. (1950). De restauratie der praeparatenverzameling uit de 18e eeuw van het Anatomisch Laboratorium te Leiden (The restauration of the collection of preparations of the 18th century of the anatomical laboratory at L.). *NTG, 94,* 205–6.

2937   — (1952). *Het Leidse kabinet der anatomie uit de achttiende eeuw. De betekenis van een wetenschappelijke collectie als cultuurhistorisch document.* (The 18th century Leyden anatomical cabinet. The significance of a scientifical collection as a cultural-historical document). Thesis Leiden (Supervisor: J. Dankmeijer). 124 pp., ill. Universitaire Pers, Leiden.
   – also as a monograph.

2938   [   ] (1725, 1943). *Index Supellectilis Anatomicae quam Academiae Batavae quae Leidae est legavit Vir Clarissimus Johannes Jacobus Rau, Rogatu Illustrissimorum et amplissimorum Academiae istius Curatorum et urbis consulum, Confectus a Bernhardo Siegfried Albino* – With English translation. *Opusc., XVII,* 184–217.

2939   GEYSKES, D. C. (with C. J. van der KLAAUW) (1934). Der heutige Zustand der anatomischen Kabinette früherer Jahrhunderte in Leiden. *Janus, XXXVIII,* 179–92, 6 ill.

2940   RICHTER, G. (1936). *Das anatomische Theater.* 150 pp., ill. Berlin. Abhandl. Gesch. Med. Naturwiss., Heft 16.
   – discusses also the former Leyden anatomical theatre. Reviewed by M. A. van Andel: *NTG, 80,* (1936), IV, 5448; *BGG, XVI,* 221.

2941   CETTO, Anna Maria (1958). Het Leidse Theatrum Anatomicum. *Ciba-Symposium, 6,* 169–72.

2942   — (1958). Le théâtre anatomique de Leyden. *Ciba-Symposium, 6,* 169–72. (French edition).

2943   A[DMUR], M. J. (1962). The Anatomical Theatre. Leiden as Kunst und
       Wunderkammer. *J. Hist. Med.*, *17*, 188. 1 pl.
       – on the engraving of the theatre by Willem van Swanenburgh (1581–1612), after a
       drawing of Jan Corn. van 't Woudt.

2944   ENDTZ, L. J. (1974). Nieuwe gegevens over het tweede Theatrum
       Anatomicum van 's-Gravenhage (New data on the second — — at
       The Hague). *NTG*, *118*, 805–10, 3 ill.

2944ª MOULIN, D. de (1972). De natuurhistorische verzameling in het voor-
       malig Theatrum Anatomicum te Rotterdam (The natural-historical
       collection in the former — — at R.). *Rott. Jbk.*, 129–39.

2944ᵇ LIEBURG, M. J. van (1974). Het anatomisch kabinet der Clinische School
       te Rotterdam (The anatomical cabinet of the Clinical School at R.)
       Rott. Jbk., 8e reeks, 2, 251–71.

2945   VIEYRA, D. (1936). Stichting van het Koninklijk Theatrum Anato-
       micum te Berlijn, in 1724 (Foundation of the Royal Theatrum Ana-
       tomicum at Berlin, in 1724). *NTG*, *80*, III, 3173–4; *BGG, XVI*, 117–8.
                                         See also 1502–07 (Ruysch)

Instruments: magnifying-glasses, microscopes and microtomes

2946   RIJKENS, R. G. (1906). Oudere en nieuwere loupen (Older and newer
       magnifying-glasses). *Natuur, XXVI*, 27.

2947   ROOSEBOOM, M. (1954). *Van vergrootglas tot oog der wetenschap*
       (From magnifying-glass till eye of science). 53 pp., ill. Rijksmuseum
       Gesch. Natuurwetenschappen, no 93. Leiden.
       – Catalogue exposition.

2948   KINGMA BOLTJES, T. Y. (1940–41). Some experiments with blown
       glasses. *Ant. van Leeuwenhoek*, 7, 61–76, 6 pl.
       – Reviewed by A. Schierbeek: *NTG, 85* (1941), IV, 4200–1; *BGG, XXI*, 149–50.

2949   RIJKENS, R. G. (1906). Uit de geschiedenis van het mikroskoop (From
       the history of the microscope). *Natuur, XXVI*, 234, 273 and 306.

2950   — (1919). De grenzen der mikroskopische waarneming van historisch
       standpunt beschouwd (The limits of microscopial observation from
       an historical point of view). *Natuur, XXIII*, 161.

2951   CROMMELIN, C. A. (1934). Tralieplaatjes van Nobert, ter beproeving
       van microscopische objectieven en ter demonstratie van interferentie-

kleuren (Trellises of N., to test microscopial objectives and to demonstrate the interference colours). *NTG, 77*, III, 3166–8; *BGG, XIV*, 149–51.

– included in a report of a meeting of the "Genootschap".

2952 ROOSEBOOM, M. (1940). Some notes upon the Life and Work of certain Netherlands Artificers of microscopic Preparations at the End of the XVIIIth century, and the Beginning of the XIXth. *Janus, XLIV*, 24–44.

2953 — (1940). Die holländischen Optiker Jan und Harmannus van Deijl und ihre Mikroskope. *Janus, XLIV*, 185–97.

2954 — (1939). Bijdrage tot de kennis der optische eigenschappen van eenige microscopen van Van Leeuwenhoek (Contribution to the knowledge of the optical properties of some microscopes of L.). *NTG, 83*, I, 63–70; *BGG, XIX*, 1–8.

2955 — (1956). *Microscopium*. 60 pp., 115 ill. Communication no 95 from the Rijksmuseum voor de Geschiedenis der Natuurwetenschappen. Leiden. f°.

2956 — (1958). Microscopie-beoefening in de 19e eeuw. Verschil van opvatting in Engeland en op het Continent (Microscopy in the 19th century. Difference of view in E. and on the Continent). *GeWiNa, 3*, 20–1.

2957 — (1965). De invoering van de micron als maateenheid in de microscopie (The introduction of the micron as unit of measure into microscopy). *Med. Blad Dienst IJkwezen, 4*, 113–7.

– The Dutchman P. Harting (1844) choose 1/1000 mM as unit in microscopy first.

2958 SNELDERS, H. A. M. (1962). De historische ontwikkeling van het microscoop (The historical development of the microscope). *Chemie en Techniek, 17*, 5–8, ill.

2959 STAR, P. van der (1952). Enige beschouwingen over 17e en 18e eeuwse enkelvoudige microscopen van het Rijksmuseum voor Geschiedenis der Natuurwetenschappen te Leiden (Observations about 17th and 18th century simple microscopes in the National Museum for the History of Science at L.). *NTG, 96*, IV, 47; *BGG, XXXII*, 47.

2960 ZINGG, Raoul (1973). Uit de beginperiode van het microscopisch onderzoek (16e en 17e eeuw) (From the beginning of microscopical investigation (16th and 17th century). I. *Image* (Roche), no *54*, 25–32, 12 ill; II. *ibidem*, no *55*, 25–31, 23 ill.

– also on Van Leeuwenhoek and Swammerdam.

2961 HARTING, P. (1866, 1970). *Das Mikroskop*. 3 vols in one, XIV + 347
pp.; VIII + 310 pp.; IX + 452 pp. Reprographical reprint of the 1866
edition. B. M. Israël, Amsterdam.
– Reviewed by G. Rosen: *J. Hist. Med.*, *XXVII* (1972), 110–1.

2962 KLAAUW, C. J. van der (1934). Oude microtomen in het Nederlandsch
historisch natuurwetenschappelijk museum te Leiden (Old microtomes
in the Dutch historical Museum of Science at L.). *NTG*, *78*, IV, 4549–
57; *BGG*, *XIV*, 187–95, 7 ill.

2963 HANEVELD, G. T. (1973). De ontwikkeling van de microtoom in het
bijzonder tijdens de periode 1865–1885 (Development of the micro-
tome, particularly in the period 1865–1885). *Sci. Hist.*, *15*, 56–60.

2964 VRIEND-VERMEER, W. (1963). Het osteotoom van Bernhard Heine (The
osteotome of —). *NTG*, *107*, II, 1930–2; *BGG*, *XLIII*, 18–20.
                    See also 1084–9 (Leeuwenhoek), 1946–9 (Zernike).

Laboratories; staining techniques, etc.

2965 HAAN, J. de (1899). Bacteriologische Laboratoria en instituten in
Nederland (Bacteriological laboratories and institutions in the Netherlands). *Alers et al.*, 110–5.

2966 IMSENECKI, A. A. (1967). Mikrobiologiia v gollandii. *Mikrobiologiia*,
36, 724–32.

2967 LUTJEHARMS, Wilh. Jan (1936). *Zur Geschichte der Mykologie. Das
XVIII. Jahrhundert*. Thesis University of Leyden. Gouda. 8°.

2968 BEVERWIJK, A. L. van (1959). The Centraal Bureau voor Schimmel-
cultures. Half a century's experience with mould cultures. *Antonie van
Leeuwenhoek*, *25* (1), 1–20.

2969 MOENS, J. (1963, 1964). Historische ontwikkeling van het gebruik van
jodium als blauwkleurend reagens in de mykologie (Historical development of the use of iodine as a blue-coloring reagent in mycology).
Sterbeeckia (Antwerp), *2* (3), 5–16 and *3* (1964), 4.

2970 PAS, P. W. van der (1970). A note on the origin of staining techniques
for microscopical preparations. *Sci. Hist.*, *12*, 63–72.
– Appendix: Bibliography of the works of Weijer Willem Muys (1682–1744). With
comments on the staining techniques of Jan Swammerdam, A. van Leeuwenhoek
and W. W. Muys.

Varia

2971 ROOSEBOOM, M. (1950). Bijdrage tot de geschiedenis der instrument-
makers in de Noordelijke Nederlanden tot omstreeks 1840 (Contribution to the history of instrument-makers in the Northern Netherlands till about 1840). *Med. Rijksmuseum Gesch. Natuurw.*, no 74,
Leiden.

2972 VOS, T. A. (1974). Wandelingen (I). Terugblik – Hulpmiddelen in de
anatomie – Ouderdom (Walks (I). Retrospect – Expedients in anatomy
– Old age). *Arts en Wereld*, 7, nr 1, 23–30, 3 ill.
– a.o. on wax-models and votive sculptures.
                                                See also 1373, 2209

Monstra

2973 BEINS, J. F. A. (1948). *Misvorming en verbeelding* (Deformation and
imagination). Thesis Groningen. Amsterdam. 8°.

2974 GEYL, A. (1905). Nog iets over den indruk, dien monsters op het
publiek maakten (Something about the impression made by monstra
on the public). *Ned. Spectator*, no 49.

2975 VIEYRA, D. (1937). Beschrijving van een misgeboorte uit het jaar 1722
(Description of an abortion from the year 1722). *NTG, 81*, I, 64;
BGG, XVII, 24.

2976 FEYFER, F. M. G. de (1907). Een scheiding van xiphopagen in. . . 1689
(Dividing a xiphopagus in. . . 1689). *NTG, 61*, I, 1720.

2977 LINT, J. G. de (1918). Historische aanteekeningen over de baring bij
diplopagi (Historical notes on childbirth with diplopagi). *NTVerl. Gyn.*,
26, 1–29.
– with a portrait of J. S. Denijs (*ca* 1681–1741).

2978 — (1916/7) Eenige merkwaardige afbeeldingen van dubbelmonstra
(Some remarkable pictures of double-monstra). *Werken Gen. Natuur-,
genees- en heelk*, IIe serie, *IX*, 73–94, 25 ill. Also in: *NTG, 61*, II,
1599–1622.

2979 LAMERS, A. J. M. (1923). Over een wanschepsel in het jaar 1595 te
's-Hertogenbosch geboren en over de gewoonte om wanschapen ge-
borenen te smoren (On a monster born at — in the year 1595 and on
the custom to smother monstra at birth). *NTG, 67*, II, 1663–7; *BGG,
III*, 317–21.

2980   VERDAM, J. (1970). Hugo de Groot over monstra (H. de G. on monstra). In *Huldigingsbundel Daniel Pont*, 440–50. A. A. Balkema, Kaapstad (S-Africa).

2980ᵃ HANEVELD, G. T. (1974). Een Nederlands schilderij van een samengegroeide tweeling (thoracopagus) uit de 17e eeuw (A Dutch painting of conjoined twins (thoracopagus) from the 17th century). *NTG, 118*, 801–5, 3 ill.
       – The painter is Everardt Crynz van der Maes (1577–1656).

2980ᵇ — (1974). De Centaurus (The Centaurus). *Arts en Wereld*, 7, no 2, 64–8, 5 ill.

E. Physiology

General

2981   LEERSUM, E. C. van (1913). Old physiological experiments. *Janus, XVIII*, 325–6, port. (of Harvey).

2982   PEKELHARING, C. A. (1907). De physiologie in Nederland in de laatste halve eeuw (Physiology in the Netherlands in the last half century). *NTG, 51*, I, 8–28.

2983   RIJNBERK, G. van (1913). Aperçu du développement de la physiologie en Hollande. *NTG, 57*, II, 611–22, 15 ill.

2984   ROOSEBOOM, M. and W. VRIEND-VERMEER (1962). *Some Dutch contributions to the development of physiology.* Souvenir of the 22th International Congress of Physiological Sciences, 10–17 September 1962. 60 pp., ill. *Rijksmuseum Gesch. Natuurw.* Comm. no *18*.

2985   PINTO, Giuseppe (1893). I fisiologi Olandesi nel XVII e XVIII secolo. *Boll. della R. Accad. Medica di Roma, XIX*, Fasc. II, 4 pp.

2986   DAGLIO, P. (1967). Il progresso della fisiologia nell'ottocento e la concezione materialistica. *Pag. Storia Med., 11* (3), 27–35.
       – Also on Jac. Moleschott.

2987   MANI, N. (1961). Darmresorption und Blutbildung im Lichte der experimentellen Physiologie des 17. Jahrhunderts. *Gesnerus, 18*, 85–146, 9 ill.
       – also on J. van Horne, J. de Wale en A. van Leeuwenhoek.

2988   BRINK, F. G. v. d. (1969). Regulatie van de maagsapsecretie en de in-
       vloed van pharmaca (Regulation of the secretion of gastric juice and
       the influence of pharmaca). *NTG, 113*, 1544–55.
       – with historical remarks.

2989   FEYFER, F. M. G. de (1926). Autostasie en geneeskunst ("Autostasy"
       and medicine). *NTG, 70*, I, 27–42; *BGG, VI*, 1–16, ill.

2990   SCHLICHTING, Th. H. (1939). De leer der spiritus of levensgeesten (The
       theory of spiritus or vital spirits). *NTG, 83*, I, 1012–25; *BGG, XIX*,
       41–54.

2991   ARIËNS KAPPERS, J. (1957). *Over de hersenvloeistof en de hersenkamers*
       (On cerebrospinal liquid and cerebral ventricles).
       – Rectorial address Groningen; with historical survey.

2992   BERTHIER, Aug. George (1914, 1920/20). Le mécanisme cartésien et la
       physiologie au XVIIe siècle. *Isis, II* (1914). 37–89; *ibid., III* (1920/21),
       21–58.

                    See also 582–8 (Descartes), 1280–2 (Moleschott), 1430–1
                    (Regius), 2136a, 2592–3.

The circulation of the blood

2993   ISRAËLS, A. H. (1860). De verdiensten der Nederlanders in het versprei-
       den en uitbreiden der Harveyaansche ontdekking (The merits of the
       Dutch in spreading and extending the Harveyan discovery). *NTG, 4*,
       361.

2994   — and C. E. DANIËLS (1883). *De verdiensten der Hollandsche geleerden
       ten opzichte van Harvey's leer van den bloedsomloop* (The merits of
       Dutch scientists with regard to Harvey's theory of the circulation of
       the blood). 135 pp. Leeflang, Utrecht.

2995   RIJKENS, R. G. (1901). Uit de geschiedenis der geneeskunde. De phy-
       siologie van den bloedsomloop (From the history of medicine. The
       physiology of the circulation of the blood). *Natuur, XXI*, 11 and 41.

2996   FEYFER, F. M. G. de (1907–1911). Geschiedenis van den bloedsom-
       loop (History of the circulation of the blood).
       I. tot Galenus (till Galen). *Med. Revue, VII* (1907), 697. II. Galenus
       (Galen). *ibid., VIII* (1908), 65; III–IV. De invloed van Galenus ge-
       durende de Middeleeuwen (The influence of Galen during the Middle
       Ages). *ibid., VIII*, 245 and 345; V. Leonardo da Vinci (1452–1518).

ibid., *VIII*, 465; VI–VII. De voorlopers van William Harvey (The pre-decessors of W.H.). *ibid.*, *VIII*, 535 and 572; IX. Zijn werk (His (Har-vey's) work). *ibid.*, *IX* (1909), 109 and 213; X. De verspreiding van Harvey's leer (The spreading of H.'s theory). *ibid.*, *IX*, 389; XI. De ontdekking der chyl- en lymphevaten (The discovery of the chyle- and lymphvessels). *ibid.*, *IX*, 477; XII–XV. Harvey's leer in Nederland (Jacob de Back en zijn werk I–III (H.'s theory in the Netherlands J. de B. and his work). *ibid.*, *X* (1910), 105 and 363; *ibid.*, *XI* (1911), 99 and 203; XVI. De ontdekker der haarvaten (The discoverer of the capillaries). *ibid.*, *XI* (1911), 563.

2997 WENCKEBACH, K. F. (1911). Harvey en de ontdekking van den bloeds-omloop (H. and the discovery of the circulation of the blood). *NTG*, *55*, I, 1444–58.

2998 ROY, P. S. (1917). Historical Development of our knowledge of the Circulation and its Disorders. The experiment of Walaeus (J. Walaeus). *Ann. Med. Hist.*, ser. 1, *I*, 230.

2999 KAISER, L. (1923). De ontdekking van den bloedsomloop (The dis-covery of the circulation of the blood). *NTG*, *67*, II, 64–5; *BGG*, *III*, 172–3.
– Review of an article by F. Lejeune (*DMW*, (1923), no 21)), discussing the contrib-ution of the Spanish veterinary surgeon Francisco de la Reina.

3000 LEERSUM. E. C. van (1913). Vesalius, Harvey and the movement of the heart. *Janus*, *XVIII*, 348–50, 2 ill.

3001 LANKHOUT, J. (1941). R. Lower's Tractatus de corde. *NTG*, *85*, I, 453–61; *BGG*, *XXI*, 16–24.

3002 LINDEBOOM, G. A. (1957). William Harvey en zijn ontdekking van de bloedsomloop (W. H. and his discovery of the circulation of the blood). *NTG*, *101*, 2209–15; *BGG*, *XXXVII*, 34–40.

3003 — (1957). The reception in Holland of Harvey's theory of the circu-lation of the blood. *Janus*, *XLVI*, 183–200.

3004 — (1964). Harvey legt zijn hand op het kloppend mensenhart (H. places his hand on the beating human heart). *NTG*, *108*, 42–3; *BGG*, *XLIV*, 24–5.
See also 905–17 (W. Harvey), 1547–51 (M. Servet), 1861–64 (J. Walaeus).

Various topics

3005   KOOPMAN, J. (1923). Bloedstolling omstreeks het jaar 1600 (Blood clot-
ting about the year 1600). *NTG*, *67*, II, 1248.

3006   SCHIERBEEK, A. (1950). *Bloed en bloedvaten. Feiten en theorieën in de
loop der tijden*. (Blood and blood vessels. Facts and theories in the
course of time). 115 pp., ill. Het Spectrum, Utrecht-Brussel.

See also 892

3007   BUESS, H. (1948). Bijdrage tot de geschiedenis van de leer der adem-
haling (Contribution to the history of the theory of respiration).
Ciba-Tdschr., no *31*, april, 1018–34, 8 ill., 6 ports.
– A list of important literature on this theme is added: *ibid*, 1035–7. And a chronological table on the development of physiology from Lavoisier till the end of the
19th century: *ibid.*, 1038–9.

See also 988

3008   JAAGER, Johan Jacob de (1865, 1970). *De Physiologische Tijd by
Psychische Processen*. Thesis Utrecht. Facsimile edition entitled:
The Reaction Time and Mental Processes. 76 pp., 8°. Translated and
edited by J. Brozek and Maarten S. Sibinga.
– Vol. XVII in the Serie: *Dutch Classics in History of Science*. B. de Graaf, Nieuw-
koop.
J. J. de Jaager was a student of F. C. Donders. His thesis was prepared under the
guidance and with collaboration of D.

3009   GLASER, Hugo (1961). *Dramatische experimenten in de geneeskunde*
(Dramatic experiments in medicine). 160 pp. Elsevier, Amsterdam-
Brussel.
– Translated from German into Dutch by E. de Gems. Reviewed by L. Elaut: *Sci.
Hist.*, *3* (1961), 205–6.

F. Nutrition

General

3010   JACOB, H. E. (1955). *Zesduizend jaar brood. De geschiedenis van ons
dagelijks brood van de Egyptenaren tot de 20ste eeuw* (Six thousand
years of bread. History of our daily bread from the Egyptians till the
20th century). Utrecht.

3011   BUREMA, L. (1953). *De voeding in Nederland van de Middeleeuwen tot*

de twintigste eeuw (Nutrition in the Netherlands from the Middle
Ages till the 20th century). Thesis University of Amsterdam (Super-
visor: B. C. P. Jansen). 327 pp., ill. Van Gorcum, Assen.
– Van Gorcum's Historische Bibliotheek, no. 43.

3012 UNGER, W. S. (1916). *De levensmiddelenvoorziening der Hollandse
steden in de Middeleeuwen* (The provision of the Dutch towns in the
Middle Ages). XV + 209 pp. A. H. Kruyt, Amsterdam.

3013 BOEKEL, P. N. (1970). De noordhollandse zuivelbereiding in het verleden en heden (Noordholland dairying in the past and present).
Voeding, 31, 607–12.

3014 HAVINGA. B. (1964). Uit de geschiedenis van het haringkaken (From
the history of the curing of herrings). *Voeding, 25*, 495–8.

3015 DRIEL, B. M. van (1919). De voeding van de overwinteraars op Nova
Zembla (The nutrition of the persons who wintered on Nova Zembla).
NTG, 63, II, 613–5.

3016 VIEYRA, D. (1936). Geneeskundige Archivalia. Krachtig voedsel voor
gezonde menschen, kan voor zieken noodlottig zijn! (Medical Records.
Strengthening nutrition for healthy people, may be fatal for patients).
NTG, 80, I, 402; *BGG, XVI*, 32.

3017 MULLER, H. C. (1918). De geschiedenis en benaming van den aardappel, en zijne verspreiding (History and name of the potato, and its distribution). *Natuur, 38*, 257–8.

3018 VANDENBROEKE, Chr (1970). De opmars van de aardappel (The advance of the patato). *Spiegel Historiael, 5*, 352–6, 5 ill. (see also 1356).

3019 [   ] (1964). De invloed van het voedsel op de gang van de geschiedenis (Influence of food on the course of history). *Gezondheidszorg, 56*,
augustus, 5–16, 4 ill.

17th and 18th century

3020 MORINEAU, M. (1970). En Hollande au XVIIᵉsiècle. In: *Pour une histoire de l'alimentation*. Armand Cohn, Paris.
– *Cahier des Annales, 28*, 107–14. Post-scriptum: De la Hollande à la France, *ibidem*,
115–25.

3021 BUREMA, L. (1967). Iets over eten en drinken in Nederland in de 17e
eeuw (Something on food and drink in the Netherlands in the 17th
century). *Voeding, 28*, 139–48.

3022 DOYER van CLEEFF, G. (1917). Verduurzaamde levensmiddelen uit de tweede helft der zeventiende eeuw (Preserved food from the second half of the seventeenth century). *Natuur, XXXVII,* 140.

3023 LINDEBOOM, G. A. (1970). De voeding in een zeventiende-eeuws studenten-internaat (The nutrition in a boarding-school for students in the 17th century). *Voeding, 31,* 339–43.

3024 [Anonym] (1956). Iets over kaas in de 17e eeuw en later (Something on cheese in the 17th century and later). *Voeding, 17,* 482.

3025 VAZ DIAS, A. M. (1937). Melkvervalsching in de 17e eeuw (Adulteration of milk in the 17th century). *NTG, 81,* I, 63–4; *BGG, XVII,* 23–4.

3026 SCHEVICHAVEN, H. D. J. van (1903). Thee, koffie en chocolade twee honderd jaar geleden (Tea, coffee and chocolate two hundred years ago). *Eigen Haard, XXIX,* 328.

3027 VANDENBROECKE, Chr. (1969). Aardappelteelt en aardappelverbruik in de 17e en 18e eeuw (Potato-growing and the consumption of potatoes in the 17th and 18th century). *T. Gesch., 82,* 49–68.

3028 LINDEBOOM, G. A. (1972). De dagelijkse kost in het Staten-College te Leiden (1731). (The daily food in the "Staten-College" at L. (1731)). *Voeding, 33,* 264–8.

19th and 20th century

3029 WEE, H. van der (1960). Voeding en dieet in het Ancien Régime (Nutrition and diet during the — —). *Spiegel Historiael, 1,* 94–101, ill.

3030 LINDEBOOM, G. A. (1966). Een pleidooi tot verbetering der volksvoeding uit de vorige eeuw (A plea for the improvement of folk-nutrition from the previous century). *Voeding, 27,* 1–5.
– Referring to: G. J. Mulder. *De voeding in Nederland, in verband tot den volksgeest,* 1847.

3031 STUIJVENBERG, J. H. van (ed.) (1969). *Honderd Jaar Margarine 1869–1969* (A century of margarine 1869–1969). 353 pp., ill., ports. M. Nijhoff, Den Haag.
– also published as: *La margarine; histoire et évolution.* Dunod, Paris 1969.

3032 JANSEN, B. C. P. (1929). *De ontwikkeling van de leer der voeding in de laatste kwarteeuw* (The development of the doctrine of nutrition in the last 25 years). 29 pp. Amsterdam-Groningen.
– Address.

3033   SCHAIK, Th. F. S. M. and C. den HARTOG (1965). Een kwarteeuw Ne-
       derlanse voeding (A quarter of a century of Dutch nutrition). *Voeding,*
       26, 340–53.

3034   JONXIS, J. H. P. (1965). Vijf en twintig jaar kindervoeding (25 years of
       children's nutrition). *Voeding, 26,* 354–9.

3035   [Anonym] (1970). Voedingswijze van zieke gevangenen in 1842 (Way of
       nutrition of ill prisoners in 1842). *Voeding, 31,* 331–3.

3036   EIJKEL, R. N. M. (1946). Uit de oude doos (Old-time notes). *Voeding,*
       7, 156–68.
       – On the work of J. Pereira (1843). *Over voedsel, voeding en spijsregel* (On food,
       nutrition and diet). Contains a.o. regimens for foundling asylums.

3037   DONATH, W. F. (1957). Samenvatting van de historische ontwikkeling
       van onderzoekingen betreffende de volksvoeding in Nederlands Indië
       rond de eeuwwisseling (Summary of the historical development of the
       investigations concerning nutrition in the Dutch East Indies about
       1900). *Voeding, 18,* 349–55.

3038   BACKER, H. J. (1914). De eerste Hollandsche beetwortel-suikerfabriek
       (1811–1814). The first Dutch beetroot-factory). *Chem. Wbl., XI,* 940.

3039   BERGHE, A. W. S. (1958). De voeding in enige psychiatrische inrich-
       tingen in Nederland van 1949–1957 (The nutrition in some mental
       asylums in the Netherlands from 1949–1957). *Voeding, 19,* 624–50.

3040   NOOT, Thomas van der (*ca* 1510, 1925). *Het eerste Nederlandsche Kook-*
       boek, Brussel (The first Dutch Cookery-book). Mart. Nijhoff, Den
       Haag.
       – Facsimile of the only known copy (in the Bayerische Staatsbibliothek, München).

3041   HERMANS, A. G. J. (1947). Onze jachtdieren in de keuken en de volks-
       geneeskunde (Our game-animals in the kitchen and in folk medicine).
       NTG, 91, III, 1815–20; *BGG, XXVII,* 28–33.

3041ᵃ BAUDET, F. E. J. M. (no d.) *De maaltijd en de keuken in de middel-*
       eeuwen (The meal and the kitchen in the Middle Ages). Leiden.
                     See also 24, 118, 1028, 1180, 1227, 1294, 1330, 1337, 1379–82
                     (Pekelharing), 1924, 2411, 2436, 2454, 2537, 2566, 2590–1,
                     2623, 2649, 2654, 2767, 3817–21 (naval medicine), 3951–3
                     (military medicine), 4048–51 (public health).

Famine; hunger

3042   ERDMAN, A. M. (1957). Hongersnood in de Bommelerwaard (Famine
in the —). *Voeding, 18*, 611–3.

3043   OOMEN, H. A. P. C. (1964). De grote hongersnood (The great famine).
Voeding, 25, 323–30.
– on the famine in Ireland 1845 and 1846.

3043ᵃ   JONGBLOET-VAN HOUTTE, G. M. A. (1966). De hongersnood van 1740
(Famine of 1740). *Spiegel Historiael, 1*, 156–64, 8 ill. cf: *ibid., 3*
(1968), 61.

3044   KRUIF, Paul de (1930). *Bezwinger des Hungers*. Leipzig–Zürich.
– German translation of the Dutch original by Curt Thesing.

3045   LINDEBOOM, G. A. (1940). De ontdekking van den partieelen honger
(The discovery of partial hunger). *Stemmen des Tijds, 29*, 868–73.
– On the discovery of beri-beri as a deficiency by Eykman and Grijns.
See also 3301

Council of Nutrition

3046   BERG, C. van den (1965). Over het ontstaan van de Voedingsorgani-
satie T.N.O. en van de voedingsraad en over het werk van deze laatste
gedurende de bezetting (On the development of T.N.O. the organization on nutrition, and the Nutrition Council and on the activities of the
latter during the Occupation). *Voeding, 26*, 299–309.

3047   EEKELEN, M. van (1965). Bij het 25-jarig bestaan van de Voedingsor-
ganisatie T.N.O. en van het Centraal Instituut voor voedingsonder-
zoek (On the 25th anniversary of T.N.O., the organization on nutrition, and of the Central Institute for nutritional research). *Voeding, 26*,
319–29.

3048   BOEKEL, P. N. (1965). De stichting tot wetenschappelijke voorlichting
op voedingsgebied een kwart eeuw oud (25th anniversary of the
Foundation for Scientific Information on Nutrition). *Voeding, 26*,
290–8.

3049   MULDER, T. (1965). 25 jaar Voedingsraad in Nederland (25 years Nutrition Council in the Netherlands). *Voeding, 26*, 310–8.

3050   SLUITER, E. (1954). De oprichting van het Nederlandsch Instituut voor
Volksvoeding en zijn eerste Directeur Prof. Dr E. C. van Leersum

(The foundation of the Netherland Institute of Nutrition and its first
Director — —). *Voeding*, *15*, 424–7, port.

3051   [Anonym] (1968). The fiftieth anniversary of the Netherlands Institute
of Nutrition 1919–1969. *Annual Report* of the Netherlands Institute
of Nutrition, 21–2. Wageningen.

– E. C. van Leersum (1862–1938) was the founder of the Institute, succeeded by
B. C. P. Jansen (1884–1962).

See also 1016–19 (B. C. P. Jansen)

Chapter VII

Pathology

In this chapter entries referring to general and special pathology have been collected. Dutch authors have paid relatively little attention to the general concepts of disease that prevailed in the past. All the more their attention has been caught by contagious and epidemical diseases that frequently occurred in the late Middle Ages and afterwards.

Further sections with references to the literature on diseases of the cardiovascular, the endocrinological and the nervous system have been inserted. The literature on case-reports is also to be found in this chapter.

A. Concepts of disease

3052 MEERLOO, A. M. (1932/33). Het ziektebegrip in verleden en heden (een kort historisch overzicht) (The concept of disease in past and present (a short historical survey)). I. *NTG, 76* (1932), IV, 5567–79; *BGG, XII,* 245–57; II. *NTG, 77* (1933), II, 2511–25; *BGG, XIII,* 136–58.

3053 SCHLICHTING, Th. H. (1949/50).Geschiedenis van het begrip ziekte, I, II, en III (History of the concept of disease).
I. *NTG, 91* (1949), III, 2987–93; *BGG, XXIX,* 39–45;
II. *NTG, 91,* IV, 3748–52; *BGG, XXIX,* 59–63.
III. *NTG, 92* (1950), IV, 2977–80; *BGG, XXX,* 38–41.
– Chapter III is entitled: Anonymus Londinensis.

3054 KUIJJER, P. J. (1948). *De ontwikkeling van het begrip tuberkel* (The development of the concept of tubercle). Thesis Amsterdam (Supervisor: H. T. Deelman). 160 pp., 13 ports., 4 ill. J. H. de Bussy, Amsterdam.

3055 LINDEBOOM, G. A. (1956). La medicina psicosomatica ed il concetto di malattia. *Med. psicosom., I,* 195–9.

3056   — (1957). From the History of the Concept of Specificity. *Janus*, *XLVI*, 12–24.

3057   — (1957). Uit de geschiedenis van het begrip specificiteit (From the history of the concept of specificity). *NTG, 101*, 357–62; *BGG, XXXVII*, 1–6.

3057ª POLAK DANIËLS, L. (1936). Ziekten en ziektenbeelden (Diseases and syndromes). In: *Jbk. R.U. Groningen*, 9–23.
    – Address.

3058   KLEIWEG de ZWAAN, J. P. (1914–16). Historische beschouwingen omtrent het wezen en het ontstaan der ziekten (Historical observations about the essence and the origin of diseases). *Med. Wbl., 21* (1914–15), 402, 414, 439, 455, 469, 478, 492, 502, 514, 522, 534, 551, 565, 575, 600; *Ibid., 22* (1915–16), 4, 17, 30, 42, 53, 65, 82, 100, 112, 121 and 131.

3059   BAUMANN, E. D. (1936). Historische Betrachtungen über die vis medicatrix naturae. *Janus, XL*, 148–70 (Das Altertum); 197–217 (Die Neuzeit).

3060   LANGEN, C. D. de (1952). *De invloed van ziekten op de ontwikkeling van oude culturen in vroeger eeuwen* (The influence of diseases on the development of ancient cultures in former ages). *MKNAW*, Akademiedagen, V, 130–47. Noord-Holl. Uitg. Mij, Amsterdam, 8°.

3061   LIGNAC, G. O. E. (1952). Quo vadis? *NTG, 96*, 2792–7.
    – with a historical introduction to pathological anatomy; ports. a.o. of Ed. and G. Sandifort.

3062   NIERSTRASZ, J. J. (1967). General Pathology and Therapy of Inflammation in the 1860s. *Janus, LIV*, 168–82.

3063   WAGENINGEN, J. van (1921). La dessication des humeurs. *Janus, XXV*, 330–4.

3064   ANDEL, M. A. van (1936). De febribus. Practijk en theorie vóór honder jaar (De febribus. Practice and theory hundred years ago). *NTG, 80*, 5428–35; *BGG, XVI*, 201–8.

3065   — (1937), Febris nautica. *NTG, 81*, 5429–38; *BGG, XVII*, 180–9.
       See also 806–9 (Gaubius), 925, 935, 2527, 2529, 2737, 5060
       and Philosophy and Ideas (2129–36a)

B. Cardiovascular diseases

3066 HOEVEN, J. van der (1921). De dissertatie anatomico-chirurgica "de aneurysmate" van Jacobus Verbrugge (The anatomical-chirurgical dissertation —— of J.V.). *NTG, 65*, II, 47–51; 728; *BGG, I*, 300–4, 340.

3067 MOULIN, D. de (1961). Some more historical notes on aneurysm. *Arch. Chir. Néerl., XII*, 277–84.

3068 LANKHOUT, J. (1934). Sénac en Corvisart: iets aangaande de leer en de behandeling der ziekten van het hart in de 18de eeuw (S. and C.: something about the theory and the treatment of the diseases of the heart in the 18th century). *NTG, 78*, IV, 5471–85; *BGG, XIV*, 223–37.

3069 NEUBURGER, Max (1923). Bijdrage tot de geschiedenis van de compenseerende hypertrophie van het hart (Contribution to the history of the compensatory hypertrophy of the heart). *NTG, 67*, II, 1632–4; *BGG, III*, 286–8.

3070 KUIJJER, P. J. (1953). De oudste ziektegeschiedenis van de tetralogie van Fallot (The oldest case-report of the tetralogy of F.) *NTG, 97*, II, 1399–1408; *BGG, XXXIII*, 33–42, 2 ill, port. (Of Eduard Sandifort (1742–1814).

3071 — (1954). L'histoire la plus ancienne de la tétralogie de Fallot. *La Presse Médicale, 62*, 199–200, 2 ill. port.

3072 HOORN, M. van (1965). Histoire des thromboses veineuses du membre supérieur. *Phlébologie, 18*, 31–44.

See also 22, 35, 36, 1514, 2533, 2546, 2681–3, 2755

3073 deleted

C. Disorders of the liver

3074 MOULIN, D. de (1971). Geel en groen zien in het verleden (Looking yellow and green in the past). *Symposium Nijmegen 1971 Pathologie van lever en galwegen*, 15–28.

D. Endocrine Glands

3075 KOOPMAN, J. (1923). Enkele oudere waarnemingen over inwendige afscheidingen (Some older observations on internal excretions). *NTG*, *67*, I, 897–8; *BGG*, *III*, 72–3.
– Review of an article of Beck (*Endocrinology* (1922), 240).

3076 — (1926, 1928, 1931). Bijdragen tot de geschiedenis der ontwikkeling van de endocrinologie (Contributions to the history of the development of endocrinology). I. Ontwikkeling der opotherapie (Development of opotherapy). *NTG*, *70* (1926), I, 2359–65; *BGG*, *VI*, 117–23. II. De pijnappelklier (The pineal gland). *NTG*, *72*, (1928), II, 1695–9; *BGG*, *VIII*, 96–100. III. Hersenaanhangsel en hersenbasis (Pituitary gland and brain base). *NTG*, *72*, II, 5458–66; *BGG*, *VIII*, 333–41. IV. De bijnier (The adrenal gland). *NTG*, *75* (1931), II, 2976–80; *BGG*, *XI*, 169–73.

3077 NIEUWENHUIS, G. (1931). Einige Anschauungen über die Funktion der Hypophyse. *Janus*, *XXXV*, 345–59.

3078 ZWAN, A. van der (1971). *Hypofysetumoren – Pituitary Tumors*. Thesis University Leyden (Supervisor: W. Luyendijk). 246 pp., ill. De Kempenaer, Oegstgeest.
– Ch. I. Historische Inleiding (Historical Introduction), 17–32.

3078ᵃ BARUCH, J. Z. (1974). Serge Voronoff en zijn apeklieren. Een verouderde verjongingskuur in historisch perspectief (— — and his monkey glands. An obsolete rejuvenation cure in historical perspective). *GG*, *5*, no. 6, 36–7.

3079 LEERSUM, E. C. van (1925). Bijdrage tot de geschiedenis der goedaardige schildklierzwelling (Contribution to the history of the benign swelling of the thyroid gland). *NTG*, *69*, II, 620–32; *BGG*, *V*, 184–96.

3080 — (1925). Contribution to the history of the simple enlargement of the thyroid gland. *Janus*, *XXIX*, 282–9, 10 ill.

3081 GREENWALD, Isidor (1960). The History of Goiter in the Netherlands. *Janus*, *XLIX*, 285–99.

See also 2507, 3298, 5276

Diabetes mellitus

3082 KOOPMAN, J. (1934). Uit de geschiedenis van den diabetes (From the history of diabetes). *NTG, 78*, II, 1973–83; *BGG, XIV*, 81–91.

3083 ELAUT, L. (1971). Vijftig jaar insuline (Fifty years insulin). *Sci. Hist.*, *13*, 177–84.

3084 [Editorial] (1972). Een halve eeuw insuline. Dr Elzas meer dan een halve eeuw diabetes specialist (Half a century insulin. Dr. E. more than half a century specialist on diabetes). *GG, 3*, 5–7, port.

3085 [Editorial] (1972). Geschiedenis van de Nederlandse insulineproduktie. Gesprek met Prof. Tausk (History of the Dutch insulinproduction. A talk with —). *GG, 3*, 7–9, port., 2 ill.

3086 KOLDITZ, W. (1972). Historische beschouwingen over diabetes-mellitus – 50 jaar na de ontdekking van insuline. Deel I. (Historical observations on diabetes mellitus – 50 years after the discovering of insulin. Part I.) *Literatuur-Dienst "Roche", XL*, no 3, 17–20, 7 ports. Part II: *Ibidem*, no 4, 25–9, ports.

See also 45, 46, 2690, 5414.

E. Deficiency Diseases

3087 KLUYVER, A. (1923). Aanteekening over het woord scheurbuik (A note on the word "Scheurbuik" (scurvy). *NTG, 67*, II, 1436–9; *BGG, III*, 235–8.
– cf: (same title): *NTG, 68* (1924), I, 57; *BGG, IV*, 23.

3088 KLEIJ, J. J. van der (1925). Over het bekend worden van de scheurbuik in de Nederlanden (On becoming known of the scurvy in the Netherlands). *NTG, 69*, II, 1573–7; *BGG, V*, 253–7.

3089 ANDEL, M. A. van (1927). De scheurbuik als Nederlandsche volksziekte (Scurvy as an endemic disease in the Netherlands). *NTG, 71*, II, 610–22; *BGG, VII*, 519–31.

3090 — (1927). Der Skorbut als niederländische Volkskrankheit. *Janus*, *XXXI*, 61–1.
– Report of a paper read at a meeting of the "Deutsche Gesellschaft für Geschichte der Medizin und der Naturwissenschaften", Düsseldorf, 19–24 September 1926.

3091 — (1927). Der Skorbut als niederländische Volkskrankheit. *Arch. Gesch. Mediz., XIX*, 82–91.

3092 AUGUSTIJN, A. H. P. (1932). *De scheurbuik in den loop der tijden* (Scurvy in the course of time). Thesis University of Amsterdam (Supervisor: Ruitinga). 113 pp. "Amstelveld", Amsterdam.

See also 788, 798, 3045, 3288–9

Rheumatism and gout

3093 TAUSK, M. (1945). *Driehonderd jaar rachitis-onderzoek. De Engelse ziekte in de geneeskunde voorheen en thans 1645–1945.* (Three hundred years of rachitis-investigation. Rachitis in medicine in the past and present 1645–1945). 78 pp., Organon, Oss.

See also 390–2

3094 BARUCH, J. Z. (1965). De historische ontwikkeling van de kennis van reumatische ziektebeelden (The historical development of the knowledge of rheumatic syndromes). *GG, 43,* 421–5.

3095 — (1965). Du développement de la connaissance des symptomes du rhumatisme. *Rhumatologie, 17,* 101–4.

3096 — (1965). De betekenis van Guillaume de Baillou voor de rheumatologie (The importance of — — for rheumatology). *Documenta Geigy,* 3–6.
– Report of the XIth Int. Congr. Rheumatology, 5–11 December 1965.

3097 KORST, J. K. van der (1970). *De strijd tegen mogendheid X* (The fight against power X). 34 pp. Dekker & Van de Vegt, Nijmegen.
– public lecture November 12, 1970, containing remarks on the history of Rheumatism and gout.

3098 GOSLINGS, J. (1971). *25 jaar reumatologie.* Rede uitgesproken ter gelegenheid van het 25-jarig bestaan van de Nederlandse Vereniging van Rheumatologen op zaterdag 30 januari 1971. (25 years of rheumatology). 23 pp.
– Oration held on the occasion of the 25th anniversary of the "Dutch Association of Rheumatologists", Saturday, 30 January 1971).

3099 — (1966). Veertig jaar rheuma-bestrijding (Forty years of the fight against rheumatism). *NTG, 110,* 1870–1.

3100 — (1967). Veertig jaar Nederlandse Vereniging tot Rheumatiekbestrijding (Fourty years of the Dutch Association for the fight against Rheumatism). *NTG, 111,* 268–71.

See also 40–42 (G. de Baillou).

3101 KLINKERT, D. (1920). Bijdrage tot de kliniek en pathogenese der jicht. Een klinisch-geschiedkundige studie (Contribution to clinic and pathogenesis of gout. A medical-historical study). *NTG, 64,* II, 2457–65.

3102 — (1921). Zur Klinik und Pathogenese der Gicht. Eine klinisch-historische Studie. *Berl. Klin. Wschr.,* no 2, 25.

3103 BAUMANN, E. D. (1921). De pathologie en therapie der jicht (Pathology and therapy of gout). *NTG, 65,* I, 108–10.

3104 WITT Jr, S. de (1964). Aspects of the history and the natural history of gout. *Acad. Med. N. J. Bull, 11* (1), 6–18.

See also 1119, 2105, 2699.

F. Contagious diseases

General

3105 GROSHANS, G. Ph. (1869). Historische aanteekeningen (historical notes). *NTG, 5,* 24, 210–54.
– This article deals with historical remarks on several diseases, as malaria fevers, contagium animatum, plague, leprosy a.o.

3106 KUIPER, J. (1899). Isoleering van besmettelijke zieken (Isolating of persons with a contagious disease); also in: *Alers et al.,* 116–24.

3107 ZUIDEN, D. S. van (1918). De contagieuse ziekte en de herbergen in Amsterdam (1618) (The contagious disease and the inns at A.) *NTG, 62,* I, 1017–8.

3108 KATE, W. ten (1936). Uit de notulen van de Staten van Overijsel. Maatregelen ter wering eener besmettelijke ziekte (From the minutes of the "States of O." Measures for the prevention of a contagious disease). *NTG, 80,* II, 1935–6; *BGG, XVI,* 75–6.

3109 FRAATZ, Paul (1929). *Beiträge zur Seuchengeschichte Westfalens und der holländischen Nordseeküste.* 68 pp., 3 fig., 2 maps. Gustav Fischer, Jena.
– Serie: *Arbeiten zur Kenntnis der Geschichte der westfälischen Medizin,* Heft 1.

3110   JONG, K. de (1939). De ontdekking van de eerste plantaardige ver-
wekker van een besmettelijke ziekte bij den mensch, het Achorion
Schönlein in 1839 (The discovery of the first vegetable causative agent
of a contagious disease in man, the — — in 1839). *GG*, *17*, 1121–2,
1 ill.

See also 5009, 5070a.

Leprosy

3111   ISRAELS, A. H. (1857). Bijdrage tot de geschiedenis der lepra in de
noordelijke Nederlanden (Contribution to the history of leprosy in the
Northern Netherlands). *NTG*, 2, 161.

3112   KETTING, G. N. A. (1922). *Bijdrage tot de geschiedenis van de lepra in
Nederland* (Contribution to the history of leprosy in the Netherlands).
Thesis University of Amsterdam (Supervisor: J. P. Kleiweg de Zwaan).
298 pp., ill. Mouton & Co. Den Haag.
– Reviewed by M. A. van Andel: *NTG*, 66 (1922), II, 576–8; *BGG, II*, 192–4.

3113   POST, A. E. (1904). *Mededeelingen over Lepra* (Informations on Leprosy). 193 pp. Van der Wiel & Co, Amsterdam. 8°.

3113ᵃ   MALET, Chr. (1974). De lepra in West-Europa gedurende de middeleeuwen (Leprosy in Western Europe during the Middle Ages). *Image*,
nr. 57, 7–15, 11 ill.

3114   KESTELOO, H. M. (1907). De leprozen te Middelburg (The lepers at
M.). *Archief*, 137–60.

3115   VEEN, S. J. van (1915). Het Zutphense leprozengild (The guild of lepers at Z.). *Gelre*, *XVIII*, 151.

3116   SCHEVENSTEEN, A. F. C. van [no d.]. *De Leprozen in de stadsrekeningen
van Antwerpen tot het einde van het Oud Regime* (The lepers in the town-
accounts of Antwerp till the end of the Old Regime). 50 pp. R. Bracke-
Van Geert, Baesrode.

3116ᵃ   — (1930). *La Lèpre dans le Marquisat d'Anvers*. Extrait du Recueil des
Mémoires couronnés de l'Académie Royale de Médecine de Belgique.
129 pp. Bruxelles. 8°.

3117   VIAENE, A. (1962). *Leprozen en leprozerijen in het oude graafschap
Vlaanderen* (Lepers and leper houses in the old county of Flanders).
47 pp., Gidsenbond, Brugge.

3118 BRUYN, J. A. de (1931). Verordening uit het jaar 1399 van het stadsbestuur te Schoonhoven betreffende de leprabestrijding en een publicatie aan de burgerij tot stichting van een nieuw leprozenhuis (Ordinance (1399) of the municipality of S. regarding the fight against leprosy and a publication to the citizens for the foundation of a new leper
house). *NTG, 75*, II, 2984–5; *BGG, XI*, 177–8.

3119 HALLEMA, A. (1957). Ordonnantie voor een dorpsleprozerie te Etten
in Noord-Brabant (Ordinance for a village leper house at E. in
Northern Brabant). *NTG, 101*, 774–7; *BGG, XXXVII*, 7–10.

3120 GOONARATNA, C. de F. W. (1971). Some historical aspects of leprosy
in Ceylon during the Dutch Period 1658–1796. *Med. Hist., 15*, 68–78.

3121 — (1973). Some descriptions of leprosy in the ancient medical literature of Ceylon. *Med. Hist., 17*, 308–15.
- With remarks on leprosy during the Dutch and Portuguese times.
        See also 2538–42 (Israel), 4402–7 (leper houses), 4850, 5005–
        6, 5035, 5052–3, 5263–8 (Medicine and Art), Dutch East
        Indies (3850–5).

PLAGUE

General

3122 MEINSMA, K. O. (1924). *De zwarte dood 1347–1352* (The black death
1347–1352). 487 pp., 3 ill. W. J. Thieme, Zutphen. 8°.

3123 NIEUWENHUIS, A. W. (1908). *The black Death of 1348 and 1349* by
F. A. Gasquet (second ed., London 1908). *Janus, XIII*, 670–2.

3124 BARUCH, J. Z. (1964). Een pestepidemie in de zeventiende eeuw naar
de beschrijving van tijdgenoten (A plague epidemic in the 17th century, after the description of contemporaries). *NTG, 108*, 1493–6;
BGG, XLIV, 28–31.

3125 — (1972). Een pest-epidemie in de zeventiende eeuw (A plague epidemic in the 17th century). *Arts en Auto, 38*, 70–1.

3126 BEEN, J. H. (1911). De gave Gods [de pest] (God's gift [the plague]).
In: *Been's Hist. Fragmenten, 1*, 93. C. Bredée, 's-Gravenhage.

3127 DIJKSTRA, J. G. (1921). *Een epidemiologische beschouwing van de Nederlandsche pest-epidemieën der XVIIde eeuw* (An epidemiological

reflection on the Dutch plague epidemics in the 17th century). Thesis University of Amsterdam (Supervisor: J. J. van Loghem). 88 pp., ill. "Volharding", Amsterdam.

– Reviewed by M. A. van Andel: *NTG, 66* (1922), I, 874–7; *BGG, II*, 81–4.

3128   LOGHEM, J. J. van (1918). Punten van vergelijking tusschen de Europesche pest in de 17e eeuw en de hedendaagsche builenpest der tropen en subtropen (Points of comparison between the European plague in the 17th century and the present bubonic plague in tropical and subtropical areas). *NTG, 62*, II, 1939–43.

3129   — (1918). The plague of the 17th century compared with the plague of our days. *Janus, XXIII*, 95–107.

3130   — (1925). Geschiedkundig Pestonderzoek (Historical investigation of the plague). *NTG, 69*, I, 1599–1602; *BGG, V*, 73–6.

3131   GODEFROI, M. J. (1886). Een merkwaardig pestboekje uit de zeventiende eeuw (A remarkable plague-book from the 17th century). *NTG, 22*, I, 53.

3132   KRUL, R. (1893). Rapport namens de commissie voor de geschiedenis der geneeskunde in Nederland. Zeven pestboekjes: 1564–1664. (Report on behalf of the commission for the history of medicine in the Netherlands. Seven plague-books: 1564–1664). *NTG, 29*, II, 916–40.

3133   PORTENGEN, J. A. (1896/97). Une théorie chinoise sur l'étiologie et la Thérapie de la peste. *Janus, I*, 461–8.

3134   — (1897–98). Historical notice about the original discovery of the bacillus of bubonic plague. *Janus, II*, 57–9.

3135   PEYPERS, H. F. A. (1903). Qu'est ce que signifie "La Modorra"? *Janus, VIII*, 247–50.

– on an epidemic disease on the Canary Islands in 1494, 1522 and 1664, probably bubonic plague.

3136   HELLINGA, W. G. and A. Querido (1960). Was the Bagford-Fragment of Kamitus "Tractatus de regimine pestilentico" printed by Claes or by Gheraert Leeu? *Gutenberg Jahrbuch, 35*, 141–3.

See also 2543, 4407a–12 (Plague houses), 5056.

Fight against plague

3137 BROUWER ANCHER, A. J. M. (1900). De pest en hare bestrijding in vroeger eeuwen (The plague and the fight against it in former centuries). *De Gids, 64* [4de serie, 18], 148–78.

3138 PEYPERS, H. F. A. (1902). La peste et son extinction par la sérothérapie. *Janus, VII,* 199–200.

3139 PUTTO, J. A. (1910). Geneeskunst in vroeger dagen (Medicine in former days). *NTG, 54,* I, 2063–70.
      – on plague and fevers.

3140 VEEN, S. J. van (1903). De pest en hare bestrijding in Gelderland, in het bijzonder te Arnhem (The plague and the fight against it in Guelderland, particularly at A.). *Gelre, VI,* 1–66.

3141 TERSTEEG, J. (1903). Enkele aanteekeningen bij de pestbestrijding in vroegeren tijd (Some notes on the fight against plague in former times). *Tijdspiegel, I,* 403.

3142 RAADT, O. L. E. de (1917). De pestbestrijding voorheen en thans (The fight against the plague – past and present). *GTNI, 57,* 342–6.

3143 LOGHEM, J. J. van (1922). Huisrat— en pestbestrijding in de 17e eeuw (House-rat and the fight against plague in the 17th century). *NTG, 66,* I, 1275–9; *BGG, II,* 85–9.

3144 BEYERMAN, J. J. (1934). Een probaat middel tegen de pest en andere besmettelijke ziekten (An efficacious remedy against plague and other contagious diseases). *NTG, 78,* II, 1569–70; *BGG, XIV,* 79–80.

3145 DITMAR, T. van (1939). Prophylaxis tegen de pest in 1666 (Prevention against plague in 1666). *NTG, 83,* I, 78; *BGG, XIX,* 16.

See also 2771–72

Local epidemics

3146 KANNEGIETER, J. Z. (1964). Pest te Amsterdam in 1602 en enkele aantekeningen over de daarop volgende epidemieën (Plage at A. in 1602 and some remarks on the subsequent epidemics). *Amstelodamum, 51,* 197–205; 221–5.

3146ᵃ BRUGMANS, H. (1922). De pest te Amsterdam (Plague at A.). *Amstelodamum, 9,* 1–3.

See also 4632a

3147   MEUNIER, L. (1903). La peste à Delft en 1557–1558, et en 1573. *Janus*, *VIII*, 200–5.

3147ª SLEE, J. C. van (1924). [Mededeling over "De Pest in Deventer, 1348–1350"] (Communication on "Plague at D. — —"). *Versl. Med. Overijsselsch Regt en Gesch.*, *42*, XIX–XX.

3148   BIJLSMA-ALTING MEES, N. (1917). De pestilencie in Oud-Dordrecht (The plague in — —). *Navorscher, LXVI*, 369–74.

3149   BUWALDA, J. M. and E. O. BUWALDA-PREY (1939). Eenige gegevens over de pest te Gouda in de 17de eeuw (Some data on the plague at G. in the 17th century). *NTG, 83*, 5663–71; *BGG, XIX*, 261–9.

3150   ANDEL, M. A. van (1913). Pestepidemieën te Gorinchem (Plague epidemics at G.). *NTG, 57*, II, 1844–62.

3151   STADERMANN, G. (1958–59). De zwarte dood in Hulst in 1625 en 1634 (The black death at H. in 1625 and 1634). *Jbk. De vier Ambachten*, Hulst, 14–28.
       – Data on plague epidemics borrowed from ordinances.

3152   NANNINGA UITTERDIJK, J. (1913). Een en ander over de pest te Kampen (Something on the plague at K.). *Versl. Med. Overijsselsch Regt en Gesch.*, *29*, 8–19.

3153   DROST, A. (1933). *De pestilentie te Katwijk (1625)* (The plague at K.) Amsterdam.

3154   PINKHOF, H. (1919). Een pest-epidemie te Oisterwijk in 1603–04 (A plague epidemic at O. in 1603–04). *NTG, 63*, II, 762.

3155   GOYARTS, C. B. (1958). De pest te Roosendaal (The plague at R.) *Jbk. Oudhk. Kring "De Ghulden Roos"* (Roosendaal), *18*, 29–36.

3156   BRUNNER, H. G. H. (1946). Pest-epidemieën van de 15e tot de 17e eeuw te Rotterdam (Plague epidemics at R. from the 15th till the 17th century). *NTG, 90*, II, 620–3; *BGG, XXVI*, 12–5.

3157   MOQUETTE, H. C. H. (1925). Pestepidemieën in Rotterdam (Plague epidemics at R.). *Rott. Jbk.*, 3de reeks, *3*, 10–52, 2 ill.

3158   WEYDE, A. J. van der (1927). Bijdrage tot de geschiedenis der pest te Utrecht (Contribution to the history of the plague at U.) *NTG, 71*, I, 3119–39; *BGG, VII*, 384–404.

See also 5056

3159 DUKES, M. N. G. (1966). De grote pestilentie in Londen (1665–66). (The great plague epidemic at L.). *Organorama, III*, no 2, 23–7.

3160 VIEYRA, D. (1936). Beschrijving der pestepidemie te Marseille in September 1720 (Description of the plague epidemic at M.). *NTG, 80*, 3567–70; *BGG, XVI*, 127–30.

Ordinances and instructions

3161 SERVAAS van ROOYEN. A. J. (1900). Oude wetten en bepalingen tegen de pest in Nederland. I. Iets over de pest in ons land (Old laws and prescriptions against the plague in the Netherlands, I. Something on the plague in our country). *Vrag. Dag, XV*, 120.

3162 ANDEL, M. A. van (1916). Plague regulations in the Netherlands. *Janus, XXI*, 410–41, ill.

3163 KATE, W. ten (1936). Geneeskundige Archivalia: Maatregelen tot wering der pest. Verzoek tot toelating als operateur der provincie. Het verbranden van veen (From medical records: Measures for the prevention of plague. Request for admittance as (operating) surgeon of the province. The burning of peat-bog). *NTG, 80*, 4043; *BGG, XVI*, 153.

3164 DOOREN, L. (1939). Een testament in pesttijd. Het ambt van ziekentrooster (1666). (A will in times of plague. The function of visitor of the sick). *NTG, 83*, 3928; *BGG, XIX*, 210.

3165 LEVELT, H. (1923). Verschillende 15de en 16de eeuwsche pestkeuren te Bergen-op-Zoom (Various plague-ordinances in the 15th and 16th century at — —). *NTG, 67*, I, 1893–5; *BGG, III*, 126–8.

3166 — (1923). De laatste Bergen op Zoomsche Pestkeure, dd 1577, October 18 (The last plague-ordinance of — —). *NTG, 67*, II, 1444–8; *BGG, III*, 243–7.

3167 DALEN, J. L. van (1900). Oude wetten en bepalingen tegen de pest in Nederland. II. Oude maatregelen in Dordrecht tegen de pest (Old laws and prescriptions against the plague in the Netherlands. II. Old measures at D. against plague). *Vrag. Dag, XV*, 125.

3168 ANDEL, M. A. van (1918). Instructiën voor pest- en sieckhuysmeesters te Gorinchem (Instructions for plague- and hospitalmasters at G.). *NTG, 62*, I, 614–21.

3169 BRUYN, J. A. de (1931). Verordeningen betreffende de pestepidemie die in de jaren 1635–1666 te Schoonhoven woedde (Ordinances regarding the plague-epidemic which was rampant in the years 1635–1666 at S.). *NTG, 75*, I, 1154–62; *BGG, XI*, 83–91.

3170 WEYDE, A. J. van der (1923). Pestkeuren in Utrecht (Plague by-laws at U.). *NTG, 67*, I, 42; *BGG, III*, 9.

3171 HULSHOF, M. H. (1939). Gebed en voorschriften tegen pest in een Utrechtsch getijdenboekje uit 1440 (Prayer and prescriptions against plague in a Utrecht breviary from 1440). *NTG, 83*, I, 533–5; *BGG, XIX*, 38–40.

3172 DONINCK, A. van (1930). Tractaten van de peste vóór de 18de eeuw in Vlaanderen (Plague treatises before the 18th century in Flandres). *NTG, 74*, II, 3431–41; *BGG, X*, 185–95.

See also 2771–72.

Sweating sickness (Sudor Anglicus)

3173 [Editorial] (1902). Une petite nouvelle contre la "suette anglaise". *Janus, VII*, 54.
– short note from the diary of G. Geldemaner Noviomagus, 1522 (with some indications of literature on the sweating sickness in the Netherlands).

3174 SCHEVENSTEEN, A. F. C. van (1932). *Un traité anversois sur la Suette anglaise.* 25 pp., 8 ill. De Coker, Antwerpen.
– with a facsimile of 8 pp.

3175 DOOREN, L. (1939). Een recept tegen de Engelsche zweetziekte, welke in de 2de helft der 16e eeuw heerschte (A prescription against the sweating sickness prevailing in the second half of the 16th century). *NTG, 83*, II, 4866–7; *BGG, XIX*, 230–1.

Syphilis

3176 FOKKER, A. A. (1860/61). Geschiedenis der syphilis in de Nederlanden (History of syphilis in the Netherlands). *NTG, 4*, (1860), 419; *ibid., 5* (1861), 451.

3177 PEYPERS, H. F. A. (1893). Lues Veterum. *NTG, 29*, II, 397–412.

3178 — (1895). *Lues medii Aevi.* Thesis University of Amsterdam (Supervisor: B. J. Stokvis). 106 pp. Amsterdam.

3179 PINKHOF, H. (1893). Een classiek boek (A classical book). *NTG, 29* (2de reeks) *37*, II, 781–7.
  – letter to the editor on the article Lues Veterum, nr 3177.

3180 — (1893). Antieke Lues? (Antique Lues?) *NTG, 29*, I, 130–4.

3181 VALK, J. W. van der (1910). *Bijdrage tot de kennis van de geschiedenis der syphilis in ons land* (Contribution to the knowledge of the history of syphilis in our country). Thesis University of Amsterdam (Supervisor: S. Mendes da Costa). 158 pp., 4 ill. Scheltema & Holkema, Amsterdam. 8°.
  – Reviewed by E. C. van Leersum: *Janus, XVI* (1911), 68–9.

3182 PEVERELLI, P. (1924). De oorsprong van de syphilis (Origin of syphilis). *NTG, 68*, I, 943–4; *BGG, IV*, 66–7.
  – report of an article of Mayo Tolman in *J. Social Hygiene*, December 1923.

3183 POSTMA, H. (1924). De oorsprong van de syphilis (Origin of syphilis). *NTG, 68*, I, 1544; *BGG, IV*, 96.
  – letter to the editor.

3184 ESSED, W. F. R. (1933). *Over den oorsprong der syphilis. Een kritisch-historische epidemiologische studie, tevens ontwerp eener nieuwe theorie* (On the origin of syphilis. A critical-historical epidemiological study, likewise draft on a new theory). Thesis Leyden (Supervisor: P. Chr. Flu). 328 pp. H. J. Paris, Amsterdam.

3185 — (1933). Syphilis en framboesia (Syphilis and framboesia). *NTG, 77*, IV, 5406–8; *BGG, XIII*, 274–6.
  – cf. *NTG, 78* (1934), II, 1992; *BGG, XIV*, 100 (letter to the ed.)

3186 LINT, J. G. de (1933). Syphilis en framboesia (Syphilis and framboesia). *NTG, 77*, II, 3987–9; *BGG, XIII*, 214–6.
  – cf: (same author and same title) *NTG, 78* (1934), I, 77–8; *BGG, XIV, 31–2.*

3187 GILS, J. B. F. van (1939). Een legende over het ontstaan van de syphilis (A legend on the origin of syphilis). *NTG, 83*, II, 3923–7; *BGG, XIX*, 205–9, 4 ill.

3188 DELPRAT, Jr, G. D. (1922). Etymology of the word "Syphilis". *Ann. Med. Hist., IV*, 211.
  – letter to the editor.

3189 [Anonym] (1939). Niet herkende syphilis (unrecognized syphilis). *NTG, 83*, I, 1031; *BGG, XIX*, 60.

3190 BEYERMAN, J. J. (1954). Een geval van syphilis vóór 319 jaar (A case of syphilis 319 years ago). *NTG*, *98*, 1379–82; 2529; *BGG*, *XXXIV*, 41–4; 81.

3191 LOON, L. van (1942). De behandeling der neurosyphilis met warme baden (Treatment of neurosyphilis with warm baths). *NTG*, *86*, III, 2173–8.

3192 MAAS, J. F. (1921). De huid- en geslachtsziekten in Nederland in de tweede helft der vorige eeuw tot aan de oprichting der Nederlandsche Vereeniging der dermatologen (Skin- and venereal diseases in the Netherlands in the second half of the previous century till the foundation of the Dutch Association of Dermatologists). *NTG*, *65*, II, 2146–63.

3193 ZUIDEN, D. S. van (1916). Een geschil over de besmettelijkheid der Spaansche pokken (anno 1696) (A dispute on the contagiousness of Spanish pox). *NTG*, *60*, I, 55–7.

3194 — (1917). Een verklaring over genezing der Spaansche pokken bij een vrouw (An explanation on the healing of Spanish pox in a woman). *NTG*, *61*, I, 43–4.

3195 BURG, C. L. van der (1904). Une relation ancienne sur la syphilis aux Indes orientales. *Janus*, *IX*, 512.

3196 DANIËLS, C. E. (1910). Lues-behandeling te Amsterdam in 1685 (Treatment of syphilis at A. in 1685). *NTG*, *54*, II, 1844–6.

3197 SCHOUTE, D. (1943). Syphilisbestrijding van overheidswege in Nederland en in Nederlandsch Indië (The fight against syphilis by the government in the Netherlands and in the Dutch East Indies). I. In Nederland: *NTG*, *87*, III, 1484–7; *BGG*, *XXIII*, 60–3. II. In Nederlandsch Indië: *NTG*, *87*, III, 1488–91; *BGG*, *XXIII*, 78–81.

3198 PRAKKEN, J. R. (1973). Hygiënisten en moralisten bij de geslachtsziektenbestrijding in de negentiende eeuw (Hygienists and moralists in the fight against venereal diseases). *NTG*, *117*, 1042–9.

3198[a] — (1974). Venereologische proeven op mensen (Venereal experiments on men). *NTG*, *118*, 795–800.

See also 1014, 1020, 1682, 3865, 4993

Cholera

3199 ANDEL, M. A. van (1938). Cholera-prophylaxis vóór honderd jaar (Cholera prophylaxis hundred years ago). *NTG*, *82*, IV, 5765–72; *BGG*, *XVIII*, 313–20.

3200 — (1939). De cholera morbus in 1832 te Gorinchem (The cholera morbus in 1832 at G.). *NTG*, *83*, II, 2619–25; *BGG*, *XIX*, 153–9.

3201 DOESSCHATE, G. ten (1952). Een cholera-epidemie te Utrecht (1832–1833) en een onbekende geneesheer (An epidemic of cholera at U. and an unknown physician). *NTG*, *96*, II, 1531–7; *BGG*, *XXXII*, 17–23.
– on an anonymous writer of a treatise on cholera in 1833.

3202 HANEVELD, G. T. (1966). Medische aspecten van de laatste cholera-epidemie in Nederland in 1866 (Medical aspects of the last cholera epidemic in the Netherlands in 1866). *GeWiNa*, no. *20*, 7–9.

3203 ADAM, H. F. (1951). Cholera-epidemie van 1866 (Cholera epidemic of 1866). *NTG*, *95*, IV, 3894; *BGG*, *XXXI*, 103.
– on a medal for good help during a cholera epidemic to an apothecary.

3204 TEIJLER, G. J. (1867). *Geschiedenis eener belangrijke cholera-epidemie welke geheerscht heeft te Jutphaas in 1866* (History of an important cholera epidemic at J. in 1866). 67 pp. Kemink & Zn, Utrecht.

3205 MELLE, M. A. van (1951). Een cholera-epidemie te Utrecht [1866] (A cholera epidemic at U.). *NTG*, *95*, IV, 3049–53; *BGG*, *XXXI*, 52–6. Also in: *Jbk. Oud-Utrecht* (1950), 130–48.

3206 SNETHLAGE, A. (1952). De cholera-epidemie van 1866 te Goes (The cholera epidemic (1866) at G.). *NTG*, *96*, II, 831; *BGG*, *XXXII*, 16.

3207 WOELDERINK, B. De cholera-epidemie van 1866 in Rotterdam (The cholera epidemic of 1866 at R.). *Rotterd. Jbk.*, 7de reeks, *4*, 302–18.

3208 SEMMELINK, J. (1885). *Geschiedenis der cholera in Oost-Indië vóór 1817* (History of the cholera in the East Indies before 1817) Utrecht.

3209 — (1885). *Histoire du choléra aux Indes Orientales avant 1817.* 169 pp. C. H. E. Breyer, Utrecht; G. Carré, Paris; A. Manceaux, Bruxelles.
– with map.

3210 GRENDEL, E. (1971). Mixtura anticholerica. *Bull. Pharm.*, no 43, augustus, 1–15, ill.

See also 4058, 5029, 5065n., 5369.

Smallpox

3211 KLEY, J. J. van der (1929). Pokkenbestrijding en pokkenbehandeling in vroeger tijd (The fight against smallpox and the treatment of smallpox in former times). *NTG, 73*, II, 4632–6; *BGG, IX*, 233–7.

3212 — (1948). Het "post of propter" van goed gevolg in de strijd tegen de pokken (The "post or propter" of success in the fight against smallpox). *GG, 26*, 209–13.

3212ª BREEN, Joh. C. (1916). Pokken te Amsterdam in het laatst der achttiende eeuw (Smallpox at A. at the end of the 18th century). *Amstelodamum, 3*, 33–5.

3213 EEGHEN, I. H. van (1969). Een Amsterdamse dokter op Urk tijdens de pokkenepidemie van 1844/1845 (An Amsterdam physician on Urk during the smallpox epidemic in 1844/1845). *Mbl. Amstelodamum, 56*, 29–38, 1 ill.
– On Corn. Everh. Heynsius (1822–86). cf: *Mbl. Amstelodamum, 56* (1969), 53.

3214 HERMANS, A. E. (1929). De pokken in Nederland in het jaar 1857 (Smallpox in the Netherlands in the year 1857). *NTG, 73*, II, 4662–3; *BGG, IX*, 263–4.

3215 BROEKSMIT, Corn. (1887). *De geschiedenis der pokken in Nederland van 1865 tot 1885* (The history of smallpox in the Netherlands from 1865 till 1885). Thesis Leyden. Rotterdam.

3215ª VIERKANT, E. K. [1902]. *Geschiedenis der pokkenepidemie te Woudsend van half Augustus 1864 tot einde Februari 1865* (History of the smallpox epidemic at W. from the middle August 1864 till the end of February 1865). Sneek, 8°.

3216 PINKHOF, H. (1932). Een pokkenepidemie onder een Indianenstam in 1837 (A smallpox epidemic among an Indian tribe in 1837). *NTG, 76* II, 1625–6; *BGG, XII*, 83–4.

3216ª JONGH, C. L. de (1972). De nomenclatuur van de pokziekte (en de syphilis). Nomenclature of smallpox (and of syphilis)). *AP*, no 9, 66–8.

3217 GREWEL, F. (1949). A cent diables la vérole. *NTG, 93*, III, 3006; *BGG, XXIX*, 58.

3218 ESSED, W. C. A. H. (1949). A cent diables la vérole. *NTG, 93*, IV, 3757–8; *BGG, XXIX*, 68–9. (letter to the editor).

3219 HERMANS, A. G. J. (1949). A cent diables la vérole. *NTG*, *93*, IV, 3758–
      9; *BGG*, *XXIX*, 69–70 (letter to the editor).

3220 LOGHEM, J. J. van (1951). Essed's Theory on the Great Pox epidemic
      in Europe. *Arch. int. Hist. Sci.*, *4* (XXX), 465–7.

> See also 1541, 1965, 2780, 3858, 3862, 3963–99 (Variation
> and vaccination), 4997, 5157n.;

Tuberculosis

3221 RIJKENS, R. G. (1902). Uit de geschiedenis der geneeskunde. De tu-
      berculose (From the history of medicine. Tuberculosis). *Natuur*, *XXII*,
      40, 76, 100 and 133.

3222 — (1905). Uit de geschiedenis der geneeskunde. De behandeling van de
      longtuberculosis (From the history of medicine. Treatment of tuber-
      culosis of the lungs). *Natuur*, *XXV*, 185 and 195.

3223 KLEIWEG de ZWAAN, J. P. (1920). Geschiedenis der tuberculose (His-
      tory of tuberculosis). *NTG*, *64*, II, 1291–1300.

3224 NOLEN, W. (1916). *Enkele bladzijden uit de geschiedenis der Phtiseologie*
      (Some pages from the history of phtiseology). *Gen. Bl.*, *XIX*, no 1,
      28 pp. Bohn, Haarlem.

3225 ZWIJNENBERG, H. A. (1923). Aanteekeningen uit de geschiedenis van
      de bestrijding der besmettelijke longziekten (Notes from the history of
      the fight against contagious lung diseases). *NTG*, *67*, II, 1676–9; *BGG*,
      III, 331–4.

3226 MOONEN, W. A. (1951). Geschiedenis der niertuberculose (History of
      renal tuberculosis). *NTG*, *95*, III, 2187–95; *BGG*, *XXXI*, 26–34.

3227 SANDRA, H. (1942–1946).
      De leer der phthisis bij oude Nederlandsche schrijvers. (The doctrine
      of phthisis in old Dutch writers).

3227[1] 1. Pieter van Foreest. *NTG*, *86*, 838–44; *BGG*, *XXII*, 48–54.

3227[2] 2. Joost van Lom. *NTG*, *86*, 1426–9; *BGG*, *XXII*, 77–80.

3227[3] 3. Rembert Dodoens. *NTG*, *86*, 1713–7; *BGG*, *XXII*, 94–8.

3227[4] 4. Johan van Heurne. *NTG*, *86*, 1960–5; *BGG*, *XXII*, 110–5.

3227[5] 5. Paul Barbette. *NTG*, *86*, 1965–6; *BGG*, *XXII*, 115–6.

3227^6 6. Johan van Beverwijck. *NTG, 86,* 2233–5; *BGG, XXII,* 121–3.

3227^7 7. Isbrand van Diemerbroeck. *NTG, 86,* 2475–7; *BGG, XXII,* 129–31.

3227^8 8. Franciscus dele Boë Sylvius. *NTG, 86,* 2477–82; *BGG, XXII,* 131–6.

3227^9 9. Steven Blankaart. *NTG, 86,* 3076–7; *BGG, XXII,* 154–5.

3227^{10} 10. Herman Boerhaave. *NTG, 87,* (1943), 648–51; *BGG, XXIII,* 26–9.

3227^{11} 11. Gerard van Swieten. *NTG, 87,* 841–7; *BGG, XXIII,* 40–6.

3227^{12} 12. Johannes de Gorter. *NTG, 87,* 1699–701; *BGG, XXIII,* 82–4.

3227^{13} 13. Petrus Camper. *NTG, 87,* 1701–5; *BGG, XXIII,* 84–8.

3227^{14} 14. E. P. Becker. *NTG, 88* (1944), 492–4; *BGG, XXIV,* 7–9.

3277^{15} 15. Conrad Gerard Ontijd. *NTG, 88,* 724–6; *BGG, XXIV,* 11–3.

3227^{16} 16. Johannes Ludovicus Conradus Schroeder van der Kolk, *NTG, 90*
        .(1946), 380–2; *BGG, XXVI,* 7–9.

3228   — (1948). *Nederlandse phthisiologie. Vijf eeuwen onderzoek naar de
       volksvijand tuberkulose* (Dutch phthisiology. Five centuries of inves-
       tigation of the enemy of the people, tuberculosis). 173 pp., 23 ill.,
       port. "De Torenlaan", Assen.

3229   MEYER, J. (1962). Twee oude proefschriften (Two old theses). *Tegen
       Tuberculose, 58,* 36–40, facs.
       – Henricus Freund. *Historia phtiseos pulmonis hereditaria,* 1826; G. van Overbeek
       de Meyer. *Over den invloed van zeereizen en het verblijf in warme luchtstreken op de
       ontwikkeling en het verloop van tuberculosis pulmonum, 1865.* (On the influence of
       sea-voyages and the stay in warm climates on the development and the course of
       — —).

3230   JONG, Zr Fr. de (1969). Uit de geschiedenis van het tuberculose-
       huisbezoek in enige West-Europese landen (From the history of visit-
       ing patients with tuberculosis in some West-European countries).
       Tegen Tuberculose, 65, 70–6; 97–9, ill.

3231   HEYNSIUS van den BERG, M. R. (1963). Enkele persoonlijke herinne-
       ringen aan de begintijd van de strijd tegen de tuberculose (Some per-
       sonal memoirs of the initial stage of the fight against tuberculosis).
       Tegen Tuberculose, 59, 21–6, ill.

3231^a SPANJAARD, R. B. (1974). Amsterdams strijd tegen t.b.c. 70 jaar (Am-
       sterdam's fight against tuberculosis 70 years). *Ons Amsterdam, 26,*
       354–63, 12 ill., port.

3232 LEE, L. van der (1963). 60 jaar tuberculosebestrijding in Rotterdam
1903–1963 (60 years of fight against tuberculosis in R.). *Tegen Tuberculose, 59,* 27–31, ill.

3233 [   ] (1964). Een pleit uit 1904 voor de bestrijding van de tuberculose (A plea from 1904 for the fight against tuberculosis). *MC, 19,*
144.

3234 WESSEL, I. (1963). 60 jaar: 50 jaar N.C.V. – 10 jaar K.N.C.V. *Tegen
Tuberculose, 59,* 4–11, ill.

– On the "*K*oninklijke *N*ederlandse *C*entrale *V*ereniging tot bestrijding van de
Tuberculose"
                                         See also 1269a, 1714, 2683, 3907.

3235 NOLEN, W. (1901). Het Congres over Tuberculose te Londen (The
Congress on Tuberculosis at L.). *NTG, 45,* II, 655–63.

– In this historical meeting lectures were delivered by R. Koch and J. Lister (cf:
NTG, 117, (1973), 630).

3236 SCHUURMANS STEKHOVEN, W. (1928). Geschiedkundig overzicht van de
verschillende methoden ter onvatbaarmaking tegen tuberculose (Historical survey of the different methods for immunization against tuberculosis). *Gen. Bl., 26,* 197–207.

3237 PRAKKEN, J. R. (1972). Het tuberculine-drama van 1890–1891 (The
tuberculin tragedy in —). *NTG, 116,* 1131–7.
                                         See also 1393, 5414, 5416.

Malaria

3238 SWELLENGREBEL, N. H. and P. J. J. HONIG (1925, 1926, 1928). Bijdrage
tot de geschiedenis der malaria in Nederland. I. en II. een onderzoek
naar de waarde der gegevens, waarvan men zich bedient ter herkenning
van de door plasmodiën veroorzaakte koorts in de geschiedkundige
overlevering. III: de juiste plaats der plasmodiose in de rij der moeras-
ziekten. IV: geen ondertitel. (Contribution to the history of malaria
in the Netherlands. I. and II: investigation into the worth of data of
which one avails oneself to recognize the plasmodian fever in historical
tradition. III: The right place of plasmodiosis in the series of paludal
diseases. IV: no subtitle.)
I: *NTG, 69,* (1925), I, 2538–55; *BGG, V,* 109–26.
II: *NTG, 70* (1926). II, 1104–20; *BGG, VI,* 233–49.
III: *NTG, 70,* II, 1864–75; *BGG, VI,* 289–300.
IV: *NTG, 72* (1928), I, 38–47; *BGG, VIII,* 1–10.

3239 RIJNBERK, G. van (1909). *Atti della Società per gli studi della Malaria*, vol. IX, 729 pp., 6 col. pl. Rome. *Janus, XIV*, 192–202.
– with notes on the history of malaria.

3240 SWELLENGREBEL, N. H. (1954). De levensgeschiedenis van een werk-hypothese (The life story of a working hypothesis). *NTG, 98*, II, 1401–8.
– on the paludal hypothesis of malaria.

See also 3294.

Typhoid fever

3241 TAAMS, J. (1932). *De historische ontwikkeling van het typhusvraagstuk* (The historical development of the problem of typhoid fever). Thesis Leyden (Supervisor R. P. van Calcar). 63 pp. Leiden.

3242 HAAS, J. H. de (1934). Bretonneau en de eerste (Fransche) literatuur over dothinentérie bij kinderen (B. and the first (French) literature on "dothinentérie" in children). *NTG, 78*, III, 3956–74; *BGG, XIV*, 167 –85.

Dysentery

3243 BAUMANN, E. D. (1926). Iets over de dysenterie in de zestiende en ze-ventiende eeuw (Something on dysentery in the 16th and 17th century). *NTG, 70*, II, 41–59; *BGG, VI*, 156–74.

3244 — (1926). Bijdrage tot de geschiedenis der dysenterie in de achttiende eeuw (Contribution to the history of dysentery in the eighteenth century). *NTG, 70*, II, 1520–34; *BGG, VI*, 257–71.

3245 — (1925). De dysenterie te Nijmegen in 1736 (Dysentery at N. in 1736). *NTG, 69*, II, 605–19; *BGG, V*, 169–83.

3245[a] MENTINK, G. J. (1970). De rode loop in Gelderland (Bloody flux in Guelders). *Gelre, LXIV*, 140.

3245[b] WENTZEL, G. (1974). Over een epidemie en een Veluwse kruidendroge-rij (On an epidemic and a Veluwe drying-house for herbs). *Ned. Hist.*, *8*, no 4, 182–6.
– on an epidemic of bloody flux on the Veluwe in the second half of the 18th century ... The drying-house is of recent date.

3246 INGELSE, P. (1935). *Oude gegevens betreffende dysenterie* (Old data concerning dysentery). Thesis Leyden 78 pp., Leiden.

3247 Putto, J. A. (1936). Oude gegevens betreffende dysenterie. Eene weinig bekende publicatie uit de achttiende eeuw (Old data concerning dysentery. A little known publication from the 18th century) *GG*, *14*, 1003–4.

3248 — (1936). Oude gegevens betreffende dysenterie (Old data concerning dysentery). *GG*, *14*, 758–60.

See also 380, 382, 5042.

Intestinal parasites

3249 Koopman, J. (1922). Een oude mededeeling over ingewandswormen (An old information on intestinal worms). *NTG*, *66*, II, 1092; *BGG*, *II*, 223.
– review of an article of Khalil (*J. trop. Med.*, 1922, no 6, 65), dealing with a manuscript of a part of Avicenna's *Canon*.

3250 Swellengrebel, N. H. and A. C. Rijpstra (1965). Over dioctophyma renale en de ontwikkeling van het inzicht in besmetting (On dioctophyma renale and the development of the understanding of infection). *NTG*, *109*, I, 30–3; *BGG*, *XLV*, 3–6, 10 ill.

3251 Jansen, J. and H. J. Over, (1968). References to liver fluke disease (fasciolosis) in the Netherlands till 1600. *It Beaken*, *(Tydskrift fan de Fryske Akademy)*, *30*, 10–2.
– see also Bidloo (104).

See also 2512, 3868

Diphteria

3252 Israëls, A. H. (1861). De geschiedenis der diphteritis, beknopt medegedeeld (History of diphteria, a condensed report). *NTG*, *5*, 203.

3253 Maathuis, R. (1938). *De diphterie in de loop der eeuwen* (Diphteria in the course of the ages). Thesis Leyden (Supervisor: Gorter). Amsterdam.

3254 Putto, J. A. (1910). Geneeskunst in vroeger dagen: hoest, keelpijn, heeschheid, kinkhoest, tering, aamborstigheid en borstkramp (Medicine in former days: cough, sore throat, hoarseness, whooping cough (pertussis), phthisis, asthma and angina pectoris). *Navorscher*, *LIX*, 454.

Influenza

3255 ANDEL, M. A. van (1929). Griep in de 16de eeuw (Flu in the 16th
century). *NTG*, *73*, II, 5744–50; *BGG*, *IX*, 328–34.

3256 HUFFEL, A. J. van (1933). De influenza in Amsterdam een eeuw geleden
(Flu at A. a century ago). *Amstelodamum*, *20*, 65.

3257 GOOYER, A. de (1968). *De Spaanse griep van '18* (The Spanish influenza in 1918). 128 pp. Philips-Duphar Nederland, Amsterdam.

3258 QUANJER, A. A. J. (1921). *De griep in Nederland in 1918 tot 1920* (Influenza in the Netherlands in – till –). Staats Uitgeverij, Den Haag.
– Publication of the National Health Council.

See also 834, 5039

Rabies canina (Hydrophobia) (and remedies for —)

3259 FEYFER, F. M. G. de (1928). Overheidszorg bij hondsdolheid in de achttiende eeuw (Governmental care about rabies canina in the 18th century). *NTG*, *72*, I, 1708–10; *BGG*, *VIII*, 109–11.

3260 DOOREN, L. (1937). Behandeling van hondsdolheid in de 18de eeuw
(Treatment of rabies canina in the 18th century). *GG*, *15*, 1128–9.

3261 BRAAT, P. (1938). Middelen tegen hondsdolheid (Remedies against
rabies canina). *NTG*, *82*, II, 2293–5; *BGG*, *XVIII*, 94–6.

3262 POLAK, M. F. (1964). Voorbehoedende behandeling tegen rabies in het
jaar 1886 (Preventive treatment against rabies, 1886). *NTG*, *108*, I,
36–40; *BGG*, *XLIV*, 18–22. Also in: *TMA*, *19* (1964), 237–43.

3263 HALLEMA, A. (1961). Een 18-eeuws Ferwerder middel tegen rabies
(An 18th century Ferwerd remedy for rabies). *NTG*, *105*, I, 39–40;
BGG, *XLI*, 7–8.

3264 HELDERS, J. (1962). Een 18e-eeuws Ferwerder middel tegen rabies
(An 18th century Ferwerd remedy for rabies). *NTG*, *106*, I, 33–4;
BGG, *XLII*, 6–7.

3265 DAMSTÉ, P. H. (1959). De Biltse drank tegen dollehondsbeet (The Bilt
draught for the bite of a mad dog). *Jbk. Oud-Utrecht*, 121–38, 1 pl.

See also 2691–92

Scabies

3266 SCHUURMANS STEKHOVEN, J. H. (1919). De geschiedenis van het schurft-
      onderzoek (History of the investigation on scabies). *NTG, 63*, I, 2144–
      7.

3267 PINKHOF, H. (1927). Een, die niet aan de schurftmijt geloofde (Some-
      one who did not believe in the sarcoptes). *NTG, 71*, I, 3150–1; *BGG,
      VII*, 415–6.
      – on W. Wildrik, the writer of a book against the belief in disease-producing in-
      sects (1781).

3268 OUDEMANS, A. C. (1927). Iets over de geschiedenis omtrent scabies en
      de acarus siro (Something on the history of scabies and the acarus
      siro). *NTG, 71*, I, 2519–25; *BGG, VII*, 369–75.

3269 LINT, J. G. de (1933). De ontdekking van den parasitairen oorsprong
      der scabies (The discovery of the parasitic origin of scabies). *NTG, 77*,
      I, 76–7; *BGG, XIII*, 27–8.

G. Diseases of the nervous system

3270 GILS, J. B. F. van (1925). De hikziekte in vroegeren tijd (The hiccup
      disease in former times). *NTG, 69*, I, 1613–4; *BGG, V*, 87–8.
      – Review of an article by Tricot-Royer.

3271 SCHULTE, B. P. M. (1966). Van "apoplexie" tot "cerebrovasculair
      accident" (From "apoplexia" till cerebrovascular accident"). *NTG, 110*
      1209–10.

3272 ZUIDEN, D. S. van (1916). Genezing van lamheid na opzettelijk besmet
      te zijn geweest door pokken (Recovery of paralysis after intentional
      infection with smallpox). *NTG, 60*, II, 2018–9.
      – Ao 1679.

3273 DONINCK, A. van (1929). Geschiedenis der behandeling van de vallen-
      de ziekte (History of the treatment of epilepsy). I. *NTG, 73*, II, 4147–
      64; *BGG, IX*, 207–24. II. *NTG, 73*, II, 4644–52; *BGG, IX*, 245–53.

3274 KAMPING, A. (1940). Een "paardemiddel" tegen vallende ziekte om-
      streeks het midden der 18e eeuw (A "kill or cure" remedy for epilepsy
      in the middle of the 18th century). *NTG, 84*, II, 1324; *BGG, XX*, 71.
      See also 2564, 3299

3275 BOLTEN, G. C. (1922). Eenige historische bijzonderheden betreffende epilepsie (Some historical details regarding epilepsy). *NTG, 66,*
I, 2156–69; *BGG, II,* 123–36.
– cf: J. H. Th. Jansen (letter to the ed.): *NTG, 66,* I, 2285.

3276 VERJAAL, A. (1960). Quelques remarques sur l'histoire de l'aphasie
frontale. *Janus, XLIX,* 130–6.

3277 MEERLOO, J. A. M. (1973). Een historische zelfbeschrijving van aphasie
(A historical self-description on aphasy). *Arts en Wereld, 6,* no 1, 15–8.
– on the short-lasting aphasy of the French physiologist Jacques Lordat (1773–
1870), in 1811.

H. Various diseases

3278 BARUCH, J. Z. (1964). Paracelsus en tijdgenoten over enkele beroepsziekten (P. and contemporaries on some occupational diseases). *T.
Soc. Geneesk.,* 42, 153–8.

3279 GEIST-HOFMAN, A. M., J. V. MEININGER and C. M. VERKROOST (1972).
Zinking, zinkingskoorts en zinkingsziekte (Catarrh, catarrhal fever and
catarrhal disease). *NTG, 116,* 23–30.

3280 VIEYRA, D. (1931). Kankerbestrijding in vroeger tijden (The fight
against cancer in former times). *NTG, 75,* IV, 5510; *BGG, XI,* 305.

3281 — (1931). Recept ter bestrijding van den kanker (Prescription for the
fight against cancer). *NTG, 75,* IV, 5018; *BGG, XI,* 281.

See also 2897, 5272a, 5303

3281ª BEUMER, H. M. (1974). Medizingeschichte des Hyperventilationssyn-
droms (Soldier's Heart). *Med. Welt,* 25 (N.F.), 471–3, port.

3282 DOESSCHATE, G. ten (1957). De geschiedenis van de Hoogteziekte
(History of altitude disease). *GeWiNa,* no. 2, 11–2.

3283 — (1957). De geschiedenis van de bergziekte (History of mountain-
sickness). *NTG, 101,* I, 1966–7; *BGG, XXXVII,* 32–3.

3284 SCHLICHTING, Th. (1956). On the history of bronchial asthma. *Proc.
Int. round table Friendship Meeting of Allergolists, Utrecht 1955,* 334–
41.
– reprint from *The Therapy of Bronchial Asthma* (ed.: W. J. Quarles van Ufford,
1956). Stenfert Kroese, Leiden.

3285 BEUMER, H. M. (1971). Allergie- und Asthmaforschung von Willem
Storm van Leeuwen (1882–1933). *Med. Welt, 22,* 1530–6, 7 ill.
See also 1600–05 (Storm van Leeuwen), 2684.

3286 — (1970). Historische ontwikkelingen rondom sarcoidosis (Historical
developments around sarcoidosis). *NedMGT, 23,* 221–8.

3287 — (1971). Medizingeschichte der Sarkoidose. Die Besnier-Boeck-
·Schaumannsche Krankheit in ihrer historischen Entwicklung. *Ärztl.
Praxis, XXIII,* 4017–22, 10 ports., 7 ill.

3288 DIEREN, E. van (1897). *Beri-beri. Eene rijstvergiftiging. Kritisch-historische bijdrage tot de kennis der meelvergiften* (Beri-beri. A rice poisoning. Critical-historical contribution to the knowledge of meal poisoning). Scheltema & Holkema, Amsterdam.
– Reviewed by C. L. van der Burg: *Janus I* (1896/97), 493–4.

3289 — (1907). *Meelvergiftigingen: Beri-beri, pellagra, kriebelziekte, erwten-
ziekte, polaranaemie, enz.* (Flour poisoning: beri-beri, pellagra, ergot-
ism, pea-disease, "polar" anaemia, etc). 470 pp., Scheltema & Holkema, Amsterdam.

3290 MENDES da COSTA, S. (1924). Lupus en zijn bestrijding in Nederland
(Lupus and the fight against it in the Netherlands). *NTG, 68,* II, 48–
52; *BGG, IV,* 171–5, 1 ill.

3290ª HILLAM, C. (translator). (1972). *An inaugural medical dissertation on
aphthae (Leyden, 1747).* Dental History Unit. Dept. of Oral Pathology,
Univ. of Birmingham.
– Thesis by J. A. Putman entitled: *De Aphthis* (23 March 1747 at Leyden). [type-
script].
See also: 2685–9; Antiquity (2678–2706); Tropical medicine
(3850–69).

I. Case-reports

3291 BOOTH, C. (1901). *Merkwaardige genezingen en ziektegevallen* (Remarkable recoveries and cases of illness). *Navorscher, LI,* 217.

3292 HAZEWINKEL, H. C. (1937). Herinnering van eene langdurige en ge-
vaarlijke kwaal en derzelver volkomene genezinge (Memory of a
protracted and dangerous disease and its complete cure). *NTG, 83,* III,
3354–6; *BGG, XIX,* 190–2.

3293 GOSLINGS-LIJSEN, J. H. (1941). Een zenuwpatiënte en haar behandeling voor twee eeuwen (A neurotic and her treatment two centuries ago). *NTG, 85,* I, 80–3; *BGG, XXI,* 8–11.

3294 WINCKEL, Ch. W. F. (1940). Een geval van malaria quartane 130 jaar geleden (A case of malaria quartane 130 years ago). *NTG, 84, III,* 3518–9; *BGG, XX,* 145–6.

3295 BOERMA, N. J. A. F. (1941). Wondergeval van Jan de Dood, een smit t'Amsterdam 1651 (The miraculous case of J. d. D., a smith at Amsterdam 1651). *NTG, 85,* III, 3631; *BGG, XXI,* 123.
- on Jan de Dood, who operated upon himself for the bladderstone. Quotation from: *Vervolgh Hist. Kroniek* van J. L. Gottfried, Leiden 1700;
See also 3414.

3296 KNAPPERT, H. E. (1921). Een ziektenverslag uit 1721 (A case report from 1721). *NTG, 65,* II, 59; *BGG, I,* 312.

3297 VEN, A. J. van de (1940). Twee onverwachte sterfgevallen in 1678 (Two unexpected deaths in 1678). *NTG, 84,* IV, 4277–84; *BGG, XX,* 161–8.
- with a postcript by M. A. van Andel.

3297ª KLAVEREN Pz, G. van and A. J. van der Weyde (1931). Een wonderlijcke genesinge [van Sophia Maria van Honthorst] aen velen tot groote verwonderinge verhaelt (A strange recovery [of — — —] told to many people to their astonishment). *Jbk. Oud-Utrecht,* 102–21.

3298 LIMBORGH, J. van (1955). Gerrit Bastiaansz. de Hals, "De Grote Boer" van Lekkerkerk. Een historisch-anthropologische studie over een reus uit de zeventiende eeuw (The "Big Peasant" from —. A histtorical-anthropological study on a giant from the 17th century). *NTG, 99,* I, 963–70; *BGG, XXXV,* 25–32, ill.

3299 RIJN, G. van (1900). De slapende boer van Stolwijk en de Rotterdamsche geneesheeren (The sleeping peasant of S. and the Rotterdam physicians). *Rotterd. Jbk.,* 1e reeks, 7, 67–87; 88–102.

3300 PENNING, C. P. J. (1928). Een geval van prostaathypertrophie in de 18de eeuw (A case of prostatic hypertrophy in the 18th century). *NTG, 72,* I, 1113; *BGG, VIII,* 80.

3301 SERVAAS van ROOYEN, A. J. (1905). Eefken Vliegen de hongerlijdster (— —, the starveling). *Alb. Nat.,* 318.

3302 TEIXEIRA de MATTOS, E. (1928). De phrenesie van de oude Jonkvrouw Jeanne de Spinosa te Rijssel, tijdsbeeld uit het begin der 17de eeuw (The phrenzy of the old noblewoman — — at R., time-picture from the beginning of the 17th century). *NTG*, *72*, II, 4958–67; *BGG*, *VIII*, 295–304.

3303 POSTMA, C. (1952). Een geval van St. Vitusdans in 1761 te Voorburg, geconstateerd door een Delftse medicus, en wat de kwakzalvers er van maakten (A case of St. Vitus' dance (chorea) in 1761 at V., diagnosed by a Delft physician, and what the quacks made of it). *NTG*, *96*, IV, 3205–9; *BGG*, *XXXII*, 42–6.

3304 GANS, O. (1968). Ein Fall von Hasenscharte (Cheiloschisis – Labium fissum – Labium leporinum) aus dem Jahre 1517. *Hautarzt*, *19*, 174–5.

J. Clinical medicine

3305 DONINCK, A. van (1929). Doctrine om d'urine te leeren kennen 1459 (Doctrine to learn to know the urine 1459). *NTG*, *73*, I, 544–54; *BGG*, *IX*, 37–47.

3306 WEIJDE, A. J. van der (1924). De inwendige geneeskunde in ons Vaderland gedurende de afgelopen 75 jaren (Internal medicine in our country during the last 75 years). *NTG*, *68*, II, 6–20; *BGG*, *IV*, 129–43, 7 ports.

3307 PEL, P. K. (1907). De klinische diagnostiek voor 50 jaar en thans (Clinical diagnostics 50 years ago and today). *NTG*, *51*, I, 19–28.

3308 VERJAAL, A. (1951). *De ontwikkelingsgang der klinische diagnostiek* (The course of development of clinical diagnostics). 46 pp. Bohn, Haarlem. 8°.

3309 SCHLICHTING, Th. H. (1952). De richting van het intellect in de ziektegeschiedenis (The trend of the intellect in the case history). *NTG*, *96*, IV, 3200–5; *BGG*, *XXXII*, 37–42.

Thermometer

3310 TJADEN MODDERMAN, R. S. (1886). De geschiedenis van den thermometer (History of the thermometer). *Alb. Nat.*, 171–86.

3311   DANIËLS, C. E. (1900). De thermometrie aan het ziekbed. Historische
       aanteekeningen (Thermometry at the sick-bed. Historical notices).
       NTG, *44*, (2de reeks *36*), II, 952–83, ill.

3312   — (1901/02). Die Thermometrie am Krankenbette. *Ztschr. diät. u.*
       physik. Therapie, *V*, Heft 5, 16 pp.
       – reprint.

3313   WAARD Jr, C. de (1914). Zur Vorgeschichte des Thermometers.
       Mitt. Gesch. Med. Naturw., *XIII*, 177.

3314   STAR, P. van der (1968). The History of Thermometry in Medicine.
       Medical Thermography. Proc. of a Boerhaave Course for post-grad.
       Medical Education, Leiden. In: *Bibl. radiol.*, no. 5, 1–7, Karger, Basel–
       New York 1969.

3315   EBSTEIN, E. (1929). Die Verdienste der holländischen Schule um die
       Entwicklung der klinischen Thermometrie. *VIme Congrès Int. d'Hist.*
       de la Méd. Leyde-Amsterdam, *1927*, 190. Anvers.

3315ª CSILLAG, J. (1963). 60 éves a húros galvanometer [Magyar] *Orv.*
       Hétil., *104*, 1617–21. port., ill.
       – also on W. Einthoven.

       Fames canina

3316   SCHRIJVER, J. (1926). Fames canina. *NTG*, *70*, I, 969–74; *BGG*, *VI*,
       49–54.

3316ª — (1926). Nog eens: Fames canina (Once again: fames canina) *NTG*,
       70, I, 2366; *BGG*, *VI*, 124.

See also 2696

Chapter VIII.

Therapeutics and Healings

It is common knowledge that in the past the most curious remedies and methods have been applied to obtain a cure of diseases or ailments. Whereas many of them belong to folk medicine, other procedures resulted from special views on the origin and character of some diseases. Blood-letting and leeches for example have been used and misused on a large scale for a long time.

A section is included referring to secret or not-secret remedies for special diseases, such as bladder stones.

Finally the literature on miraculous healings is put together in a section.

A. General

3317 LINDEBOOM, G. A. (1956). La thérapeutique en perspective historique. *Atti del XIV congresso internazionale di storia della Medizina, Roma-Salerno, 13–20 September 1954.*

3318 D[OOREN], L. (1936). Orgaan-therapie omstreeks 1580 (Organ-therapy about 1580). *GG, 14*, 524–5.

3319 FÜLÖP-MILLER, René (1947). *De triomf over de pijn* (The triumph over pain). 385 pp. Allert de Lange, Amsterdam.
– Dutch translation by C. C. Bender; reviewed by D. Schoute: *NTG, 92* (1948), IV, 3207; *BGG, XXVIII,* 10.

3320 BOERMA, N. J. A. F. (1939). Intraveneuse toediening van geneesmiddelen in ouden tijd (Intravenous administration of remedies in ancient times). *NTG, 83,* IV, 5292; *BGG, XIX,* 253.

See also 2561, 3838

B. Homoeopathy

3321 KNUFMAN, C. J. F. L. (no d.) *De geschiedkundige ontwikkeling en betekenis der homoeopathie* (The historical development and significance of homoeopathy). 87 pp. Zaandam.

3322 STOKVIS, B. J. (1888). *Voordrachten over homoeopathie, gehouden aan de Amsterdamsche Universiteit* (Lectures on homoeopathy, delivered in the Amsterdam University). *79* pp. Bohn, Haarlem.

3323 HAER, P. van der (1906). *De homoiopathie. Eene historisch-kritische beschouwing* (Homoeopathy. A historical-critical dissertation). Thesis Leyden. 112 pp. 8°.

3324 FEYFER, F. M. G. de (1926). De wijsgeerige achtergrond der homoeopathie (Proeve eener historische synthese). Philosophical background of homoeopathy (A specimen of a historical synthesis)) *NTG, 70,* I, 1400–10; *BGG, VI,* 69–79.

3325 BIER, August (*ca.* 1926). *Welk standpunt moeten wij ten opzichte van de homoeopathie innemen?* (Which point of view do we have to take with respect to homoeopathy?). Zwolle.
– Translation of the German edition: *Wie sollen wir uns zur der Homöopathie stellen?* (München, 1925).

3326 JONGH, D. K. de (1943). *Critische beschouwingen over de Homoeopathie. Ontstaan, ontwikkeling en wezen van dit therapeutische stelsel* (Critical observations on Homoeopathy. Origin, development and essence of this therapeutic system). Thesis University of Amsterdam. X + 479 pp. Amsterdam. 8°.
– with historical survey.

3327 VOS, T. A. (1948). Kennis van het gelijke door het gelijke (Knowledgement of the same by the same). *Hermèneus, 19,* 91–2.

3328 — (1973). Geschiedkundige bijdragen. I. Kennis van het gelijke door het gelijke (Historical contributions. I. Knowledge of the same by the same). *Arts en Wereld, 6,* no 3, 33–4.

3329 RIET, A. van 't (1973). Homoeopathie, moderne geneeswijze uit de achttiende eeuw (Homoeopathy, modern cure from the 18th century). *GG, 4,* 235–7.

3330 ARON, W. (1970). Hahnemann et Spinoza; une étude comparée de leur psychologie. *Rev. Hist. Méd. hébraique*, *23*, 11–3.

> See also 889–90 (Hahnemann), 967, 1331–51 (Paracelsus), 2075.

C. Miracles (and the belief in them)

3331 SERVAAS van ROOYEN, A. J. (1905). Een jaar van wonderen (A year of miracles). *Alb. Nat.*, 277.

3332 RIJNBERK, G. van (1914). Hedendaagsch mirakelgeloof (Miracle-belief to-day).

3332[1] 1. Inleiding (Introduction). *NTG*, *58*, I, 1347–52.

3332[2] 2. Sterrewichelarij (Astrology). *ibid.*, 1431–7; letter to the editor: *ibid.*, 1501–2.

3332[3] 3. Over eenige mediamieke verschijnselen: De "Telekinesiën". (On some mediumistic phenomena: Telekinesis). *ibid.*, 1511–5; letters to the ed.: *ibid.*, 1571; 1676–7.

3332[4] 4. Over eenige mediamieke verschijnselen. De "Teleplasiën" (On teleplastic phenomena). *Ibid.*, 1757–62; letter to the ed.: *ibid.* 1837–8.

3332[5] 5. over somnabulisme (On somnabulism). *ibid.*, 1969–73.

3332[6] 6. Over dierlijk magnetisme (On animal magnetism). *ibid.*, 1974–81.

3332[7] 7. Denkende dier (Thinking animal). *ibid.*, 2135–41.

3332[8] 8. Denkende dier: het aandeel der menschen (Thinking animal: the share of mankind). *ibid.*, 2231–8.

3332[9] 9. De wichelroede: De leer (The dowsing-rod: The doctrine). *ibid, II*, 805–10.

3332[10] 10. De wichelroede. Een poging tot verklaring (The dowsing-rod. An attempt at explanation). *ibid.*, 885–92.

3332[11] 11. Samenvatting en besluit (Summary and conclusion). *ibid.*, 1405–8; letter to the ed.: *ibid.*, 1466.

3333 NOLEN, W. (1919). De wonderen der geneeskunst (The miracles of medicine). *NTG*, *63*, I, 1468–82; 1708.

3334   BOEKELMAN, W. A. (1919). De wonderen der geneeskunst (The miracles of medicine). *NTG*, *63*, I, 1607–8.

3335   BALEN, A. van (1919). Wonderen der geneeskunst (Miracles of medicine). *NTG*, *63*, I, 1608.

3336   LINDEBOOM, G. A. (1966). Het wonder in de geneeskunde (The Miracle
in medicine). *Soteria*, *X*, 160–6.

3336ᵃ   FOX, J. (1959). Middeleeuwse wondergenezingen (Miraculous healings in the Middle Ages). *Amstelodamum*, *46*, 139.

3337   TJADEN MODDERMAN, R. S. (1905). Het rozenwonder van den heiligen
Franciscus (The miracle of roses of St. Franciscus). *Alb. Nat.*, 109.

3338   SLOOTMANS, C. (no d.). *De St. Geertruydsbronne. Legende en historie*;
(The St. Geertruyds-source. Legend and history). Bergen op Zoom.
– To the water of this source healing power was attributed; reviewed by M. A. van
Andel: *NTG*, *75* (1931), I, 1154; *BGG*, *XI*, 83.

3339   MENDELS, J. I. H. (1937). Een Maria-legende (A Maria legend). *NTG*,
81, 602–3; *BGG*, *XVII*, 36–7.
– Appearance of Maria as a helper at a hopeless delivery.

3340   JANSMA, J. R. (1921). Verschijnselen, waargenomen aan het lijk van
Maria van Valckenisse (Phenomena, observed on the corpse of —— ——).
NTG, *65*, I, 1252–8.

3341   BURGER, D. (1959). Ce que disent des témoins oculaires sur la pluie
de sang à Bruxelles, le 6 Octobre 1646. *Janus*, *XLVIII*, 203–7.

D. Fontanels, blood-letting, leeches, Spanish fly

3342   BLÖTE, H. W. (1924). Over de toepassing van de fontanel bij longtering
(On the application of the fontanel to phthisis). *NTG*, *68*, II, 2254–5;
BGG, *IV*, 291–2.

3343   HERMANS, A. G. J. (1942). De bloedzuiger als vriend en vijand (The
leech as a friend and as an enemy). *NTG*, *86*, I, 151; *BGG*, *XXII*, 27.

3344   GILS, J. B. F. (1942). De bloedzuiger als vriend en vijand (The leech
as a friend and as an enemy). *NTG*, *86*, I, 22–7; *BGG*, *XXII*, 1–6.

3345   — (1946). Spaansche vlieg (Spanish fly). *NTG*, *90*, II, 377–80; *BGG*,
XXVI, 4–7.

3346 HIJMANS, H. (1925). De kooplieden en het aderlaten (Merchants and blood-letting). *NTG*, *69*, I, 1133–4; *BGG*, *V*, 66–7, 1 ill.

3347 ANDEL, M. A. van (1932, 1933). De aderlating in theorie en practijk (Blood-letting in theory and practice). I. De humoraal-pathologie (Humoral pathology). *NTG*, *76*, IV, 4648–68; *BGG*, *XII*, 181–201. II. De astrologie (Astrology). *NTG*, *76*, IV, 5164–79; *BGG*, *XII*, 224–39. III. Hygiëne en Techniek (Hygiene and technics) *NTG*, *77* (1933), I, 1015–21; *BGG*, *XIII*, 61–7.

E. Resuscitating of drowned persons; fumigator

3348 EYSSELSTEIN, G. van (1911). Erste Hilfe bei Ertrunkenen nach dem Schriftstellen des Altertums. *Janus*, *XVI*, 577–88.

3349 ARRIAS, E. (1910). Vergeten en te vergeten methodes tot het bijbrengen van drenkelingen (Methods for resuscitating drowned persons, forgotten and to be forgotten.). *NTG*, *54*, II, 2203–4;

3350 NIEMEYER, A. (1910). Een vergeten methode tot het bijbrengen van drenkelingen (A forgotten method for resuscitating drowned persons). *NTG*, *54*, II, 1780–1.

3351 LEERSUM, E. C. van (1910). Een vergeten methode tot het bijbrengen van drenkelingen (A forgotten method for resuscitating drowned persons). *NTG*, *54*, II, 1544–8.
– natural heat: a young, naked person (woman) laid against the drowned person.

3352 — (1911). Een bijkans vergeten methode tot het bijbrengen van drenkelingen (A nearly forgotten method for resuscitating drowned persons. *NTG*, *55*, I, 1926–9.

3353 BAIS, W. J. (1911). Natuurlijke warmte bij drenkelingen (Natural warmth with drowned persons). *NTG*, *55*, I, 59.

3354 BITTER, H. (1915). Voorschriften voor het opwekken der levensgeesten bij schijndode drenkelingen in de 18de eeuw (Instructions for resuscitating apparently dead drowned persons in the 18th century). *Navorscher*, *LXIV*, 379.

3355 LANGEVELD, C. H. J. (1941). Hoe men 170 jaar geleden een drenkeling behandelde. Rechterlijk archief van Hardingsveld 1773 (How a drowned person was treated 170 years ago. Judicial archive of H.). *NTG, 85,* IV, 4202; *BGG, XXI,* 151.

3356 GORTER, R. A. (1950). De oudste methodes tot het opwekken der levensgeesten (The oldest methods for resuscitating). *NTG, 94,* I, 37–40; *BGG, XXX,* 1–4.

3357 KOOPMAN, J. (1929). De vrees voor schijndood in het verleden (The fear of apparent death in the past). *NTG, 73,* II, 5725–30; *BGG, IX,* 309–14.

3358 GORTER, R. A. (1952). De tabaksrookclysteer "van Gaubius" (The fumigator "of G."). *NTG, 96,* IV, 3196–3200; *BGG, XXXII,* 33–7, ill.

3359 — (1953). *De tabaksrook-klisteer voornamelijk als reanimator* (Fumigator mainly for resuscitation). 169 pp., 66 fig. and ill. Maatschappij tot Redding van Drenkelingen, Amsterdam.
– with summary in English.

3360 — (1956). Nog eens de tabaksrook-klysteer "van" Gaubius (Once again the fumigator "of G".). *NTG, 100,* IV, 3458–60; *BGG, XXXVI,* 77–9, 2 ill.

3361 — (1957). De oudste tabaksrook-klisteer "machine" (The oldest fumigator (machine). *Het Reddingswezen, 46,* (2), ill.

3362 HERMANS, A. G. J. (1953). De tabaksrookclysteer "van Gaubius" (The fumigator "of G."). *NTG, 97,* II, 1412–3; *BGG, XXXIII,* 47–8.

3363 DOOREN, L. (1935). Geneeskundige Archivalia (Medical archives) *NTG, 79,* IV, 5660–1; *BGG, XV,* 246–7.
– on the fumigator with drowned persons. Letter to the editor.

3364 ELAUT, L. (1960). Een origineel hulpmiddel om de levensgeesten op te wekken (An original expedient for resuscitating). *Het Vlaamse Kruis, 33,* 57–63, ill.
– on the Dutch translation (by Jan Bernard Jacobs, 1734–90) of a small French work by J. J. Gardane, wherein the use of a clyster with tobacco smoke is recommended.

Life-saving service

3365 MYNLIEF, C. J. (1907). Het reddingswezen 1857–1907 (Life-saving service 1857–1907). *NTG, 51,* I, 73–85.

3366 — (1909). Die "Maatschappij tot redding van drenkelingen" in Amsterdam und ihre historische Bedeutung für die Entwicklung des Rettungswesens. *Janus, XIV,* 876–89, 3 ill.

3367 BREEN, J. C. (1909). De Maatschappij tot redding van drenkelingen (The Society for rescuing drowned persons). *Navorscher, LVIII,* 291.

3368 SNUIF, M. G. (1934). Uit de kinderjaren van de Maatschappij tot redding van drenkelingen (From the infancy of the Society for rescuing drowned persons). *NTG, 78,* II, 1560–7; *BGG, XIV,* 70–7.

3368ª RINGOIR, D. J. B. (1974). Maatschappij tot Redding van Drenkelingen (The Society for rescuing drowned persons). *AP.* no 16–17, 63–76, 4 ill.

See also 1987, 4634.5, 5489.

F. Hydrotherapy and mud baths

3369 BURG, C. L. van der (1899). Inrichtingen voor hydrotherapie in Nederland (Institutions for hydrotherapy in the Netherlands). *Alers et al.* 27–9.

3370 — (1899). Inrichtingen volgens Kneipp (Kneipp Institutions). *Alers et al.* 40–1.

3371 VAREKAMP, H. (1911). Over de geschiedenis van het baden (On the history of bathing). *NTG, 55,* II, 1780–92.

– Address delivered to the "Dutch Association for Thalassotherapy", 24 September 1911 at Scheveningen.

3372 HERMANIDES, C. H. (1935). Het begin der thalassotherapie in Nederland (The start of the thalassotherapy in the Netherlands). *NTG, 79,* III, 3737–43; *BGG, XV,* 161–7.

3373 NUYENS, B. W. Th. (1928). Een vliegend blaadje uit de 16de eeuw, als reclame voor de badplaats Pyrmont (A pamphlet from the 16th century, as advertisement for the watering place P.) *NTG, 72,* I, 2190–5; *BGG, VIII,* 113–8.

3374 REYS, J. H. O. (1917). *De Rockanje-Radium-Modder en haar therapie* (The Radium-mud at R. and its therapy). 24 pp., ill. Rora, Rockanje.

– After the discovery by E. H. Bücher (1913) the application of the radio-activity of lake "De Waal", in R. was started in 1916 in "Huys Walesteyn" a bath-house for taking radium-mud baths. On the radio-activity of the mud several notes in *NTG.* cf: *NTG, 62* (1918), I, 371–2 and 641–2.

See also 2491, 2711

G. Physical therapy

3375 BARUCH, J. Z. (1959). Geschiedenis van de Physische Therapie (History of Physical Therapy). *Ned. T. Heilgymn. Massage en Physiotechn.*, *69*, 93–9.

3376 ARNTZENIUS, A. K. W. (1899). De geschiedenis der pneumatische inrichtingen in Nederland (History of the pneumatic institutions in the Netherlands). *Alers et al.*, 86–8.

3377 BAART de la FAILLE, J. M. (1899). Inrichtingen voor mechanotherapie in Nederland (Institutions for mechano-therapy in the Netherlands). *Alers et al.* 130–4.

3378 EIJKMAN, P. H. (1899). Physiatrische inrichtingen (Physiatric institutions). *Alers et al.* 164–7.

3379 ALIMONDA, Nino and Francesco de (1899). *Het menschelijk organisme en zijne genezing door middel van electriciteit. Theorie en Praktijk* (The human organism and its cure by means of electricity. Theory and Practice). XXVIII + 230 pp., 1 pl. Rotterdam. 2nd ed.
– From the Italian original translated into German by the authors and from the German translated into Dutch by D. Kouwenhoven.

See also 1268–9 (Metzger).

H. Bloodtransfusion

3380 [Anonym] (1942). Uit de geschiedenis der bloedtransfusie (From the history of blood-transfusion). *NTG*, *86*, III, 2238; *BGG, XXII*, 126.
– a small note on a blood-transfusion with sheeps blood (from the diary of S. Pepys (1632–1703).

3381 HEFTING, H. (1942). *De Geschiedenis van de Bloedtransfusie* (History of blood-transfusion). Thesis University of Amsterdam (Supervisor: G. van Rijnberk). 85 pp., ill. H. J. Paris, Amsterdam.

3382 MOULIN, D. de (1958). Some remarks on the early history of blood-transfusion. *Arch. chir. néerl.*, *10*, 176–83.

3383 LINDEBOOM, G. A. (1940). Een bloedtransfusie op paus Innocentius VII? (A blood-transfusion to Pope —?). *Org. Chr. Ver. Natuur- en Geneesk.* no 1., 29–38.

3384 — (1954). The Story of a Blood-Transfusion to a Pope. *J. Hist. Med.,* IX, 455–9.

I. Sympathic cure

3385 BAKKER, C. (1924). Over een paar gevallen van sympatische genees-wijze (On some cases of sympathic cure). *NTG, 68,* I, 2622–7; *BGG, IV,* 117–22.

3386 — (1924). Wat is "poudre de sympathie"? (What is — —?) *NTG, 68,* I, 928–34; *BGG, IV,* 51–7.

3387 ZUIDEN, D. S. van (1940). Sympathische genezing (Sympathic cure). *NTG, 84,* II, 2050; *BGG, XX,* 105.

See also 3718–9 (Hypnosis)

J. Remedies

For urinary calculus

3388 HELLINGA, G. (1923). Een geheim geneesmiddel uit de 18de eeuw (A secret remedy from the 18th century). *NTG, 67,* II, 2297–9; *BGG, III,* 355–7.
– a remedy for the stone in the kidneys and in the urinary bladder.

3389 HOEVEN, J. van der (1935). De medicijnen van juffrou Joanna Stephens tegen den steen in de blaas (The remedies of — — for the stone in the bladder). *NTG, 79,* II, 2659–64; *BGG, XV,* 131–6, ill.

3390 ANDEL, M. A. van (1935). Geneesmiddelen tegen den steen der nieren en der blase (Remedies for the stone in the kidneys and in the bladder). *NTG, 79,* III, 3307–12; *BGG, XV,* 152–7.

3391 STIGCHEL, J. W. B. van der (1935). Geneesmiddelen tegen den steen der nieren en der blase (Remedies for the stone in the kidneys and in the bladder). *NTG, 79,* IV, 4658–9; *BGG, XV,* 211–2.
– Letter to the editor.

See also (3412–25) surgery.

For constipation

3392 KEIL, Gundolf (1966). Das "costelic laxatijf" Meister Peters van Dordt. Untersuchungen zum Drogen-Einblattdruck des Spätmittelalters. *SA, 50*, 113–35.

3393 DOOREN, L. (1939). Lotterdranck als laxans in de 14de eeuw ("Lotterdranck" as a laxative in the 14th century). *NTG, 83*, III, 3928; *BGG, XIX*, 210.

For various diseases and ailments

3394 RHIJN Jr, W. P. van (1919–20). Behandeling van blindheid in 1607 (Treatment of blindness in 1607). *Med. Wbl., 26*, 119.

3395 HERMANS, A. G. J. (1952). Behandeling van slangebeet (Treatment of a snake-bite). *NTG, 96*, II, 1546; *BGG, XXXII*, 32.

3396 POSTMA, C. (1960). Middel tegen hoofdzweer, anno 1824 (A remedy for ulcer of the head). *Bull. Pharm, no 21*, febr. p. 3 of the cover.

3397 ZUIDEN, D. S. van (1915). Genezing van waterzucht door een geheim middel omstreeks 1750 (Recovery from dropsy by a secret remedy about 1750). *NTG, 59*, II, 2245–50.

3398 — (1915). Van een oolijken dominee en een oud recept (On a sly clergyman and an old prescription). *NTG, 59*, II, 1450.

See also 4850

K. Treatment of lunatics

3399 RHIJN Jr, W. P. van (1919–20). Een staaltje van behandeling van krankzinnigen in het jaar 1600 (A sample of the treatment of lunatics in the year 1600). *Med. Wbl., 26*, 11.

3400 BREUKINK, H. (1921–22). Overzicht van de opvatting en de behandeling van geesteszieken in oude tijden (Survey of the conception and the treatment of mental patients in former times).
I. *NTG, 65*, I, 3076–94; *BGG, I*, 243–61, 21 ill.
II. *NTG, 65*, II, 2806–14; *BGG, I*, 438–46, 10 ill.
III. *NTG, 66* (1922), II, 1076–91; *BGG, II*, 207–22, 18 ill.

3401 ARIËNS KAPPERS, C. U. (1927). Overzicht van de geschiedenis der therapie van geestes- en zenuwziekten en haar tegenwoordigen stand (Survey of the history of the therapy of mental and nervous diseases and its present position). *NTG*, *71*, II, 1947–62; *BGG*, *VII*, 649–64.

3402 — (1929). L'Histoire de la thérapie des maladies nerveuses et mentales et son état actuel. *Livre mémorial du VIme congrès d'hist. de la Médecine*, 18–23 Juillet 1927 Leyde-Amsterdam. "De Vlijt" Antwerpen.

3403 SPEIJER, N. (1941). De behandeling van geesteszieken met kunstmatig opgewekte epileptische insulten in de 18e eeuw (Treatment of mental patients by means of artificially provoked epileptic fits in the 18th century). *NTG*, *85*, II, 1481–4; *BGG*, *XXI*, 46–9.

See also 4283–4305 (mental nursing).

Chapter ix

Surgery

Just as in other countries, till the eighteenth century most surgeons were barber-surgeons. Only relatively lately has surgery became a separate and independent profession. At the end of the Middle Ages and in the beginning of the new era surgeons were often gathered in the same guild with such craftsmen as shoemakers or carpenters.

In fact, for a long time most surgeons were illiterate men who made their living from their barber-shop wherein minor operations, such as blood-letting, the dressing of ulcers and wounds, and cupping, were performed. Major operations were decided on only after the advice of a doctor. The cutting for the stone in the urinary bladder was performed by specialists. Some towns or provinces had an appointed lithotomist.

Surgery was taught at the universities only theoretically until the end of the eighteenth century. This teaching was destined for the physicians. Teaching of practical surgery was provided by the town councils in consultation with the surgeon's guilds.

These guilds also provided teaching of anatomy for apprentice surgeons and midwives. Such a teacher was called praelector or sometimes professor. There were often prominent men among these teachers, occasionally who became professors in a university. At Harderwijk the professor of medicine also taught anatomy to future surgeons.

In 1555, King Philip II of Spain, then already count of Holland, granted a privilege to the Amsterdam surgeon's guild to perform a dissection of the corpse of an executed criminal. Later public anatomy lessons, organized by university professors or the surgeons' guilds came into use. The magistrates and the older surgeons had their seat in the first rows of the anatomical theatre.

In Leyden public anatomies were performed by the professor of anatomy and took place in the university anatomical theatre. The first public anatomy in Leyden was performed by Peter Paaw, in 1598.

The surgeon's guild was directed by a board (the "Overlieden"). At Leyden the president of the guild was usually a professor of the University.

The guilds had a surgeon's room at their disposal for their meetings. Such surgeon's rooms are still present at Gouda and at Enkhuizen. There the guild had a chest with books on surgery, and a chest with instruments; often some paintings adorned the walls.

The examination of the future surgeons was held before the board of the guild assisted by the lecturer.

For dislocations sometimes the help of the hangman was requested.

A. General

3404 KORTEWEG, J. A. (1907). De ontwikkeling der Heelkunde gedurende de laatste halve eeuw (The development of surgery during the last half century). *NTG*, *51*, I, 28–35.

3405 KOCH, C. F. A. (1924). De heelkunde van 1849 (Surgery in 1849). *NTG*, *68*, II, 21–4; *BGG*, *IV*, 144–7.

3406 DEELMAN, H. T. (ed.) (1925). *Surgery: a hundred years ago*. Extracts from the Diary of Dr C. B. Tilanus, afterwards Professor of Surgery at the University of Amsterdam Edited by —, Professor of Pathology at the University of Groningen. Translated from the Dutch by Joseph Bles. 156 pp., Geoffrey Bles, London.
– reviewed by G. C. Delprat: *NTG*, *70* (1926), I, 43–5; *BGG*, *VI*, 17–9.

3407 LANZ, Otto (1925). *De oorlogswinst der heelkunde* (The wargain of surgery). Amsterdam. 8°.
– Rectorial address.

3408 WITTEBOL, Paul (1971). *Het denken van de heelmeester* (The thinking of the surgeon). 16 pp., 1 ill. F. van Rossen, Amsterdam.
– Inaugural address University of Utrecht, October 4, 1971; with a picture of a master-diploma of a surgeon's pupil.

3409 ROGGE, C. W. L. (1967). Sanguis et Ecclesia. *Ned. T. Med. Stud.*, febr., 7 pp., 3 ill.

3410 MOULIN, D. de (1960). Praehistorische chirurgie (Prehistoric surgery). *GeWiNa*, no. *8*, 8.

3411 FÉRIZ, Hans [1964, 1965]. Schedelchirurgie in het oude Peru (Skull surgery in ancient Peru). *Organorama*, *I*, no 1, 18–21; *ibid.*, *II.* (1965), 18–23, ill.

See also 2216a, 2737–41 (Medieval medicine), 3943, 4583–4632 (Guilds), 5003–4 (Local medicine.)

B. Cutting for the stone

3412 GEYL, A. (1911). Enkele mededeelingen en opmerkingen over de twee oudste methoden van steensnijding (Some information and remarks on the two oldest methods of cutting for the stone). *NTG*, *55*, I, 280–5.

3413 AVALON, J. (1922). Une auto-opération au XVIIe siècle. *Bull. Soc. Fr. Hist. Méd.*, *XVI*, 309–11, ill.
      – on Jan de Dood – see N. Tulp (1652). *Observationes Medicae* book IV, Observ. 31. Amsterdam.

3414 LINT, J. G. de (1928). Comment Jan de Doot, forgeron, s'opéra d'un calcul de la vessie. *Aesculape*, *18*, 50–3, 4 ill;   *See also 3295*

3415 WEIJDE, A. J. van der (1924). Iets over steensnijding en steensnijders (Something on lithotomy and lithotomists). *NTG*, *68*, II, 655–66; *BGG*, *IV*, 191–202, 6 ports.

3416 STAVEREN, C. van (1934). *"Aentekeningen omtrent operatiën van den Steen"* ("Notices on operations for the stone"). Thesis Amsterdam (Supervisor: M. W. Woerdeman). 127 pp., 8 ill. Van Gorcum, Assen.

3416ᵃ FOURNIER, M. (1974). Van de steen gesneden (Cutting for the stone). *Spiegel Historiael*, *9*, 80–7. 12 ill. Also published as *Med. Rijksmuseum Gesch. Natuurwtsch.*, no 146, Leiden.

3417 VEN, A. J. van de (1935). Een steensnijding in 1653 (Stone-cutting in 1653). *NTG*, *79*, III, 3300–7; *BGG*, *XV*, 145–52.

3418 — (1935). Een steensnijding in 1653. II. Medische adviezen. (Stone-cutting in 1653. II. Medical advices). *NTG*, *79*, III, 3750–60; *BGG*, *XV*, 174–84.

3419 MOULIN, D. de (1971). Cutting for the stone in the early Middle Ages. *BHM*, *XLV*, 76–9.

3420 GEIST-HOFMAN, A. M. (1969). In twee reizen (In two stages). *Arts en Auto*, *35*, 1561–3.

3421   WOUDSTRA, D. (1970). Als de roep van een vreemde vogel... (As the
       call of a rare bird...). *Arts en Auto*, *36*, 214.
       – a note on Camper's proposal to perform the operation for the stone in the bladder
       in two stages.

3422   SERMES, J. (1726, 1943). *Aanmerkingen over de twee manieren van steen-*
       snijden van de heren J. J. Rau en J. Douglas (Comments on the two
       methods of Lithotomy of Mr —— and Mr ——). With English trans-
       lation. *Opusc.*, *XVII*, 218–55.

3423   DENYS, J. (1730, 1943). *Op hoe veelerhande wyzen den steen uit de blaaze*
       wordt gehaald (On the various manners in which the stone is removed
       from the bladder). With English translation. *Opusc.*, *XVII*, 256–89.

3424   FRANCKEN, J. H. (1733, 1943). *Over het steensnyden, zo boven als onder*
       het schaambeen (On the Excision of stones, both above and below the
       pubic bone). With English translation. *Opusc.*, *XVII*, 290–345.

3425   ZUIDEN, D. S. van (1916). Een contract tusschen steensnijders (1694).
       (A contract between lithotomists (1694)). *NTG*, *60*, II, 1422.

                    See also 66–70 (J. de Beaulieu), 483, 2778, 3388–91, 5490.

C. Fractures and amputations

3426   GEYL, A. (1911). De ontdekking van de breuk van den hals van het
       dijbeen door den Amsterdamschen chirurgijn Borst in 1680 (The dis-
       covery of the fracture of the neck of the femur by the Amsterdam sur-
       geon — in 1680). *NTG*, *55*, II, 1613–9.

3427   KATE, W. ten (1937). Langdurige invaliditeit tengevolge van onder-
       beenbreuk (Uit de notulen van de Staten van Overijssel) (Lasting in-
       validity caused by a fracture of the leg. (From the minutes of the
       States of O.)) *NTG*, *81*, II, 1965; *BGG*, *XVII*, 95.

3428   KULSDOM, M. E. (1954). Fractuurbehandeling door een chirurgijn in
       het begin der achttiende eeuw (Roelof Roukema te Leeuwarden) (Treat-
       ment of a fracture by a surgeon in the beginning of the 18th century
       (R. R., at L.)). *NTG*, *98*, I, 29–34; *BGG*, *XXXIV*, 3–8.

3429   LOON, L. van (1935). De geschiedenis der hardwordende verbanden
       bij fractuurbehandelingen (History of plaster of Paris bandages in the
       treatment of fractures). *NTG*, *79*, IV, 5163–4; *BGG*, *XV*, 226–7.
       – included in a report of a meeting of the "Genootschap".

3430   — (1935). *Historisch overzicht van de fractuurbehandeling der lange*
        pijpbeenderen (Historical survey of the treatment of the fractures of
        the long bones). Thesis Leiden (Supervisor: W. F. Suermondt). 205 pp.,
        ill. Zomer en Keuning, Wageningen.

3431   JONAS, A. F. (1956). The history of plaster of Paris bandages. *Surg.*
        gynec. Obstet., *102*, 249–52.
        – Also on A. Mathijsen (with port.).
                                                    See also 1239–55 (A. Mathijsen).

3432   WEIJDE, A. J. van der (1923). Het afzetten van een been in 1652 (The
        amputation of a leg in 1652). *NTG*, *67*, II, 905; *BGG*, *III*, 220.
        – Resolution of the Utrecht City Fathers on a proposed amputation of the leg of a
        woman of 29 years.

D. Wounds

3433   EYKEL, R. N. M. (1911). Eenige grepen uit de geschiedenis der wond-
        behandeling (Analecta from the history of the treatment of wounds).
        Med. Rev., *XI*, 311 and 371.

3434   VERAART, B. A. G. (1925). *Over antisepsis als eisch voor aseptisch wond-*
        beloop (On antisepsis as a demand for aseptic woundhealing). Thesis
        University of Amsterdam. H. J. Koersen, Amsterdam.
        – Reviewed by J. G. de Lint: *NTG*, *69* (1925), II, 2110–2; *BGG*, *V*, 279–81; and by
        T. Bijleveld: *NTG*, *69*, II, 1607–8.

3435   CROES, Felix (1940). *Schotwonden in de 16e eeuw* (Shot-wounds in the
        16th century). Thesis University of Amsterdam (Supervisor: G. van
        Rijnberk). 140 pp., facs. Holdert & Co, Amsterdam.
        – Facsimile of the chapter on Shot-wounds in Vigo's *Chirurgia*, Roma 1513.
                                                    See also 2706, 5414

E. Ligature

3436   PRINS, K. (1900). De ligatuur vóór A. Paré (The ligature before —).
        NTG, *35*, II, 797.
        – A protest against this article was published as a pamphlet by H. F. A. Peypers:
        De ligatuur voor A. Paré (Protest tegen de ten name van Dr K. Prins staande kritische-
        historische bijdrage.) This pamphlet was added to the *NTG*; a copy is bound up in
        Janus, 1901 (copy of the U.B. Amsterdam, nr: G.T. 435).

3437   MOULIN, D. de (1955–56). Historical notes on vascular surgery:
I. Vascular suture and lateral ligation in the pre-antiseptic era. *Arch. chir. néerl.*, 7, 218–26.
II. Development of vascular suture in the 19th century, after the introduction of antisepsis. *Ibid.*, 321–30.
III. Development and applications during the first fifteen years of the twentieth century. *Ibid.*, 8, (1956), 31–42.

F. Special operations

3438   PENNING, C. P. J. (1929). Waarneming over een intussusceptio intestinorum, of de inkokering, van den eenen darm in den anderen, door dr. J. van der Hout, te Haarlem (Observation of an intussusceptio intestinorum, or invagination of one gut into another by — —, at H.). *NTG*, 73, I, 2177–80; *BGG*, *IX*, 127–30.

3439   HERMANS, A. G. J. (1963). Aambeien, fistels, bistouri royal (Hemorrhoids, fistulas, bistoury royal). *NTG*, 107, I, 965; *BGG*, *XLIII*, 7.

3440   BEYERMAN, J. J. (1966). Operatie van een doofstom meisje van 17 jaar in 1827 (Operation of a deaf and dumb girl of 17 years in 1827). *Numaga*, 13, 46.
– The operation was performed by Dr E. André of Brussels.

3441   BALEN BLANKEN, G. C. van (1924). Een stuk uit de oude doos van West-Friesland (operatie van hazenmond) (An ancient report from West-Friesland (operation of a hare-lip)). *NTG*, 68, II, 2257; *BGG*, *IV*, 294.
– report; certificate of a successful operation for hare-lip.

3442   HOEVEN, J. van der (1925). Een hazelip-operatie in het begin der 19de eeuw (An operation for a hare-lip in the beginning of the 19th century). *NTG*, 69, I, 44–51; *BGG*, *V*, 16–23, 3 ill.

3443   DOOREN, L. (1936). Een medisch wonderkind in 1648 (A medical child prodigy). *GG*, 14, 1146.
– on the operation of a hare-lip at Schiedam by a 16 year old surgeon: Mr Johannes Schrader.

3444   RHIJN Jr, W. P. van (1918–19). Merkwaardige operatieve geneeswijze in 1627 (Remarkable operative cure in 1627). *Med. Wbl.*, 25, 10.

3445   LINT, J. G. de (1930). De Pruysiaansche messenslikker (The Prussian knife-swallower). *NTG*, 74, II, 3442–7; *BGG*, *X*, 196–201, 3 ill.

3446 — (1930). La taille stomacale en 1635, d'un paysan, qui avait avalé son couteau. *Aesculape, 20,* 223–6, 4 ill.

3447 ROOSEBOOM, M. and J. J. P. ZAAIJER (1942). Van den Prussiaenschen mes-inslicker (On the Prussian knife-swallower). *NTG, 86,* I, 568–70; *BGG, XXII,* 32–4.

3448 ARTELT, Walter (1969). Die Operation des preuszischen Messerschluk-kers und ihre Folgen. *Mediz. Hist. J., 4,* 231–49.

3449 ROEGHOLT, M. N. (1966). Niertransplantatie in 1908 (Transplantation of a kidney in 1908). *NTG, 110,* 1877; cf: *NTG, 110,* 2006.
– On an auto-transplantation of a kidney of a dog into the left groin by Prof. Zaa-yer. The dog died in 1917 at a normal age. From the autopsy a notarial act was made.

3450 KOLFF, W. J. (1965). First clinical experience with the artificial kidney. *Ann. Int. Med., 62,* 608–19.   *See also* 1421.

G. Surgical instruments

3451 LINT, J. G. de (1927). Instrumentafbeelding in handschriften van Guy de Chauliac (Pictures of instruments in the manuscripts of — —). *NTG, 71,* I, 724–49; *BGG, VII,* 117–42, ill.

3452 — (1927). Representations in the Utrecht Manuscript of Guy de Chauliac of Instruments for the Reduction of the Uvula. *Ann. Med. Hist.,* ser. 1, *IX,* 408–10.   *See also* 506

3453 KLAAUW, C. J. van der (1939). Het eertijds verplichte instrumentarium van den heelmeester (The former obligatory cabinet of instruments of the surgeon). *NTG, 83,* III, 3343–53; *BGG, XIX,* 179–89, ill.

3454 DANIËLS, C. E. (1908). Bijdrage tot de geschiedenis van den catheter (Contribution to the history of the catheter). *NTG, 52,* I, 1251.
– Quotation from: J. B. van Helmont. *Dageraad ofte Nieuwe Opkomst der Ge-neeskonst,* Amstelod., 1660).

3455 MOONEN, W. A. (1969). Iets over de geschiedenis van de catheter (Something on the history of the catheter). *NTG, 113,* 1201.
– cf: *NTG, 113* (1969), 1401, letter to the editor by G. A. Lindeboom.

3456 HANEVELD, G. T. (1964). Uit de geschiedenis van het tourniquet (From the history of the "tourniquet"). *Ned. MGT, 17,* 63–5.

3457 EIJDE, A. J. van der (1927). Iets over kunsthanden, instrumenten voor bultenaars en bulten (Something on artificial hands, instruments for hunchbacks and hunches). *NTG*, *71*, II, 661–3; *BGG*, *VII*, 570–2.

3458 SWANE, J. A. W. (1962). Het instrumentarium van den chirurgijn (The cabinet of instruments of the surgeon). *Brabants Heem*, *14*, 153.
– Description of surgical instruments (1680), from a document of the municipal records of Eindhoven.

3459 MÜLLER, I. und E. PÜSCHEL (1973). Die "Sanitätskiste", Cista militaris oder "Feldkast" des Wilhelm Fabry aus Hilden (1560–1634). *Dtsch. Apoth. Ztg.*, *113*, 147–9; 171–6; 339–42., ill.
– on the contents of a field-surgeon's box, as seen by Fabry, during his journey to Holland, in the army of Count Maurice of Nassau (1567–1625).
See also 1560, 2677

H. Surgeons (general)

3460 KNAPPERT, L. (1905). Chirurgijns en barbiers (Surgeons and barbers). *Leids Jbk.*, *II*, 56.

3461 GEYL, A. (1911). Iets over veldscheerders (Something on barber-surgeons). *NTG*, *55*, II, 1235–9.

3462 ENKLAAR, D. Th. (1924). Van zwervende dichters en reizende meesters (From wandering poets and travelling masters]. *Groot Nederland*, I, 612–41.
– Reviewed by M. A. van Andel: *NTG*, 68 (1924), II, 74–6; *BGG*, II, 210–2.

3463 P[UTTO], J. A. (1935). Dokters en chirurgijns te velde in vroegere jaren (Physicians and barber-surgeons in former years). *GG*, *13*, 1077–9.

3464 ROEKEL, G. van (1940). De Chirurgijns: Helpers der menschheid in vroeger tijd (Surgeons: helpers of mankind in former times). *NTG*, *84*, IV, 4298–9; *BGG*, *XX*, 182–3.

3465 ANDEL, M. A. van (1941). *Chirurgijns, Vrije Meesters, Beunhazen en kwakzalvers. De chirurgijnsgilden en de practijk der heelkunde (1400–1800)*. (Surgeons, Free Masters, Bunglers and Quacks. The guilds of surgeons and the practice of surgery). 193 pp., ill. Van Kampen & Zn., Amsterdam. 2nd ed.

3466 ROETEMEIJER, H. J. M. (1973). De chirurgijns te land en ter zee (Surgeons by land and sea). *Unieschakel* (Periodical of the "Nederlandsche Scheepvaart Unie"), no 8, 12–5.

3466ᵃ [   ] (1916). De Heelmeesters in Stad en Lande in de 18e eeuw (The surgeons in "Town and Country" in the 18th century). *Groningen, 1*, 250–2.

3467 BIK, J. G. W. F. (1962). De getekende dagen der chirurgijns (The marked days of the surgeons). *Jbk. Dodonaea, 30*, 544–57.

3468 — (1964). De getekende dagen der chirurgijns (The marked days of the surgeons). *NTG, 108*, I, 21–7; *BGG, XLIV*, 3–10.
– letter to the editor (with the same title) by A. G. J. Hermans: *NTG, 108*, 1496; *BGG, XLIV*, 31.

3469 HELLINGA, G. (1927). De gasthuischirurgijns en de algemeene wijk-vergadering (The hospital surgeons and the general district-meeting). *NTG, 71*, II, 2730–3; *BGG, VII*, 701–4.

3470 — (1926). Een en ander over de positie der 17e en 18e eeuwsche gast-huis-chirurgijns in Amsterdam (Something on the position of the hos-pital surgeons in the 17th and 18th century at A.). *NTG, 70*, II, 30–41; *BGG, VI*, 145–56.

3471 KALFF, S. (1914). Amsterdamsche chirurgijns (Amsterdam surgeons). *Telegraaf*, 25 januari, and foll.

3472 VLES, A. B. van der (1918). De Amsterdamsche Chirurgijns (Heel-meesters) van 1730–1829 (The Amsterdam Surgeons from — —). *Ned. Leeuw, XXXVI*, 276, 320 and 353.

3473 [Anonym] (1961). Middeleeuwse chirurgen (Medieval surgeons). *Periodiek, 16*, 161–5.

3474 ROOSBROECK, R. van (1968). Zestiende eeuwse chirurgen aan het werk (Sixteenth century surgeons at work). *Periodiek, 23*, 64–70; 92–9.

3475 BITTER, H. (1914). Stadsoperateurs en steensnijders in de 17de en 18de eeuw te Haarlem (Town-surgeons en lithotomists at H. in the 17th and 18th century). *NTG, 58*, II, 568–76,

3476 ANDEL, M. A. van (1919). De heelmeester in de 18de eeuw (The sur-geon in the 18th century). *NTG, 63*, II, 1663–9.

3477 HALLEMA, A. (1954). Hoe een halfbakken chirurgijn in 1801 te Breda werd geweerd (How a "half-baked" surgeon was refused admittance at B.). *NTG, 98*, I, 710–2; *BGG, XXXIV*, 31–3.

3478 KULSDOM, M. E. van (1955). De Landschapsmedici en operateurs van Friesland in de 18e eeuw. Lijkschouwen aan het Hof (The regional physicians and surgeons of F. in the 18th century. Coroners at Court). *NTG, 99,* II, 1582–91; *BGG, XXXV,* 42–51.

3479 PUTTO, J. A. (1936). Keur en ordonnantie tot maintien van den chirurgijn en van de vroedvrouw van Esselicherwoude. In dato 26 september 1729. Bij den hove van Holland geaggreëert en geapprobeert den 2en November 1729 (Charter and ordinance maintaining the surgeon and the midwife of E. Dated 26 September 1729. At the Court of Holland aggregated and approbated 2nd November 1729). *GG, 14,* 1128–30.

3480 BOLT, M. (1918). Een vrouwelijke chirurg in de 17e eeuw (A female surgeon from the 17th century). *NTG, 62,* I, 1312–5;

3481 VEEN, S. J. van (1915). Chirurgijn-Vleeschhouwer (1636). (A surgeon-butcher). *Gelre, XVIII,* 84.

3482 DANIËLS, C. E. [1913]. Een dominé-operateur in de zeventiende eeuw en nog iets (A reverend-surgeon in the 17th century and something else). *Populair wetenschappelijk Nederland,* no 7, ill.

3483 ANDEL, M. A. van (1919). Een chirurgijn-kermisreiziger (A surgeon-showman). *NTG, 63,* II, 1016–20.

3484 BAKKER, C. (1922). Drie chirurgijns, tevens schout en gerechtsbode (Three surgeons, at the same time sheriff and usher). *NTG, 66,* I, 1284–7.

3485 PINKHOF, H. (1931). Koninklijke bejegening van een chirurgijn (Royal treatment of a surgeon). *NTG, 75,* I, 1163; *BGG, XI,* 92.

3486 BRAAT, P. (1938). Verbod aan chirurgijn een tapperij te houden (Prohibition to a surgeon to keep a gin-shop). *NTG, 82,* II, 2295; *BGG, XVIII,* 96.

3487 BIJL, W. F. Th. van der (1930). Zondagsrust in vroeger tijden (Sunday-rest in former times). *NTG, 74,* II, 3917; *BGG, X,* 235.
– Resolution of the surgeons of Veere that on Sunday the barbers should not shave.

3488 WEIJDE, A. J. vander (1924). Eed voor een heelmeester in 1811 (Oath for a surgeon in 1811). *NTG, 68,* II, 1258; *BGG, IV,* 221.

3489 HALLEMA, A. (1962). Een gewantrouwde chirurgijn in 1577. De gewonde vader van Mr Johan van Oldenbarnevelt eiste vrije artsenkeuze

(A distrusted surgeon in 1577. The wounded father of — — required free choice of physicians). *NTG, 106,* I, 484–5; *BGG, XLII,* 16–7.

3490　BREEN, J. C. (1920). Een barbierswinkel in 1669 (A barbershop in 1669). *Jbk. Amstelodamum, XVIII,* 1.

3491　EMEIS Jr, M. G. (1972). Pruikebollen – Chirurgijns (Wig-blocks – Surgeons). *Ons Amsterdam, 24,* 66–70, 6 ill.

3492　RADBILL, S. X. (1936). The barber surgeons among the early Dutch and Swedes along the Delaware. *Bull. Inst. Hist. Med., IV,* 718–43, 6 ill.

3493　WITTOP KONING, D. A. (1956). Scheerbekkens met opschriften (Barber's basins with inscriptions). *Bijdr. Med. Rijksmuseum Volkenkunde, 21,* 18–9.

> *See also* 2468, 4633.21, 5440–3 (Museums), further: Medieval medicine, Local medicine, Medical profession.

Hangman

3494　BITTER, H. (1914). De beul te Haarlem als chirurgijn in de 17de en 18de eeuw (The hangman as a surgeon in the 17th and 18th century at H.). *Maandbl. t.d. Kwakz.,* afl. 3, 5 and 9.

3495　FOKKER, A. A. (1870). De scherprechter-ledenverzetter (The executioner-setter of limbs). *NTG, 6,* II, 177.

3496　ZUIDEN, D. S. van (1917). Scherprechter chirurgijn (The executioner surgeon). *NTG, 61,* II, 1436.

3497　ANDEL, M. A. van (1932). De chirurgijn in dienst der justitie (The surgeon in service of the judicature). *NTG, 76,* II, 2224–8; *BGG, XII,* 90–4.

3498　— (1936). Beul en geneeskunde (Hangman and medicine). *NRC,* 1 november.

3499　WITT HUBERTS, F. de [no d.]. *De beul en zijn werk* (The hangman and his work). 222 pp., ill. Andr. Blitz, Amsterdam.

3500　ANDEL, M. A. van (1925). Onze collega de beul (Our colleague the hangman). *NTG, 69,* II, 2100–8; *BGG, V,* 269–77.

Chapter x

Obstetrics and Gynaecology

Obstetrical aid must have been poor in the Middle Ages and still long thereafter. Many women died in childbed who now could have been saved. The midwives mostly came from the lower classes; they were often plain and illiterate women and their help was frequently inexpert.

In the seventeenth century, towns of a certain size – not only Amsterdam but also such towns as Kampen or Gouda – began to make sincere efforts to care for the education of their midwives. A local doctor was appointed to teach midwifery to the apprentices, and also to the qualified midwives. Among the teachers who earnestly tried to enhance the level of midwifery in their towns, we find Fred. Ruysch and Peter Camper. The former made regulations for the education and examination of the midwives.

In the rural districts the practice of midwifery was perhaps worse than in the towns. However from her diary it appears that the excellent midwife Schraders, practising in Friesland, had a very low maternal and infant mortality rate. When delivery did not make progress and lasted one or more days, the midwife would call a surgeon. If he thought that a major operation was indicated, the city-doctor had to give his consent.

An often used obstetrical instrument was the speculum matricis, detested by the surgeon-obstetrician Van Solingen. In the seventeenth century the socalled Roonhuysian secret – a kind of obstetrical spoon – came into use with several doctors. Caesarian section, when performed, resulted mostly in the death of the woman. In the eighteenth century symphysiotomy, first advocated in France, was also performed several times in our country. In the nineteenth century artificial premature labour was introduced.

As rhachitis was endemic in Holland, deformations of the pelvis making a normal delivery very difficult or even impossible were not rare. Hendrik van Deventer was one of the first to study the pathology of the female pelvis, also one of the first to write a useful textbook of obstetrics.

A. General studies, surveys, etc.

3501 TREUB, Hector (1887). *De verdiensten der Nederlanders op het gebied van de bekkenleer* (The merits of the Dutch in the field of the theory of the (female) pelvis). 35 pp. Van Doesburgh, Leiden.
– Inaugural address, delivered on January 26, 1887.

3502 GEYL, A. (1893). Historische kantteekeningen (Historical marginal notes). *NTVerl. Gyn.*, *4*, 253–72.

3503 — (1906, 1907). Bemerkungen um und ueber die *"Geschichte der Geburtshuelfe"* von Dr Heinrich Fasbender (Jena, 1906). *Janus, XI*, 607–16; *ibid, XII* (1907), 34–43; 114–21; 164–73.

3504 DANIËLS, C. E. (1914–15). Bijdrage tot de geschiedenis der verloskunde. I–II. (Contribution to the history of obstetrics). I. *NTG*, *58*, I, 1667–73; II. *NTG*, *59*, (1915), 1006–15.
– a.o. on the Ms of G. F. Mohr. *Die Gebährende Frau*, Frankfurt 1750.

3505 — (1915–16). Beiträge zur Geschichte der Geburtshilfe, I, II, III. *Janus, XX*, 41–6; 489–504; *ibid., XXI* (1916), 167–8.

3506 FREMERY, N. C. de (1793, 1922). *De mutationibus figurae pelvis, praesertim iis, quae ex ossium emollitione oriuntur* – with Dutch translation. *Opusc., IV*, 214–340.

3507 TUSSENBROEK, Catharine van (1911). *De ontwikkeling der aseptische verloskunde in Nederland* (The development of aseptic obstetrics in the Netherlands). 296 pp., 8 ports. Bohn, Haarlem. 8°.

3508 — (1912). Vijf en twintig jaren verloskundig onderwijs (25 years of obstetrical teaching). In: *Feestbundel... Hector Treub* (1912), 1–6. S. C. van Doesburgh, Leiden.

3509 [HIST] [pseudonym] (1915). Uit de geschiedenis der verloskunde (From the history of obstetrics). *Ned. Mndschr. Verl. Vrouwenz. en kindergeneesk., IV*, 204.

3510 BEEKENKAMP, T. (1909). Verloskundige praxis ten plattenlande. Verslag van – en opmerkingen over 1500 partus (Obstetrical practice in the country. Report of – and remarks on 1500 deliveries). *NTVerl. Gyn., 19*, 191–256.

3511 DROGENDIJK, A. C. (1963). Toen moeder worden nog gevaarlijk was; een stukje historie van de verloskundige hulp door de eeuwen heen (When becoming a mother was still dangerous; a little bit of the history of obstetrical care through the centuries). *Spreekuur Thuis, 5*, 396–9 and 482–5.

3512 ZUIDEN, D. S. van (1915). Iets over de verloskunde in het einde der 17de eeuw (Something on obstetrics at the end of the 17th century). *NTG, 59*, I, 1450–3.

3513 RIJKEN, J. (1959). Verloskunde in de 17de en 18de eeuw (Obstetrics in the 17th and 18th century). *GG, 37*, 99–104.

3514 DANIËLS, C. E. (1912). Bijdrage tot de geschiedenis der Verloskunde in Nederland in 1750 (Contribution to the history of obstetrics in the Netherlands in 1750). In: *Feestbundel ... Hector Treub* (1912), 121–8. S. C. van Doesburgh, Leiden.

3515 SCHRIPSEMA, J. (1936). *Bijdrage tot de kennis van de ontwikkeling der verloskunde in de 18e eeuw* (Contribution to the knowledge of the development of obstetrics in the 18th century). Thesis Groningen (Supervisor: J. L. B. Engelhard). 92 pp., ill. Pet, Gasselternijveen.

3516 GEYL, A. (1896). Bijdragen tot de kennis van de geschiedenis der obstetrie en gynaekologie in ons vaderland, vooral met het oog op de verdiensten der Hollanders van de 18e eeuw (Contributions to the knowledge of the history of obstetrics and gynaecology in our country; especially in view of the merits of the Dutch in the 18th century). *NTVerl. Gyn., 7*, 82–167.

3517 TREUB, H. (1899). Verloskunde en gynaecologie in de laatste 50 jaren (Obstetrics and gynaecology in the last 50 years). *NTG, 35*, 123–37.

3518 NIJHOFF, G. C. (1907). Bijdrage tot de geschiedenis der praktische verloskunde en gynaecologie in Nederland 1850–1860 (Contribution to the history of the practical obstetrics and gynaecology in the Netherlands 1850–1860). *NTG, 51*, 36–47.

3519 PIERCE RUCKER, M. (1946). Leaves from a Bibliotheca Obstetrica. *BHM, XIX*, 177–99, 13 ill.
   – with a.o. a title page (dated 1685) from S. Jansen. *Korte en Bondige Verhandeling, van de Voortteeling en 't kinderbaren met den aenkleve vandien*. Amsterdam, Timotheus Hoorn, 1688.

3520 KULSDOM, M. E. (1950). Vagitus uterinus. *NTG, 94*, II, 2617–21; *BGG, XXX*, 26–30.

3521 WICHERS, P. (1901). *Een overzicht der obstetrie in Frankrijk in de zeventiende eeuw* (A survey of obstetrics in France in the 17th century). Thesis Groningen. 8°.

3522 NIJHOFF, G. C. (1924). Het onderwijs in de verloskunde en de uitoefening der verloskunst in Nederland gedurende de laatste 75 jaren (The teaching of obstetrics and the practice of obstetrics in theNetherlands during the last 75 years). *NTG, 68*, II, 25–32; *BGG, IV*, 148–55.

3523 LINT, J. G. de (1916). Oude obstetrisch-anatomische afbeeldingen en de platen van Jenty (Old obstetrical-anatomical pictures and the plates of —). *NTVerl. Gyn., 25*, 107–22, 4 ill. See also 2929.

3524 HUFFMANN, J. W. (1970). The great eighteenth century obstetric atlases and their illustrator [Jan van Riemsdijk (fl. 18th cent.)] *Obstet. Gynec., 35*, 971–6, ill. See also 1444

> See also 484–6, 601–13 (H. v. Deventer), 835–56 (R. de Graaf), 989–92a (J. v. Hoorn), 1731–9 (H. Treub), 2143a, 2756a, 4451–52a, 5013–21 (local medicine).

B. Generation, fertility and infertility

3525 RAVESTEIN, Th. L. W. van (1946). *Studies over de follikelrijping*. Histologisch onderzoek over de follikel van De Graaf in de praeovulatiephase, klinisch onderzoek over de oorlogsamenorrhae te 's-Gravenhage in 1944 en 1945, met een inleiding over de geschiedenis van het onderzoek van de follikel van De Graaf (Studies on the maturation of the follicle ... with an introduction on the history of the examination of the follicle of De Graaf). Thesis University Utrecht (Supervisor: J. Boeke). 127 pp., port. (R. de Graaf). E. Ydo, Leiden.

3526 FIRENZE, P. (1964). Il secolo di Galileo e il problema della generazione. *Physis, VI*, 141–204, 18 ill., ports.

– Summary: The XVII century – the century of Galileo – is the period in which the problem of generation was actually posed. Fabrizi (1600), Aromatari (1625), Harvey (1651), Steno, (1667, 1675), Redi (1668, 1684), Malpighi (1669, 1681), Swammerdam (1669, 1672), (De Graaf (1672), Van Leeuwenhoek (1677, 1685), Borelli (1680).

3527 HERMANS, A. G. J. (1954). Stoornissen in de spermatogenese (Disturbances in spermatogenesis). *NTG, 98, IV*, 3590–1; *BGG, XXXIV*, 103–4.

– on aphrodisiacs and drugs enhancing generation power.

3528 FRANCESCHINI, P. (1965). Luci e ombre nella storia delle trombe di Falloppia. *Physis*, *VII*, 215–50.

– Also on Reinier de Graaf (1641–73).

3529 SCHIERBEEK, A. (1952). Het probleem der bevruchting in de loop der tijden (The problem of fertilization in the course of time). *MKVAW*, *XIV* (12), 1–30.

3530 BOERMA, N. J. A. F. (1942). Merkwaardige vruchtbaarheid (Remarkable fertility). *NTG*, *86*, II, 1098; *BGG*, *XXII*, 71.

3531 BUISSINK, J. D. (1971). Regional differences in marital fertility in the Netherlands in the second half of the nineteenth century. *Popul. Stud.*, *5*, 353–74.

3532 PUTTO, J. A. (1936). Een geval van onvruchtbaarmaking in 1094 (A case of sterilization in 1094). *GG*, *XIV*, 1004.

3533 MEUWISSEN, J. H. J. M. (1965). *Huwelijksonvruchtbaarheid. Een onderzoek in Ghana* (Marital infertility in Ghana). Thesis Nijmegen (Supervisor: L. A. M. Stolte). 130 pp., ill. Dekker & Van de Vegt, Nijmegen-Utrecht.

– with an English summary.

See also 899a, 1122–24, 1132, 1626, 5478.

C. Virginity, conception, anticonception, sexuality

3534 BAUMANN, E. D. (1935). *Medisch-Historische Studiën inhoudende: Over de teekenen van den maagdom. Exotische Psychosen. Psychosen en primitieve Kultuur* (Medical-Historical Studies, containing: On the signs of virginity. Exotic Psychoses. Psychoses and primitive Culture). 58 pp. Misset, Arnhem.

3535 — (1940). *Historische Betrachtungen über das Koïtus-Konzeptions-Problem.* 99 pp. Misset, Arnhem.   See also 1845

3535ᵃ THIERY, M. (1973). De historische ontwikkeling van de intra-uteriene anticonceptie (Historical development of intra-uterine anti-conception). *Sartonia*, no 21, 4–22, ill. See also 1015

See also 2381, 2598, 2630a, 2648.

3536 LINT, J. G. de (1916). "Venus minzieke Gasthuis" ("Venus love-sick hospital"). *NTVerl. Gyn.*, *25*, 273–81, 1 ill.

– on the book with the same title (Amsterdam, 1687, by J.V.E.), dealing with the sexual life of married people.

3537 P[UTTO], J. A. (1936). Sodomie in de vereenigde gewesten (Sodomy in the united regions). *GG, 14,* 88–91.

3538 GEYL, A. (1891). Wat werd in vroegeren tijd onder castratie verstaan? (What was, in former days, understood by castration?) *NTG, 27,* I, 267–8.

3539 PINKHOF, H. (1922). Steinach vegetabilis. *NTG, 66,* I, 71–3; *BGG, II,* 24–6, ill.
   – prescriptions of Tobias Katz (see: *NTG, 58* (1914), I, 2026–8), for deficiencies of the male semen a.s.o.

3540 OUDSCHANS DENTZ, Fred. (1941). Het mysterie van den "kapokdocter" James Barry, die een vrouw was (The mystery of the capokdokter — —, who was a woman). *NTG, 85,* III, 3253–5; *BGG, XXI,* 97–9, ill.

3541 SCHIERBEEK, A. (1942). Over de invoering van de tekens ♂ and ♀ voor mannelijk en vrouwelijk (On the introduction of the signs ♂ and ♀ for male and female). *NTG, 106,* I, 34; *BGG, XLII,* 7.

3542 ZWAN Jr, A. van der (1962). Antiek Hermafroditisme (Ancient Hermaphroditism) *G&W, 60,* 219–35.

3543 BAUMANN, E. D. (1934). Vervrouwelijking bij de primitieven (Feminizing with the Primitives). *Mensch & Maatsch., 10,* 118–33.

D. Pregnancy

3544 VIEYRA, D. (1933). Zwanger of niet zwanger (Pregnant or not pregnant) *NTG, 77,* I, 1033–5; *BGG, XIII,* 79–81.

3545 NIJHOFF, G. C. (1927). De eerste jaren van het onderzoek door middel van het gehoor in de verloskunde (The first years of examination by means of hearing in obstetrics). *NTG, 71,* I, 750–6; *BGG, VII,* 143–9.
   – on the auscultation of the abdomen in pregnancy.

3546 VALCKENIER SURINGAR, J. (1927). Het "verzien" (Versehen, Maternal Impression, Influence de l'imagination maternelle). *NTG, 71,* I, 1179–90; *BGG, VII,* 176–87.

3547 BEINS, J. F. A. (1948). *Misvorming en verbeelding* (Deformation and imagination). Thesis University Groningen (Supervisor: J. J. Th. Vos). Amsterdam.

3548 STURKOP, St. (1909). *Bijdrage tot de kennis der zwangerschapslusten* (Contribution to the knowledge of pregnancy appetites). Thesis University Amsterdam. 120 pp., ill.

3549 HERMANS, A. G. J. (1943). Over wanlusten (On fancies). *NTG, 87*, II, 657; *BGG, XXIII*, 35.

3550 KLEIJ, J. J. van der (1925). Bevalling ten Hove, Anno 1601 (Delivery at Court). *NTG, 69*, I, 638–40; *BGG, V*, 202–4.

3551 BOSCH, N. H. van den (1940). Een verlossing in 1803 (A delivery in 1803). *NTG, 84*, II, 1324–5; *BGG, XX*, 71–2.

3552 DONGEN, J. A. van (1956). Het sluitlaken (The obstetric binder). *NTG, 100*, II, 1806–11.

3553 ZWAN, A. van der (1964). Uit de geschiedenis der geneeskunde. I. De kraamvrouw (From the history of medicine. I. The woman in childbed). *Gezondheidszorg*, 56, sept., 4–10, 3 ill.

3553[a] HOUTZAGER, H. L. (1974). Eclampsie, en de gedachten hierover in de 17e eeuw (Eclampsia and some 17th century thoughts on it). *AP*, no 16–17, 95–8.

3554 ENGELENBURG, W. van (1903). Beschützung der Wöchnerinnen in vorigen Jahrhunderten. *Janus, VIII*, 463.

3555 ROEKEL, G. van (1940). Onschendbaarheid van het kraamhuis (Inviolability of the maternity house). *NTG, 84*, III, 3519; *BGG, XX*, 146.

3556 SALOMONSON, J. G. (1925). *Het stillen van pijn tijdens de normale baring. Een historisch-kritische studie.* (Allaying of pain during normal labour. A historical-critical study). Thesis University Amsterdam (Supervisor: A. H. M. J. van Rooy).

3557 — (1926). Barenspijn en haar bestrijding in den loop der tijden (Labour pains and the fight against it in the course of times). *NTG, 70*, II, 2367–82; *BGG, VI*, 125–40.

3558 EPS, L. W. Statius van (1954). *Over de baringspijn (Anthropologisch en Historisch).* (On labour pains. Anthropological and historical). 235 pp., ill. Thesis University Amsterdam. Amsterdam.

3559 GEYL, A. (1891). Kleine bijdragen tot de historie der keering (Small contributions to the history of version). *NTG, 27*, 465–72.

3560   KLEIWEG de ZWAAN, J. P. (1914). Zoogen door meisjes? (Suckling by girls?). *NTG*, *58*, II, 144–6.

– on breast-feeding by girls, who had never been pregnant; by Minangkabau-Malayans at Talouk (Sumatra) and on analogous cases in other countries. cf: *NTG*, *58*, II, 580 (letter to the editor).

See also 269, 560, 2344, 2432, 2785i, 5008, 5050, 5386

E. Abortion, premature birth, multiple birth

3561   BRENKMAN, C. J. (1912). *Historisch-critische beschouwingen over abortus* (Historical-critical observations on abortion). Thesis University of Amsterdam (Supervisor: H. Treub). 104 pp.

3562   RÖMER, R. (1909). Die Abortiva der Malaien auf der Ostküste Sumatra's. *Janus*, *XIV*, 890–7.

3563   LINT, J. G. de (1918). Historische aanteekeningen over de baring bij diplopagi (Historical notes on the delivery at diplogenesis). *NTVerl. Gyn.*, *26*, 1.

3564   WEIJDE, A. J. van der (1926). Een geval van tweelinggeboorte na den dood der moeder (A case of the birth of twins after the death of the mother). *NTG*, *70*, I, 63–4; *BGG*, *VI*, 178–9.

3565   LINT, J. G. de (1935). Meervoudige geboorten (Multiple births). *NTG*, *79*, IV, 4648–54; *BGG*, *XV*, 201–7.

3566   — (1935). Vijflingen (Quintuplets). *NTG*, *79*, IV, 4272–83; *BGG*, *XV*, 185–96.

3566ª   NIEROP, Leonie van (1959). De keuren tegen "Het ombrengen van jonggeboren kinderen" in de 17de en 18de eeuw (The by-laws against "Dispatching of new-born children" in the 17th and 18th century). *Amstelodamum*, *46*, 154–6. *See also* 2979.

See also 2248, 4633.16.

F. Instruments

3567   GEYL, A. (1907). Het verloskundig instrumentarium (The obstetrical cabinet of instruments). *Cat. Gesch. Tent. Nat. en Geneesk. Leiden*, 148.

3568 NIJHOFF, G. C. (1924). Iets uit de geschiedenis der verlostang (Something on the history of the forceps). *NTG, 68*, I, 49–51; *BGG, IV*, 15–7.

3569 BOERMA, N. J. A. F. (1937). Iets uit de geschiedenis van de verloskundige tang (Something on the history of the forceps). *NTG, 81*, I, 52–60; *BGG, XVII*, 12–20.

3570 — (1924). Een hefboom (Vectis) (A lever (Vectis)). *NTG, 68*, I, 926–7; *BGG, IV*, 49–50, 1 ill.

3571 — (1936). De oudste geschiedenis van de verloskundige tang (The oldest history of the forceps). *NTG, 80*, II, 2622–3; *BGG, XVI*, 95–6, ill.
      – included in a report of a meeting of the "Genootschap".

3572 NIJHOFF, G. C. (1929). Tang, hefboom of speculum matricis? (Forceps, lever or speculum matricis). *NTG, 73*, I, 2622–34; *BGG, IX*, 137–49, 1 ill.

3573 BOERMA, N. J. A. F. (1903). *Catalogus van de geschiedkundige verzameling verloskundige instrumenten der Universiteits-Vrouwenkliniek te Groningen* (Catalogue of the historical collection of the obstetrical instruments of the gynecological clinic of the University of G.). Groningen. 8°.

3574 SCHRIPSEMA, J. (1936). De verloskundige tang, met naschrift van N. J. A. F. Boerma (The forceps, with postscript by —) *NTG, 80*, IV, 5047–8; *BGG, XVI*, 197–8.

3575 ELAUT, L. (1965). Hoofdmomenten in de struktuur van de verlostang en het aandeel dat Nederlanders in de ontwikkeling daarvan hebben gehad (Principal moments in the structure of the forceps and the part that the Dutch have had in its development). *Sci. Hist, 7*, 57–91.

3576 KLAAUW, C. J. van der (1940). Het eertijds verplichte instrumentarium van den vroedmeester (The formerly obligatory cabinet of instruments of the accoucheur). *NTG, 84*, IV, 4814–23; *BGG, XX*, 189–98.

3577 — (1942). Het eertijds verplichte instrumentarium van de vroedvrouw (The formerly obligatory cabinet of instruments of the midwife). *NTG, 86*, IV, 2790–6; *BGG, XXII*, 140–6.

3578 GILS, J. B. F. van (1941). De twee strikken uit de verlostasch (The two ties from the obstetrical bag). *NTG, 85*, II, 1912–3; *BGG, XXI*, 66–7, pl.

Roonhuysian secret

3579 NUYENS, B. W. Th (1905). De geschiedenis van het Roonhuysiaansch geheim (The history of the Roonhuysian secret). *Ned. Spectator*, 364.

3580 GEYL, A. (1905). *De geschiedenis van het Roonhuysiaansch geheim* (History of the Roonhuysian secret). 238 pp., ill. M. Boogaerdt, Rotterdam.

3581 — (1906). Die Geschichte des Roonhuysschen Geheimnisses. Friedrich Ruysch und die soziale und ethische Bedeutung des Geheimnisses. *Janus, XI*, 253–67; 292–313.

3582 — (1910). Een Roonhuysiaan tegenover een sterk vernauwd bekken (A Roonhuysian facing a much narrowed pelvis). *NTG, 54*, II, 1982–3.

3583 ZUIDEN, D. S. van (1915). Iets over het Roonhuysiaansch geheim (Something on the Roonhuysian secret). *NTG, 59*, I, 703–4.

3584 — (1916). Nog meer over het Roonhuysiaansch geheim (Something more on the Roonhuysian secret). *NTG, 60*, I, 939–40.

3585 SCHLICHTING, Th. H. (1956). Het Roonhuysiaans geheim (The Roonhuysian secret). *NTG, 100*, IV, 3448–54; *BGG, XXXVI*, 67–73.

3586 BOERMA, N. J. A. F. and B. W. Th. NUYENS (1926). Het zwaartepunt van het "Roonhuysiaansch geheim" I en II (The crux of the "Roonhuysian secret" I and II). *NTG, 70*, II, 64–5; *BGG, VI*, 179–80.

See also 1481, 1917, 3587a

G. Obstetrical operations

General

3587 NIJHOFF, G. C. (1907). Over den ouderdom van verloskundige operaties (On the age of obstetrical operations). *Med. Revue*, 7, 1–12; 81–91; 229–37.

3587ᵃ [Anonym] (1974). Classic pages in obstetrics and gynecology. H. van Roonhuyze: "Heelkonstige aanmerkingen betreffende de gebreeken der vrouwen". *Amer. J. Obstet. Gynec., 118*, 564.

Caesarean section

3588 ADRIANI, D. H. N. (1890). *Beknopte geschiedenis der keizersnede van 1869–1890* (Condensed history of the caesarean section from 1869–1890). Thesis University Groningen. 166 pp.

3589 POLL, C. N. van der (1905). M. Lanverjat's: sectio caesarea per vaginam (M.L.'s caesarean section per vaginam). *Med. Wbl.*, 18 febr..

– M. Lanverjat. *Nouvelle méthode de pratiquer l'opération césarienne et parallèle de cette opération et de la section de la symphyse des os pubis.* Paris, 1788. German translation 1790.

3590 KULSDOM, M. E. (1962). Uit de geschiedenis der keizersnede (From the history of the caesarean section). *NTG, 106,* I, 1194–1201; *BGG, XLII,* 21–8.

3591 HERMANS, A. G. J. (1963). Uit de geschiedenis van de keizersnede (From the history of the caesarean section). *NTG, 107,* I, 964–5; *BGG, XLIII,* 6–7.

3592 LINT, J. G. de (1921). Le flamand Pierre Joseph van Baveghem et l'Opération Césarienne. *Lib. mém. du 1er Congrès de l'hist. de l'art de guérin.* Anvers.

3593 SCHOO, H. J. M. (1912). Stier's wreedheid (Cruelty of a bull). In: *Feestbundel ... Hector Treub,* 499–528, S. C. van Doesburgh, Leiden.

See also 5281

3594 BRAAK, H. E. G. ter (1934). Een keizersnede in het jaar 1861 (A caesarean section in the year 1861). *NTG, 78,* III, 3975; *BGG, XIV,* 186.

3595 VIEYRA, D. (1936). Beschrijving eener postmortale keizersnede door een pastoor (Description of a post-mortal caesarean section by a priest). *NTG, 80* III, 3174; *BGG, XVI,* 118.

3596 NIJHOFF, G. C. (1921). Histoire d'un foetus, conçu dans la Trompe droite de Faloppe, ou il séjourna pendant quinze Mois et treize Jours, et dont il fut tiré par l'Opération Césarienne, ou proprement dit par l'incision du ventre qui n'est encore jamais arrivé de la sorte, faite par Rudolph Frédéric Hoffmann, Chirurgien Aide-Major, du 33 Rég. d'Inf. Légère, en Garnison à Charlemont, *Janus, XXV,* 341.

– R. F. Hoffmann (1769–1844) performed this operation in 1813. In 1824 he settled as a medical practitioner at Vugt (near Bois-le-Duc).

See also 5184

Symphysiotomy

3597 FEYFER, F. M. G. de (1914). Zur Geschichte des Schamfugenschnittes in Holland (bis 1840). *Janus, XIX*, 312–27; 341–79.

3598 — (1912). Een en ander uit de geschiedenis der schaambeensnede in Nederland (Something on the history of symphysiotomy in the Netherlands). *Med. Revue, XII*, 181, 295, 379, 501.

3599 LINDEBOOM, G. A. (1972). De symfysiotomie in Nederland (The symphysiotomy in the Netherlands). *NTG, 116*, 759–60.
– letter to the editor (short survey).

3600 ENDTZ, L. J. (1972). Symfysiotomie in Nederland (Symphysiotomy in the Netherlands). *NTG, 116*, 759.
– letter to the editor (symphysiotomy by J. C. Damen).

3601 BONN, A. (1776, 1934). *Over het maaksel van de beweeglijke loswording van beenvereenigingen van het bekken, enz.* (On bone joints of the pelvis becoming mobile and loose). *Opusc., XII*, 33–64.

3602 HASSELMAN, D. (1798, 1934). *Berigt aangaande ene gelukkige verlossing, door middel van de doorsnijding der schaambeenderen* (Report concerning a successful delivery, by means of symphysiotomy). *Opusc., XII*, 187–90.

3603 MUNSTER, J. van (1804, 1934). *Een zestal verloskundige operatiën, zo omtrent het verlossen van vrouwen door de sectio symphysis ossi pubis ...* (Six obstetrical operations and observations, concerning the delivery of women by symphysiotomy). *Opusc., XII*, 191–218.

3604 GROSHANS, G. R. F. (1778, 1934). *Waarneeming eener operatie der doorsnede van de kraakbeenige vereeniging der schaambeenderen* (Observation of an operation of symphysiotomy). *Opusc., XII*, 65–70.

3605 MICHELL, J. P. (1781, 1934). *Onderzoek aangaande het nut van de kraakbeen-sneede in moeijelijke verlossingen* (Examination concerning the usefulness of symphysiotomy in difficult deliveries). *Nadere opheldeeringen over de historie en het nut van de schaambeensnede in moeielijke verlossingen* (Further explanation on the history and the usefulness of symphysiotomy) *Opusc., XII*, 71–113; 115–48.

3606 BLEULAND, C. (1792, 1934). *Verhaal van de doorsnijding van de kraakbeenige vereeniging der schaamtebeenderen* (Account of symphysiotomy). *Opusc., XII*, 175–86.

3607 WIJ, G. J. van (1805, 1934). *De uitvoerlijkheid en nuttigheid der schaam-beendoorsnijding* (The practicability and usefulness of symphysiotomy). *Opusc.*, *XII*, 219–44.

3608 SALOMON, G. (1813, 1934). *Verhandeling over de nuttigheid der schaam-beensnede* (Treatise on the usefulness of symphysiotomy). *Opusc.*, *XII*, 245–354.

3609 HALDER, A. (1815, 1934). *Waarneming eener verlossing door middel der sectio synchrondosis ossium pubis* (Observation of a delivery by means of the — — —). *Opusc.*, *XII*, 355–62.

3610 BAL, J. (1822, 1934). *Waarneming wegens eene verlossing door de schaambeensnede* (Observation of a delivery by symphysiotomy) *Opusc.*, *XII*, 363–70.

3611 WAGENINGE, P. J. van (1831, 1934). *Schaambeensnede* (Symphysio-tomy). *Opusc.*, *XII*, 371–83.

See also 487

H. Customs

3612 POLL, C. N. van de (1902–03). Het een en ander omtrent bijgeloof, volksgewoonten enz. bij zwangerschap, baring en in het kraambed (Something on superstition, popular customs, etc. at pregnancy, delivery and in childbed). *T. prakt. Verl.*, *6*, 161–5; 186–90; 193–8; 209–14; 225–7; 245–8; 257–62; 273–9.

3613 SWAAK, A. J. (1964). Gebruiken en gewoonten rondom huwelijk en zwangerschap (Usages and customs relative to marriage and preg-nancy). *Gezondheidszorg*, *56*, no 5, 11–5, ill; no 6, 11–5, ill.
– in Old Brabant.

3614 GEYL, A. (1903). Das "Kraamkloppertje" (The "Childbed-knocker"). *Janus*, *VIII*, 585–6.

3615 KLEIWEG de ZWAAN, J. P. (1915–16). De couvade – het mannenkraam-bed (The man-childbed). *Med. Wbl.*, *22*, 197 and 213.

3616 JOSSELIN de JONG, J. P. B. (1922). De couvade (The man-childbed). *MKNAW*, afd. Letterk., *54*, serie B, no 4.

3617 MELCHIOR, A. (1962). *Van bruidegom tot kraamheer* (From bride-groom to father of the child). 208 pp. Gottmer, Haarlem.

3618   LUNSINGH SCHEURLEER, Th. H. (1971/72). Enkele oude Nederlandse kraamgebruiken (Some old Dutch childbed customs). *Antiek, 6,* 297–332, 41 ill.

3618ª   LEVELT, H. (1920). Het wegen van kinderen in de Roomsche Kerk (Weighing of children in the Roman-catholic Church). *Taxandria, 27,* no 9–10, 249 ff.

– A devotional custom. Reviewed by A. J. M. Lamers: *NTG, 65* (1921), I, 671–2; *BGG, I,* 85–6.

See also 5079

I. Midwives and Accoucheurs

General

3619   BERG, H. van den (1901). Eenige historische bizonderheden over de vroedvrouwen van vroegeren tijd (Some historical details on midwives in former times). *Ned. T. prakt. Verl., 4,* 20–2.

3620   GEYL, A. (1911–12). Beschouwingen en mededeelingen over vroedvrouwen uit de 15de tot en met de 18de eeuw (Observations and informations on midwives from the 15th up to and including the 18th century). *Med. Wbl., XVIII,* 227, 266, 279, 318, 341, 368, 377, 401, 414 and 425.

– also as a reprint, 131 pp.

3621   REEUWIJK, Adr. Joh. van (1941). *Vroedkunde en vroedvrouwen in de Nederlanden in de 17e en 18e eeuw* (Obstetrics and midwives in the Netherlands in the 17th and 18th century). Thesis University Amsterdam (Supervisor: M. A. van Bouwdijk Bastiaanse). 76 pp. ill. Amsterdam. 8°.

3622   SNAPPER, I. (1963). Midwifery, past and present. *Bull. N. Y. Acad. Med., 39,* 503–32.

3623   GILS, J. B. F. van (1938). De Kapiteinse (The wife of the captain). *NTG, 82,* III, 3871;, *BGG, XVIII,* 144–5.

– Formerly in some parts of the Netherlands a midwife was called "Kapiteinse" (Wife of a captain). Explanation.

3624   — (1942). Beroemde vroedvrouwen (Famous midwives). *NTG, 86,* I, 573–9; *BGG, XXII,* 37–43;

– letter to the editor (under same title) by M. J. W. Stassen: *NTG, 86,* IV, 2483; *BGG, XXII,* 137.

3625 GROSHEIDE, F. W. and A. EIKELENBOOM (1912). De geschiedenis van Anna Doornbosch, de Oranjegezinde vroedvrouw (The history of — —, the Orangist midwife). *Navorscher, LXI*, 1 and 170.

3626 GEYL, A. (1896–7). Catharina Gertruyt Schraders. Investigatrice du caractère anatomique de la Placenta praevia. *Janus, I*, 537–40.

3627 NUYENS, B. W. Th. (1926). Het dagboek van vrouw Schraders. Een bijdrage tot de geschiedenis der verloskunde in de 17e en 18e eeuw (The diary of Mrs. —; A contribution to the history of obstetrics in the 17th and 18th century). *NTG, 70*, II, 1790–1801; *BGG, VI*, 93–104.

3628 DROGENDIJK, A. C. (1935). Het dagboek van Vrouw Waltman, vroedvrouw in de 19de eeuw te Dordrecht (The diary of Mrs. —, midwife at D. in the 19th century). *NTG, 79*, IV, 5163; *BGG, XV*, 226.
– included in a report of a meeting of the "Genootschap".

3629 — (1936). Het dagboek van vrouw Waltman, vroedvrouw in de 19de eeuw te Dordrecht (The diary of Mrs. —, midwife at D. in the 19th century). *NTG, 80*, I, 981–8; *BGG, XVI*, 33–40.

See also 3479, 4633.15, 5010, 5012, 5032.

Professional Training

3630 GEYL, A. (1897). Over de opleiding en maatschappelijke positie der vroedvrouwen in de 17ᵉ en 18ᵉ eeuw (On the training and social position of the midwives in the 17th and 18th century). *Med. Wbl.*, reprint 87 pp. 8°.
– reviewed by C. E. Daniëls: *Janus, II* (1897–8), 292–4.

3631 — (1912). Rond de examens der mannelijke verloskundigen te Utrecht (About the examinations of the accoucheurs at U.). In: *Feestbundel ... Hector Treub*, 149–70. S. C. van Doesburgh, Leiden.

3632 SNOO, K. de (1914). *De ontwikkeling van het vroedvrouwenonderwijs te Rotterdam* (The development of the teaching of midwives at R.). 64 pp., ill. Rotterdam.

3633 PUTTO, J. A. (1938). Het ambt van "Kraamverzorgster" (vroedvrouw) in Leiden voor 350 jaren (The office of "obstetric nurse" (midwife) at L. 350 years ago). *GG, 16*, 286–7.

3634 — (1964). 't Ampt van de Kraem-versorghsters ruim 300 jaar geleden (The office of the obstetric nurse before 300 years). *GG, 42*, 44.
– a short note quoted from *Keuren der Stadt Leyden*, Hackes en Leffen, Leiden 1653, 121–3.

3635 WIJNDELTS, J. W. (1918). Een vroedvrouwen-eed in de 16de eeuw (A midwifes' oath in the 16th century). *NTG*, *62*, I, 1260.

See also 4450–52a

Local

3636 POST, C. R. (1956). De Amsterdamse vroedvrouw uit de 18ᵉ eeuw (The Amsterdam midwife from the 18th century). *NTG*, *100*, I, 167–74; *BGG*, *XXXVI*, 1–8, 2 ill.

3637 BITTER, H. (1915). Vroedvrouwen en leerling-vroedvrouwen te Haarlem in de 17de en 18de eeuw (Midwives and aspirant midwives at H. in the 17th and 18th century). *NTG*, *59*, II, 2197–2207.

3638 BERGER, J. A. (1931). Ordonnantie en reglement op de vroedvrouwen der stad Middelburg (Ordinances and regulations for midwives of M). *NTG*, *75*, I, 77–81; *BGG*, *XI*, 13–8.

3639 BIJL, W. F. Th. van der (1929). Sprokkels uit oude archivalia – Smertbrief van Willem Humanssone (Gleanings from old files – Smart-letter of — —). *NTG*, *73*, I, 1132; *BGG*, *IX*, 92.
   – two notes, the first concerns the search for a midwife by the Zealand town Veere, whereas the second is a surgeon's certificate on a wound.

3640 THEUNISZ, Joh. (1940). Voordracht, benoeming, instructie en eed voor een stadsvroedvrouw te Zwartsluis in 1795 (Nomination, appointment, instruction and oath for a city-midwife at Z. in 1795). *NTG*, *84*, II, 1721–2; *BGG*, *XX*, 88–9.

3641 WATTEL, J. (1963). De karpelsvroedvrouwen van het Hoogeveen in de 18de eeuw (The regional midwives of H. in the 18th century). *Nwe. Drentse Volksalmanak*, *81*, 77–99.

3642 HALLEMA, A. (1955). Vroedvrouwen in stad en dorp in het westen van Noord-Brabant. Hoe stads- en dorpsbesturen zorgden voor verloskundige hulp gedurende de 16ᵉ tot de 18ᵉ eeuw (Midwives in town and village in the West of Northern Brabant. How the local governments of towns and villages did provide for obstetrical care during the 16th till the 18th century). *NTG*, *99*, III, 2660–7; *BGG*, *XXXV*, 85–92.

3643 HOEVEN, J. van der (1937). Medisch tuchtrecht; onderzoek naar de leiding van een bevalling door een vroedvrouw; bestraffing (Medical disciplinary code; investigation of the management of a delivery by a midwife; punishment). *NTG*, *81*, III, 4268–73; *BGG*, *XVII*, 160–5.

Chapter XI

Ophthalmology

In earlier times eye-operations were performed by journey-men or special surgeons, who where familiar with the technique of couching for cataract. Spectacles were already used by some persons in the fourteenth century.

In the nineteenth century the famous Dutch physiologist Donders became one of the founders of modern ophthalmology; he was one of the first to use the ophthalmoscope.

A. General

3644 ZEEMAN, W. P. C. (1957). Zur Geschichte der Augenheilkunde in den Niederlanden. *Ophthalmologia, 134*, 100–19.

3645 [   ] (1942). *Hoofdfiguren uit de geschiedenis der optica* (Leading figures from the history of optics). Publ. by the "Genootschap voor Geschiedenis der Geneeskunde, etc.".
– addresses delivered at the Symposium on this subject (May 31, 1942), by Crommelin, Kramers, Colenbrander and Van Heel).

3646 HOEVE, J. van der (1924). De ontwikkeling der oogheelkunde gedurende het tijdperk 1849–1924 (The development of ophthalmology during the period — —). *NTG, 68*, II, 33–42; *BGG, IV*, 156–65.

3647 HOORN, Willem van (1972). *Ancient and modern theories of visual perception.* Thesis University Leiden (Supervisor: A. M. J. Chorus). 281 pp., ill. University Press Amsterdam.

3648 ROCHAT, G. F. (1924). Het oudste Duitse leerboek der oogheelkunde (The oldest German textbook of ophthalmology). *NTG, 68*, I, 47–8; *BGG, IV*, 13–4.
– by Bartisch, 1583.

3649 STRAUB, M. (1908). Eine bisher nicht veröffentlichte Schrift von Christiaan Huygens über das Auge und das Sehen. *Klin. Monatsbl. Augenheilk.*, *46*, 295.

3650 VOS, T. A. (1973). Geschiedkundige bijdragen. VI. Beschouwingen over het zien (Historical contributions. VI. Observations on vision). *Arts en Wereld*, *6*, nr 10, 25–40, 8 ill.

3651 DOESSCHATE, G. ten (1938). Uit de geschiedenis der oudste stadia van de perspectiefleer (From the history of the oldest stages of the doctrine of perspective). *NTG, 82*, III, 3341–53; 3856–67; *BGG, XVIII*, 116–40.

3652 — (1940). *De derde Commentaar van Lorenzo Ghiberti in verband met de middeleeuwse optiek* (The third Commentary of — — in view of medieval optics). Thesis University of Utrecht. Hoorne N. V. Utrecht.

3653 — (1946). Het zien (Vision). 48 pp. *Problemen der Natuurwetenschap in hun historische ontwikkeling*, deel I. Het Spectrum Utrecht-Brussel.

3654 — (1947). De schijnbare kromming van rechte lijnen (The apparent curve of right lines). *NTG, 91*, IV, 2841–52; *BGG, XXVII*, 54–65.

3655 — (1957). De idee van de wiskundige eenvoud in de middeleeuwse optiek (The idea of mathematical simplicity in medieval optics). *NTG, 101*, II, 1655–9; *BGG, XXXVII*, 22–6, 1 ill.

3656 HALBERTSMA, K. T. A. (1949). *A history of the theory of colours.* 267 pp., Swets & Zeitlinger, Amsterdam.

3657 BOUMAN, M. A. (1961). Developments in the physiology of color vision since Einthoven. *NTG, 105*, II, 1540–4.
   – address delivered at the Einthoven-Symposium June 25th, 1960.
         See also 57–8, 262–4 (Boerhaave), 488–91 (P. Camper), 655–94 (F. C. Donders), 831, 998, 1397, 1525, 1892–4 (H. Weve), 2490, 2600, 2621–2, 2715, 4673–4, 4724, 5185, 5399

B. Refraction

3658 RISNERUS, Frid. (1918). *Opticum cum annotationibus Will. Snelli ed J. A. Vollgraff.*, Pars I. Gandavi. 8°.

3659 WAARD, C. de (1935). Le manuscrit perdu de Snellius sur la réfraction. *Janus, XXXIX*, 51–73, 7 ill.

3660 VOLLGRAFF, J. A. (1936). Snellius' notes on the reflection and refraction of rays. *Osiris, I*, 718–25. *See also* 693

C. Optotypes

3661 VRIEND–VERMEER, W. (1963). Honderd jaar optotypen van Snellen (Hundred years optotypes of —). *NTG, 107*, 1, 963–4; *BGG, XLIII*, 5–6, 1 ill.
– Herman Snellen (1834–1908). 1877 professor of ophthalmology at Utrecht.

3662 TANNENBAUM, S. (1971). The eye chart and Dr Snellen. *J. Amer. optom. Ass., 42*, jan., 89–90.

3663 FARRELL, G. (1963). Hermann Snellen and the letter E. *Ophthal. Opt., 3*, 119–21, port. *See also* 4459, 5399

3664 PERGENS, Ed. (1917). Optotypes. *Janus, XXII*, 406–8. [French].
– Pergens, a contributor to *Janus*, died on April 11, 1917, was a specialist on optotypes, and in his memory the introduction was reprinted which he wrote to the *Catalogue* of the exhibition organized on the occasion of the Dutch Congress of Natural Sciences and Medicine at Leyden (1907). See: E. C. van Leersum *Janus, XII* (1907), 319.

D. Eye-diseases

3665 MENDELS, J. I. H. (1937). Waarneming van een oogziekte in een familie op het eiland Wieringen 1795 (Observation of an eye-disease in a family on the island W.). *NTG, 81*, IV, 5837–8; *BGG, XVII*, 223–4.

3666 SCHOUTE, G. J. (1914). Een oud boekje (A little old book). *NTG, 59*, II, 706–8.

– Translation of Guillemeau. *Des maladies de l'oeil qui sont un nombre de cent treize auxquelles il est subject*, Paris 1585. Translated by Carolus Battus (Carel Baten), edited in 1597 by Abraham Caen at Dordrecht.

3667 ROEKEL, G. van (1939). Een oogheelkundige bij de gratie van den magistraat. (An ophthalmologist by the grace of the magistrate). *NTG, 83*, IV, 4867; *BGG, XIX*, 231.
– On Albertje Hesselink at Groningen, who cured in special cases some eye-diseases (1772)..
See also 1035, 4307

Strabismus

3668 HALBERTSMA, K. T. A. (1939). Honderd jaren scheelzienoperatie (1839–1939). (A century of operations for strabismus). *NTG, 83,* IV, 5274–81; *BGG, XIX,* 235–42.

3669 ESSO Bzn, l. van (1937). De eerste operatie van strabismus in Nederland (The first operation for strabismus in the Netherlands). *NTG, 81,* I, 603–4; *BGG, XVII,* 37–8;

Cataract, Glaucoma and Trachoma

3670 JUDA, M. [1897]. Het aandeel, dat de Nederlanders hebben gehad in de ontwikkeling der methode van de staaroperatie (The part of the Dutch in the development of the method of the operation for cataract). *Ned. Oogheelk. Bijdr., I.*
– Reviewed by E. Pergens: *Janus, III* (1898), 286.

3671 HALBERTSMA, K. T. A. (1937). Uit de ontwikkelingsgeschiedenis van de staaroperatie (From the history of the development of the operation for cataract). *NTG, 81,* I, 591–601; *BGG, XVII,* 25–35.

3672 ROEKEL, G. van (1939). Een staar-operatie in 1599 (An operation for cataract in 1599). *NTG, 83,* IV, 4867–8; *BGG, XIX,* 231–2.

3673 VOS, T. A. (1971).|Cataractchirurgie (Cataract surgery). *Arts en Wereld, 4,* no 2, 9–20; no 3, 8–13; no 5, 11–8; no 6, 7–15; no 7, 9–14.

3674 ANDEL, M. A. van (1924). Oogmeesters en staarstekers (Eye-masters and cataract-couchers). *NRC,* 25 maart.   See also 403

3675 VOS, T. A. (1947). Glaucoomgeschiedenis (History of glaucoma). *NTG, 91,* IV, 2945–6.

3676 — (1948). Over het woord glaucoom (On the word: glaucoma). *Hermèneus, 20,* 152–6.

3677 DOESSCHATE, G. ten (1936). Uit de geschiedenis van de kennis van het trachoom (From the history of the knowledge of trachoma). *MGT, 25,* 22–33; 45–52.

3678 VOS, T. A. (1973). Geschiedkundige bijdragen. IV. Blindheid, een symptoom (! of ?) (Historical contributions. IV. Blindness, a symptom (! or ?)). *Arts en Wereld, 6,* no 6, 43–54, 11 ill.

3679 JACOBS, A. A. (1968). *De lectuurvoorziening van blinden en slechtzienden in Nederland. Beschouwing bij gelegenheid van het vijftigjarig bestaan van Blindenbibliotheek Le Sage Ten Broek, Nijmegen* (Provision with reading-matter for blind persons and persons with poor eyesight in the Netherlands. Reflection on the occasion of the 50th anniversary of the library for the blind — —). 22 pp., Nijmegen.

E. Spectacles

3680 FEYFER, F. M. G. de (1921). Het eerste meniscus-glas (The first meniscus-glass). *NTG, 65*, II, 705–10; *BGG, I*, 317–22.

3681 WEVE, H. (1929). Beitrag zur Geschichte der Hohlgläser. *Janus, XXXIII*, 23–40, 11 ill.

3682 MODDERMAN, R. S. Tjaden (1904). De oudste brillen (The oldest spectacles). *Alb. Nat.*, 350.

3683 WEVE, H. J. M. (1929). Zur Geschichte der Brille in den Niederlanden. *VIme Congrès Int. d'Hist. Méd. Leyde-Amsterdam 1927*, 127–32, 6 ill. Anvers.

3684 PERGENS, Ed. (1908). Die Geschichte der stenopäischen Brille In: *Zwanzig Abhandlungen zur Geschichte der Medizin. Festschrift Hermann Baas in Worms zum 70. Geburtstage gewidmet*, 131–50 Hamburg-Leipzig.
– Reviewed by M. Quix: *Janus, XIV* (1909), 140–1.

3685 RIJKENS, R. G. (1918). Uit de geschiedenis van het optisch glas (From the history of optical glass). *Natuur, 38*, 112–7, 2 ill., port. (of E. Abbe).

3686 SCHEVENSTEEN, A. van (1923). Bijdrage tot de bibliographie der brillen (Contribution to the bibliography of spectacles). *NTG, 67*, II, 1661–3; *BGG, III*, 315–7.

3687 VOS, T. A. (1947). De Bril en de Oudheid (Spectacles and Antiquity). *Hermèneus, 18*, 138–40.

3688 — (1973). Geschiedkundige bijdragen. VIII. Optische hulpmiddelen (Historical contributions. VIII. Optical expedients). *Arts en Wereld, 6*, no 12, 20–36, 16 ill.

3689 HAAS, E. H. (1958). De uitvinding van de bril (The invention of spectacles). *NTG, 102*, II, 2171; *BGG, XXXVIII*, 32.

3690 HELLINGA, G. (1929). [A fill-up]. *NTG*, *73*, I, 2186; *BGG*, *IX*, 136.
      – On "Kittelsteene Brillen" (On spectacles of ground pebble). From the *Amsterdam Courant*.

3691 WEVE, H. J. M. (1927). Korte mededeeling betreffende een verdichte brillengeschiedenis (Short information concerning an invented history of spectacles). *NTG*, *71*, I, 3140–2; *BGG*, *VII*, 405–7.

3692 WEVE, H. J. M. (1928). Wie alt sind die Lentriculargläser? *Janus*, *XXXII*, 227–30.

See also 1730a, 5286–7.

F. Lenses

3693 CROMMELIN, C. A. (1929). *Het lenzenslijpen in de 17de eeuw* (Grinding of lenses in the 17th century). 45 pp. 29 ill. H. J. Paris, Amsterdam.
      – also on the lenses of Van Leeuwenhoek, who also used small globes of melted glass. Reviewed by F. M. G. de Feyfer: *NTG*, *75* (1931), I, 1152–3; *BGG*, *XI*, 81–2.

G. Ophthalmological instruments

3694 WEIJDE, A. J. van der (1923). De oogspiegel (The ophthalmoscope). *NTG*, *67*, II, 2289–91; *BGG*, *III*, 347–9.

3695 HALBERTSMA, K. T. A. (1951). Het eeuwfeest van de oogspiegel (1851–1951). The centenary of the ophthalmoscope). *NTG*, *95*, IV, 3413–20; *BGG*, *XXXI*, 58–65, 3 ill., port.

3696 SNELLEN Sr, H. (1902). De oogspiegel sedert een halve eeuw (The ophthalmoscope since half a century). *NTG*, *38* (2de reeks), I, 306–12.

3697 DOESSCHATE, G. ten (1952). Een eeuw ophthalmoscopie (A century of ophthalmoscopy). *NTG*, *96*, II, 819–25; *BGG*, *XXXII*, 4–10.

3698 SETERS, H. W. van (1946). Anatomische oogmodellen uit de 17de en 18de eeuw (Anatomical eye models from the 17th and 18th century). *NTG*, *90*, IV, 1320–30; *BGG*, *XXVI*, 39–49.

3699 PERGENS, Ed. (1909). Zur Geschichte der anatomischen Augenmodelle und der schematischen Augen zu optischen Berechnungen. *Janus*, *XIV*, 435–56, 19 ill.

See also 1913, 2953, 3451–2.

Chapter XII

Various other Disciplines

In this chapter the literature is collected that refers to specialisms that have mainly developed as a separate discipline in the last hundred years. Of course, the roots of some of these disciplines are to be found in earlier times.

A. Neurology and Psychiatry

3700 VALKENBURG, C. T. van (1958). De ontplooiing van de neurologie sinds 1900 (The development of neurology since 1900). *NTG, 102*, I, 1155–8; *BGG, XXXVIII*, 7–10.

3701 SCHULTE, B. P. M. (1966). Een mechanistische ziekteleer van het zenuwstelsel in de eerste helft van de 18de eeuw (A mechanistic doctrine of the pathology of the nervous system in the first half of the 18th century). *MKVAW, XXVIII*, no 7, 3–16. 5 ill., 1 port.

3702 LENSHOEK, C. H. (1968). *Enkele historische beschouwingen over de neurochirurgie in Nederland* (Some historical reflections on neuro-surgery in the Netherlands). 18 pp., Wolters-Noordhoff Groningen. – Valedictory address. *See also* 85.

3703 ROTHSCHUH, K. E. (ed.) (1964). *Von Boerhaave bis Berger. Die Entwicklung der kontinentalen Physiologie im 18. und 19. Jahrhundert mit besonderer Berücksichtigung der Neurophysiologie*. Vorträge des Internationalen Symposions zu Münster/Westf. 18–20. September 1962. Medizin in Geschichte und Kultur, Bd 5, VIII + 254 pp., ill. G. Fischer, Stuttgart.

3704 EVRARD, A. K. (1955). *Korte inleiding tot de geschiedenis der psychiatrie* (Short introduction to the history of psychiatry). Wereldbibliotheek, Amsterdam.

3705 BEEK, H. H. (1969). *Waanzin in de Middeleeuwen. Beeld van de gestoor-de en bemoeienis met de zieke* (Madness in the Middle Ages. Picture of the mentally deranged and the care of the sick). 327 pp., ill., 16 col. pl. G. F. Callenbach, Nijkerk – De Toorts, Haarlem.
 – The author (1921–69) wrote this splendidly illustrated book as a thesis, but died about a month before his graduation. Foreword written by J. Bastiaans.

3706 MESDAG, M. J. (1922–23) *Bibliographie van de werken van Nederland-sche schrijvers op het gebied der neurologie en psychiatrie en aanver-wante vakken* (Bibliography of the works of Dutch writers in the field of neurology and psychiatry and related disciplines). Bohn, Haarlem.
 – Subsequent volumes without author's name 1935–1937.

3706ᵃ STERREN, H. A. van der (1974). De hallucinaties van Orestes (The hallucinations of —). *Arts en Wereld, 7,* no 3, 65–9. De Hallucinaties van Ajax en Heracles (The hallucinations of — and —). *Ibidem,* no 4, 44–7.

3706ᵇ BARUCH, J. Z. (1973). Een psychiatrische waarneming door Friedrich Schiller (A psychiatric observation by — —). *GG, 4,* 288–9.

3707 KLEY, J. J. van der (1943). De kliniek der dementia paralytica in de afgeloopen 150 jaren (Clinic of dementia paralytica in the last 150 years). *GG, 21,* 563–9; *ibid., 22,* 1–7.

3708 BOOY, Joh. (1966). Over de ontwikkeling der psychiatrie in de laatste zestig jaar (On the development of psychiatry in the last sixty years). In: *De vooruitgang van de geneeskunde in onze eeuw,* 226–39. J. H. de Bussy, Amsterdam.

3709 LANKHOUT, J. (1939). Algemeene grondbeginselen der hedendaagsche affectpsychologie bij Spinoza (Basic elements of present-day affect-psychology in S.). *NTG, 83,* I, 523–9; *BGG, XIX,* 28–34.

3710 BAUMANN, E. D. (1932). *De Goddelijke waanzin. Vier studies over de ekstase* (The divine madness. Four studies on ecstasy). 113 pp. Van Gorcum, Assen.
 – reviewed by M. A. van Andel: *NTG, 77* (1933), III, 3055–6; *BGG, XIII,* 170–1.

3711 — (1934). Kollectieve waandenkbeelden (Collective fallacies). *Haagsch Mbl., XXII,* 491–502.

3712 DIEREN, E. van (1922). Twee ten onrechte beroemd geworden krank-zinnigen: Charles Fourier en Graaf St. Simon (Two lunatics who be-came famous wrongly: — — and Count — —). *NTG, 66,* I, 503–4; *BGG, II,* 60–1.

3713 SPEYER, N. (1938). Overzicht van de geschiedenis van den zelfmoord in Nederland (met bibliographie van Nederlandsche schrijvers over het zelfmoord-vraagstuk). (Survey of the history of suicide in the Netherlands (with a bibliography of Dutch writers on the problem of suicide). *NTG, 82*, II, 1599–1608; *BGG, XVIII*, 70–9. See also 5349

3714 HES, J. Ph. (1972). Psychiatric care of Jews in Holland from the beginning of the nineteenth century to World War II. *Koroth, 6*, (1–2), 58–61 [Hebrew;] XXI–XXVII [English].

3715 LOGHEM, J. J. van (1951). Harlekijn en de psychiater (Harlequin and the psychiatrist). *NTG, 95*, II, 1383; *BGG, XXXI*, 25.

3716 JORDAN, H. (1935). Gehirn und Seele. *SA, 27*, 250–66.

3717 REE, Chr. van der (1974). Ontwikkelingslijnen in de sociale psychiatrie: verleden, heden en toekomst (Development in social psychiatry: past, present and future). *T. Soc. Geneesk., 52*, 812–7; 838.
II. HART de RUYTER, Th. De bijdrage van de kinderpsychiatrie in de ontwikkeling van de sociale psychiatrie (Contribution of children's psychiatry to the development of social psychiatry). *Ibidem*, 818–25.
III. BAAN, P. A. H. Vijf-en-twintig jaar sociale psychiatrie; hoe verder? (25 years of social psychiatry; how further?) *Ibidem*, 826–32.
– Addresses delivered on the occasion of the 25th anniversary of the "Stichting voor de geestelijke gezondheid in de provincie Drenthe", on 28 February 1973 at Assen.

3717ᵃ MEININGER, J. V. (1974). Uit de geschiedenis van de anthropologische psycho-somatiek (From the history of anthropological psychosomatics). In: *Circa Tiliam*, 165–210. Brill, Leiden.

> See also 84–5, 253–9 (Boerhaave), 412–5, 502, 883, 1532–8 (Schroeder van der Kolk), 1918–20 (C. Winkler), 2210, 2275, 2455, 2693–5, 2700–4 (Antiquity), 3302, 3399–3403 (Remedies), 4283–4305 (mental nursing), 4413–40 (Lunatic asylums), 5382.

Hypnosis

3718 VIËTOR, W. P. J. (1964). Hypnosis in the Netherlands. A historical survey of the Dutch literature about 1900. Part I. Van Renterghem and Van Eeden. *Brit. J. med. Hypnot., 15* (3), 30–2.

3719 RINGELBERG, J. (1968). Enkele hoofdlijnen uit de geschiedenis der hypnose in Nederland (Main features from the history of hypnotism in the Netherlands). *NTG, 112*, 137–40.

B. Pediatrics

3720 CAULFIELD, E. (1928). A full view of all the diseases incident to children (also recording an early case of infantile cerebral hemorrhage the earliest pediatric anthology). *Ann. Med. Hist.*, s. l, *X*, 409–16, 1 ill.

– with chapters on: "Boerhaave on the diseases of children" and on "Franciscus dele Boë Sylvius: upon the Thrush".

3721 BENEDUM, J. (1971). Uit de geschiedenis van de kindergeneeskunde (From the history of pediatrics). *Image*, no 44, 28–36, 12 ill.

3722 CREVELD, S. van (1967). De ontwikkeling van de kindergeneeskunde in de laatste 75 jaren (Development of pediatrics in the last 75 years). *Mndschr. Kindergeneesk.*, *35*, 109–24.

3723 LEENDERS, E. and W. K. SIEBER (1970). Congenital megacolon observation by Frederick Ruysch. 1691. *J. Pediatr. Surg.*, *5*, 1–3.

See also 117, 119, 478, 533, 1469, 2462, 2742, 3034, 3973, 4453–5, 5289

C. Otorhinolaryngology

3724 KAN, P. Th. L. (1907). *De keel-, neus- en oorheelkunde in hare ontwikkelingsgeschiedenis* (Otorhinolaryngology in its history of development) 43 pp. Kooyker, Leiden.

– Inaugural address May 22, 1907 Leiden.

3725 BURGER, H. (1924). De keel- neus- oorheelkunde in de laatste 75 jaren (Otorhinolaryngology in the last 75 years). *NTG*, *68*, II, 43–7; *BGG*, *IV*, 166–70.

3726 HAVERKAMP, A. D. (1947, 1950²). *De ontwikkeling der oorheelkunde in Nederland in de negentiende eeuw, in het bizonder door de pioniers Van der Broek, Symons en Swaagman* (The development of otology in the Netherlands in the nineteenth century, particularly by the pioneers — —, —, and —). Thesis University Leiden (Supervisor: P. H. G. van Gilse). 217 pp., 30 ill. Leiden.

3727 EGMOND, A. A. J. van (1938). Iets over de ontwikkeling van de oorheelkunde (Something on the development of otology). *NTG*, *102*, II, 2407–10.

3728 [   ] (1968). *Gedenkboek. Nederlandse keel-, neus-, oorheelkundige vereniging. 75. 1893–1968* (Memorial volume. Dutch Association of Otorhinolaryngology. 75.) 80 pp., ill., ports. Ellerman Harms N.V. Amsterdam.

3729 KYLSTRA, P. H. (1973). Enige Nederlandse bijdragen tot de vocaalanalyse (Some Dutch contributions to the vocal analysis). *Sci. Hist.*, *15*, 12–21, ill.

3730 LUYENDIJK-ELSHOUT, A. M. (1973). The Cavity of the Nose in Dutch Baroque Medicine. *Clio. Med.*, *8*, 295–303, 1 ill.

See also 1030, 1554

Laryngeal instruments

3731 GILSE, P. H. G. van (1949). Wie vond de keelspiegel uit? (Who invented the laryngoscope?). *NTG*, *93*, II, 1358; *BGG*, *XXIX*, 28.

3732 VRIEND-VERMEER, W. [1965]. De laryngoscoop (The laryngoscope). *Organorama*, *II*, 23–6.

See also 801

D. Anaesthesiology

3733 COHEN, Ernst (1907). *Das Lachgas. Eine chemisch-kulturhistorische Studie.* 31 ill., Col. pl. W. Engelmann, Leipzig.

3734 HAMMES, Th. (1907). Historische bijdrage omtrent de invoering der narcose in de heelkunde en Dr William T. G. Morton's aandeel daarin (Historical contribution concerning the introduction of narcosis in surgery and the part of —— in it). *T. Tandhk.*, *XIV*, 118 and 184.

3735 DANIËLS, C. E. (1908). De waarheid in de geschiedenis van de anaesthetische werking van chloroform (The truth in the history of the anaesthetical action of chloroform). *NTG*, *52*, I, 266–9.

3736 SANDRA, H. (1940). Van narcose in vroegere eeuwen (On narcosis in former centuries). *NTG*, *84*, IV, 4285–92; *BGG*, *XX*, 169–76.

3737 LINDEBOOM, G. A. (1946). Honderd jaar narcose (A century of narcosis). *Org. Chr. Ver. Nat. Geneesk.*, *44*, 127–31.

3738 — (1946). De slaap ter verdooving (The sleep to anaesthesia). *Voortgang*, *I*, 1 (september).

3739 SCHOUTE, D. (1947). Over de invoering der narcose in ons land honderd jaar geleden (On the introduction of narcosis in our country hundred years ago). *NTG*, *91*, II, 941–6; *BGG*, *XXVII*, 9–14.

3740 HALBERTSMA, K. T. A. (1947). Het eeuwfeest der aethernarcose (Centenary of the narcosis with ether). *GG*, *25*, 327–31; 346–51.

3741 VOORHOEVE, H. C. (1949). Anaesthesie, door middel van zuurstofgebrek in vroeger tijden (Anaesthesia, by means of lack of oxygen in former times). *NTG*, *93*, II, 1350–7; *BGG*, *XXIX*, 20–7.

3742 KLEIN, S. A. (1964). De Historie van de Ontdekking der Narcose (History of the discovery of narcosis). *GeWiNa*, no 15, 16–9.

3743 RITSEMA VAN ECK, C. R. (1969). Geschiedenis van de anaesthesie in Nederland (History of anaesthesia in the Netherlands). *NTG*, *113*, 1763–8.

E. Orthopedics

3744 MOL, W. (1972). De ontwikkeling van de orthopedie in deze eeuw (The development of orthopedics in this century). *GG*, *3*, 16–9, port.

3745 PEPPINK, H. J. (1925). Über eine Methode aus dem Jahre 1778 zur Heilung eines Klumpfuszes. *DMW*, *50*, no 12.
       – on Jacob van der Haan who invented a new apparatus for the treatment of clubfoot.

See also 1297

F. Radiology

3746 COBBEN, J. (1959). Nederlandse pioniers in de radiologie (Dutch pioneers in radiology). *J. Belge Radiol.*, *42*, 738–45.
       – on K. A. Wertheim Salomonson (1864–1922), H. Eykman (1862–1914) and Nicolaas Voorhoeve (1879–1927).

3746[a] WIT, R. de and T. de ROO (1974). Description of an antique Radium goblet; a dangerous curiosity. *Med. Hist.*, *18*, 299–303.
       – on a radium goblet about 1920.

3746[b] WYLICK, W. A. H. van (1974). Beiträge aus den Niederlanden zur Entwicklung der Röntgenologie und Beziehungen auf röntgenologischem Gebiet zwischen den Niederlanden und Deutschland. *Med. Techn. Radiol.*, *5*, 78–88, 4 ill., 1 port.

See also 1457–68b (Röntgen)

G. Endocrinology

3746[c] JONGH, S. E. de (1968). Recollections of the heyday of experimental endocrinology under Laqeur at the Amsterdam Polderweg. *Acta Endocr.* (Kobenhavn), *57*, 1–15.

H. Dermatology

3747 ELAUT, L. (1958). De eerste geïllustreerde dermatologische verhandeling (The first illustrated dermatological treatise). *NTG*, *102*, II, 1749–53; *BGG, XXXVIII*, 13–7.
– on the book of J. L. Alibert (1768–1837). *Description des maladies de la peau* (1806).

3748 VANDEWIELE, Leo J. (1971, 1972). Een onbekend middelnederlands traktaat over huidziekten (An unknown Middle Dutch treatise on skin-diseases). *Farm. T. Belg.*, *48*, 126–39, ill. Also in: *Bull. Pharm.*, no 44 (febr. 1972), 23–36.

3748[a] NATER, J. P. (1974). Grepen uit de geschiedenis van de moderne dermatologie (Analecta from the history of modern dermatology).
I. Huidartsen, huidziekten en huidpatienten (Dermatologists, skin-diseases and skin patients). *Arts en Wereld*, *7*, no 5, 5–13.
– a.o. on J. J. Planck (1738–1807), R. Willan (1757–1812) and Th. Bateman (1778–1821).
II. De ontwikkeling van de dermatologie in Frankrijk (Development of dermatology in France). *Ibid.*, *7*, no 6, 5–10. (port. of J. L. Alibert (1768–1837)), ill.
III. De eerste afbeeldingen van huidziekten in de moderne dermatologie (The first pictures of skin-diseases in modern dermatology). *Ibid.*, *7*, no 7, 20–4.
IV. De ontwikkeling van het begrip allergie (Development of the con-

cept of allergy). *Ibid.*, 7, no 8, 16–20 (port. of Bela Schick (1877–1967). – a.o. on Portier (1866–?), Pirquet (1874–1920).

V. Ferdinand von Hebra en de ontwikkeling van het begrip eczeem (— — and the development of the concept of eczema) *Ibid.*, 7, 27–30, 2 ill.

3748ᵇ PRAKKEN, J. R. (1974). The development of dermatology in the Netherlands. *Brit. J. Derm.*, *91*, 225–33, 2 ports, 2 ill.

See also 4674a, 5288

I. Dental surgery

3749 BISSELING, G. H. (1921). Uit de geschiedenis der tandheelkunde (From the history of dentistry). *T. Tandh, XXVIII*, 773; also in: *NTG*, *65*, II, 1174; *BGG, I*, 341.

3750 — (1922). Die "Zene Arztney van 1530" in verband met Tandheelkunde uit Hollandsche werken omtrent dien tijd (The "Zene Arztney of 1530" in view of dental surgery from Dutch works in that time). *T. Tandh., XXIX*, 349; also in: *NTG, 66*, I, 2170–80; *BGG, II*, 137–47.

3751 — (1922). Uit een oud kruidboek (From an old herbal). *T. Tandh., XXIX*, 592.

3752 — (1922). Uit "de aanmerkingen van Hendrik Ulhoorn" (From "the notes of — —). *T. Tandh., XXIX*, 428; *NTG, 66*, II, 2608-20; *BGG, II*, 352–64.

3753 — (1922). Tandheelkundige aankondigingen uit Nederlandsche Couranten van vroeger (Dental announcements from Dutch papers in the past). *T. Tandh., XXIX*, 28, 53 and 118.

3754 — (1923). Tandheelkundige bevindingen bij menschapen (Dental (surgical) findings with man-apes). *T. Tandh., XXX*, 200.

3755 MOULIJN, J. A. (1931). Pierre Fauchard, de grondlegger der moderne tandheelkunde (— —, the founder of modern dentistry). *NTG, 75*, II, 1770–8; *BGG, XI*, 93–101, ill.

3756 BISSELING, G. H. and S. W. F. MARGADANT (1923). *Libellus de dentibus* van Bartholomeus Eustachius (*Libellus de dentibus* by — —). *T. Tandh., XXX*, 351, 462, 572 and 687.

3757 HAMER, A. A. H. (1921). Een stukje geschiedenis (A small piece of history). *T. Tandh.*, *XXVIII*, 139.

3758 HASSELT, A. G. J. C. van (1911). Uit de oude doos (Old history). *T. Tandh.*, *XVIII*, 518.

3759 DENTZ, Th. (1912, 1914). Herinneringen (Memories). *T. Tandh.*, *XIX*, 76; *ibid.*, *XXI*, 109.

3760 — (1921). Uit de oude doos (Old history). *T. Tandh*, *XXVIII*, 963.

3761 STEDEHOUDER, L. J. (1969). Historische kanttekeningen. Uit een encyclopedie Ao 1778 (Historical marginal notes. From an encyclopaedia, 1778). *T. Tandh.*, *LXXVI*, 69, 145, 348 and 440.
   - on the entries "tandkas", "tandtrekken", "tandpijn" in: Egbert Buys. *Woordenboek voor konsten en wetenschappen*, 1778.

3762 WILLEMSE, L. M. (1924). Het planteeren van Tanden en Kiezen (Implantation of Teeth and Molars). *T. Tandh.*, *XXXI*, 818, 12 ill.
   - with a historical introduction, a.o. on A. Paré.

3763 BOERMA, N. J. A. F. (1942). De tandtechniek in het Oosten omstreeks 1600 (Dental technics in the East about 1600). *NTG*, *86*, III, 1717; *BGG*, *XXII*, 98.

3764 MAAR, F. E. R. de (1960). Prothetische tandheelkunde in Amsterdam in het midden van de 19e eeuw (Prothetic dental surgery at A. in the middle of the 19th century). *T. Tandh.*, *LXVII*, 634–8, ill.

3765 — (1964). Prothetic dentistry in Amsterdam in the middle of the nineteenth century. *Revue Hist. Art. dent.*, *I*, no 4, 18–29, ill.

3765ᵃ — (1974). An Amsterdam toothmaker of 1843 In: *Proc. XXIII Int. Congr. Hist. Med. London 2–9 Sept. 1972*, Vol. II, 960–1. The Wellcome Institute of the History of Medicine, London.
   - on Mr Grader van der Maas [Abraham Grader] (1800–64).

3766 PROUDLER, R. T. (1956). Recruitment to the profession (An account of a tooth extraction, performed by J. Gyon and H. Kaau-Boerhaave, recorded in "The Memories of Catherine the Great"). *Brit. dent. J.*, *100*, 145–6.

3767 MARGADANT, G. D. (1961). Vijftig jaar A.T.V. (50 years "Amsterdamsche Tandheelkundige Vereniging" (Amsterdam Association of Dentistry)). *T. Tandh. LXVIII*, 748–51.

3768   LINDEN, J. van der (1965). Historisch overzicht van de middelen voor het speekselvrijhouden van de mondholte (Historical survey of the means to keep the oral cavity free from saliva). *T. Tandh. LXXII*, 575–84.

3769   SCHIJNDEL, L. J. A. van (1969). De opkomst van de vrouwelijke tandarts in Nederland (The rise of the female dentist in the Netherlands). *T. Tandh., LXXVII*, 268–75.

3770   BUISMAN, P. H. (1969). De ontwikkelingsgang der tandheelkunde in ons land. Het tijdperk der tandmeesters (The development of dentistry in our country. The period of the tooth-masters). *T. Tandh., LXXVI*, 166–99. cf: *ibid.*, 610–1.

3771   MAAR, F. E. R. de (1969). Prothèse dentaire à Amsterdam au milieu du siècle. *Rev. Franç. Odontostomat.*, *16*, 1219–30.

3772   DEENIK, B. Z. (1969). Driekwart eeuw collegiale kopij: van mond- tot zetspiegel (Three quarters of a century of copy from colleagues: from mouth-glass to type area). *Ned. T. Tandheelk.*, *76*, 257–62.

3773   VISSER, J. B. (1969). Het tijdschrift 75 jaar (The periodical 75 years). *Ned. T. Tandheelk.*, *76*, 163–5.

3774   MAAR, F. E. R. de (1968). Wie introduceerde het zilveramalgaam in de tandheelkunde? (Who did introduce silver amalgam in dentistry?). *Sci. Hist.*, *10*, 68–78.

Dental instruments and old books

3775   — (1960). The Kalman Klein Collection. *Fed. dent. int. sub-Committee dent. hist. circ.*, Letter no 4, 3–6.

3776   — (1961–3). The Kalman Klein Collection. *Janus, L*, 66–70, ill.
– The Collection of Mr Kalman Klein, who practised dentistry at The Hague and died in 1947, comprises and extensive library of rare dental books, a few hundred dental prints and engravings and a curious collection of old dental instruments. It was bought by Utrecht University in 1960.

3777   — (1965). Het instrumentenkistje van Marie Louise, aartshertogin van Oostenrijk, hertogin van Parma, Piacenza en Guastalla (Box of instruments of — —, archduchess of Austria, duchess of Parma, — and —). *T. Tandh.*, 72, 393–406,

See also 115, 746–7, 787, 1118, 1307, 1561, 1692a, 1818–20 (Vesalius), 2364, 2424–5, 3908, 4063, 4672a, 5290, 5367–8.

J. Forensic medicine

3778 ZUIDEN, D. S. van (1917). Een merkwaardige rechterlijke lijkopening in 1679 (A remarkable judicial autopsy in 1679). *NTG, 61*, I, 566–7.
– The Hague. Rechterlijk Archief, no 639. (Judicial Archive).

3779 FIJN van DRAAT, G. A. B. (1919). Een gerechtszitting in 1790 (A session of the Court in 1790). *NTG, 63*, II, 568–9.

3780 PENNING, C. P. J. (1930). Eenige merkwaardige vonnissen (Some remarkable sentences). *NTG, 74*, II, 3918; *BGG, X*, 236.

3781 KULSDOM, M. E. (1952). Geneeskunde en recht in de 18de eeuw (Medicine and justice in the 18th century). *NTG, 96*, II, 1527–42; *BGG, XXXII*, 23–8.

3782 HALLEMA, A. (1963). Ontwikkelingsgang van de lijkschouwingsrapporten te Amsterdam, voornamelijk in de tweede helft van de 16e eeuw (Development of the autopsy reports at A. particularly in the second half of the 16th century). *NTG, 107*, II, 1922–30; *BGG, XLIII*, 10–8.

3783 HERMANS, A. G. J. (1964). Lijkschouwingsrapporten te Amsterdam (Autopsy reports at A.). *NTG, 108*, I, 40; *BGG, XLIV*, 22.
– Letter to the editor.

3784 BROEKSMIT, C. (1927). Boetebepalingen van toegebrachte verwondingen. Tarief volgens de grootte en diepte der wonden (Provisions of fines for inflicted injuries. Rate according to the size and deepness of the wounds). *NTG, 71*, II, 94–6; *BGG, VII*, 498–500.

3785 HULST, J. P. L. (1922). De geschiedenis van de longproef en van hare beteekenis voor de gerechtelijke geneeskunde en rechtspraak (History of the lung-test and of its significance for forensic medicine and justice). I. (till 1800): *NTG, 66*, II, 57–74; *BGG, II*, 151–68. II (from 1800 till now): *NTG, 66*, II, 2058–80; *BGG, II*, 251–68.
– On the floating of the lungs of a dead, newborn child as a sign of having lived.

3786 HILL, Boyd H. (1961–3). Frisian law and the foetus. *Janus, L*, 55–9.

3787 ROEKEL, G. van (1940). De guillotine (The guillotine). *NTG, 84*, I, 52; *BGG, XX*, 19.

See also 1500, 2562, 2744, 3355, 3494–3500 (Hangman).

K. Veterinary medicine

3788   WESTER, J. (1939). *Geschiedenis der Veeartsenijkunde* (History of veterinary medicine). 574 pp. Utrecht. 8°.
– from Antiquity till *ca* 1920.

3789   MEY, G. J. W. van der (1968). Over de aanvang der veeartsenijkunde
in Nederland (On the beginning of veterinary medicine in the Netherlands). *Sci. Hist.*, *10*, 79–86.

3790   WEIJDE, A. J. van der (1930). Geneeskundigen als veeartsen (Physicians as veterinary surgeons). *NTG*, *74*, I, 2257–9; *BGG*, *X*, 136–8.

3791   WELLEN, J. W. (ed.) (1971). *Veterinary works in the Netherlands*. 314
pp., ill. Ministry of Agriculture and Fisheries, The Hague.
– Commemorating the centenary of the State Veterinary Service. Historical survey,
12–7.

3792   ZWIJNENBERG, H. A. (1923). De beteekenis van den arts Alexander
Numan voor de diergeneeskunde (The significance of the physician
— — to veterinary medicine). *NTG*, *67*, II, 2279–89; *BGG*, *III*, 337–47.

3793   BRUINS, L. H. (1941). *Leven en werken van Gerrit Reinders, de grondlegger van de immunologie* (Life and Works of G. —, founder of immunology). Thesis University Groningen (Supervisor: A. B. F. A. Pondman). 200 pp., port. De "Marne", Leens.
– also as a monograph; G. Reinders (1737–1815), a Groningen peasant, a fighter
against cattle-plague.

3794   BOERMA, N. J. A. F. (1908). Eenige bladzijden uit de geschiedenis van
de inenting tegen de veepest in de achttiende eeuw (Some pages from
the history of vaccination against cattle-plague in the 18th century).
Gron. Volksalm., *20*, 208–27.

3795   FABER, J. A. (1962). Cattle-plague in the Netherlands during the
eighteenth century. *Med. Landbouwhogesch. Wageningen*, *62* (11), 1–7.

3796   — (1966). De veepest in Nederland in de achttiende eeuw (Cattle-
plague in the Netherlands in the eighteenth century). *Spiegel Historiael*,
1, 67–74, 10 ill.

3797   HENDRICX, M. (1962). Oude recepten om paarden te genezen en vissen
te vangen (Old prescriptions to heal horses and to catch fishes). *Limburg*, *41*, 259–61.

3798 VRIEND, H. J. de (ed.) (1972). *The Old-English "Medicina de quadru-pedibus"*. Thesis University Groningen. 106 + 162 pp., ill. Gianotten, Tilburg. 4°.

– with an introduction and notes by —, and with Latin text.

3799 KOK, J. (1934). Het veterinair instrumentarium der Arabieren in de Middeleeuwen (The cabinet of instruments of the Arabs in the Middle Ages). *NTG, 78*, IV, 5066; *BGG, XIV*, 212.

– included in a report of a meeting of the "Genootschap".

See also 475, 2785n., 3910, 5347.

Chapter XIII

Naval and Tropical Medicine

In 1602 the Dutch "Oost-Indische Compagnie" (East Indian Company) was founded, in 1621 the West Indian Company. The ships of the first sailed via Cape Town to the isles of what became the Dutch East Indian Archipel, India, Japan and Australia; the fleet of the latter did business with North America, South America and the Antilles.

The ships of these companies had on board a naval chaplain ("ziekentrooster") and a surgeon who had at his disposal a chest with instruments and another with a choice of drugs. Many surgeons and also some doctors lived for years in tropical areas (Gerard de Bondt, Willem Piso). They described the diseases they observed there, native methods of treatment (e.g. Moxa) and brought home medicinal herbs unknown in Europe. In this way they were the pioneers in the field of tropical medicine to which later on many others made noteworthy contributions.

On the long voyages especially to the East scurvy often developed among the crew, of which sometimes half or more had died before Cape Town was reached where the remaining seamen found relief by fresh fruit.

The medical service on the fleet of the East Indian Company has been studied notably by Schoute.

In this chapter are also included entries bearing on the history of medical missionary activities.

A. Naval medicine

General

3800 SCHOUTE, D. (1929). *De geneeskunde in den dienst der Oost-Indische Compagnie in Nederlandsch-Indië* (Medicine in the service of the East India Company in the Dutch Indies). 347 pp. De Bussy, Amsterdam.

– reviewed by A. W. Nieuwenhuis: *Janus, XXXIII* (1929), 400–1; and by M. A. van Andel: *NTG, 73,* (1929), II, 5156–7; *BGG, IX,* 296–7; and by G. van Rijnberk: *NTG, 73* (1929), II, 5721–4; *BGG, IX,* 305–8.

3801   POP, G. J. (1866–68, 1922). *De geneeskunde bij het Nederlandsche zeewezen* (Dutch naval medicine). Weltevreden. 8°.

– reprint of articles in the *Geneesk. T. Zeemacht,* edited by L. S. A. M. von Römer.

3802   LEUFTINK, A. E. (1952). *De geneeskunde bij 's lands oorlogsvloot in de 17de eeuw* (Medicine in the Dutch Navy in the 17th century). Thesis University Groningen (Supervisor: J. J. Th. Vos). 135 pp., ill., ports. Van Gorcum, Assen.

– also as a monograph.

3803   — (1963). *Chirurgijns Zeekompas. De medische verzorging aan boord van de Nederlandse zeeschepen gedurende de Gouden Eeuw* (The surgeon's sea-compass. Medical care on board the Dutch sea-going vessels during the Golden Age). 72 pp., ill. Ned. Gist- en Spiritusfabriek, Delft; Wereldvenster, Baarn. ²1965: De Branding, Antwerpen.

3804   — (1966). Varende chirurgijns (Sailing surgeons). *GeWiNa,* no 19, 6.

3805   HULLU, J. de (1912). Zieken en doctors op de schepen der O.I. Compagnie (Patients and physicians on the ships of the East India Company). *Bijdr. Taal-, Land-, en Volkenkunde Ned.-Indië, 67,* 28 pp.

3805ᵃ BRUGMANS, H. (1928). Zieke en gewonde matrozen (Ill and wounded sailors). *Amstelodamum, 15,* 14.

3806   [   ] (1903). Reglement voor de opleiding van studenten in de geneeskunde aan de Nederlandse Universiteiten tot officier van gezondheid bij de Zeemacht (Vastgesteld bij Kon. Besluit van 6 Mei 1886, no 41). (Regulation for the training of medical students at the Dutch Universities for medical officer in the Navy). (Royal Decree, May 6, 1886, no 41). no pl. 8°.

see also 2727–32 (Roman medicine), 1993–2001 (naval surgeons), 4634.6.

Medical service

3807   ALERS, C. (1899). Eenige aanteekeningen omtrent den geneeskundigen dienst bij Hr. Ms. Zeemacht in de laatste 50 jaren (Some remarks concerning the medical service of the Royal Navy in the last 50 years). *Alers et al.,* 1–15.

3808   HAVER DROEZE, J. J. (1921). De geneeskundige dienst bij de Neder-
landsch-Oost-Indische Compagnie (The medical service of the Dutch
East-India Company). *NTG, 65*, I, 2535–60; *BGG, I*, 193–218.

3809   METS, C. (1964). De Geneeskundige Dienst der Zeemacht als onder-
deel van de Geneeskundige Dienst der Landmacht (The medical service of the Navy as a unit of the Medical Service of the Land-forces).
NedMGT, 17, 262–8.

Nursing

3810   PORTENGEN, J. A. (1897–98). Treatise on the nature of injuries, which
may be sustained in future naval warfare. *Janus, II*, 306–12.

3811   GIJSBERTI HODENPIJL, A. K. A. (1918). Ziekten aan boord van schepen
der O.I. Compagnie in de eerste helft der 18de eeuw (Diseases on board
ships of the East-India Company in the first half of the 18th century).
NTG, 62, I, 636–9; 972–6.

3812   PUTTO, J. A. (1937). Zorg voor gewonde en zieke schepelingen in de
achttiende eeuw (Care of wounded and ill sailors in the 18th century).
GG, 15, 68–70.

3813   HANEVELD, G. T. (1959). Een Spaans hospitaalschip uit de zestiende
eeuw (A Spanish floating hospital from the 16th century). *NedMGT, 12*,
116–9.

Hygienics

3814   ODERWALD, J. (1914). Hygiëne bij de scheepvaart, voorheen en thans
(Hygiene on board ships, past and present). *Vrag. Dag, XXIX*, 706.

3815   — (1940). Zorg voor de gezondheid aan boord van zeilschepen in de
19de eeuw (Care of health on board sailing-vessels in the 19th century).
NTG, 84, I, 416–23; *BGG, XX*, 20–7.

3816   ANDEL, M. A. van (1931). Geneeskunde en hygiëne op de slavensche-
pen in den Compagniestijd (Medicine and hygiene in the slaveships
in the time of the Company). *NTG, 75*, I, 614–37; *BGG, XI*, 21–44, 3
ill.

3816ᵃ ROESSINGH, M. P. H. (1967). De watervoorziening op de schepen van
de V.O.C. (Water supply in the ships of the United East India Company). *Spiegel Historiael, 2*, 20–6, 8 ill.

Nutrition

3817 GIJSBERTI HODENPIJL, A. K. A. (1922). De scheurbuik (scorbuut) op 's compagnieschepen uit het Vaderland komende in het jaar 1730(Scurvy in the ships of the Company, coming from the Netherlands in 1730). *NTG, 66*, I, 496–501; *BGG, II*, 53–8.

3818 ANDEL, M. A. van (1926). Citroenen en sinaasappelen als scheurbuikmiddel op de schepen van de Vereenigde Nederlanden (Lemons and oranges as a remedy for scurvy in the ships of the United Netherlands). *NRC*, 18 december.

3818ª HULLU, J. de (1910). De voeding op de schepen der Oost-Indische Compagnie (Nutrition in the ships of the Dutch East-India Company). *Bijdr. Taal-, Land-, en Volkenkunde Ned.-Indië, 65*, 22 pp.

3819 BOLT, N. A. (1926). Verstrekking van citroenen op Hollandsche schepen in de 17de eeuw (Providing of lemons in Dutch ships in the 17th century). *NTG, 70*, II, 1127; *BGG, VI*, 256.
– letter to the editor.

3820 MANTZ, J. J. C. (1957). Over de voeding op Nederlandse koopvaardijschepen (On nutrition in Dutch merchant vessels). *Voeding, 18*, 498–505.

3821 GEMEREN, M. C. van and J. C. LUCAS (1958). Voeding en hygiëne aan boord van Nederlandse haringloggers (Nutrition and hygiene on board Dutch herring-drifters). *Voeding, 19*, 189–226.

Pharmacy

3822 GIJSBERTI HODENPIJL, A. K. A. (1919). Opdracht in de 17de eeuw aan apothekers en chirurgijns der vloot (17th century order to apothecaries and surgeons of the fleet). *NTG, 63*, II, 1743.

3823 VIEYRA, D. (1936). Lijst van geneesmiddelen en instrumenten voor heelmeesters op koopvaardijschepen der stad Amsterdam in het jaar 1796 (List of drugs and instruments for surgeons in trading ships of the city of Amsterdam in the year 1796). *NTG, 80*, II, 1931–5; *BGG, XVI*, 71–5.

3824 BRANS, P. H. (1958). Beiträge zur Geschichte der Schiffs-pharmazie in den Niederlanden und in Niederländisch Indiën. *Veröfftl. Int. Gesellsch. Gesch. Pharm., 13*, 59–83.

3825   — (1963). Mitarbeiter der "Oost-Indische Compagnie" aus deutschen Ländern. *Dtsch. Apoth. Ztg.*, *103*, 905–10.

3826   — (1963). De geneesmiddelenvoorziening bij de Admiraliteiten en bij
de Oost-Indische Compagnie (Provision of drugs at the Admiralties
and at the East India Company). *Ph. W. 98*, 596–608; *Bull. Pharm.*,
no 31, november, 12–13.

B. Tropical medicine

General

3827   REDDY, D. V. S. (1951). Seventeenth Century Dutch Writers on Tropical Medicine and Tropical Herbs. *J. Hist. Med.*, *VI*, 258–60.

3828   ANDEL, M. A. van (1938). Deutsche und Niederländer als Pioniere
der Tropenmedizin im 17. Jahrhundert. *Klin. Wschr.*, *17*, 24–7, 6 ill.
– also on W. Piso, W. ten Rhijne and C. Bontekoe.

3829   — (1924). Dutch naturalists of the 17th century and the materies
medica of tropical America. *Janus*, *XXVIII*, 219–31, ill.
– The article deals with Monardes (Spanish), Dutch translation of the works of Jean
de Léry and Jospeh Acosta, and the great work of W. Piso and Georg Marcgraf
(*Historia Naturalis Brasiliae*, 1648).

3829ª   RÖMER, L. S. A. M. von (ed.) (1921). *Historische Schetsen. Een inleiding tot het vierde congres der Far Eastern Association of Tropical Medicine te houden te Batavia van den 6den tot den 13den Augustus 1921*
(Historical sketches. An introduction to the 4th Congress of the
— — — — to be held at B. from 6th till 13th August 1921). XI +
335 pp. 218 ill., (many ports). Javasche Boekhandel en Drukkerij,
Batavia.

> See also 379–86 (J. Bontius), 1395–9 (W. Piso), 1435–9 (W.
> ten Rhijne), 2213.

Dutch East Indies

3830   STEEGE, Joac. van der (1779, 1921). *Geneeskundige berichten* (Medical
tidings). Javasche Boekhandel, Rijswijk-Batavia.
– A reprint of the original from the "Verhandelingen van het Bataviaasch Genoot-
schapvan Kunsten en Wetenschappen", on the occasion of the Congress of the Far
Eastern Association of Tropical Medicine (Batavia, 1921), with an introduction
by L. S. A. M. von Römer.

3831 HOGENDORP, Mr W. van (1780, 1921). *Geneeskundige Propaganda-ge-schriften* (Medical propaganda-writings). Javasche Boekhandel, Rijswijk-Batavia.
– Reprint of two articles from the "Verh. Bataviaasch Genootschap Kunsten en Wetenschappen". The second article deals with variolation.

3832 STOKVIS, B. J. (1883). Discours d'ouverture du congrès international de médecine des colonies, Amsterdam September 1883.
– The speaker dwells upon Dutch tropical physicians, such as Bontius, Piso, etc.

3833 SIRKS, M. J. (1915). *Indisch natuuronderzoek; een beknopte geschiedenis van de beoefening der natuurwetenschappen in de Nederlandse Koloniën* (Indian natural science; a brief history of the practice of natural sciences in the Dutch Colonies). Thesis University Utrecht. 303 pp., ill., ports. Amsterdam.

3834 MEYERHOFF, M. and H. C. ROGGE (1939). Medizinisches aus Reisebeschreibungen nach Niederländisch-Indien im siebzehnten Jahrhundert. *Janus, XLIII*, 92–122.

3835 HONIG, P. and F. VERDOORN (ed.) (1945). *Science and scientists in the Netherlands Indies.* I–XXIII and 491 pp., 134 ill. New York City, Board for the Netherlands Indies, Surinam and Curacao.
– Reviewed by A. Wolsky: *Arch. Int. Sci., 5* (1948), 218–20.

3836 SCHOUTE, D. (1931). Het tijdvak Daendels – Raffles en de geneeskunde in Nederlandsch-Indië (The period Daendels – Raffles and medicine in the Dutch Indies). *NTG, 75*, IV, 5893–5902; *BGG, XI*, 313–22.

3837 — (1935). *De geneeskunde in Nederlandsch-Indië gedurende de negentiende eeuw* (Medicine in the Dutch East Indies during the 19th century). 381 pp. G. Kolff, Batavia.
– Essays previously published in the *Geneeskundig Tijdschrift voor Nederlandsch-Indië*, 1934 and 1935.

3838 — (1937). *Occidental therapeutics in the Netherlands East Indies during three centuries of Netherlands settlement 1600–1900.* Netherlands Indies Public Health Service. Kolff & Co, Batavia.
– Reviewed by B. W. Th. Nuyens: *NTG, 81* (1937), IV, 4698–4700; *BGG, XVII*, 177–9.

3839 GIJSBERTI HODENPIJL, A. K. A. (1922). Het gebruik van inlandsche geneesmiddelen in den Compagniestijd (The use of native drugs during the time of the Company). *NTG, 66*, II, 1651–4; *BGG, II*, 237–40.

3840 KLEIWEG de ZWAAN, J. P. (1914–15). Bestanddeelen van het menschelijk lichaam als versterkende middelen voor planten en dieren,
volgens de opvattingen der inlanders in onze Oost (Elements of the
human body as restoratives for plants and animals, according to the
ideas of the natives in the Dutch East Indies). *Med. Wbl.*, *21*, 346, 365
and 371.

3841 BRANS, P. H. (1952). De pharmaceutische verzorging bij de O.I. Compagnie (The pharmaceutical care of the East India Company). *NTG*,
96, II, 830–1; *BGG*, *XXXII*, 15–6.
– included in a report of a meeting of the "Genootschap".
See also 396, 2856–7.

Batavia [Djakarta]

3842 BLEEKER, P. (1844). Bijdragen tot de geneeskundige topographie
van Batavia (Contributions to the medical topography of B.) I. Ge-
steldheid van grond en lucht (Character of the soil and air) II. Vege-
tatie en derzelver producten (Vegetation and its products) *Natuur- en
Geneeskundig Archief voor Neerland's Indië*, *1*, 1–80 (I) and 169–220
(II). Batavia.

3843 — (1844). Bijdrage tot de kennis der genees- en artsenijmengkunde onder de Chinezen in het algemeen en onder die te Batavia in het bijzonder (Contribution to the knowledge of medicine and pharmacy among
the Chinese generally and particularly among those at B.) *Natuur- en
Geneesk. Arch. Ned. Indië*, *1*, 257–84.

3844 SWAVING, C. (1878). Batavia's sanitaire geschiedenis onder het bestuur
van de Oost-Indische Maatschappij (Sanitary history of B. under the
government of the East-India Society). *NTG*, *14*, II, 1.

3845 KALFF, S. (1910). Bataviasche Doctoren uit de 17de eeuw (Batavian
physicians from the 17th century). *Ind. Gids*, *XXXII*, 1136 and 1284.

3846 GORKOM, W. J. van (1913). *Ongezond Batavia. Vroeger en nu.* (Un-
healthy Batavia. Past and present). Batavia.

3847 GIJSBERTI HODENPIJL, A. K. A. (1918). Verbetering in de behandeling
der zieken van het hospitaal te Batavia in 1743 (Improvement of the
treatment of the sick in the hospital at B. in 1743). *NTG*, *62*, II, 399–
405.

3848 — (1919). Een inspecteur van den gezondheidsdienst te Batavia in

het midden der 18de eeuw (An Inspector of the public health service at B. in the middle of the 18th century). *NTG, 63*, II, 444–51.
– on the desirability to appoint a sanitary inspector at B. in view of the high mortality rate.

3849 — (1920). De toestand in de beide hospitalen te Batavia in 1768 (The situation in both hospitals at B. in 1768). *NTG, 64*, II, 249–55.

Diseases

3850 THIEL, P. H. van (1971). History of the control of endemic diseases in the Netherlands overseas territories. *Ann. Soc. belge Méd. trop.*, 51, 443–57.

3851 SITANALA, J. B. (1938). Geschiedenis der lepra in Ned.-Indië (History of leprosy in the Dutch East Indies). *Mndschr. locale Gezondh.*, *1*, 103–7; also in: *T. Kon. Aard. Gen.*, (2), *56* (1939) no 1, 157.

3852 BROES van DORT, T. (1897). Een en ander over de Lepra in Nederland en zijn Koloniën (Something on leprosy in the Netherlands and its Colonies). *NTG, 33*, I, 292–6 and 384–91; II 407–21 and 650–1.
– with historical introduction; reviewed by C. E. Daniëls: *Janus, II*, (1897–98), 183–4.

3853 — (1898). *Historische studie over Lepra, voornamelijk in verband met het voorkomen dezer ziekte in Nederlandsch-Oost-Indie* (Historical study on leprosy, mainly in relation to the occurrence of this disease in the Dutch East Indies). Van Hengel, Rotterdam; Kolff & Co, Batavia
– Reviewed by M. S. Gutteling: *NTG, 35* (1899), 97–8.

3854 KLEIWEG de ZWAAN, J. P. (1914–15). De lepra in Nederlandsch-Indië (Leprosy in the Dutch East Indies). *Med. Wbl.*, *21*, 227, 238 and 247.

3855 SOEST, A. H. van (1959). De Karo-Bataks en lepra (The — — and leprosy). *NTG, 103*, I, 738–9.　　　　　　　　*See also* 1435, 3120–1

3856 BEYLON, David (1780, 1921). *Knokkelkoorts* (Breakbone fever). Javasche Boekhandel, Rijswijk-Batavia.
– reprint of an article from the "Verhandelingen van het Bataviaasch Genootschap van Kunsten en Wetenschappen (1780), republished on the occasion of the Congress of the Far Eastern Association of Tropical Medicine, Batavia 1921. Introduction by L. S. A. M. von Römer.

3857 BURG, C. L. van der (1901). Dengue, *Janus, VI*, 359.

3858 PEYPERS, H. F. A. (1901). Remarque à propos de l'ouvrage du Dr
      Schenke (*Die Krankheiten der warmen Ländern*, II. Aufl.) et: Die Pest
      und Ihre Geschichte (Antwort an Dr Schenke). *Janus*, *VI*, 170–2;
      340–6.

3859 SCHOUTE, D. (1935). Enkele volksplagen in het verleden van Neder-
      landsch-Indië (Some popular plagues in the past of the Dutch East
      Indies).
      1. Pokken (Smallpox). *NTG*, *79*, I, 42–57; *BGG*, *XV*, 1–16.
      2. Syphilis. *NTG*, *79*, I, 455–71; *BGG*, *XV*, 21–37.
      3. Cholera. *NTG*, *79*, I, 890–906; *BGG*, *XV*, 52–68.
      4. Lepra (Leprosy). *NTG*, *79*, II, 1587–1604; *BGG*, *XV*, 74–91.
      5. De bestrijders der plagen (The fighters against the plagues). *NTG*,
      79, II, 2089–2106; *BGG*, *XV*, 101–18.

3860 LOGHEM, J. J. van (1912). The first plague-epidemic in the Dutch
      Indies. *Janus*, *XVII*, 153–90, 3 ill.

                                              See also 617, 1020, 3288–9
3861 deleted

3862 GIJSBERTI HODENPIJL, A. K. A. (1918). Pokken epidemie te Kaap de
      Goede Hoop in 1735 (Smallpox epidemic at Cape Good Hope in —).
      NTG, *62*, II, 1434–8.

3863 [   ] (1963) Early European Medicine in India. Jacob Bontius and
      his writings on diseases and herbs of the East Indies. *BDHM Hyder-
      abad*, *I*, 118–28, port.

3864 DALEN, H. van (1951). *Ontwikkeling onzer kennis der gele koorts*
      (Development of our knowledge of yellow fever). Thesis University
      Utrecht. 124 pp. Utrecht.

3865 SLUIS, Isaac van der (1969). *The Treponematosis of Tahiti. Its Origin
      and Evolution. A Study of the Sources*. Thesis University Amsterdam
      (Supervisor: J. R. Prakken). 178 pp. B. M. Israël, Amsterdam.

3866 BOOTH, C. C. (1964). The first description of tropical sprue (William
      Hillary). *Gut*, *5*, 45–50.

3867 HERMANS, E. H. (1927). Enkele beschouwingen over de geschiedenis
      van de framboesia tropica (Some observations on the history of — —).
      NTG, *71*, I, 1191–8; *BGG*, *VII*, 188–95.

3868 KUENEN, W. A. (1909). Die Aetiologie und Diagnose der Amoebiasis.
      Janus, *XIV*, 542–69.
      – historical remarks, 544–8.

3869 STATIUS VAN EPS, L. W. and E. LUCKMAN-MADURO (eds). (1973). *Van scheepschirurgijn tot specialist. 333 jaar Nederlands-Antilliaanse geneeskunde* (From naval surgeon to specialist. 333 years of Dutch Antilles medicine). 196 pp., fig. Van Gorcum, Assen. *See also* 1444a
– Reviewed by J. R. Prakken: *NTG, 118* (1974), 521.

C. Medical mission

3870 GAAY FORTMAN, N. A. de (1908). *De geschiedenis der medische zending* (History of medical mission). 415 pp. Callenbach, Nijkerk.
– on missionary work in North and South America and on all American Missionary Societies in and outside America during the 19th century.

3871 SILLEM- [GAYMANS, Aug.] (1910). *Wat melaatschen te danken hebben aan de zending* (What lepers owe to the mission). 41 pp. ill. Amsterdam. 4°.

3872 DAKE, W. J. L. (1972). *Het medische werk van de zending in Nederlands-Indië* (The work of the medical mission in the Dutch East Indies). Vol. I, 235 pp., fig. J. H. Kok, Kampen.
– Reviewed by M. F. Polak: *NTG, 117* (1973), 1164.

3873 KRAMER, Rijk (1937). Herinneringen en ervaringen uit de eerste 12 jaren van de medische Zending te Solo, naar aanleiding van haar zilveren jubileum 1 November 1912 – 1 November 1937 (Memories and experiences of the first 12 years of medical mission at S. with reference to its silver jubilee — —). *G&W, 35,* 161.

Chapter XIV

Military Medicine

For its eighty years' war with Spain (1568–1648) the young Dutch Republic needed a rather big army with field surgeons in its service. The King-Stadtholder Willem III improved the medical and pharmaceutical service with the help of Govert Bidloo, who acted as general inspector. After the Napoleontic area the military medical service was reorganized and a military medical school was established at Utrecht in order to provide a special training for the medical officers.

In this chapter are also included sections on military hospitals, military pharmacy, the transport and nursing of wounded soldiers and on the Red Cross.

A. General

3874 Vos, J. H. J. (no d.). *De zorg voor de gezondheid in het leger met een naschrift over de Spaansche griep* (Health care in the Army with a postscript on the Spanish flu). Serie: Kleine Boekerij, no 4. Zaltbommel. 8°.

3875 Fransen, J. W. P. (1918). *Eerste heelkundige behandeling van oorlogsgewonden* (First surgical treatment of war-casualties). Leiden. 8°.

3876 Braat, P. (1938). Reglement voor de Meesters-Chirurgijns te velde 1677 (Regulations for the Master-surgeons). *NTG, 82*, IV, 5774–5; *BGG, XVIII*, 322–3.
– Groot Placaatboek deel III, 1383 (February 20, 1677).

3876ᵃ Verdoorn, J. A. (1972). *Arts en oorlog. Medische en sociale zorg voor oorlogsslachtoffers in de geschiedenis van Europa. Inleiding in de medische polemologie* (Physician and war. Medical and social care of war victims in the history of Europe. Introduction to medical polemology). 2 vols; I. Van de antieke wereld tot de twintigste eeuw (From antiquity till the 20th century). VIII + 474 pp. II: Van de eerste wereldoorlog tot de tegenwoordige tijd (From the first world war till the present time). 435 pp. Stichting Uitgeverij Lynx, Amsterdam.

See also 3802

B. Education

3877 DONDERS, F. C. (1867). *De kweekschool voor militaire geneeskundigen in verband beschouwd met de Staatsbegrooting voor het dienstjaar 1867 en met de regeling van het hooger onderwijs* (The training college for military physicians considered in relation to the State-budget for the year of service 1867 and to the regulations for higher education). Utrecht. 8°.
– with an answer to some objections.

3878 [   ] (1913). Reglement voor de opleiding van studenten aan de Nederlandsche Universiteiten tot officier van gezondheid bij de landmacht (Regulation for the training of students, at the Dutch Universities, for medical officer in the Army). 's–Gravenhage. 8°.

3879 HOITINK, A. W. J. H. (1949). *De militaire school voor hygiene en preventieve geneeskunde* (The Militairy School for hygiene and preventive medicine). 's-Gravenhage. 8°.

3880 BROEK, P. van den (1964). De School Geneeskundige Dienst (The School Medical Service). *NedMGT, 17*, 342–5, ill.

3881 JONG, C. de (1964). De militaire school voor hygiene en praeventieve geneeskunde (The military school for hygiene and preventive medicine). *NedMGT, 17*, 345–52, ill.

See also 2237

C. Army Medical Corps

3882 DOELEMAN, Frans (1955). *De medische geschiedenis van een infanteriebataljon der Koninklijke Landmacht gedurende drie jaar actieve dienst op Java 1946–1950* (Medical history of an infantery batallion of the Royal Army during three years of active service on Java). Thesis University Utrecht. 235 pp., Van Gorcum, Assen.
– with a summary in English.

3883 PUTTERS, H. (1969). 100 jaar Geneeskundige Troepen. Voorwoord van de voorzitter der Jubileum Commissie (100 years of Medical Troops. Preface of the chairman of the Jubilee-Committee). *NedMGT*, *22*, 4–5.

3884 BERG, T. van den (1969). 100 jaar geneeskundige troepen 1869 – 7 april – 1969 (100 years of Medical Troops). *NedMGT*, *22*, 6–13.

3885 BINSBERGEN, J. van (1969). Honderd jaar Geneeskundige Troepen (Hundred years Medical Troops). *Arts en Auto*, *35*, 9.

3886 GEELEN, H. J. van [1969]. *Van Hospitaalsoldaten tot geneeskundige troepen* (From ambulance-men to medical troops). 125 pp., no pl. no d.
– Edited on the occasion of the 100th anniversary of the Regiment Medical Troops; with a foreword by H.R.H. Prince Bernhard.

3887 BAKEMA, K. L. (1969). Voorwoord van de Inspecteur Geneeskundige Dienst der Koninklijke Landmacht. 100 jaar geneeskundige troepen 1869–1969 (Preface of the Inspector of the Medical Service of the Royal Forces. 100 years medical troops). *NedMGT*, *22*, 3.

See also 5079a

D. Medical and Sanitary Services

3888 DOMMELEN, G. F. van (1857). *Geschiedenis der militaire geneeskundige dienst in Nederland met inbegrip van die zijner zeemacht en overzeesche bezittingen vanaf den vroegsten tijd tot op heden* (History of the Military Medical Service in the Netherlands, including that of the Navy and the overseas possessions from the earliest times up to the present). Nijmegen. 8°.

3889 WIJN, J. W. (1954). Stukken betreffende de geschiedenis van de Militair-Geneeskundige Dienst (Papers concerning the history of the Military Medical Service). *NedMGT*, *7*, 291–3.

3890 QUANJER, A. A. J. (1899). De Militair Geneeskundige Dienst in Nederland in de laatste vijftig jaren (The Military Medical Service in the Netherlands in the last fifty years). *Alers et al*, 16–20.

3891 — (1907). De militair-geneeskundige dienst voor vijftig jaar en thans (The Military Medical Service fifty years ago and now). *NTG*, *43*, I, 51–9.

3892 ROMEYN, D. (1913). *Onze militair geneeskundige dienst voor 100 jaren en daaromtrent* (Our military medical service 100 years ago). 73 pp., port. (of S. J. Brugmans). Bohn, Haarlem. 8°.

3893 DORNICKX, Ch. G. J. (1931). Een en ander over den militair genees-kundigen dienst hier te lande in het eind der 18e eeuw (Something on the military medical service in our country at the end of the 18th century). *NTG, 75,* III, 4056–62; *BGG, XI,* 237–43.

3894 ENKLAAR, W. F. (1916). *Over reorganisatie van den Militairen Genees-kundigen Dienst* (On the reorganization of the Military Medical Service). 23 pp. A. Hooiberg, Epe.

3895 KARBAAT, J. (1960). De Militair Geneeskundige Dienst vroeger en nu (The Military Medical Service past and present). *Mil. Spectator, 129,* 403.

3896 — (1964). Invloed van de M.G.D. op de ontwikkeling van de wes-terse geneeskundige wetenschap in Japan (Influence of the Military Medical Service on the development of western medical science in Japan). *NedMGT, 17,* 371–2.

3897 ROMEYN, J. A. (1908). Een roemvolle bladzijde uit de geschiedenis van den geneeskundigen dienst van het leger der Vereenigde Staten van Noord-Amerika (A glorious page from the history of the military medical service of the United States of North America). *MGT, 12,* 179–82.

3898 SIESTROP, J. G. (1935). Schetsen uit vroegere oorlogen. Hygienische maatregelen door den Engelschen Militair Geneeskundigen Dienst tijdens den Krimoorlog genomen (Sketches from former wars. Hygienic measures taken by the English Army Medical Corps during the Crimean War). *MGT, 24,* 156–8.

3899 — (1937). De Militair Geneeskundige Dienst op de Citadel van Ant-werpen tijdens het beleg in 1832 (The Military Medical Service on the Citadel of Antwerp during the siege in 1832). *MGT, 26,* 52–66, 3 ill.

3900 STOLTZ, T. (1939). Honderd vijf en twintig jarig bestaan van den Ge-neeskundigen Dienst der Koninklijke Landmacht (125th anniversary of the Medical Service of the Royal Land-forces). *MGT, 28,* 77.

3901 [Anonym] (1940). Honderd en vijf en twintig jarig bestaan van de in-spectie van den Geneeskundigen Dienst der Landmacht (125th anniversary of the Inspection of the Medical Service of the Land-forces). *MGT*, *29*, 1–2.

3902 [   ] (1964). Herdenking van het 150-jarig bestaan van de inspectie van de militair geneeskundige dienst op 14 October 1964 in de Juliana van Stolbergkazerne te Amersfoort (Commemoration of the 150th anniversary of the Inspection of the Military Medical Service on October 14, 1964 in the Barracks "Juliana van Stolberg" at A.). *NedMGT*, *17*, 353–67, 7 ill.

3903 SCHRAM, J. J. L. J. (1964). Militaire keuringen 150 jaar geleden en nu (Military medical examinations 150 years ago and now). *NedMGT*, *17*, 368–71.

3904 ROMEYN, D. (1913). Der militär-Sanitätsdienst in Niederland vor hundert Jahren. *Janus, XVIII*, 477–506.

3905 MEERBEECK, Lucienne van (1956–1959). Le Service sanitaire de l'Armée espagnole des Pays-Bas à la fin du XVIme et au XVIIme siècle). *Rev. int. d'Hist. Militaire*, *5*, 479–93, ill.

3906 BRANGER, J. D. (1964). De dienst militair röntgenologisch borstonderzoek in de periode 1954–1964 (The Service of military X-ray examination of the chest during the period — —). *NedMGT*, *17*, 312–6, fig.

3907 BOTENGA, S. P. (1964). De wording en ontwikkeling van de strijd tegen de tuberculose bij de Koninklijke Land- en Luchtmacht (The origin and development of the fight against tuberculosis in the Royal Land- and Air Forces). *NedMGT.*, *17*, 179–86.

3908 DEKKER, A. A. (1964). De ontwikkeling van de militair tandheelkundige verzorging (The development of military dental care) *NedMGT*, *17*, 303–7, 4 ill.

3909 KROEZE, R. C. (1964). Iets over de historie van de Milva geneeskundige dienst (Something on the history of the Women's Military Medical Service). *NedMGT*, *17*, 308–12, ill.
   – Milva: Military Women's Section.

3910 BRAAK, A. J. (1964). De geschiedenis van de militair veterinaire dienst in Nederland en in Nederlands Oost-Indië, van 1815 tot heden (History of the military veterinary service in the Netherlands and in the Dutch East Indies, from 1815 up tot the present). *NedMGT*, *17*, 297–303, ill.

3911 STIGTER, H. (1964). De ontwikkeling van de Geneeskundige Dienst bij de Luchtstrijdkrachten (The development of the Medical Service of the Air Forces). *NedMGT, 17*, 271–80.

3912 WERFF, J. van der (1957, 1958). Uniformen en officieren van de geneeskundige dienst van het Nederlandse leger in verleden en heden (Uniforms and officers of the medical service of the Dutch Army past and present). *NedMGT, 10*, 389–98, 1 col. pl., 1 ill; *ibid., 11*, 20–9; 49–58; 147–55; 205–14; 235–48.

> See also 1972–92 (military surgeons and physicians), 2727–32 (Antiquity), 3807, 3809, 4725, 4632n., 5075.

E. Surinam and the Dutch Antilles; Africa

3913 KARBAAT, J. (1963). De bijdrage van de MGD aan de opbouw van Suriname (The contribution of the Military Medical Service to the upbuilding of Surinam). *Mil. Spectator, 132*, 235.

3914 — (1964). De invloed van de militair geneeskundige dienst op de ontwikkeling van de openbare gezondheidszorg in Suriname. I. en II. (Influence of the military medical service on the development of public health in Surinam). *NedMGT, 17*, 165–71, ill.; 193–200, facs.

3915 — (1964). De historie van de militair geneeskundige dienst in Suriname (History of the military medical service in Surinam). *NedMGT, 17*, 273–80, 4 ill.

3916 — (1964). *Sociaal-geneeskundige beschouwingen over de personeelsleden van de troepenmacht in Suriname en hun gezinnen* (Socio-medical observations on the personnel of the medical troops in S. and their families). Thesis University Leiden (Supervisor: P. Muntendam). 242 pp., ill. Broos, Amsterdam.
– with some historical pictures.

3917 — (1960). 200 jaar Militair Hospitaal in Paramaribo (1760–1960) (200 years Military Hospital at P.). *NedMGT, 13*, 355–64, 4 ill.

3918 HANEVELD, G. T. (1964). De geschiedenis van de militair geneeskundige dienst op de Nederlandse Antillen (History of the military medical service on the Dutch Antilles). *NedMGT, 17*, 281–6, ill.

3919 WILKENS, J. Th. (1964). De Geneeskundige Dienst van het Konink-

lijk Nederlands Indische Leger (The Medical Service of the Royal
Dutch Indies Army). *NedMGT, 17*, 268–70.

3920   KARBAAT, J. (1964). De Militair Geneeskundige Dienst in Afrika
(The Military Medical Service in Africa). *NedMGT, 17*, 372–7, ill.

F. Hospitals

3921   ROMEYN, J. A. (1913). Hoe het er voor 200 jaren in de garnizoenshospi-
talen uitzag (On the situation in the military hospitals 200 years ago).
MGT, 17, 25–31.

3922   LIJFERING, K. A. (1964). Het gewestelijk militair hospitaal te Assen,
in de loop der tijden (The regional military hospital at A. in the course
of time). *NedMGT, 17*, 327–30, ill.

3923   SCHMELZER, L. (1964). Het militair Sanatorium te Amersfoort (The
military Sanatorium at A.). *NedMGT, 17*, 339–41.

3924   HOLST, J. G. E. van (1964). Het gewestelijk militair hospitaal te Amersfoort (The regional military hospital at A.) *NedMGT, 17*, 330–1.

3925   SIEMENS, J. L., J. D. BRANGER and A. M. LATERVEER [1949]. *Ter herdenking van het 60-jarig bestaan van de Militaire Ziekeninrichting
te Arnhem* (In commemoration of the 60th anniversary of the Military
Hospital at A.) 76 pp., ill. Uitgave van Mil. Ziekeninrichting, Arnhem.

3926   DUYN, P. den (1964). Het gewestelijke militair hospitaal Arnhem door
twee eeuwen heen (The regional military hospital at A. through two
centuries). *NedMGT, 17*, 323–7, ill.

3927   BROEK, P. van den (1964). Militaire Hospitalen in de Hofstad (Military
Hospitals in the Court Capital [The Hague]). *NedMGT, 17*, 321–3.

3928   PENNING, C. P. J. (1941). Het voormalige militair hospitaal te Harderwijk en iets over het koloniaal werfdepot en de eerste 500 hervisitatiën
van 1843–1866. (The former military hospital at H. and something on
the colonial recruiting depot and the first 500 re-visitations from — —).
NTG, 85, I, 876–83; *BGG, XXI*, 25–32.

3929   BOERMAN, J. (1964). Korte geschiedenis van het oude militaire hospi-
taal Springweg (Short history of the old military hospital Springweg).
NedMGT, 17, 316–20, 4 ill.
– On the "Duitsche Huis" at Utrecht.

3930 PRAAG, S. W. van (1938). Een nieuw Militair Hospitaal te Utrecht (A new Military Hospital at U.). *MGT, 27,* 81–5, 4 ill.

3931 BOERMAN, J. (1964). Geschiedenis van de Militair Geneeskundige Dienst. Militair Hospitaal Dr. A. Mathijsen (History of the Military service. Military hospital — —). *NedMGT, 17,* 121–3.

3932 — (1968). Het geestelijk-sociaal verzorgingscentrum in het Militair Hospitaal "Dr. A. Mathijsen" (The mental-social care-centre in the Military Hospital — —). *NedMGT, 21,* 117–9.

3933 BERG, T. van den (1964). Het militair revalidatie-centrum (The military revalidation centre). *NedMGT, 17,* 337–9.

G. Pharmacy

3934 STADELMANN von ESCHOLMATT, J. H. (1964). De geschiedenis van de militair pharmaceutische dienst (History of the military pharmaceutical service). *NedMGT, 17,* 287–91, fig.

3935 ITALLIE, E. J. van (1938). Uit de geschiedenis der militaire pharmacie in Nederland (From the history of military pharmacy in the Netherlands). *Ph. W., 75,* no 37, 46.

3936 GRENDEL, E. (1966). Enkele kanttekeningen bij de geschiedenis van de militaire apothekers in Nederland (Some marginal notes to the history of the military apothecaries in the Netherlands). *Ph. W., 101,* 187–92, 3 ill; also in: *Bull Pharm.,* no 36, 13–8.

3937 KOSTER, I. (1917/18). Het Rijks-magazijn van geneesmiddelen (The State storehouse for drugs). *Onze neutraliteit, 2,* no 2, 265–70.

3938 STEKELENBURG, N. J. (1964). Het Rijksmagazijn van geneesmiddelen (The State storehouse for drugs). *NedMGT, 17,* 332–6, 3 ill.

H. Transport and nursing

3939 KROMHOUT, J. H. (1877). *La voiture – tente – ambulance.* La Haye. f°.
3940 PUTTERS, H. (1964). Het gewondenvervoer in de loop der tijden (The transport of wounded persons in the course of time). *NedMGT, 17,* 377–81, ill.

3941 MENSONIDES, P. C. (1908). Het draagbaar spoorwegmaterieel aange-
wend ten dienste van het vervoer van zieken en gewonden in oorlogs-
tijd (The portable railway-material applied for the use of the transport
of the sick and wounded in war time). *MGT, 12*, 57–116.

3942 JURRIAANSE, A. (1902). *Veldambulances en wondbehandeling* (Field-
ambulances and treatment of wounds). Thesis University Leiden. Leiden.

3943 WINTERS, V. M. E. (1931). *Oorlog en heelkunde. Bijdrage tot de kennis
der oorlogschirurgie.* I. Transport van gewonden. II. Wondbehandeling
(War and surgery. Contribution to the knowledge of war surgery. I.
Transport of wounded persons. II. Treatment of wounds). Thesis
University Amsterdam. ill. Kerkrade. 8°.

3944 SALM, A. J. (1917). De oorsprong der ambulances bij de legers en van
het Roode Kruis (Origin of the ambulances of the armies and of the
Red Cross). *NTG, 61*, I, 117–20.
  – letters to the editor (with same title): by E. C. van Leersum: *Ibid.*, 407–8; by T.
  Kuiper: *ibid.*, 408–9; by D. L. Stibbe: *ibid.*, 571.

3945 ROMEYN, D. (1900). Met de 1ste Nederlandse Roode Kruis-ambulance
naar Zuid-Afrika. Terugblik. (With the first Dutch Red Cross ambulance to South-Africa. A retrospective view). *MGT, 4*, 212–32.

3946 RIJKENS, R. G. (1900). De verpleging der gewonden in den oorlog
(Nursing of wounded persons in the war). *Natuur, XX*, 23, 59, 68, 112
and 138.

3947 KRUL, R. (1903). Voor onze zieke en gekwetste soldaten. Oprakeling
uit Hage's geschiedenis (For our sick and wounded soldiers. Digging
up the history of The Hague). *Tijdspiegel, II*, 288.

3948 GEYL, A. (1909). Vorschläge zu organisierter Hilfe für Verwundete
und Kranke in Kriegszeiten während der letzten Hälfte des 18. Jahrhunderts. *Arch. Gesch. Mediz., II*, 101–12.

3949 STEEN van OMMEREN, L. van den (1916). Overzicht van den vooruitgang in de verpleging te velde en in de militaire hospitalen in de afgelopen 25 jaren (Survey of the progress of nursing in the field and in
the military hospitals in the last 25 years). Amsterdam.
  – Reprint of: Herdenkingsbundel van het *T. v. Ziekenverpleging.*

3950 KOPPERT, G. (1965). Van houten krib tot stalen bedspiraal (From
wooden crib to steel bedspiral). *NedMGT, 18*, 284–7, 5 ill.

I. Nutrition

3951 SOLY, H. (1971). Een Antwerpse Compagnie voor de levensmiddelen-
bevoorrading van het leger in de Nederlanden in de zestiende eeuw
eeuw (An Antwerp company for supplying provisions for the army in
the Netherlands in the 16th century). *Bijdr. Gesch.*, *86*, 350–62, 67 refs.

3952 JULIUS, C. F. (1901). Een en ander over voeding (Something on nutrition). *Org. Ver. ter beoef. krijgswtsch.*, Verslag 1900–01, 7. Den Haag.

3953 KRUL, W. F. J. M. (1921). Drinkwaterzuivering bij de oorlogvoerende
legers (Water purification in the belligerent armies). *Polyt. Wbl.*,
no 46.

J. Red Cross

3954 VERSPYCK MIJNSSEN, J. C. (1915/16). Ontstaan en werking van het
informatiebureau van het Nederlandse Rode Kruis (Origin and functioning of the inquiry office of the Dutch Red Cross). *Org. Ver. beoef.
Krijgswtsch.*, 303–39.

3955 [   ] (1959). *Ontstaan en ontwikkeling van het Rode Kruis* (Origin
and development of the Red Cross). Ned. Roode Kruis.

3956 QUANJER, A. A. J. (1917). Het Nederlandsche Roode Kruis (The
Dutch Red Cross). *Eigen Haard, XLIII*, 505.

3957 MANDERE, H. Ch. G. J. van der (1917). *Geschiedenis van het Nederlandsche Roode Kruis 1867 – 19 Juli – 1917* (History of the Dutch Red
Cross — —). ill. Amsterdam. 8°.
– with a foreword by A. A. J. Quanjer.

3958 — (1921). *Het Nederlandsche Roode Kruis van 1917–1920* (The Dutch
Red Cross from — —). ill. Amsterdam. 8°.

3959 LINDEBOOM, G. A. (1940). Het Roode Kruis (The Red Cross). *Stemmen des Tijds, 29*, 47–55.

3960 BEELAERTS van BLOKLAND, H. (1947). *Enkele hoofdpunten uit de geschiedenis van het Nederlandsche Roode Kruis* (Some main points from
the history of the Dutch Red Cross). Den Haag.

3961 ROMBACH, J. H. (1967). Nederlanders en het Rode Kruis (The Dutch and the Red Cross). *Spiegel Historiael*, 2, 466–74, ill.

3962 VERSPYCK, G. M. (1967). *Het Nederlandsche Roode Kruis (1867–1967)* (The Dutch Red Cross). XIV + 392 pp., ill. no pl.

See also 5414, 5415

Chapter xv

Preventive Medicine and Public Health

For a long time preventive medicine remained restricted to variolation and vaccination against smallpox.

For centuries the care of public health was mainly a matter of municipal governments. Later on the provinces appointed a provincial medical supervisor (archiater) who, for example, had to advise in case of epidemics. Moreover, sometimes special medical care was provided by the province: Paulus de Wind was lithotomist of Zealand.

Under the French rule a strong tendency to centralisation became apparent, the local guilds being liquidated. In the earlier nineteenth century local and regional committees of medical supervision were set up, and in 1865 state medical supervision was regulated by the laws of the famous liberal statesman Thorbecke (1798–1872).

In most cities there were hospitals, orphanages and almshouses for elderly people. In the eighteenth century sick-funds are already heard of.

Already in the fifteenth century in some towns there was supervision of the quality of food. In the towns where no rain- or pumpwater was available in sufficient quantity, reliable drinking water was often not easily obtainable. The water of the canals into which sewers drained was sometimes used. The custom of burying in the churches was abandoned gradually in the nineteenth century.

On the whole our knowledge of the early history of hygiene and public health is still poor.

A. Preventive medicine

Variolation and vaccination

3963 PENNING, C. P. J. (1940). Lady Mary Worthley Montagu en de variolatie (— — — and variolation). *NTG, 84*, I, 41–8; *BGG, XX*, 8–15, port.

3964 HOGENDORP, W. van (1779, 1921). *Geneeskundige propagandageschriften* (Medical propaganda-writings). 114 pp., port. Reprint Javasche Boekhandel & Drukkerij, Batavia.
– for the promotion of variolation.

3965 EPKEMA, E. (1906). Inenting (1785). (Variolation). *Gelre, IX,* 304.

3966 HOEVEN, J. van der (1921). Letters of Thomas Schwenke on the inoculation of smallpox. *Janus, XXV,* 325.

3967 — (1921). Eenige brieven van Thomas Schwencke over de inoculatie der kinderpokken (Some letters of — — on the inoculation of smallpox). *NTG, 65,* I, 1258–62; *BGG, I,* 109–13.

3968 PINKHOF, H. (1929). Galante propaganda voor de inoculatie (Gallant propaganda for inoculation). *NTG, 73,* II, 3588; *BGG, IX,* 200.

3969 DOOREN, L. (1937). Verbod van vaccinatie in 1785 te Zaltbommel (Prohibition of vaccination [variolation] in 1785 at Z.). *GG, 15,* 1225.

3970 PUTTO, J. A. (1937). Verbod van inenten tegen pokken in 's-Gravenhage in 1765 (Prohibition of inoculation against smallpox at The Hague in 1765). *GG, 15,* 1129.

3970ᵃ WIERSUM, E. van (1933). Briefwisseling Rotterdam-Kaapstad over de inenting (Correspondence R. – Cape Town on vaccination) *Rott. Jbk., 24* (vierde reeks, N.S. I), 7–11 (with port. of S. de Monchy).
– between S. de Monchy (1716–94). and R. Tulbagh, governor of the Cape Colony 1751–71).

See also 887, 1286

3971 POSTMA, C. (1951). Bijdrage tot de geschiedenis van de koepokinenting in Nederland (Contribution to the history of vaccination in the Netherlands). *NTG, 95,* II, 1377–80; *BGG, XXXI,* 19–22.
– The extensive narrative does not concern vaccination (as the title suggests), but inoculation.

3972 PLESSER-GINZBURG, R. (1967). Een 18e eeuws responsum over de inenting tegen pokken (An 18th century responsum by Salomo Saruco on vaccination). *Stud. Rosenthaliana* (Assen), *I,* 107–9.

3973 STEEGE, J. van der (1779, 1921). *Bericht nopens den aart der kinderziekten te Batavia tot hoe verre men met de inenting derzelve gevorderd is en wat daarbij is waargenomen* (Piece of information concerning the character of children's diseases at B., on the progress of their variolation and what has been observed). 58 pp., Batavia.
– Reprint 1921.

3974 CAPADOSE, A. (1823). *Bestrijding der vaccine, of vaccine aan de begin-selen der godsdienst, der rede en der ware geneeskunde getoetst* (Fight against vaccine, or vaccine tested to the principles of religion, of sense and of true medicine). XVI + 330 + IV pp. Sulpke, Amsterdam.
– The author was against vaccination, not only on medical, but also on religious grounds.

3975 — (1825). *Ernstige en herhaalde waarschuwing ... tegen de ongeoorloof-de en verderfelijke koepokinenting ...* (Serious and repeated warning ... against the unallowed and pernicious vaccination...) XII + 185 + I pp. J. H. den Ouden, Amsterdam.

3976 HEUSDEN, A. J. M. van (1824). *Verdediging der vaccine tegen de bestrij-ding van A. Capadose* (Defence of vaccine against the fight of —). IV + 89 + II pp., W. van Vergen & Co, Breda.

3977 BERG, H. van den (1896). *Edward Jenner en zijn tijd, benevens de ge-schiedenis der vaccinatie* (E. J. and his time, and the history of vacci-nation). 47 pp. L. A. Laurey, Haarlem.
– The author was director of the "parc vaccinogène" at Haarlem.

3978 [Esculaap] (pseudonym) (no d.). *Jenner en de vaccinatie. Eenige ver-bijsterende hoofdstukken uit de geschiedenis der geneeskunde. Een boek voor Arts en Leek* (J. and vaccination. Some bewildering chapters from the history of medicine. A book for physician and layman). 409 pp., ill. De Anti-vivisectie Stichting, Den Haag.

3979 PEYPERS, H. F. A. (1900). Jenner, Benjamin Jesty et les découvertes simultanées de la vaccination. *Janus, V*, 580–3, port. (of Jesty).

3980 DANIËLS, C. E. (1896). Edward Jenner. Rede gehouden ter herdenking van den 14den Mei 1796, den dag waarop Edw. Jenner de eerste koe-pok-inenting van arm op arm verricht heeft (E.J. Address delivered in commemoration of 14th May 1796, the day when J. did the first vacci-nation from arm to arm). *NTG, 32*, 2de reeks: I, 789–806, ill., port.

3981 — (1896). Twee spotprenten betreffende de vaccinatie (Two caricatures concerning vaccination). *NTG*, 2de reeks, *34*, I, 807–8.

3982 HALBERTSMA, K. T. A. (1946). *Edward Jenner en de ontdekking der vaccinatie* (E.J. and the discovery of vaccination). port. Delft. 8°.
– Address.

3983 RIJKENS, R. G. (1913). Uit de geschiedenis der koepokinenting (From the history of vaccination). *Natuur, XXIII*, 161.

3984   DROGENDIJK, A. C. (1937). Grepen uit de geschiedenis der pokken en hun bestrijding (Analecta from the history of small-pox and the fight against it), *GG, 15*, 595–604; 691–701; 750–60; 763–73.

3984ᵃ VERJAAL, A. (1973). De geschiedenis van de pokkenvaccinatie (History of small-pox vaccination). *GeWiNa*, no 32, 5–6.

3985   KLEIJ, J. J. van der (1930). Pokken in vroeger tijd: de inenting (Small-pox in former times: vaccination). *NTG, 74*, I, 1084–91; *BGG, X*, 73–80.

3986   ANDEL, M. A. van (1932). De ontdekking der vaccinatie (The discovery of vaccination). *NTG, 76*, III, 3308; *BGG, XII*, 140.

3987   LINT, J. G. de (1932). De ontdekking der vaccinatie (The discovery of vaccination). *NTG, 76*, III, 3867–8; and 4242; *BGG, XII*, 155–6.

3988   IDSINGA, J. (1899). Mededeelingen omtrent Koepok-Inenting in Nederland, gedurende de laatste vijftig jaren (Communications concerning vaccination in the Netherlands, during the last fifty years). *Alers et al.*, 135–44.

3989   SANDRA, H. (1937). Sprokkelingen betreffende de inenting tegen pokken in ons land omstreeks 1800 (Gleanings concerning the vaccination in our country about 1800). *NTG, 81*, II, 2644–52; *BGG, XVII*, 103–11.

3990   PUTTO, J. A. (1937). Stuipen na inenting tegen pokken voor ruim honderd jaar? (Convulsions after vaccination a good hundred years ago?). *GG, 15*, 13–5.

3991   EIJKEL, R. N. M. (1938). Napoleon I en de vaccinatie tegen de pokken (— and vaccination against smallpox). *GG, 16*, 936.

3992   PUTTO, J. A. (1938). De bevordering der inenting tegen pokken onder de regering van Koning Lodewijk Napoleon (The promotion of vaccination under the reign of King — —). *GG, 16*, 369–71.

3993   PINKHOF, H. (1912). Een Amsterdamsch inentingsmanifest in 1808 (An Amsterdam vaccination-manifesto in 1808). *NTG, 56*, I, 1584.

3994   VIEYRA, D. (1936). Het aandeel van twee Amsterdamsche geneeskundigen in de inenting met "Koeipokstof" in 1800 (The part of two Amsterdam physicians in the vaccination with vaccine in 1800). *NTG, 80* III, 4325–30; *BGG, XVI*, 171–6.
– A. M. Valencijn van de Lande and H. de H. Lemon (*ca* 1750–1823).

3995 BITTER, H. (1916). Pokken en inenting te Amsterdam vóór ruim 100 jaar (Smallpox and vaccination at A. a good 100 years ago). *NTG, 60*, I, 1291–6.

3996 VELDHUYZEN, W, F. [1957]. *Honderd en vijftig jaar pokkenpreventie.* De geschiedenis van het Amsterdamsch Genootschap ter bevordering der koepokinenting voor minvermogenden 1803–1953 (Hundred and fifty years of smallpox prevention. History of the Amsterdam Association for the promotion of vaccination for the poor —). 85 pp., facs. Scheltema & Holkema, Amsterdam.
– After Veldhuyzen's death in 1954 Th. H. Schlichting finished the book.

3997 BRONDGEEST, P. Q. (1896). *De koepokinenting te Utrecht 14 Mei 1796 – 14 Mei 1896* (The vaccination at U.). Utrecht.

3998 HALLEMA, A. (1933). Eenige wettelijke bepalingen betreffende de vaccine-therapie voor sociaal-behoeftigen een eeuw geleden in Friesland (Some provisions concerning the vaccination therapy for the poor in F. a century ago). *NTG, 77*, II, 2526–31; *BGG, XIII*, 151–6, 1 ill., port.

3999 VELDHUYZEN, W. F. (1954). Het Amsterdamsch Genootschap ter bevordering der koepokinenting van minvermogenden (1 November 1803 – 1 November 1953) (The Amsterdam Society for the promotion of vaccination of the poor). *NTG, 98*, III, 2514–20; *BGG, XXXIV*, 66–72, 1 ill.
– with pictures of two medals.

4000 TESCH, J. W. (1956). Genootschap ter Bevordering der Koepokinenting, Rotterdam. Onder de zinspreuk: ne pestis intret vigila (Society for the Promotion of vaccination. Under the device — — —). *NTG, 100*, IV, 3454–8; *BGG, XXXVI*, 73–7.

4000ª GADEYNE, G. (1972). De maatregelen ter bevordering van de vaccinatie uitgevaardigd door het centraal bestuur in het Schelde-departement (1800–1814) (Measures for the promotion of vaccination issued by the Central Board in the Schelde department —). *Ann. Gesch. Oudhk. Kring Ronse*, 217–28.

4001 BURG, C. L. van der (1905). Contribution à l'histoire de la vaccination aux Indes orientales néerlandaises. *Janus, X*, 24–8.

4002 SCHOUTE, D. (1942). De reis van Jenner's koepokstof van Europa naar Oost-Azië (The voyage of J.'s vaccine from Europe to East Asia). *NTG, 86*, III, 2229–33; *BGG, XXII*, 117–21.

4003   OUDSCHANS DENTZ, Fr. (1943). Maatregelen tegen de pokken en de toepassing van Jenner's koepokstof in Suriname in het begin van de 19e eeuw (Measures against smallpox and the application of J.'s vaccine in Surinam in the beginning of the 19th century). *NTG, 87,* II, 1090–1; *BGG, XXIII,* 53–4.

> See also 486, 1678, 1679, 1744, 1965, 2743, 3211–20 (smallpox), 3831, 5371, 5372, 5383, 5395, 5396, 5414.

B. Public health

General – rehabilitation

4004   GILS, J. B. F. van (1940). Gezondheidszorg in "Utopia" (Public health in —). *NTG, 84,* III, 3510–6; *BGG, XX,* 137–43.

– cf: letter to the editor with same title by Th. H. Schlichting: *NTG, 84,* IV, 3903; *BGG, XX,* 160.

4005   HEKMAN, J. (1930). Ziekenzorg in Nederland (Care of the sick in the Netherlands). *G&W,* 54–77.

4006   ROGIER, L. J. (1961). *Een kwarteeuw geestelijke en lichamelijke gezondheidszorg* (25 years of mental and physical public health). Ubbergen – Nijmegen.

– Memorial volume published on the occasion of the 25th anniversary of the St. Maarten's clinic and the Pedological Institution at Ubbergen.

4007   ZWAN, A. van der (1964–1966). Uit de geschiedenis der geneeskunde (From the history of medicine). II, III and IV. De zieke (The patient) *Gezondheidszorg, 56,* 12 dec., 6–11, 3 ill; *57,* 1 jan. 3–6, ill.; *57,* 2 febr., 5–8. V and VI. De zenuwzieke (The mental patient) *57,* 12 dec., 2–8, 2 ill; *58* (1966), 1 jan.; VII and VIII. De stervende (The dying person) *58,* no 2, 2–7; no 3, 2–3.

4007ᵃ REMIJNSE, J. G. (1939). *De Sociale Geneeskunde en de artsen* (Social Medicine and the physicians). 24 pp. Oosthoek, Utrecht.

– inaugural address, 13 november 1939; J.G.R. (1878–1971), originally a surgeon, was the second professor of social medicine in the Netherlands.

4008   QUERIDO, A. (1968). *The development of socio-medical care in the Netherlands.* IX + 118 pp. Routledge & Paul, London; Humanities Press, New York.

> See also 551–4 (Coronel), 2743, 5022, 5054, 5163a, 5165

4009 VENEMA, F. B. (1962). The development of rehabilitation services in the Netherlands. *Rehabilitation*, no 43, 37–41.

4010 MULDER, R. D. (1963). Volksgezondheid en volksaard in Drenthe in de eerste helft van de 19e eeuw (Public health and national character in D. in the first half of the 19th century). *Nieuwe Drentse Volksalmanak, 81*, 48–74.

4011 VERDOORN, J. A. (1965). *Volksgezondheid en sociale ontwikkeling. Beschouwingen over het gezondheidswezen te Amsterdam in de 19de eeuw* (Public health and social development. Observations on sanitation at A. in the 19th century). 449 pp., 16 fig. Het Spectrum, Utrecht-Amsterdam. Aula boeken, no 199.

Statistics

4012 HAAKSMA TRESLING, J. (1901). Herinneringen aan een oud register en een terugblik op de medische statistiek van Nederland in de vorige eeuw (Memories of an old register and a retrospective view on medical statistics of the Netherlands in the last century). *NTG*, 2de reeks *37*, II, 518.

4013 ZEEMAN, J. (1899). Sterfte-statistiek (Statistics of mortality). *Alers et al.*, 181–93.

4014 DROOGLEVER FORTUYN, H. J. W. (1924). De sterftelijn in de laatste driekwart eeuw (Statistics of mortality in the last three-fourths century). *NTG, 68*, II, 53–63; *BGG, IV*, 176–86.

4015 HOOGENDOORN, D. (1973). De statistiek van de doodsoorzaken in 1901 en in 1970 (Statistics of the causes of death in 1901 and in 1970). *NTG, 117*, 1003–6.

4016 VIEYRA, D. (1936). Honden, inenting en geboortelijsten in Amsterdam in het jaar 1796. Adres van het Collegium Medicum (Dogs, vaccination and birth lists at A., 1796. Address of the — —). *NTG, 80*, II, 2618–21; *BGG, XVI*, 91–4.

4017 HAAS, J. H. de (1968). 75 jaar zuigelingensterfte (75 years of infant mortality). *NTG, 112*, 248.

4018 DUPAQUIER, J. (1965). Evolution démographique et progrès économique aux Pays Bas: vue perspective. *Ann. Démog. hist.* (Etud. et Chron.), 199–226.
  – Analysis of a paper by J. A. Faber *et al.*

See also 4992, 5050, 5067–8, 5073

Poor relief, sick-fund system, municipal health care

4019 HELLINGA, G. (1932). De geschiedenis der geneeskundige armverzorging buiten de gasthuizen te Amsterdam (History of the medical poor relief outside the hospitals at A.) *NTG*, *76*, IV, 4219–35; *BGG, XII*, 157–73 and *NTG*, *77* (1933), 528–43; *BGG, XIII*, 37–52.

See also 4634

4020 PUTTO, J. A. (1936). Geneeskundige armverzorging onder de Bataafsche Republiek (Medical poor relief under the Batavian Republic). *GG*, *14*, 44–7.

4021 SAUER, H. C. (1935). *Geneeskundige Verzorging van den minvermogenden zieke in Nederland* (Medical care of the poor in the Netherlands). 165 pp. H. J. Paris, Amsterdam.
– Chapter I. History (from Middle Ages up to the present).

4022 VOORST van BEEST, C. van (1955). *De Katholieke Armenzorg te Rotterdam in de 17e en 18e eeuw* (The Roman-catholic poor relief at R. in the 17th and 18th century). Thesis. 148 pp. Den Haag.

4023 PHILIPS, Grete (1969). Brugse armenzorg in de 16de eeuw (Poor relief at Bruges in the 16th century). *Spiegel Historiael*, *4*, 19–24, 8 ill.

4024 BERGER, J. A. [no d.] *De geschiedenis van het Ziekenfondswezen in Nederland* (History of the Sick-Fund System in the Netherlands). 207 pp., F. vande Velde, Vlissingen.

4025 DROGENDIJK, A. C. (1948). Wettelijke regeling van het ziekenfondswezen in het verleden (Legal regulation of the sick-fund system in the past). *Ziekenfondsgids*, *2*, 76–80; 89–95; 144–7; 155–9.

4026 — (1951). Uit het verleden van het ziekenfondswezen (From the past pf the sick-fund system). *Soc. Zorg*, *13*, 5 maart.

4027 — (1962). Ontstaan, groei en ontwikkeling van het ziekenfondswezen (Origin, growth and development of the sick-fund system). *Ziekenfondsgids*, *16*, 48–53.

4028 GODEFROI, L. S. (1963). *Het ziekenfondswezen in Nederland. Ontwikkeling en perspectieven* (Sick-fund system in the Netherlands. Development and perspectives). X + 264 pp. M. Nijhoff, Den Haag.
– Geschriften Prof. Mr. B. M. Teldersstichting, no 10.

4029 LEDEBOER, L. V. (1958). Medical care insurance in the Netherlands. *Bull. int. Soc. Secur. Ass.*, *11*, 397–413.

4030 — (ed.) (1960). *Kort overzicht van de ontwikkeling van de Nederlandse ziekenfondsverzekering* (Short survey of the development of Dutch medical care insurance). 55 pp. Amsterdam.

4031 PUTTO, J. A. (1964). Zorg voor ziekte en ongeval vóórdat onze sociale verzekeringswetten van kracht werden (Care of disease and accident before our laws of social insurance came into force.) *GG*, *42*, 161–2.

4032 WIBAUT, F. (1951). Een ziekenfonds ten plattenlande in 1785 (A sick-fund in the country in —). *MC*, *6*, 94–106.
– With photostatic reprint of the regulations of the sick-fund of Tienhoven and Oud-Maarseveen.

4033 DAM, C. van (1965). De ziekenfondsen in de Zaanstreek (The sick-funds in the "Zaan-region". *Noord-Holland*, *10*, 83–8.

4034 NIEUWENHUIZEN, J. P. van (1965). De geneeskundige praeventie in de Zaanstreek (Medical prevention in the "Zaan-region"). *Noord-Holland*, *10*, 88–92.

4035 BERGER, J. A. (1930). Een rapport omtrent het ziekenfondswezen in Amsterdam in 1842 (A report concerning the sick-fund system at A. in —). *NTG*, *74*, I, 2259–61; *BGG*, *X*, 138–40.

4036 — (1931). Een rapport over het Ziekenfondswezen in 1849 (A report on the sick-fund system in —). *NTG*, *75*, II, 1792–1806; *BGG*, *XI*, 115–29.

4037 ABEELEN, E. L. J. van den (1946–50?). Een en ander uit de Geschiedenis van het Haagse Ziekenfondswezen (Something from the History of the The Hague Sick-Fund System). 20 articles: *Ziekenfonds*, *20*, (1946), 11–2; 24–5; 56–7; 73, 76; 87–8; 112. *21* (1947), 24–5; 27; 76; 91–2; 99–100. *22* (1948), 8; 16; 23–4; 32; 40; 59–60; 74; 90; 122–3.
– The series has been continued

4038 ROMIJN, W. (1955). *Welvaart en Gezondheid* (Welfare and Health). 301 pp. De Beursdrukkerij, Amsterdam.
– Published on the occasion of the 60th anniversary of the general sick-fund "Ziekenzorg" at Amsterdam.

4039 HALLEMA, A. (1941). Iets over organisatie van de geneeskundige dienst en de inrichting der zogenaamde medische politie ten plattelande gedurende de 18e eeuw (Something on the organisation of medical service and the structure of the so-called medical police in the country during the 18th century). *NTG, 85*, III, 3608–14; *BGG, XXI*, 100–6.

4039ᵃ WITTOP KONING, D. A. (1951). Het 50-jarig bestaan van de Gemeentelijke Geneeskundige Gezondheidsdienst (The 50th anniversary of the municipal medical health service). *Amstelodamum, 38*, 26–7.
  – at Amsterdam.

4039ᵇ SMULDERS, A. J. M. (1974). De Gemeente en de gezondheidszorg. Verleden, heden, toekomst (The Municipality and public health care. Past, present, future). *MC, 29*, 1205–16, 14 ill.
  – Address delivered May 1974 on the occasion of the silver jubilee of A. J. M. Smulders, medical superintendent of the municipal medical and health service at Breda.

4040 PUTTO, J. A. (1960). De GG en GD van 's-Gravenhage onder zijn eerste directeur (The municipal medical and health service of The Hague under its first director). *GG, 38*, 193–8.
  – Dr. G. W. Boland (?–1938).

4041 [Anonym] (1965). 50 jaar G.G. en G.D. in Utrecht (Fifty years of Municipal medical service and public health service at U.) *Voeding, 26*, 564–5.

Drinking-water and food

4042 HALBERTSMA, H. P. N. (1899). Historische schets der drinkwaterleidingen in Nederland (Historical sketch of the drinking-waterworks in the Netherlands. *Alers et al.*, 158–63.

4043 LINDEBOOM, G. A. (1946). Over de drinkwatervoorziening in Nederland (On the drinking-water supply in the Netherlands). *Stemmen des Tijds, 35*, maart, 222–36.

4044 HERMANS, A. G. J. (1962). Water en waterleidingbedrijven (Water and water companies). *NTG, 106*, I, 483–4; *BGG, XLII*, 15–6.

4045 WITTOP KONING, D. A. (1960). Het drinkwateronderzoek door de Maatschappij in 1843 (The examination of drinking-water by the [Pharmaceutical] Association). *PhW., 95*, 770–4.

4046 DANIELS, C. E. (1899). Het drinkwater in Amsterdam (The drinking water at A.). *Alers et al.*, 66–8.

4047 BARNOUW, P. J. (1899). Baden en zwemmen (Bathing and swimming). *Alers et al.*, 54–7.

4048 DHONT, (1899). Abattoirs en vleeschkeuring (Abattoirs and meat inspection). *Alers et al.*, 173–6.

4049 REICHER, L. Th. (1899). Een en ander over de keuring van voedingsmiddelen in Nederland gedurende de laatste vijftig jaren (Something on the inspection of articles of food in the Netherlands during the last fifty years). *Alers et al.*, 145–9.

4050 HARDON, H. J. (1958). Het begin van het overheidstoezicht op voedingsmiddelen in 1858 (The beginning of the State-supervision of articles of food in —). *Voeding, 19*, 283–92.

4051 ANDEL, M. A. (1912). Onze gemeentelijke keuringsdienst over vier eeuwen (Our municipal food-inspection department during four centuries). *Nieuwe Gorinchemse Courant*, 8 December.

See also 3953

C. Hygiene

General

4052 HEEDERIK, G. J. (1959). Hygiëne in oude tijden (Hygiene in ancient times). *Voeding, 20*, 185–9.

4053 CEUSTER, P. de (1961–62). Uit de geschiedenis van de hygiëne (From the history of hygiene). *Ons Heem, 16*, 1–4.

4054 SNIJDERS, A. J. C. (1903). De gezondheidsleer, voorheen en thans (Hygiene, past and present). *Tijdspiegel, III*, 238.

4055 SLOBBE, J. F. van (1937). *Bijdrage tot de geschiedenis en de bestrijding der prostitutie in Amsterdam* (Contribution to the history of and the fight against prostitution at A.). Scheltema & Holkema, Amsterdam.

4055ª LINDEBOOM, G. A. (1941). Blanke kolonisatie in Suriname, hygienisch beschouwd (White colonisation in S. hygienically considered). *Stemmen des Tijds, 30*, 575–86.

See also 754, 1445, 3814–16 (naval medicine), 4995, 5022, 5025, 5045, 5057, 5468–9.

Housing and schoolhygiene

4056 TELLEGEN, J. W. C. (1899). Arbeiderswoningen en woninghygiene in Nederland (Working-class houses and housing hygiene in the Netherlands). *Alers et al.*, 151–7.

4057 KRUSEMAN, J. (1940). *De Volkshuisvesting onder de woningwet. Geschiedkundig overzicht en herinneringen* (Housing of the people under the housing act. Historical survey and memories). Haarlem.

4057ᵃ WILLEMSEN, J. Th. W. (1969). *De Volkshuisvesting in Arnhem 1829–1925* (Housing of the people at A. — —). 144 pp., ill. Gemeentearchief, Arnhem.

4058 MOMMAAL, D. (1966). Over de huisvestingsomstandigheden ten tijde van de laatste cholera-epidemie in Nederland in 1866 (On the housing conditions at the time of the last cholera epidemic in the Netherlands, 1866). *GeWiNa*, no 20, 5–7.

4059 TUSSENBROEK, Cath. van (1899). Schoolhygiëne in Nederland (School hygiene in the Netherlands). *Alers et al*, 44–53.

4059ᵃ LOJENGA, W. J. (1942). *De hygiene van het schoolgebouw met name van het schoolgebouw ten plattelande* (Hygiene of the school-building, particularly of the rural school). Thesis Groningen. 213 pp., 55 ill. Van Gorcum, Assen.

4059ᵇ JANSEN, D. (1926). Schoolgebouw en schoolvertrek vóór 1800 (School-building and class-room before 1800). *Oudhk. Jbk.*, 3–27, ill.

4060 BERGINK, A. H. (1965). *Schoolhygiëne in Nederland in de negentiende eeuw* (School hygiene in the Netherlands in the 19th century) 136 pp., 5 ill. Marko Meubelen, Veendam. pr. pr.

4061 PUTTO, J. A. (1959). Uit de geschiedenis van de Haagse Schoolartsendienst (From the history of the School Medical Service at The Hague). *T. Soc. Geneesk.*, *37*, 421.

4062 [Anonym] (1930). Five years of municipal infant welfare, 1922–1926. Published by the Municipal health service of Amsterdam. 1 map. Amsterdam. 8°.

4063 MAAR, F. E. R. de (1965). Twintig eeuwen mondhygiene (Twenty centuries of oral hygiene). *GeWiNa*, no *18*, 16–7.

4064 SCHAGEN, K. H. and J. P. KRAMER (1968, ²1971). *Historisch overzicht van de lichamelijke opvoeding* (Historical survey of physical training). 2 vols. Nijgh & van Ditmar, 's-Gravenhage.

– Vol. I: Van de oudheid tot en met de Franse tijd (From Antiquity till the French time (S.). Voll. II: De negentiende en twintigste eeuw (The 19th and 20th century) (K.).

See also 3844

Industry

4065 RUYSCH, W. P. (1899). Nijverheidshygiëne (Industrial hygiene). *Alers et al*, 168–72.

4066 BIERSTEKER, K. (1968). Luchtverontreiniging in Haarlem in 1608 (Air pollution at H., 1608). *NTG, 112*, 33.

4067 ROMEYN, D. (1909). De regeling van de eerste hulp bij spoorwegongelukken in Nederland, voorheen en thans (The arrangement of first aid at railway-accidents in the Netherlands, past and present). *Gen. Crt.*, 8 febr., 25 juli.

Antisepsis, quarantine

4068 PEYPERS, H. F. A. (1896/97). Un ancien pseudo-précurseur de Pasteur ou le système d'un médecin anglois sur la cause de toutes les maladies (1726). *Janus, I.*, 56–66; 121–31; 251–62.

– on a critic of the hypothesis of the microbial cause of diseases.

4069 SALTET, R. H. (1899). Ontsmettingen in Nederland (Disinfections in the Netherlands). *Alers et al.*, 83–5.

4070 WEYDE, A. J. van der (1931). Ontsmetting van goederen door hooge temperatuur omstreeks 1830 (Disinfection of goods by high temperature about —). *NTG, 75*, IV, 5902–4; *BGG, XI*, 322–4.

4071 PUTTO, J. A. (1937). Quarantaine maatregelen voor twee honderd jaar (Quarantine-measures two hundred years ago). *GG, 15*, 540–2.

4072 — (1937). Quarantaine maatregelen in Nederland vóór een kleine twee honderd jaren (Quarantine-measures in the Netherlands about two hundred years ago). *GG, 15*, 1059–61.

Cemeteries

4073 WEIJDE, A. J. van der (1930). Over begraafplaatsen en begraven in het bijzonder te Utrecht (On cemeteries and burying particularly at U.). *Jbk. Oud-Utrecht*, 85–113.

4074 ROEKEL, G. van (1940). Het verzet tegen buitenbegraafplaatsen (The resistance against outside-cemeteries). *NTG, 84*, I, 839–41; *BGG, XX*, 54–6.

D. State medicine

4075 MIDDENDORP, A. A. (1878). *Het Geneeskundig Staatstoezicht en de geneeskundige stand* (Medical State supervision and medical profession). 38 pp. Scheltema & Holkema, Amsterdam.

4076 WEIJDE, A. J. van der (1923). Toezicht op de uitoefening der geneeskunde in 1817 (Supervision of the practice of medicine). *NTG, 67*, II, 902–4.

4077 BOERMA, N. J. A. F. (1938). Het ambtelijk toezicht op de artsen in de 16e eeuw (Official supervision of the physicians in the 16th century). *NTG, 82*, II, 2297; *BGG, XVIII*, 98.

4078 BERG, C. van den (1965). Een eeuw Staatstoezicht op de volksgezondheid (A century of State-supervision of public health). *T. Soc. Geneesk., 43*, 682–8.

4079 QUERIDO, A. (1965). *Een eeuw Staatstoezicht op de Volksgezondheid* (A century of State-supervision of public health). 295 pp. Staatsuitgeverij, 's-Gravenhage.

4080 STAL, P. L. [1965]. *Honderd jaar Staatstoezicht op de Volksgezondheid* (A century of State-supervision of public health). 44 pp. no pl. no d.

4081 K[UYVENHOVEN], L. M. (1965). Honderd jaar Staatstoezicht op de Volksgezondheid (A century of State-supervision of public health). *PhW., 100*, 856–9.

4082 VELDE, G. C. J. van der (1967). Gezondheidszorg te Nijmegen in de periode 1816–1865. De werkzaamheden van de "Plaatselijke Commissie van Geneeskundig Toevoorzigt" (Public health at N. during the period — —. The activities of the "local Committee of medical supervision"). *Numaga*, *14*, 5-39.

Supervision, legal measures.

4083 Dozy, J. P. (1899). Organisatie der Medische Politie, Provinciale Commissie, enz. (Organization of Medical Police, Provincial Committee, etc.). *Alers et al.*, 125-9.

4084 Juten, W. J. F. (1906). Gezondheidsmaatregelen in de 18de eeuw (Sanitary measures in the 18th century). *Taxandria, XIII*, 13.

4085 Putto, J. A. (1936). Geneeskundige staatsregeling onder de Bataafsche Republiek (Medical constitution during the Batavian Republic). *GG, 14*, 67-9.

4086 — (1936). Een plan voor geneeskundige voorziening van de commissie van geneeskundig bestuur in het departement van den Rhijn, resideerende te Arnhem, onder de Bataafsche Republiek (1802) (A plan for medical provision of the committee of medical management in the department of the Rhine, residing at A., under the Batavian Republic). *GG, 14*, 977-81.

4087 Cannegieter, D. (1954). *Honderdvijftig jaar Gezondheidswet* (Hundred and fifty years health law). Assen.

4088 Muntendam, P. (1965). Een eeuw geneeskundige wetgeving (A century of medical legislation). *NTG, 109*, 1032-3.

See also 1323a

Chapter XVI

Medical Education

Before the foundation of Leyden University (1575) there was no opportunity to study medicine in the Northern Netherlands. For that purpose the young men went to Louvain or, preferably, to Italy. In the earlier seventeenth century several Dutch doctors took their degree in one of the northern Italian universities, especially Padua or Bologna, later on the Dutch universities were preferred.

The university of Leyden was, for political reasons, founded in great haste: the first letter of prince William of Orange (surnamed the Silent) dates from 29 December 1574, and the university was opened in state on 8 February 1575. Whereas Leyden had the academy of the provinces Holland and Zeeland, the Frisians founded their own academy at Franeker in 1585, Groningen followed in 1614 and Utrecht in 1636. The university of Guelders was opened at Harderwijk in 1648, and in 1655 Nijmegen founded a university that never flourished and closed down in 1672. The universities of Franeker and Harderwijk (where Boerhaave and Linnaeus had taken their degrees) were closed by Napoleon about 1811. Actually Harderwijk having mostly only one professor of medicine could not provide a complete medical education, but many foreigners, especially Scandinavians, came there to take their degree only.

Leyden had undoubtedly the best Medical Faculty though it has known periods of decline. The study took mostly not more than two years, during which some theses had to be defended twice in public. After that the student could apply for the final examination and the graduation that usually followed immediately. In the presence of the Vice-Chancellor a printed thesis had to be defended publicly or privately (before the Senate). The grade of doctor of medicine granted at the same time the license of practising medicine.

Bedside teaching was announced by Willem van der Straaten at Utrecht at his inaugural oration at Utrecht of 17th March 1636. It has been provided at Utrecht for some years, but soon it was totally neglected. At Leiden it was delivered in the Caecilia Hospital from 1637 by two professors alternatively, but from 1744, though announced at the *Series Lectionum*, it was actually not delivered for some 45 years.

Several towns in the Dutch Republic founded an illustrious School or Atheneum: Amsterdam in 1632, Deventer in 1630, Bois-le-Duc in 1636, Utrecht in 1634, Dordrecht in 1635, Middelburg in 1650. An illustrious school had not the privilege to grant grades. Sometimes, if there was a prominent physician in the town, they had a medical professor for a shorter or longer time (f.e. Bois-le-Duc), but on the whole the medical teaching in the Illustrious Schools was of little importance. The Illustrious School of Amsterdam was elevated to the status of university in 1877.

In 1818 a new law created the possibilitiy of establishing Clinical Schools. Soon Amsterdam, Rotterdam, Alkmaar and Middelburg opened a clinical school. They provided only practical education and different restricted licenses, for example to practise as a surgeon or a physician in the country as a so-called "plattelandsheelmeester" or – geneesheer". The law of 1865 regulating the supervision of medicine put an end to their existence.

The Free University at Amsterdam, founded in 1880, got a medical faculty in 1950. About the same time the new Catholic University at Nijmegen, founded in 1923, opened a medical faculty. In Rotterdam a Medical School was founded in 1948 and incorporated into the new Erasmus University in 1972. A new medical school has just been founded at Maastricht.

After 1865 only one general qualification for practising medicine was granted, that of "arts" (physician). The "arts" as such has not the grade of doctor medicinae; in order to obtain this grade he has to write and to defend a thesis, something which, in fact, only a small number of physicians are doing.

The teaching of practical surgery was, as already said, for a long time provided by individual surgeons under the supervision of their guilds. At the universities surgery was only taught theoretically to the students of medicine by the professor of anatomy. Not before the second half of the nineteenth century full professors of theoretical and practical surgery were appointed. About the same time obstetrics became an academical discipline.

A. General

4089 SCHWENGEN, M. (1907). De ontwikkeling van het hooger onderwijs in de Middeleeuwen (The development of higher education in the Middle Ages). *Annuarium R.K. Stud. Ned.*, 31–188.

4090 SNAPPER, I. (1956). *Meditations on Medicine and Medical Education.*

Past and Present. 138 pp. Grune & Stratton, New York–Londen. 8°.
– Chapter II: The Influence of Boerhaave of Leyden on Medicine in the U.S.A., 50–91.

4091 Vos, T. A. (1972). Arts en Wereld in vroeger tijden. 4. Over medisch onderwijs (Physician and world in former times. 4. On Medical education). *Arts en Wereld, 5,* nr 9, 8–23, 10 ill.

4092 Bekkering, D. H. (1972). The history of biomedical education in the Netherlands. *Med. biol. Engng, 10,* 579–83.

4093 Lagrange, E. (1967). Guillaume 1 et l'Enseignement Supérieur en Belge. *Janus, LIV,* 256–61.

4094 Weijde, A. J. van der (1930). Bijdrage tot de kennis van den toestand van het Hooger Onderwijs in België in het midden der 16de eeuw (Contribution to the knowledge of the situation of higher education in Belgium in the middle of the 16th century). *NTG, 74,* II, 5393–4; *BGG, X,* 293–4.
– a proposal for the teaching in the Medical Faculty at Louvain, anno 1557.

4095 Langen, C. D. de (1938). Medical Training in the Netherlands Indies. *Med. Life, 45,* 23–31; also in: *Bull. Kon. Inst. Amsterdam.*

4096 — (1951). Honderd jaren Westers geneeskundig onderwijs in Indonesië (A century of western medical education in Indonesia). *NTG, 95,* III, 2862–3.

See also 3876–81 (Military medical education); 4127–32 (Leiden University).

B. Bedside teaching and clinical instruction

4097 Kroon, J. E. (1912). First clinical instruction in Holland. *Janus, XVII,* 443–7.

4098 Leersum, E. C. van (1916). Bijdrage tot de geschiedenis van het klinisch onderwijs in de Nederlanden (Contribution to the history of clinical instruction in the Netherlands). *NTG, 60,* II, 2139–50.

4099 Lindeboom, G. A. (1970). Medical Education in the Netherlands 1575–1750. In: C. D. O'Malley (ed.) *The History of Medical Education.* UCLA Forum Med. Sci. no 12, University of California Press, Los-Angeles – London., 201–16.

4100 SCHOUTE, D. (1941). Uit het verleden van ons academisch onderwijs aan het ziekbed (From the past of our academic education at the sickbed). *NTG*, *85*, II, 1468–74; *BGG*, *XXI*, 33–9.

4101 CASTIGLIONI, A. (1938). Una pagina di storia dell'insegnamento clinico (da Padova a Leida) (A page from the history of bedside-teaching). *NTG*, *82*, IV, 4878–90; *BGG*, *XVIII*, 246–58.

C. Universities and Academies

General

4102 BANNENBERG, G. P. J. (1953). *Organisatie en bestuur van de Middeleeuwse Universiteit* (Organization and government of the medieval university). Thesis University Nijmegen (Fac. of Arts). 183 pp. Janssen, Nijmegen.

4103 RIDDER-SYMOENS, Hilde de (1970). De structuur van de Middeleeuwse universiteit (The structure of the medieval university). *Spiegel Historiael*, *5*, 345–51, 7 ill.

4104 STRUBBE, E. I. (1971, 1972). Het ontstaan van de Middeleeuwse Universiteiten (Origin of the medieval universities). *Spiegel Historiael*, *6*, 650–8, 6 ill; Studie en studenten aan de Middeleeuwse universiteit (Study and students at the medieval university). *Ibid.*, *7*, 18–25, 7 ill.; Boemelen en zingen aan de Middeleeuwse universiteit. (Being on the spree and singing at the medieval university). *Ibid.*, *7*, 98–103, 7 ill.

4105 HOFSTEE, N. F. (1950). *Organisatie en bestuur der Universiteit. Een vergelijking tussen Amerika, Engeland en Nederland* (Organization and government of the University. A comparison between America, England and the Netherlands). Assen.

4106 POELHEKKE, J. J. (1961). Nederlandse leden van de Inclyta Natio Germanica Artistarum te Padua 1553–1700 (Dutch members of the — — — at P.). *Med. Ned. Hist. Inst. Rome*, *31*, 263–73, ill.

4107 HULSMAN, J. C. (1969). *Disciplina vitae scipio. Over de Universiteiten in Nederland* (On the Universities in the Netherlands). 31 pp., ill. Van Lindonk, Amsterdam.
   – printed for Merck Sharp & Dohme Nederland, Haarlem.

4108 Vos, T. A. (1972). Arts en wereld in vroeger tijden. 2 en 3. Over Universiteiten (Physician and world in former times. 2 and 3. On Universities). *Arts en Wereld*, *5*, no 5, 13–25, 5 ill; *Ibid.*, no 6, 15–24.

4109 Br[ouwer], W. (1972). Van Salerno tot Maastricht (From Salerno till M.). *Metamedica*, *51*, 222–3.
– At Maastricht a new medical school is being founded.

4109ᵃ Wülfrath, Karl (1938). Die niederländischen Hochschulen als Erben der alten Universität Köln. *De Vlag*, *II*, 111.

4109ᵇ Schneppen, Heinz (1960). *Niederländische Universitäten und deutsches Geistesleben von der Gründung der Universität Leiden bis ins späte 18. Jahrhundert.* 164 pp. Neue Münstersche Beiträge zur Geschichtsforschung, Bd. 6. Aschendorffsche Verlagsbuchhandlung, Münster.
– Reviewed by H. H. Eulner: *SA*, *45*, (1961), 189.

Students general

4109ᶜ Wolf, Karl (1930). Pfälzische Studenten im 17. Jahrhundert auf niederländischen Universitäten. *Mannheimer Geschichtsblätter.*

4109ᵈ — (1939). Altpreuszische Studenten auf niederländischen Hochschulen im 17. Jahrhundert. In: Ekkehard. *Mitteilungsblatt deutscher genealogischer Abende*, *15*, no 1–3.

4109ᵉ Vrankrijker, A. C. J. [no d.]. *Vier eeuwen Nederlandsch Studentenleven* (Four centuries of Dutch student-life). 372 pp. Boot, Voorburg. 4°.

Leyden (founded 1575).

General

4110 [   ] (1875). *Album Studiosorum Academiae Lugduno Batavae MDLXXV – MDCCCLXXV*, accedunt nomina curatorum et professorum per eadem secula. LVII + 1440 columns + 279 pp. Hagae comitum apud Martinum Nijhoff.

4111 Kroon, J. E. [1925] *Album studiosorum Academiae Lugduno-Batavae MDCCCLXXV – MCMXXV.* 462 pp. Sijthoff, Leiden. 4°.
– with a foreword by A. J. Blok, vice-chancellor.

4112 Siegenbeek van Heukelom-Lamme, C. A. (1941). *Album Scholasticum*

Academiae Lugduno-Batavae MDLXXV – MCMXL. 237 pp. Brill, Leiden. 4°.

– list of the professors and readers with data of birth, death, appointment, etc.

4113   [   ] (1925). *Pallas Leidensis MCMXXV.* 365 pp. Leiden

– Memorial volume Leyden University on faculties, buildings, student-life, academy printers, centenaries.

4113ᵃ BLOK, P. J. and W. MARTIN (1932). *De Senaatskamer der Leidsche Universiteit.* Hare geschiedenis benevens een volledige catalogus der geschilderde portretten (The Senate room of Leiden University. Its history and a complete catalogue of the painted portraits). 156 pp. (2nd edition) 18 ports. S. C. van Doesburgh, Leiden.

4114 SCHÖFFER, I. (ed.) (1973). *Icones Leidenses. De portretverzameling van de Rijksuniversiteit te Leiden* (The collection of portraits of Leyden University). 302 pp., 464 ports. Universitaire Pers, Leiden.

– compiled by order of the "Stichting Historische Commissie voor de Leidse Universiteit".

4115 SIEGENBEEK, Matthijs (1829–32). *Geschiedenis der Leidsche Hoogeschool van hare oprigting in den jare 1575 tot het jaar 1825* (History of Leyden University from the foundation in 1575 till the year 1825). 2 vols. Leiden. 8°.

4116 SCHOTEL, G. D. J. (1875). *De academie te Leiden in de 16de, 17de en 18de eeuw* (Leyden University in the 16th, 17th and 18th century). 410 pp., ill. Haarlem. 4°.

4117 MOLHUYSEN, P. C. (1913–24). *Bronnen tot de geschiedenis der Leidsche Universiteit* (Sources to the history of Leyden University). 7 vols: I (1574–1610); II (1610–1647); III (1647–1682); IV (1682–1725); V (1725–1765); VI (1765–1795); VII (1795–1811). Rijks Geschiedkundige Publicaties no: 20, 29, 38, 45, 48, 53 and 56. M. Nijhoff. Den Haag. 4°.

– This monumental work offers an excerpt of the "Acta Senatus" and of the Book of Resolutions of the Governors, added are 1188 documents and a list of all the graduations.

4118 — (1924). De voorrechten der Leidsche Universiteit (The prerogatives of Leyden University). *MKNAW*, vol. 58, serie B, no 1, 32 pp. Noord-Holl-Uitg. Mij, Amsterdam.

4119 WITKAM, H. J. (1969). *Introductie tot de dagelijkse zaken van de Leidse Universiteit van 1581 tot 1596* (Introduction to the daily affairs of Leyden University from — till —). 223 pp. pr. stencilled for the author, Rapenburg 21, Leiden.

4120 — (1970–1974). *De dagelijkse zaken van de Leidse Universiteit van 1581 tot 1596* (The daily affairs of Leyden University). Vol. I–X. Leiden.

4121 JURRIAANSE, M. W. (1965). *De stichting der Leidsche Universiteit* (Foundation of Leyden University). E. J. Brill, Leiden.

4122 WOLTJER, J. J. (1965). *De Leidse Universiteit in verleden en heden* (Leyden University: past and present). 114 pp., 16 ill. Universitaire Pers, Leiden.

4123 MOURIK, B. A. van [1949]. *Universitas Leidensis. Een document van het leven der Leidse Universiteit* (A document of the life of Leyden University). 189 pp., 100 photogr. Batteljee & Terpstra, Leiden. 4°.
– the book was made at the instigation of the Governors. Letterpress and summary also in French and English.

4124 LUYENDIJK-ELSHOUT, A. M. and J. DANKMEIJER (1970). La faculté de médecine de l'université de Leyde. *Médecine Europ.*, *11*, 70–4.

4125 JORISSEN, W. P. (1909). *Het Chemisch (thans anorganisch chemisch) Laboratorium der Universiteit te Leiden 1859–1909 en de chemische Laboratoria dier Universiteit vóór dat tijdperk en hen, die er in doceerden* (The Chemical (presently anorganic chemical) Laboratory of Leyden University 1859–1909 and the chemical Laboratories of that University before that period and those who lectured therein). A. W. Sijthoff, Leiden.

4126 HENIGER, J. and J. W. van SPRONSEN (1969). Driehonderd jaar scheikunde in Leiden (Three hundred years of chemistry at L.). *Chem. Wbl.*, *65*, no 32, (8 aug.) 17–21, 27, 6 ill.

See also 2884–5, 2933–43 (Anatomical theatres)

Medical Education

4127 GEYL, A. (1911). Bijdrage tot de geschiedenis van het geneeskundig onderwijs in Leiden in de 2de helft der 16de eeuw (Contribution to the history of medical education at L. in the second half of the 16th century). *NTG*, *55*, II, 824–32 and 1178.

4128 KROON, J. E. (1911). De geschiedenis van het geneeskundig onderwijs te Leiden (History of medical education at L.) *NTG*, *55*, II, 1034.
– letter to the editor.

4129 — (1911). *Bijdragen tot de geschiedenis van het geneeskundig onderwijs aan de Leidsche Universiteit 1575–1625* (Contributions to the history of medical education at Leyden University — —) Thesis University Leyden (Supervisor: E. C. van Leersum). 153 pp. S. C. van Doesburgh, Leiden. 4°.

4130 BARGE, J. A. J. (1934). Het geneeskundig onderwijs aan de Leidsche Universiteit in de 18de eeuw (The medical education at Leyden University in the 18th century). *NTG, 78,* I, 47–68; *BGG, XIV,* 1–22.

4131 — (1937). *De stichting van het academisch klinisch onderwijs te Leiden voor 300 jaren* (The foundation of university clinical education at L. 300 years ago). 32 pp., ill. Stenfert Kroese, Leiden.
– memorial address.

4132 NUYENS, B. W. Th. (1937). De stichting van het Academisch Clinisch Onderwijs te Leiden voor 300 jaren plechtig herdacht (The foundation of University clinical education 300 years ago solemnly commemorated). *NTG, 81,* IV, 5448–9; *BGG, XVII,* 199–200.

4133 GIJSBERTI HODENPIJL, A. K. A. (1917). Een advies der geneeskundige faculteit te Leiden uit de achttiende eeuw (An advice of the medical faculty at L. from the 18th century). *NTG, 61,* I, 1680–2.

4134 PROBST, Chr. (1971). Ärztliche Forschung am Krankenbett im Zeitalter der Aufklärung. Gezeigt am Beispiel der Leydener und der Wiener Schule. In: *Festschrift für Hermann Heimpel zum 70. Geburtstag am 19. September 1971,* 568–98. Vandenhoeck & Ruprecht, Göttingen.

4135 MULDER, J. and A. J. Ch. HAEX, (1963). Van universitaire armenpolikliniek tot universitair diagnostisch centrum voor inwendige geneeskunde (From university outpatient department for the poor to a university diagnostic centre of internal medicine). *MC, 18,* 819–21.
See also 378, 786, 5143

4136 SURINGAR, G. C. B. (1860). De twee eerste hoogleeraars in de geneeskunde te Leiden. (The two first professors of medicine at Leiden.) *NTG, 4,* 641.

4137 — (1861). Over de beoefening der voorbereidende en hulpwetenschappen bij de medische studie aan de Leidsche hoogeschool, gedurende de de eerste halve eeuw van haar bestaan inzonderheid over den aanvang en de eerste lotgevallen van het botanische onderwijs (On the study of the preparative and auxiliary sciences at the medical study at Leiden

University, during the first half century of its existence, particularly on the beginning and first vicissitudes of botanical education). *NTG*, 5, 121.

4138   — (1861). De vroegste geschiedenis van het ontleedkundig onderwijs te Leiden. (The earliest history of anatomical education at L.). *NTG*, 5, 385.

4139   — (1861). De medische faculteit te Leiden, in het begin der zeventiende eeuw. (The Medical Faculty at L., in the beginning of the 17th century). *NTG*, 5, 641.

4140   — (1862). Stichting der School voor Klinisch Onderwijs te Leiden, onder Heurnius en Screvelius, in het jaar 1637. Toestand der overige medische studievakken aan de Leidsche Hoogeschool, omstreeks het midden der zeventiende eeuw. (Foundation of the School for clinical education at L., under Heurnius and Screvelius, in 1637. Situation of the other medical subjects at Leiden University, about the middle of the 17th century). *NTG*, 6, 515–32.

4141   — (1863). Het geneeskundig onderwijs van Albert Kyper en Johannes Antonides van der Linden. De ontleedkundige school van Johannes van Horne (The medical teaching by — and —. The anatomical school of — —). *NTG*, 7, 193–206.

4142   — (1863). Chemiatrische school van Sylvius. De Verdiensten van dien hoogleeraar als ontleedkundige, en zijn praktisch-geneeskundig onderwijs in het Akademische Ziekenhuis te Leiden (1658–1672). (Chemiatric school of —. The merits of this professor as an anatomist, and his practico-medical teaching in the University Hospital at L.). *NTG*, 7, 497–510.   *See also* 1705–10 (Sylvius)

4143   — (1864). Invloed der Cartesiaansche Wijsbegeerte op het Natuur- en Genees-kundig onderwijs aan de Leidsche Hoogeschool (Influence of Cartesian philosophy on the physical and medical education at Leyden University). *NTG*, 8, 153–70.

4144   — (1864). De Medische Faculteit te Leiden op het einde der zeventiende en in het begin der achttiende eeuw, Lucas Schacht en diens ambtgenooten. Anatomisch onderwijs van Drelincourt, Nuck en Bidloo (The Medical Faculty at L. at the end of the 17th century and in the beginning of the 18th century, — — and his colleagues. Anatomical teaching by — — —). *NTG*, 8, 561–86.

4145 — (1865). De Leidsche hoogleeraren in de Natuurkundige Weten-schappen, inzonderheid in de Kruid- en Scheikunde, na den dood van Sylvius en vóór Boerhaave's benoeming tot Professor Chemiae (1672–1718) (The Leyden professors of Natural Science, particularly of Bo-tany and Chemistry, after the death of — and before B.'s appointment to — — —). *NTG*, *1* (2nd series), II, 275–306.

4146 — (1866). De Leidsche Geneeskundige Faculteit in het begin der acht-tiende eeuw. Boerhaave en zijne Ambtgenooten (The Leyden Medical Faculty in the beginning of the 18th century. B. and his Colleagues). *NTG*, *2*, II, 1–39.

4147 — (1866). Het Theoretisch-geneeskundig Onderwijs van Boerhaave. De Klinische Lessen door hem en zijn ambtgenoot Herman Oosterdijk Schacht gegeven (The theoretical-medical teaching by —. The Clinical Lectures given by him and by his colleague — —). *NTG*, *2*, II, 199–225.

4148 — (1866). Verval van het Klinisch Onderwijs na den dood van Boer-haave. Adriaan van Roijen als hoogleraar in de Kruid- en Geneeskun-de. Waardering van het dynamisch element in de theoretische leer van Gaubius en Frederik Winter. Pieter van Musschenbroek als hoog-leraar in de Physica (Decline of the clinical instruction after the death of B. A. van R. as a professor of Botany and Medicine. Appraisal of the dynamic element in the theoretical doctrine of G. and F.W., P.v.M. as a professor of Physics). *NTG*, *2*, II, 256–83.

4149 — (1867). De School van Bernhard Siegfried Albinus (The School of — —). *NTG*, *3*, II, 1–21.

4150 — (1867). Het bijeenbrengen eener verzameling van Natuurlijke voor-werpen voor het akademisch onderwijs, omstreeks het midden der acht-tiende eeuw. Eerste afzonderlijke lessen over de natuurlijke history, door den hoogleeraar Allamand, en over de Zoölogie door Le Francq van Berkhey (Gathering of a collection of natural objects for academi-cal teaching about the middle of the 18th century. First special lectures on natural science, by — —, and on zoology by — —). *NTG*, II, *3*, 265–84.

4151 — (1868). Vertegenwoordiging der Pathologische Anatomie door Gualtherus van Doeveren en Eduard Sandifort. Hunne ambtgenooten Frederik Bernhard Albinus en David van Roijen (Representation of pathological anatomy by — — and — —. Their colleagues — and — —). *NTG*, *4*, II, 1–24.

4152   — (1869). Herstelling van het Klinische Onderwijs in 1787. Aankoop van een daarvoor bestemd afzonderlijk gebouw in 1797. De Praktisch-geneeskundige lessen van Oosterdijk en Paradijs, benevens de Heelkundige Kliniek en het Praktisch-verloskundig Onderwijs door Meinard Simon de Pui. Het Theoretisch Onderwijs der drie genoemde hooglee-raren (Reestablishment of clinical instruction in 1787. Purchase of a building, destined for that purpose in 1797. The Practical-medical Lectures by — and —, and the surgical and practico-obstetrical teaching by M. S. de Pui. The theoretical teaching of the three professors mentioned). *NTG*, 5, II, 121–56.

4153   — (1870). Het Onderwijs in de Natuurkundige Wetenschappen aan de Leidsche Hoogeschool, gedurende het dertigjarig tijdvak van 1785–1815 (The teaching of Natural Science at Leyden University, during the period 1785–1815). *NTG*, 6, II, 1–75.

4154   SIMON THOMAS, P. H. (1909). *Het onderwijs in de verloskunde aan de Leidsche Hoogeschool gedurende het tijdvak 1791–1900.* (Teaching of obstetrics at Leyden University during the period (1791–1900). ill. Leiden.   *See also* 1416

Students

4155   COLENBRANDER, H. T. (1925). De herkomst der Leidsche Studenten (The provenance of Leyden students). In: *Pallas Leidensis MCMXXV*, 275–303. Leiden.

4156   BLANKEN, G. H. (1869). *Het aantal studenten aan de Hoogeschool te Leiden van 1775 tot en met 1868* (The number of students at Leyden University from 1775 till 1868). 189 pp. Leiden.
   – Blanken was bedell at the University; with addition of the names of professors in that period.

4157   KLAAUW, C. J. van der (1931). De studentenbevolking van de faculteiten der geneeskunde en der wis- en natuurkunde sinds 1818, in het bijzonder te Leiden (The student-population of the faculties of medicine and of the faculties of mathematics and physics since 1818, particularly at L.). *NTG*, 75, II, 2381–90; *BGG*, XI, 157–66, ill.

4158   INNES SMITH, R. W. (1932). *English-speaking students of Medicine at the University of Leyden.* 258 pp. Edinburgh – London. 8°.
   – foreword by John D. Comrie; portrait of Arch. Pitcairne.

4159 UNDERWOOD, E. ASHWORTH (1969). English-Speaking Medical Students at Leyden. *Nature*, *221*, no 5183, 810–4.

4160 ROOK, Arthur (1973). Cambridge medical students at Leyden. *Med. Hist.*, *XVII*, 256–65.

4161 HOFMEIER, H. K. (1962). Westfälische Studenten der Rechten, Medizin und Theologie an der Universität zu Leiden 1575–1813: ein Beitrag zu den kulturellen Beziehungen zwischen den Niederlanden und Deutschland. *Beitr. Gesch. Dortmunds u.d. Grafschaft Mark*, *58*, 59–90, ill.

4162 TEUTSCH, Fritz (1881). Die Studirenden aus Ungarn und Siebenburgen auf der Universität Leyden von 1575–1870. In: *Archiv des Vereins für siebenbürgische Landeskunde*, N.F. *XVI*, 204–26, Hermannstadt.

4163 STEENIS, [   ] van (1955). Leids studentenleven in de zeventiende eeuw (Leyden student life in the 17th century). *N.T. Med. Stud.*, *1*, 112–3.

Franeker (founded 1585).

4164 FOCKEMA ANDREAE, S. J. and Th. J. MEIJER (ed.) (1968). *Album Studiosorum Academiae Franekerensis (1585–1811, 1816–1844)*. I. Naamlijst der studenten (List of names of the students). 539 pp. T. Wever, Franeker.
    – Vol. II has not yet been published.

4165 MEIJER, Th. J. (ed.). (1972). *Album Promotorum Academiae Franekerensis (1591–1811)*. 159 pp. T. Wever, Franeker.

4166 BOELES, W. B. S. (1878, 1879). *Frieslands Hoogeschool en het Rijks Athenaeum te Franeker* (The Friesland Academy and the State Athenaeum at F.). 2 vols (in one binding). Vol. I: 506 pp., Vol. II: 854 pp., ports. H. Kuipers, Leeuwarden.

4167 NAPJUS, J. W. (1927). De Geneeskundige Faculteit van de Hoogeschool en het Rijks Athenaeum te Franeker 1585–1843 (The Medical Faculty of the Academy and the State Athenaeum at F.) *NTG*, *71*, II, 1003–27; *BGG*, *VII*, 577–601.
    – in a long series of articles Napjus later dealt with several professors of medicine of Franeker Academy. These are listed in the biographical part of the present work under the names of the professors in question.

4168 GALAMA, S. H. M. (1954). *Het wijsgerig onderwijs aan de hogeschool te Franeker 1581–1811* (The philosophical education at Franeker Academy). Thesis University Leyden.

4169   MEINSMA, J. J. (1968). Het scheikundig onderwijs aan Frieslands Hoge-
       school en Rijksathenaeum te Franeker (1585–1843) (The chemical
       teaching at Friesland Academy and the State Athenaeum) *De Vrije
       Fries*, *48*, 30–52, 3 ill.

4170   BECKER, Georg (ed.) (1943). *Die deutschen Studenten und Professoren
       an der Akademie zu Franeker*. Soest.

4171   KALMA, J. J. (1957). *Ostfriesische Studenten in Franeker*. Leeuwarden.
                        See also 11, 27, 28, 371, 509, 559, 561, 794, 903n., 954, 1055,
                        1256, 1304, 1452, 1921, 1922, 2879.

Groningen (founded 1614)

4171ᵃ NAUTA, G. A. (1910). Waar studeerden de Groningers vóór de stich-
       ting hunner Academie? (Where did the inhabitants of Groningen study
       before the foundation of their Academy?). *Gron. Volksalm.*, *22*, 1–27.

4171ᵇ [   ] (1968). *Effigies et vitae professorum Academiae Groningae et
       Omlandiae cum historiola fundationis eiusdem Acad. Groningae*. Gro-
       ningen.
       – Facsimile of the first edition (1654) with Dutch translation.

4172   [   ] (1915). *Album studiosorum Academiae Groninganae*. 711 pp.
       Wolters, Groningen. 4°.
       – Published by: Historisch Genootschap Groningen.

4173   JONCKBLOET, W. J. A. (1864). *Gedenkboek der Hoogeschool te Gro-
       ningen ter gelegenheid van haar vijfde halve eeuwfeest* (Memorial Volume
       on the occasion of the 250th anniversary of Groningen University).
       Groningen.

4174   DIJK, Is. van, J. W. MOLL, G. C. NIJHOFF et al. (1914). *Academia Gro-
       ningana MDCXIV–MCMXIV*. 578 pp., 63 ill. P. Noordhoff, Gronin-
       gen, 4°.
       – Memorial volume edited on the occasion of the 3rd centenary of Groningen
       University.
       p. XIII–XXIV, 1–238: J. Huizinga. Geschiedenis der Universiteit gedurende de
       derde eeuw van haar bestaan (History of the University during its third centenary).
       p. 258–337: G. C. Nijhoff. De hoogleeraren in de faculteit der geneeskunde aan de
       Groningsche Hoogeschool van 1614–1914 (The professors of medicine at Groningen
       University).

4175 FENEMA, C. H. van (1909). *Het Academie-gebouw te Groningen 1614–1909* (The Academy-building at G.). 59 pp., ill., facs. Groningen. 4°.

4176 BRUGGENCATE, B. ten and H. de BUCK (1930). *De Rijksuniversiteit te Groningen* (Groningen University). 127 pp., ill. Groningen. 4°.

4177 VISSER, Elizabeth (ed.) (1966). *Universitas Groningana MCMXIV–MCMLXIV.* Gedenkboek ter gelegenheid van het 350-jarig bestaan der Rijks-Universiteit Groningen uitgegeven in opdracht van de Academische Senaat (Memorial Volume on the occasion of the 350th anniversary of Groningen University, edited by the Academical Senate). 288 pp., ill. J. B. Wolters, Groningen.

4178 EBELS-HOVING, B. (1965). Some remarks on the history of Groningen University. *J. Path. Bact.*, 89 (1), 415–20.

4179 MACLEAN, J. (1972). Science and theology at Groningen University (1698–1702). *Ann. Sci.*, 29, 187–201.

4180 ROGGE, C. W. L. (1964). Academia Groningae instituta. *N.T. Med. Stud.*, 10, 118–23.   See also 1299, 2821, 2881–2

Utrecht (founded 1636).

4181 deleted

4182 [   ] (1886). *Album Studiosorum Academiae Rheno-Traiectinae MDCXXXVI–MDCCCLXXXVI*, accedunt nomina curatorum et professorum per eadem secula. XLVI + 590 + 59 pp. Ultraiecti apud J. L. Beyers et J. van Boekhoven.

4183 KETNER, Frans (ed.) (1936). *Album promotorum, qui inde ab anno MDCXXXVIo usque ad annum MDCCCXVum in Academia Rheno-Trajectina gradum doctoratus adepti sunt, Societas cui nomen "Provinciaal Utrechtsch Genootschap van Kunsten en Wetenschappen" componendum edendumque curavit, atque Academiae Rheno-Trajectinae trecesimo die natali donum obtulit.* Trajecti ad Rh. VIII + 278 pp. 8°.

4184 CITTERT-EYMERS, Joh. G. van (ed.) (1963). *Album promotorum der Rijksuniversiteit Utrecht 1815–1936, en Album promotorum der Veeartsenijkundige Hoogeschool, 1918–1925.* 350 pp. Leiden. 4°.
   – Publication of the Utrecht University Museum: sequel to previous item.

4185 WYNNE, J. A. (1886). *De Utrechtsche Hoogeschool in vorige eeuwen* (Utrecht University in former centuries). 46 pp. Utrecht.
   – Address.

4186 LONCQ, C. Jzn, G. J. (1886). *Historische schets der Utrechtsche Hooge-school tot hare verheffing in 1815* (Historical sketch of Utrecht University till its elevation in —). 340 pp. Utrecht.

4187 KERNKAMP, G. W. (1914). *De Utrechtsche Hoogeschool in den Fran-schen tijd* (Utrecht University in the French time). Haarlem.

4188 — *et al.* (1936). *De Utrechtsche Universiteit 1636–1936.* 3 vols. Utrecht. 4°.
I. De Utrechtsche Academie 1636–1815. XII + 392 pp.
II. De Utrechtsche Universiteit. VII + 410 pp.
III. Het Derde Eeuwfeest der Utrechtsche Universiteit, Juni 1936 (The 3rd centenary). 131 pp.
– with numerous facs., ports, ill., after old originals.

4189 BIERENS de HAAN, J. *et al.* (1936). *Het Utrechtsch Studentenleven, 1636–1936.* (Utrecht student life). 594 pp., ill. Utrecht
– Companion volume to the previous item.

4190 VREDENBURCH, Baron W. C. A. van (1914). *Schets van eene geschie-denis van het Utrechtsche studentenleven* (Sketch of a history of Utrecht student life). 316 pp., 14 pl. A. Oosthoek, Utrecht.

4191 SCHMITZ, Machteld M. (1969). Studentenleven in de 17de en 18de eeuw (Student life in the 17th and 18th century). *Spiegel Historiael, 4,* 216–223, 8 ill.
– Mostly on Utrecht student life.

4192 BÁNKI, Ö. (1940). De Utrechtse Universiteit in de Hongaarsche be-schavingsgeschiedenis (Utrecht University in the history of Hungarian civilization). *Jbk. Oud-Utrecht, 13,* 87–117, ill.

4193 DOESSCHATE, G. ten (1963). *De Utrechtse Universiteit en de geneeskunde 1636–1900* (Utrecht University and medicine — —). 180 pp., ill., ports. B. de Graaf, Nieuwkoop;

4194 PINA, Luis de (1959). Ojuramento dos médicos na Universidade de Utreque no século XVIII. *Imprensa medica* (Lisboa), *23,* 201–8.
– on the doctor's oath at Utrecht University in the 18th century. The oath is printed in Th. Janssonius ab Almeloveen's "Hippocratis Aphorismi", Leipzig, 1756.

4195 COHEN, E. (1941). Chemisch-historische aantekeningen VIII: De che-mie te Utrecht in de loop der eeuwen (Chemical-historical notes: Chemistry at U. in the course of the centuries). *Chem. Wbl., 38,* 299.

4196 LESKY, Erna (1960). Paris und Utrecht von einem Rokitansky-Schüler gesehen. *Wiener klin. Wschr.*, 72, 237–9.
– Letter from the young Dutch physician H. van Leeuwen to Carl von Rokitansky (1804–78).

4197 DOESSCHATE, G. ten (1953). De studie in de geneeskunde te Utrecht in de eerste helft van de negentiende eeuw (The study of medicine at U. in the first half of the 19th century). *NTG*, 97, II, 1142–8; *BGG*, *XXXIII*, 23–30.

4198 BEUMER, H. H. (1965). Het klinisch geneeskundig onderwijs te Utrecht in de 17de eeuw (Clinical medical teaching at U. in the 17th century). *Jbk. Oud-Utrecht*, 38, 25–9, ill.

4199 MEULDER, A. B. J. de (1914). De Rijks-Veeartsenijschool te Utrecht (The State Veterinary School at U.). *Eigen Haard*, XL, 104.

4200 OFFRINGA, C. (1971). *Van Gildestein naar Uithof – 150 jaar diergenees-kundig onderwijs in Utrecht* (From "Gildestein" to "Uithof" – 150 years of veterinary teaching at U.). 351 pp., ill. Published by the Veterinary Faculty of the University.
– Reviewed by A. Willems: *Sci. Hist.*, *14* (1972), 154–63.

4201 EVERS, G. A. (ed.) (1937, 1941, 1951). *Lijst van gedrukte geschriften over de Rijksuniversiteit te Utrecht. Proeve eener Bibliographie* (List of published writings on Utrecht University. Specimen of a bibliography). 3 vols. A. Oosthoek, Utrecht.
Vol. I: 1634–1936, 245 pp.
Vol. II: Addition to the years 1634–1936; continuation on the years 1936–1941, 76 pp.
Vol. III: Addition to the years 1634–1941; continuation on the years 1941–1951, 73 pp.
– These volumes contain a wealth of references dealing with the history of Utrecht University, its buildings, Faculties, Institutes, Laboratories, professors, lectors, students, graduations, orations a.s.o.
See also 123, 903n., 1607, 2888–88a

Harderwijk

4202 EPEN, D. G. van (1904). *Album Studiosorum Academiae Gelro-Zut-phanicae MDCXLVIII–MDCCCXVIII*, accedunt nomina curatorum et professorum per eadem secula cura. J. Hoekstra, Den Haag.

4203 BOUMAN, Hermannus (1844–47). *Geschiedenis van de voormalige Gel-*

dersche hoogeschool en hare hoogleeraren (History of the former Guelders Academy and its professors). 2 vols. Utrecht.

4204 VEEN, J. S. van (1898). Uit de uitwendige en inwendige geschiedenis der voormalige Geldersche hoogeschool (From the external and internal history of the former Guelders Academy). *Gelre, I,* 1–70.
– with two stamps.

4205 — (1906). Bijdrage tot de geschiedenis der Harderwijksche School (Contribution to the history of the Harderwijk School). *Gelre, 9,* 271–7.

4206 IDENBURG-SIEGENBEEK VAN HEUKELOM, O. C. D. (1934). De laatste jaren der Hoogeschool van Harderwijk (The last years of Harderwijk Academy). *Gelre, 37,* 253.

4207 KOCH-de MEYER, G. (1964). De Illustre Hogeschool van Harderwijk en haar boekenschat (The Illustrious Academy of H. and its treasure of books. *West-Vlaanderen, 13,* 112–6, ill.

4208 WITTOP KONING, D. A. (1961). Inleiding over de Gelderse Hogeschool (Introduction on the Guelders Academy). *GeWiNa,* no 10, 12.

4209 — [1965]. De hogeschool van Harderwijk (The Academy of H.). *Organorama, 2,* no 3, 17–21.

4210 LINDEBOOM, G. A. (1968/9). Het lesrooster van het Athenaeum te Harderwijk voor het zomerseizoen van het jaar 1646 (The time-table of the Athenaeum at H. for the summer-season, 1646). *Gelre, LXIII,* 99–102.

4211 LENNEP, M. J. van (1966). Harderwijkse gepromoveerden uit de Friese gewesten (Harderwijk graduates from the Frisian regions). *De Vrije Fries, 47,* 196–205.
– List of students hailing from Groningen and East-Friesland who graduated at H. in the years between 1659 and 1811.

4212 HAAN, A. A. M. de (1960). *Het Wijsgerig Onderwijs aan het Gymnasium Illustre en de Hogeschool te Harderwijk 1599–1811* (The Philosophical teaching at the — — and the Academy at H.). Thesis University Leyden. XIV + 198 pp., 5 pl. Harderwijk. 8°.

4213 PICKÉE, J. A. (1958). Iets over het onderwijs in de exacte vakken aan de Harderwijker Hogeschool en het Athenaeum te Deventer (Something on the teaching of exact sciences at Harderwijk Academy and the Athenaeum at D.) *GeWiNa,* no 3, 7–17.

4214   MEINSMA, J. J. (1973). Het scheikundig onderwijs aan de voormalige
       Hogeschool (1648–1811) en het Rijksathenaeum (1815–1818) te Har-
       derwijk (Chemistry at the former Academy and the State Athenaeum at
       H.). *GeWiNa*, no 31, 17–9.   See also 123, 153, 1163–64, 1484

       Nijmegen (founded 1655).

4215   MEER VAN KUFFLER, J. C. F. van (1890). De voormalige illustre school
       en academie te Nijmegen (The former illustrious school and academy
       at N.). *Tijdspiegel, II*, 154–77.

4216   ROGGE, Y. H. (1900). De Academie te Nijmegen. *Oud-Holland, 18*,
       153–80.

4217   SASSEN, F. L. R. (1955). De kwartierlijke Hogeschool te Nijmegen
       (The quarterly Academy at N.). *Numaga, II*, 57–67. Also in: *Universi-
       teit en Hogeschool*, I, 203–9.

4218   — (1962). Levensberichten van de hoogleraren der kwartierlijke Hoge-
       school te Nijmegen (Biographical notices of the professors at the quar-
       terly Academy at N.). *Numaga, IX*, 104–27, 3 ports.

4219   BRINKHOFF, J. M. G. M. (1969). De kwartierlijke academie (The quar-
       terly Academy). *Numaga, XVI*, 230–4.

4220   LINDEBOOM, G. A. (1969). Het eerste lesrooster (1656) van de kwartier-
       lijke Universiteit te Nijmegen (The first time-table (1656) of the quar-
       terly University at N.). *Numaga, XVI*, 395–401, ill.

4221   HERMESDORF, B. H. D. (1971). Rumoer in de Nijmeegse Kwartierlijke
       Akademie (Clamour in the Nijmegen Quarterly Academy). *Numaga,
       XVIII*, 24–8.

4221ª MANNING, A. F. (ed.). (1974). *Katholieke Universiteit Nijmegen 1923–
       1973* ([Roman-]Catholic University Nijmegen — —) 511 pp., Ambo,
       Bilthoven.   See also 1755, 2886.

       Athenaeum (1632) and University (1877) of Amsterdam

4222   [   ] (1882). *Album Academicum van het Athenaeum Illustre en van
       de Universiteit van Amsterdam*, bevattende de namen der hoogleeraren
       en leeraren van 1632 tot 1882 en der studenten van 1799 tot 1882
       (Album Academicum of the Athenaeum Illustre and of the University

of A., containing the names of professors and teachers from 1632 till 1882 and of the students from 1799 till 1882). 170 pp. Van Munster & Zn, Amsterdam. 4°.

– contains also a list of the professors of the Clinical School (1828–66) who were at the same time professores honorarii at the Athenaeum.

4223 [   ] (1913). *Album Academicum van het Athenaeum Illustre en van de Universiteit van Amsterdam*, bevattende de namen der curatoren, hoogleeraren en leeraren van 1632–1913, der Rectores Magnifici … van 1877 tot 1913, der leden van den Ill. Senatus Studiosorum Amstelodamensium van 1851 tot 1913, en der studenten van 1799 tot 1913 (Album Academicum of the — — and of the University of A., containing the names of curators, professors and teachers from — till —, of the — — … from — till —, members of the — — — from — till — and of the students from — till —). 522 pp. (with appendices). R. W. P. de Vries, Amsterdam.

– Edited by the Amsterdam Students Corps.

4224 STERCK, J. F. M. (1921). Van Kloosterkerk tot Athenaeum. Memorieboek en geschiedenis van het St. Agnesklooster te Amsterdam 1397–1599 (From Conventual Church to Athenaeum. Memorial volume and history of the St. Agnes monastery at A.). *Bijdr. Gesch. Bisdom Haarlem*, 66 pp.

4225 EEGHEN, I. H. van, W. Gs HELLINGA and H. de la FONTAINE VERWEY (1957). *Het illustre begin van het Athenaeum*. Drie opstellen. Ter inleiding van de tentoonstelling ingericht … ter gelegenheid van het 325-jarig bestaan van de instelling voor hoger onderwijs te Amsterdam (The illustrious beginning of the Athenaeum. Three essays. Introduction to the exposition … organized on the occasion of the 325th anniversary of the institution for higher education at A.). 29 pp. Noord-Holl. Uitg. Mij., Amsterdam.

4226 [   ] (1927). *Van Athenaeum tot Universiteit. Geschiedenis van het Athenaeum Illustre in de negentiende eeuw* (History of the Athenaeum Illustre of A. in the 19th century). 186 pp., ill. Stadsdrukkerij Amsterdam. 4°.

– Edited by Curators of the University of A.; in an introduction the foundation of the Athenaeum in 1632 is discussed.

4227 BRUGMANS, H. *et al.* (1932). *Gedenkboek van het Athenaeum en de Universiteit van Amsterdam 1632–1932* (Memorial Volume of the Athenaeum and University of A.). 719 pp., ports., ill. Stadsdrukkerij, Amsterdam. 4°.

– p. 163–290: W. P. C. Zeeman *et al.* De Geneeskunde. De Geschiedenis van het ge-neeskundig onderwijs aan Athenaeum en Universiteit van Amsterdam (Medicine. History of medical education at the — and the University of A.).

4228 [   ] (1933). *Verslag van de viering van het 3de eeuwfeest van de Universiteit van Amsterdam* (Report of the celebration of the 3rd centenary of the University of A.). 174 pp., ill. sm. f°.

4229 LINDEBOOM, G. A. (with N. Th. de BRUIJNE). (1972). De benoeming van een hoogleraar in de heelkunde (J. A. Korteweg) aan de Universiteit van Amsterdam in 1889 (The appointment of a professor of surgery (— —) in the University of A., 1889). *NTG, 116,* 1137–44, 3 ill., port.

4230 HELLINGA, G. and J. GROEN (1953). Bijdrage tot de geschiedenis van het onderwijs in de algemene ziektekunde en van de Stichting van het Laboratorium voor Algemene Pathologie aan de Universiteit te Amster-dam (Contribution to the history of teaching of pathology and of the Foundation of the Laboratory for general pathology at the University of A.). *Gen. Bl., 45,* 65–106, port. (of J. van Geuns).

4230ᵃ ARKEL, C. G. van (1973). Het Laboratorium voor Artsenijbereid-kunde van de Universiteit van Amsterdam van 1882–1972 (The La-boratory for pharmacy of Amsterdam University from —). *PhW, 108,* 272–5; also in: *Bull. Pharm,* no 48, 26–30, ill.

4231 GROOT, A. W. de [1945]. *De Universiteit van Amsterdam in oorlogs-tijd* (Amsterdam University in war-time). 154 pp. Amsterdam.

4232 EEGHEN, I. H. van [1953] *De historische verzameling der Universiteit van Amsterdam (1923–1953)* (The historical collection of Amster-dam University). 16 pp.
– with a photograph of a pencil-drawing by I. G. Keber, 1862: "Morgenbezoek Prof. C. B. Tilanus met zijn studenten op zaal 5 van het Oude Mannenhuis".
See also 1450, 2876–8a

Free University Amsterdam (founded 1880)

4233 RULLMANN, J. C. (1930). *De Vrije Universiteit, haar ontstaan en haar bestaan 1880–1930. Ter gelegenheid van haar halve eeuwfeest historisch geschetst* (The origin and existence of the Free University. On the occasion of the 50th anniversary, a historical survey). Amsterdam.

4234 ROELINK, J. (1955). *Vijfenzeventig jaar Vrije Universiteit 1880–1955.* Gedenkboek bij het vijfenzeventig-jarig bestaan der Vrije Universiteit te Amsterdam (Seventy-five years Free University. Memorial volume

on the occasion of the 75th anniversary of the Free University at A.).
228 pp., ill., ports. Kok, Kampen.

– The Medical Faculty of the Free (Protestant) University was founded in 1950.

4235   NAUTA, D., H. SMITSKAMP and W. J. WIERINGA (ed.) (1955) *Gegevens betreffende de Vrije Universiteit*. Ter gelegenheid van haar 75-jarig bestaan ... (Data concerning the Free University. On the occasion of the 75th anniversary ...). 140 pp. Kok, Kampen.

– p. 80–8: list of theses; p. 89–133: Matriculation list from 1930–1955.

4235ᵃ   HAM, A. A. G. (1972). De eerste "Vrije Universiteit" (1617–19) op de Keizersgracht te Amsterdam (The first "Free University" (1617–19) on the — at A.). *AP*, no 9, 71–6, 1 ill.

– This academy was founded by Samuel Coster (1579–1665), physician at Amsterdam.

Foreign Universities

4236   FLORKIN, Marcel (1967). La Faculté de médecine de Liège sous le régime hollandais. *Chron. Univ. de Liège*, 39–52.

4237   SONDERVORST, F. A. (1959). Die Universität zu Löwen. Aus der Geschichte der Brabanter Katholischen Universität. *Grünenthal Waage, I*, 66–72, ill.

4238   ESSEN, L. van der (1927). *L'Université de Louvain*. Bruxelles.

4239   [   ] (1930). *L'académie Royale des Sciences. Les Universités et les écoles techniques supérieures aux Pays-Bas et aux Indes Néerlandaises.* 103 pp., ill. S. C. van Doesburgh, Leiden.

4240   WAART, A. de, J. F. van HOYTEMA and S. P. SLAGTER *et al.* (1926). *Ontwikkeling van het Geneeskundig Onderwijs te Weltevreden 1851–1926*. Uitgegeven bij het 75-jarig bestaan van de School tot opleiding van Indische artsen (S.T.O.V.I.A.) (Development of medical education at W. Edited on the occasion of the 75th anniversary of the School for training of Indian physicians). 371 pp., ill. Weltevreden. 8°.

4241   KAISER, W. and H. KROSCH (1969). Nordrheinische und niederländische Ärzte des 18. Jahrhunderts als Absolventen der Medizinischen Fakultät Halle. In: W. Kaiser u. C. Beierlein (ed.) *In Memoriam Hermann Boerhaave 1668–1738*, 101–24.

4242   RIJNBERK, G. van (1924). Het eerste eeuwfeest der Accademia medico-

physica te Florence 1824–1924 (The first centenary of the — — at F.).
NTG, *68*, II, 677–8; *BGG*, *IV*, 213–4.

– Note on the special issue of *Lo Sperimentale*, May 1924, commemorating the first
centenary of the Florence Academy of Medicine and Science.

D. Illustrious Schools (Athenaea)

Breda

4243 NAUWELAERTS, M. A. (1945). *De oude Latijnse School van Breda* (The
old Latin School at B.) 226 pp. Prov. Genootsch. Kunsten en Wetenschappen, 's-Hertogenbosch.

4244 LANGEDIJK, D. (1934, 1935). "De Illustre Schole ende Collegium Auriacum" te Breda ("The Illustrious School and the Collegium Auriacum"
at B.). *Taxandria*, *41*, 257–70; 290–300; 328–36; *ibid.*, *42* (1935), 28–
39; appendices on 72–98 and 128–35.

4245 ALPHEN, G. van (1951). De Illustre School te Breda en haar boekerij
(The Illustrious School at B. and its library). *T. Gesch.*, *64*, 277–314.

4246 LINDEBOOM, G. A. (1971). De Illustre School te Breda (The Illustrious
School at B.). *Spiegel Historiael*, *5*, febr., 95–100, ill.

4247 SASSEN, F. L. R. (1962). Het wijsgerig onderwijs aan de Illustre School
te Breda 1646–1669 (The teaching of philosophy at the Illustrious
School at B.). *MKNAW*, N.R. 25, no 7, 106 pp. Noord-Holl. Uitg.
Mij, Amsterdam. 8°.

4247[a] — (1966). Levensberichten van de Hoogleeraren der Illustre School
te Breda (Biographical notices of the professors of the Illustrious School
at B.). *Jbk. "De Oranjeboom"*, *19*, 123–57.

4247[b] KOT, Stanislaw (1954). Polen in Breda in de 17e eeuw (Poles at B. in
the 17th century). *Jbk. "De Oranjeboom"*, *VII*, 91–114, 3 facs (of
titlepages).

– Translated from Polish into Dutch by T. Eekman; on Polish calvinistic students,
who studied at the Illustrious School; only a few of them studied medicine.

See also 408

Deventer

4248 AREND, J. P. (1831). *Het tweede eeuwfeest van de stichting der door-
      luchtige school te Deventer plegtig gevierd op den 16den van Sprokkel-
      maand 1830* (The second centenary of the foundation of the Illustrious
      School at D. celebrated on February 16, 1830). 81 pp. Deventer.

4249 SLEE, J. C. van (1916). *De Illustre school te Deventer 1630–1878. Hare
      geschiedenis, hoogleeraren en studenten, met bijvoeging van het Album
      Studiosorum* (The Illustrious School at D. History professors, stu-
      dents, adding the *Album Studiosorum*). 289 pp., 2 ports. M. Nijhoff,
      Den Haag.

4250 — (1916). *De Illustre school te Deventer 1630–1878. Register op het
      Album Studiosorum* (The Illustrious School at D. Register to the — —).
      XXIX pp. M. Nijhoff, Den Haag. 8°.

4251 BECKER, Karl (1943). Das Athenaeum in Deventer und seine Bezieh-
      ungen zum Reich. In: *Ewiges Volk*, no 1. Soest.

's-Hertogenbosch (Bois-le-Duc)

4252 HAAS, M. de (1926). *Bossche scholen van 1629 tot 1795* (Schools at
      Bois-le-Duc from 1629 till 1795). Thesis University of Amsterdam
      (Supervisor: H. Brugmans). XIII + 275 pp. 's-Hertogenbosch.

4253 SASSEN, F. L. R. (1970). Studenten aan de Illustre School te 's-Herto-
      togenbosch 1636–1810. Ter reconstructie van het *Album Studiosorum*
      (Students of the Illustrious School at Bois-le-Duc. For reconstruction
      of the — —). *MKNAW*, afd. Letterkunde, n.r. deel *33*, no 2., 108
      pp. Noord-Holl-Uitg. Mij, Amsterdam.

Maastricht

4254 — (1972). De Illustre School te Maastricht en haar Hoogleraren(1683–
      1794) (The Illustrious School at M. and its professors). *MKNAW*,
      afd. Letterkunde, n.r. deel *35*, no 1, 92 pp. Noord-Holl. Uitg. Mij,
      Amsterdam.
      – with 16 biographies of professors who served this School.
      – For Amsterdam- *see* Universities (4222–28).

E. Clinical Schools

General

4255 WITTOP KONING, D. A. (1953). De geschiedenis van de klinische scholen (History of the clinical schools). *Bull. Pharm.*, *VII*, Umschlag.

Alkmaar

4256 BRUINVIS, C. W. (1915). *De geneeskundige school te Alkmaar 1827–1865* (The clinical school at A.). 31 pp. no pl. pr. pr.
– Reviewed by F. M. G. de Feyfer: *Janus*, *XXI* (1916), 58.

Amsterdam

4257 RIJNBERK, G. van (1928). De clinische school van Amsterdam 1828 – 1 September – 1867. (The clinical school at A.). *NTG*, *72*, II, 4219; *BGG*, *VIII*, 229.

4258 HELLINGA, G. (1928). De voormalige Amsterdamsche Clinische School en het Binnengasthuis 1828 – 1 September – 1867 (The former Amsterdam Clinical School and the Inner Hospital). *NTG*, *72*, II, 4220–69; *BGG*, *VIII*, 230–79.

4258ª BRUGMANS, H. (1928). De klinische school en het Binnengasthuis (The clinical school and the Inner Hospital). *Amstelodamum*, *15*, 90–1.
– at Amsterdam.

4259 — (1934). Een critiek op de regeling van den stedelijken geneeskundigen dienst en op zekere toestanden in de heel- en verloskundige afdeeling der Amsterdamsche clinische school (Criticism of the regulation of the municipal medical service and of certain situations in the surgical and obstetrical department of the clinical school at A.). *NTG*, *78*, III, 3579–83; *BGG*, *XIV*, 159–63.

4260 — (1953). Het gebouw der voormalige genees-, heel- en verloskundige school aan de Kloveniersburgwal (1839–1867) (The building of the former medical, surgical and obstetrical school on the — —). [Amsterdam]. *NTG*, *97*, I, 621–5; *BGG*, *XXXIII*, 11–5, 2 ill.

Hoorn

4261 WITTOP KONING, D. A. (1950). De geneeskundige school te Hoorn
      (The clinical school at H.) *NTG, 94,* II, 1287–90; *BGG, XXX,* 22–5.

Middelburg

4262 MAN, J. C. de (1902, 1904). *De geneeskundige school te Middelburg
      1825–1866* (The clinical school at M.). 2 vols. Vol. I: 221 pp. Vol. 2:
      154 pp. D. G. Kröber, Middelburg. 8°.
      – with short biographies of lecturers and pupils.

Rotterdam

4263 SIMON THOMAS, P. H. (1913). De Rotterdamsche geneeskundige school
      1828–1866 (The Rotterdam clinical school). *Rott. Jbk,* 2de reeks, *1,*
      44–73.

4264 KRAMER, P. H. (1931). De clinische school te Rotterdam (The Rot-
      terdam clinical school). *GG, 9,* 101–22, 5 ports, 1 ill.

4265 LINDEBOOM, G. A. (1965). De Clinische School te Rotterdam (1828–
      1866) (The clinical school at R.). *NTG,* 109, II, 2095–8; *BGG, XLV,*
      36–9, 1 ill.

4266 FLIERINGA, H. J. (1969). *De geschiedenis van de "Stichting Klinisch
      Hoger Onderwijs" te Rotterdam, 1950–1967.* (History of the "Foun-
      dation Clinical Education" at R.). 2 vols. no pl.

                              See also 1296, 2887, 2944a, 2944b

Chapter XVII

Nursing and Hospitals

Before the time of the Reformation the sick in the Netherlands were nursed by nuns; charity was practised by rich people by way of doing good works. In the following centuries nursing in the hospitals was mostly left to ill-bred women. Sick-nurses ("diaconessen") came from pastor Fliedner's houses in Germany to the Netherlands in the first half of the nineteenth century, and in the second half girls from the higher classes began to devote themselves to nursing in the hospitals not without resistance (Jeltje de Bosch Kemper).

The history of nursing lunatics is listed apart. The fate of mental patients has for a long time been miserable. In the nineteenth century Schroeder van der Kolk as inspector of the lunatic asylums achieved a considerable improvement and, as in other countries, many modern lunatic asylums have been built since then.

In this chapter are also collected entries bearing on leper houses, orphanages, maternity homes etc.

A. Nursing

General

4267 ALERS *et al.* (1899). *De Ziekenverpleging en de zorg voor de openbare gezondheid in de laatste 50 jaren* (Nursing and care of public health in the last 50 years). 193 pp. Van Rossen, Amsterdam. 8°.

– a publication of the *Nederlands Tijdschrift voor Geneeskunde*, being the collected articles that had appeared in the *Catalogus der Historisch-Geneeskundige Tentoonstelling te Arnhem, Juli 1899*. The 30 articles on different kinds of medical services, hospitals, clinics, mental care. etc. are also listed separately in this bibliography.

4268 BOSCH KEMPER, J. de (1899). Geschiedkundig overzicht der ziekenverpleging in Nederland gedurende de laatste vijftig jaren (Historical survey of nursing in the Netherlands during the last fifty years). *Alers et al.*, 58–65.

4269   BARGER, G. J., H. FRANSSEN and J. TEVES Tzn (1902). *Onze Kranken.* Drie verhandelingen aangaande de historie, de verplichting en de practijk der ziekenverpleging (Our patients. Three treatises concerning the history, the obligation and the practice of nursing). 57 pp. J. H. Kok, Kampen.

4270   VERNÈDE, C. H. (1927). *Geschiedenis der ziekenverpleging* (History of nursing). 400 pp., 112 ill. Bohn, Haarlem.

4271   DANE, Corrie (1966). *Geschiedenis van de Ziekenverpleging. Een kort overzicht ten dienste van de opleiding tot verplegende* (History of nursing. A short survey at the service of the training of nurses). 119 pp., ill. De Tijdstroom, Lochem. ²1967.

4272   BINNENKADE, C. (1973) *Honderd jaar opleiding tot verpleegkundige in Nederland, 1872–1972* (Hundred years of training of nursing in the Netherlands, —). Thesis Free University of Amsterdam (Supervisor: A. C. Drogendijk Sr). 135 pp. Stafleu, Leiden.

4273   MEIJ-de LEUR, A. P. M. van der (1971). *Van Olie en Wijn. Geschiedenis van verpleegkunde, geneeskunde en sociale zorg* (On Oil and Wine. History of nursing, medicine and social care). 253 pp., ill. Agon-Elsevier, Amsterdam-Brussel.

4274   BRINK-POORT, Martha van (1963) *Anna Reynvaan.* 24 pp. Int. Arch. Vrouwenbeweging.
       – Anna Reynvaan (1844–1920) one of the founders of modern nursing in the Netherlands.

4274ª NATER, P. J. (1974). Nurse Edith Cavell. Mysteries rond de dood van een verpleegster (— —. Mysteries around the death of a nurse). *Arts en Wereld*, 7, no 9, 83–9, ill.
       – on E. Cavell (1865–1915), an English nurse who became matron of a School of nursing near Brussels. She was executed by a German firing-squad in World War I for her part in the resistance movement.

4275   RIJPSTRA-VERBEEK, M. (²1968). *Dienend in het wit; het levensverhaal van Zuster F. Meyboom* (Serving in white; biography of nurse — —). 232 pp. De Tijdstroom, Lochem.

4276   MEYBOOM, F. (1970). *Grepen uit de geschiedenis van zorgen en verzorgen* (Analecta from the history of nursing). 158 pp. Agon-Elsevier, Amsterdam-Brussels.

4277 BREMER, J. J. C. B. (1972). *De Ziekenhuispatient. Een hoofdstuk uit de medische psychologie* (The hospital patient. A chapter from medical psychology). 196 pp., 26 ill. 2nd ed. Medische reeks: Mens en Gezin, II. Nijmegen.
– Chapter 5 deals with medical care (60 pp.).

4278 BERESTEYN, E. A. van (1934). *Geschiedenis der Johanniter-orden in Nederland tot 1795* (History of the orders of the knights of St. John in the Netherlands till 1795). 104 pp., ill. Van Gorcum, Assen.
– Historical sketch.

4279

4280 TOURS, J. A. (1889). Iets over de Vereeniging voor Ziekenverpleging te Amsterdam en over pleegzusters (Something on the Association of Nursing and on nurses). *Eigen Haard, XV*, 325–7, 338–40, 344–6.

4281 DATEMA, Sicco (1972). *Met de zuster op stap. Een eeuw ziekenverpleging in Oosterbeek zonder winst-oogmerk* (A century of non-profit nursing at O.). 93 pp., ill. Oosterbeek. 8°.

4282 [   ](1925). *In Zilverkrans. Gedenkboek, uitgegeven ter gelegenheid van het 25-jarig bestaan van het Groene Kruis* (In a silver garland. Memorial volume, edited on the occasion of the 25th anniversary of the "Green Cross").

4282ᵃ [   ] (1916). *De vooruitgang op medisch en verplegingsgebied in de laatste 25 jaren. Herdenkingsbundel bij de voltooiing van zijn 25en jaargang, uitgegeven door het Tijdschrift voor Ziekenverpleging* (The progress in medicine and nursing in the last 25 years. Memorial volume at the completion of its 25th volume, published by the — — —). 168 pp. J. H. de Bussy, Amsterdam.
– comprises many articles on different fields of medicine, nursing, etc.

See also 3810–13 (naval medicine), 3939–50 (military medicine), 5509a

Mental nursing

4283 HILBERS, J. J. T. (1922). Geschiedenis der krankzinnigenverpleging (History of mental nursing). *NTG, 66*, I, 504–5; *BGG, II*, 61–2.

4284 LEERSUM, E. C. van (1927). Kleine bijdrage tot de geschiedenis der krankzinnigenverpleging hier te lande (A small contribution to the history of mental nursing in our country). *NTG, 71*, II, 1402–3; *BGG, VII*, 642–3.

4285   VEEN, S. J. van (1904). Behandeling van krankzinnigen (1432–'89) (Treatment of lunatics). *Gelre, VII*, 317.

4286   [G.E.] (1909). Krankzinnigenverpleging in de XVIe eeuw (Mental nursing in the 16th century). *Navorscher, LVIII*, 549.

4287   DOOREN, L. (1939). Behandeling van krankzinnigen (1432–1489). (Treatment of lunatics). *NTG, 83*, I, 1027–8; *BGG, XIX*, 56–7.

4288   DEVENTER, J. van (1901). *Krankzinnigenverpleging in de eerste helft der vorige eeuw* (Mental nursing in the first half of the last century). 203 pp. Van Heteren, Amsterdam.

4289   KOENEN, J. (1930). Sprokkels uit oude boeken. Guislain's *Traité sur l'aliénation mentale et sur les hospices des aliénés* (Gleanings from old books. Guislain's — — —). In: *Tweede Jbk. Ver. R.K. Gestichten en Inrichtingen voor krankzinnigen en zwakzinnigen.*
       – Reviewed by M. A. van Andel: *NTG, 76* (1932), II, 2230; *BGG, XII*, 96.

4290   BREUKINK, H. (1921, 1922, 1926). Overzicht van opvatting en behandeling van geesteszieken in oude tijden (Survey of conception and treatment of mental patients in ancient times).
       I. *NTG, 65*, (1921), I, 3076–94; *BGG, I*, 243–61, 21 ill.
       II. *NTG, 65*, II, 2806–14; *BGG, I*, 438–46, 10 ill.
       III. *NTG, 66*, (1922), II, 1076–91; *BGG, II*, 207–22, 21 ill.
       IV. *NTG, 70*, (1926), II, 2560–7; *BGG, VI*, 319–26, 5 ill.

4291   BERGER, J. A. (1931). Een tarief voor de verpleging in het gesticht no 2 te Middelburg (A tariff for nursing in the asylum no 2 at M.). *NTG, 75*, I, 643–6; *BGG, XI*, 50–3.
       – on the tariffs of the lunatic asylum.

4292   WAP, J. J. (1931). Geneeskundige Archivalia (Medical Records). *NTG, 75*, I, 1162–3; *BGG, XI*, 91–2.
       – refers to the previous item; letter to the editor.

4293   VEERMAN, W. (1971). Krankzinnigenzorg in Middelburg (Mental care at M.). *Zeeuws T., 21*, 132–3.

4294   BRUYN, J. A. de (1931). Overeenkomst tusschen de stad Schoonhoven en een harer burgers, aangaande onderhoud en verpleging van een krankzinnige (Agreement between the city of S. and one of its citizens, concerning support and nursing of a lunatic). *NTG*, *75*, II, 2379; *BGG*, *XI*, 155.

4295 WEIJDE, A. J. van der (1929). De arbeidstherapie in "het geneeskundig gesticht voor krankzinnigen te Utrecht" voor omstreeks 100 jaren (Labour-therapy in "the lunatic asylum at U." about 100 years ago). *Jbk. Oud-Utrecht*, [7], 177–82.

4296 — (1931). De behandeling der krankzinnigen in vroeger tijd te Utrecht (Treatment of lunatics at U. in former times). *NTG*, *75*, IV, 5002–14; *BGG*, *XI*, 265–77.

4297 MULDER, R. D. (1963). De zorg voor krankzinnigen en geestelijk gestoorden in Drenthe in vroeger eeuwen (The care of lunatics and mental patients in D. in former centuries). *Nieuwe Drentse Almanak*, *81*, 124–32.

4298 KATE, W. ten (1937). Uit de notulen van de Staten van Overijsel. Verpleging van krankzinnigen 15 Maart 1734 (From the minutes of the States of Overijsel. Nursing of lunatics, March 15, 1734). *NTG*, *81*, *II*, 1462; *BGG*, *XVII*, 83.

4299 ANDEL, M. A. van (1933). Krankzinnigenverpleging in Nederlandsch Indië (Mental nursing in the Dutch East Indies). *NRC*, 23 April.

4300 DONINCK, A. van (1929). Het gebruik der boeien bij de behandeling der krankzinnigen in vroeger tijd. Colonie-Gheel (België) (The use of fetters and wristlets at the treatment of lunatics in former times. Colony-Gheel (Belgium). *NTG*, *73*, I, 1732–7; *BGG*, *IX*, 105–10.

4301 — (1930). Ste-Dimphna-cultus en gezinsverpleging. Met een plaat (Ste-Dimphna-cult and boarding out. With a plate). *NTG*, *74*, II, 5928–35; *BGG*, *X*, 307–14, ill.
– on mental nursing at Gheel; with 2 ill. of medals: Ste Dymphna.
See also 4413–40 (lunatic asylums).

4302 — (1932). Gezinsverpleging in vroegere tijden te Gheel. De duivel-banning (Boarding out of lunatics at G. Exorcism). *NTG*, *76*, II, 2219–24; *BGG*, *XII*, 85–90.

4303 — (1933). Gezinsverpleging te Gheel. Het vraagstuk der infirmerie (Boarding out at G. The question of the infirmary). *NTG*, *77*, I, 544–51; *BGG*, *XIII*, 53–60.

4304 VERAGHTERT, Karel (1970). Naar een moderne gezinsverpleging te Geel (1790–1860) (Towards modern boarding out at G.). *Ann. Belg. Ver. Hosp. Gesch.*, 8, 55–72.

4305 — (1971). De Geelse gezinsverpleging als regionale welvaartsfaktor (1795–1860). (The boarding out at G. as a regional factor of prosperity). *Bijdr. Gesch.*, *54*, 3–30.

> See also 1538, 3399–3403 (Treatment) 4425–29b, 4533, 4633.7, 4680.

Varia

4306 SNELLEN Sr, H. (1899). De oogheelkundige verpleging in Nederland gedurende de laatste 50 jaren (Ophthalmological nursing in the Netherlands during the last 50 years). *Alers et al.*, 69–82, 5 ill.

> See also 813

4307 ROEKEL, G. van (1940). Vondelingen verzorging (Care of foundlings). *NTG*, *84*, I, 435–6; *BGG*, *XX*, 39–40.

4308 VOUTE, A. (1908–1910). Bijdrage tot de kennis der verzorging van het gezonde en zieke kind in de tweede helft der achttiende eeuw (Contribution to the knowledge of the care of the healthy and sick child in second half of the 18th century). *Med. Wbl.*, *15* (1908–09), 553 and 565; *ibid.*, *16* (1909–10), 25, 37 and 49.   See also 754

4309 SCHMIDT, J. (1915). *Weezenverpleging bij de Gereformeerden in Nederland tot 1795* (Orphan's maintenance with the Calvinists in the Netherlands till —). 288 pp. Utrecht. 8°.

B. Hospitals

General

4310 WORTMAN, J. L. C. (1915). Het ziekenhuis voorheen en thans. (The hospital past and present). *NTG*, *59*, I, 1313–34.

4311 ROEKEL, G. van (1940). Volk bij den weg in vroeger tijd, de oorsprong der gasthuizen (Travellers in former times, the origin of the hospitals). *NTG*, *84*, IV, 3902–3; *BGG*, *XX*, 159–60.

4312 SCHOUTE, D. (1920). Geschiedenis van het ziekenhuiswezen (History of the system of hospitals). *NTG*, *64*, I, 444–5.
– included in a report of a meeting of the "Genootschap".

4313 DROGENDIJK, A. C. (1962). Het ziekenhuiswezen voorheen en thans (The system of hospitals past and present). *Spreekuur Thuis*, *4*, 744–7; *ibid.*, *5*, (1963), 54–7.

4314 BONENFANT, Paul (1965). Hôpitaux et bienfaisance publique dans les anciens Pays-Bas des origines à la fin du XVIIIe siècle. *Ann. Soc. belge d'Hist. Hospitaux, 3*, 1-44.

4315 SPANJE, N. P. van (1899). Ziekenhuizen in Nederland gedurende de laatste vijftig jaar (Hospitals in the Netherlands during the last fifty years). *Alers et al.*, 89-109, 3 ill.

4316 QUERIDO, A. (1960). *Godshuizen en Gasthuizen* (Charitable Institutions and hospitals). 215 pp., ill. E. M. Querido, Amsterdam.

4317 FENEMA, C. H. van (1913). Het administratieboek van een ziekenhuis als genealogische bron (The administration book of a hospital as a genealogical source). *Ned. Leeuw, XXXI*, 280.

4318 WEE, Herman van der (1966). Les archives hospitalières et l'étude de la pauvreté aux Pays-Bas du XVe au XVIIIe siècle. *Revue du Nord, 48*, 5-16.

4319 PUTTO, J. A. (1936). Een hospitaalreglement uit de achttiende eeuw (A hospital regulation from the 18th century). *GG, XIV*, 69.

4320 HALLEMA, A. (1933). Welke instrumenten en toestellen de doktoren in onze vaderlandsche hospitalen en ziekenhuizen een eeuw geleden gebruikten (On the instruments and apparatuses, used in our national hospitals a century ago). *Ziekenhuiswezen, 6*, no 6, 15 pp., 10 ill.

See also 3849, 3921-33 (military hospitals).

Local Hospitals

Amersfoort

4321 BEURDEN, A. F. van (1924). *Het Sint Elisabeth's Gast- of Ziekenhuis te Amersfoort* (St. Elisabeth's hospital at A.). Amersfoort.
– with woodcuts of Victor van Schoonhoven van Beurden; reviewed by D. Schoute: *NTG, 70* (1926), I, 1410-1; *BGG, VI*, 79-80.

Amsterdam

4322 BERNS, A. W. C. (1883). *De gasthuizen van Amsterdam van de 14e eeuw tot op heden* (The hospitals of A. from the 14th century up to the present). 79 pp. Van Heteren, Amsterdam.
– Reviewed by G. D. L. Huet: *NTG, 19* (1883), 411-7.

4323 — (1886). *De wenschelijkheid van één Gasthuis voor Amsterdam* (The desirability of *one* hospital for A.). 117 pp. Van Heteren, Amsterdam.

4324 TILANUS, J. W. R. (1907). De vernieuwing der stedelijke ziekenhuizen te Amsterdam in de 19de eeuw. Historische schets (The renovation of the municipal hospitals at A. in the 19th century. Historical survey). *NTG*, *51*, I, 85–112, 17 ill.

4325 WORTMAN, J. L. C. (no d.). *De Amsterdamsche Ziekenhuizen* (The hospitals of A.). 169 pp., 176 ill. Alg. Periodieken Mij, Lochem.
– Dutch and English text.

4326 HELLINGA, G. and G. C. DELPRAT (1932). De Gasthuizen (The Hospitals). In: *Gedenkboek van het Athenaeum en de Universiteit van Amsterdam 1632–1932*, 415–74. Stadsdrukkerij, Amsterdam.
– Hellinga deals with the history of the period 1669–1883; Delprat with that of 1883–1932.

4326ᵃ HELLINGA, G. (1927). Amsterdamsche hulpziekenhuizen (Amsterdam auxiliary hospitals). *Amstelodamum*, *14*, 8.

4327 — (1936). Amsterdamsche hulpziekenhuizen (The auxiliary hospitals of A.). *NTG*, *80*, I, 391–8; *BGG*, *XVI*, 21–8.

4328 — (1923). Nog iets over de Amsterdamsche gasthuizen (More about the Amsterdam hospitals). *NTG*, *67*, II, 886–901; *BGG*, *III*, 201–16.

4329 — (1924). Een en ander van oudsher ingeslopen misbruiken bij het opnemen van zieken in de Amsterdamsche gasthuizen, en de daartegen genomen maatregelen (Something on abuses crept in of old, in admitting patients to the Amsterdam hospitals, and the measures against it). *NTG*, *68*, II, 2230–9; *BGG*, *IV*, 267–76.

4329ᵃ — (1927). Schets van de opkomst, bloei en opheffing van het Amsterdamsche Gasthuisbestuur (Sketch of the rise, flourishing and dissolution of the Amsterdam Hospital board). *Jbk. Amstelodamum*, *24*, 107–32.

4330 — (1927). Gasthuistoestanden in den "goeden ouden tijd" (Hospital conditions in the "good old days"). *NTG*, *71*, II, 97–108; *BGG*, *VII*, 501–12.

4331 — (1928). Een stukje gasthuisgeschiedenis uit het midden der negentiende eeuw (A bit of hospital history from the middle of the 19th century). *NTG*, *72*, I, 562–6; *BGG*, *VIII*, 38–42.

4332 — (1929). De afschaffing van het z.g. poort- of stuiversgeld voor de Amsterdamsche gasthuizen (The abolition of the so-called gate- or penny money for the Amsterdam hospitals). *NTG, 73*, II, 3575–9; *BGG, IX*, 187–91.

4333 — (1930). De Amsterdamsche gasthuizen en het geneeskundig onderwijs (1862–1871). (The Amsterdam hospitals and medical education). *NTG, 74*, I, 2906–13; *BGG, X*, 164–71.

4334 — (1932, 1933). De Amsterdamsche gasthuizen beoordeeld door vreemdelingen (The Amsterdam hospitals judged by foreigners). *NTG, 76*, (1932), II, 2800–14; *BGG, XII*, 105–19; *NTG, 77* (1933), II, 1410–24; *BGG, XIII*, 85–99.

4334[a] [Anonym] (1932). Vreemdelingen over onze gasthuizen in vroeger tijd (Foreigners on our hospitals in former times). *Amstelodamum 19*, 77–8.

4334[b] HELLINGA, G. (1943). Het toezicht houdend en dienst-personeel der Amsterdamsche gasthuizen in vroeger tijden (Superintending and domestic staff of the Amsterdam hospitals in former times). *Ziekenhuiswezen, XVI*, 174–9; 181–9; 209–29; 251–61; 281–3.

4334[c] — (1948). Uit de geschiedenis der Amsterdamsche gasthuizen. De Sleutel-, Paasch- en Gedachtenismaaltijden; presenten uit de apotheek (From the history of the Amsterdam hospitals. The Key-, Eastern and Memorial meals; gifts from the chemist's shop). *Ziekenhuiswezen, 21*, 82–6, ill.

St. Pietersgasthuis (Binnengasthuis) (St Peter's Hospital (Inner Hospital))

4335 HELLINGA, G. (1923). Een en ander uit de geschiedenis der Amsterdamsche gasthuizen (het Sint Pieters-gasthuis en pesthuis) (Something from the history of the hospitals at A. (the St. Peter's hospital and the plague-house). *NTG, 67*, I, 43–7; *BGG, III*, 10–4.

4336 — (1923). De Amsterdamsche gasthuizen en de slag bij Doggersbank (The Amsterdam hospitals and the battle at D.). *NTG, 67*, I, 2395–3005; *BGG, III*, 129–39.

4337 — (1927). Eenige mededeelingen uit de geschiedenis der voormaligen Amsterdamsche Kraamzaal (Some communications of the former lying-in room at A.). *NTG, 71*, II, 1963–8; *BGG, VII*, 665–70.

4338   — (1929). Een en ander over het aandeel van het Amsterdamsche St. Pietersgasthuis en het in vroeger tijden "logheeren, cureeren ende accomodeeren" van zieke en gewonde soldaten en matrozen (Something on the part of the Amsterdam St. Peter's Hospital and the "lodging, healing and accomodating" of ill and wounded soldiers and sailors in former times). *NTG, 73*, I, 1720–31; *BGG, IX*, 93–104.

4339   — (1929). Een en ander over de overeenkomsten, aangegaan gedurende het tijdvak 1651–1699 tusschen regenten van het Amsterdamsche St. Pieters gast- en Pesthuis en cureerders (Something on the agreements, made during the period — — between the Governors of the St Peter's Hospital and Plague-house and the healers). *NTG, 73*, II, 4141–6; *BGG, IX*, 201–6.

4340   — (1930). *Geschiedenis van het St. Pieters- of Binnengasthuis* (History of the St Peter's- or Inner Hospital). 135 pp., ill. Stadsdrukkerij, Amsterdam. 4°.

4341   — (1933). De beteekenis van het Amsterdamsche St. Pietersgasthuis voor het ontleedkundig onderwijs in ons land in vroeger tijden (The significance of the Amsterdam St. Peters Hospital for anatomical teaching in our country in former times). *NTG, 77*, III, 3042–52; *BGG, XIII*, 157–69.

4342   — (1934). Sprokkelingen uit het gasthuisarchief (Gleanings from the archive of the hospital). *NTG, 78*, II, 1983–8; *BGG, XIV*, 91–6.

4343   — (1938). Mededeelingen uit de oudste geschiedenis van het Amsterdamsche St. Pietersgasthuis (Communications from the oldest history of the Amsterdam St. Peter's Hospital). *NTG, 82*, II, 2281–91; *BGG, XVIII*, 82–92.

4344   — (1939). Regeling van de geneeskundige verzorging in het Amsterdamsche St. Pietersgasthuis (Regulation of the medical care in the Amsterdam St. Peter's Hospital). *NTG, 83*, I, 514–22; *BGG, XIX*, 19–27.

4345   — (1939). Van "verbanthuys" tot dubbele chirurgische cliniek (From "dressing-house" to double surgical clinic). *NTG, 83*, IV, 4857–64; *BGG, XIX*, 221–8.

4345ᵃ   — (1962). Een en ander over bayerds in het algemeen en overdien van het Amsterdamsche St. Pietersgasthuis in 't bijzonder (Something on night-shelters in general and in particular on those of the Amsterdam St Peter's Hospital). *Jbk Amstelodamum, 23*, 93–104, ill.

4345[b] BALBIAN VERSTER, J. F. L. de (1930). Het Sint Pieters of Binnengast-huis (The St. Peter of Inner Hospital). *Amstelodamum, 17,* 91–2.

4346 DIJKHUIZEN, Sietzo (1971). Het Binnen Gasthuis in Amsterdam: ... Daar is altijd getimmerd ...! (The Inner Hospital at A. ... there has always been carpentering ...!) *Arts en Auto, 37,* 607–15, ill.

4347 HALLEMA, A. (1937). Een debat in het Amsterdamsche St-Pieters- of Binnengasthuis voor twee en halve eeuw terug (A debate in the Amsterdam St. Peter's- or Inner Hospital two and a half centuries ago). *Ziekenhuiswezen, 10,* no 5, 8 pp.
– on remarkable pamphlets in this hospital and on a French physician P. Guenellon Jr? who was practising there.

4348 ROETEMEIJER, H. J. M. (1970). Het Binnengasthuis (The Inner Hospital). *Ons Amsterdam, 22,* 198–205.

See also 4258, 4258a

Wilhelmina Hospital

4348[a] HELLINGA, G. (1928). Oproep voor een gediplomeerd geneeskundig assistent aan het Buitengasthuis in 1842 (A call for a qualified medical assistant in the Outer Hospital in 1842). *Amstelodamum, 15,* 15–6.

4349 HELLINGA, G. (1940). Een sombere bladzijde uit de geschiedenis van het voormalige Amsterdamsche Buitengasthuis (A dark page from the history of the former Amsterdam Outer Hospital). *NTG, 84,* I, 424–34; *BGG, XX,* 28–38.

4350 QUERIDO, A. (1961). *Het Wilhelmina Gasthuis te Amsterdam. Geschiedenis en voorgeschiedenis* (The Wilhelmina Hospital at A. History and previous history). 336 pp., ill. De Tijdstroom, Lochem.

4351 LEIDERITZ, A. F. (1966). 75-jarig jubileum Wilhelmina Gasthuis te Amsterdam (75th anniversary of the Wilhelmina Hospital at A.). *T. Ziekenverpl., 19,* 346–9.

Various Amsterdam Hospitals

4352 STOLK, L. (1923). *Geschiedenis van het Onze Lieve Vrouwe Gasthuis* (History of the Holy Virgin Hospital). 102 pp., ill. no pl. 8°.

4352[a] [Anonym] (1948). Onze Lieve Vrouwe Gasthuis 1898–1948 (The Holy Virgin Hospital — —). *Amstelodamum, 35,* 154–5.

4353 [   ] (1958). *Aspecten van Caritas en Geneeskunde. Gedenkschrift bij het zestigjarig bestaan van het Onze Lieve Vrouwe Gasthuis te Amsterdam* (Aspects of Charity and Medicine. Memorial volume on the occasion of the 60th anniversary of the Holy Virgin Hospital at A.). 330 pp., ill., ports. Proost & Brandt, Amsterdam.

4354 FUCHS, J. M. [1967]. *Verzorgen en verplegen. Evangelisch-Lutherse bejaardenzorg. Luthers Diaconessenhuis, Amsterdam* (Tending and nursing. Evangelic-Lutheran care for the aged. Lutheran Deaconesses' Institution —). XV + 135 pp., Veenman, Wageningen.

4355 [   ] (1965). *Een eeuw Emma Kinderziekenhuis* (A century Emma Children's Hospital). 36 pp., ill. De Arbeiderspers, Amsterdam. – 1865-1965.

4356 [ROELFS, Jan] (1972). *Weesperplein 1. Vijfentwintig jaar Gemeenteziekenhuis 1947-1972* (25 years Municipal Hospital). 32 pp. Bureau Voorlichting Gem. Amsterdam.

4357 POST, C. R. (1973). The Antoni van Leeuwenhoek Hospital. *Arch. Chir. Neerl.*, *XXV*, 335-40, 6 ill.

4357ᵃ [Anonym] (1938). Het Burgerziekenhuis (The Citizens' Hospital). *Amstelodamum*, *25*, 11-3; 27.

Arnhem

4358 KNOTTNERUS, A. (1909). *Nederlands-Hervormd Diaconessenhuis te Arnhem 1884-1909* (Dutch Reformed Deaconesses' Institution at A.). 35 pp., ill.

Breda, Delft, Deventer

4359 BREKELMANS, F. A. (1951). *Het Bredasche Gasthuis. Geschiedenis van het Oud-Mannenhuis met de daarmee in 1798 verenigde gestichten* (The Breda Hospital. History of the Home for aged men and of the asylums united with it in 1798). 201 pp. Breda. (pr. pr.)

4360 BOURICIUS, L. G. N. (1928). Eenige grepen uit de geschiedenis van het St. Joris gasthuis te Delft (Analecta from the history of the St. Joris Hospital at D.). *NTG*, *72*, I, 553-61; *BGG*, *VIII*, 29-37.

4361 OOSTERBAAN, D. P. (1954). *Zeven eeuwen. Geschiedenis van het Oude en Nieuwe Gasthuis te Delft* (Seven centuries. History of the Old and New Hospital at D.). 457 + LXIX pp., ill., ports. Gaade, Delft.

4362 [   ] [1950]. *Gedenkboek ter gelegenheid van het 75-jarig bestaan van het St Josef Ziekenhuis te Deventer (1875–1950)* (Memorial volume on the occasion of the 75th anniversary of the St Josef Hospital at D.). No pl.

Dordrecht

4363 DROGENDIJK, A. C. (1949). Het Diaconessenhuis (The Deaconesses' Institution). *Eeuwfeestnummer Med. blad*, Afd. Dordrecht, 24 November.

4364 — (1960). 50 jaar Ver[eniging] van Diaconessenarbeid in Dordrecht en omstreken (50 years "Association of Deaconesses' work" at D. and its environs). *Med. blad.*, Afd. Dordrecht, 29 April.

4365 [   ] (1968). *Het Gemeenteziekenhuis van Dordrecht vernieuwd.* (The renovation of the Municipal Hospital at D.). 43 pp., ill. Gemeente Delft.
– p. 1–25: Th. E. Jensma. Geschiedenis van het Heilig Sacramentsgasthuis te Dordrecht (History of the Holy Sacrament Hospital).

Groningen

4365ª EVERS, G. A. (1904). Het Typographen-Gasthuis te Groningen (The Typographers Hospital at G.). *Het Noorden, 1*, 229, 268, 361, 384, 6 pl.

4365ᵇ FEITH, J. A. (1907). Wandelingen door het oude Groningen. XV. Ziekenhuizen (Walks through old G. XV. Hospitals). *Gron. Volksalm., 18*, 1–25.

4365ᶜ EYSSELSTEYN, G. van (1907). *Het Algemeen Provinciaal-, Stads- en Academisch Ziekenhuis te Groningen* (The General Provincial-, Municipal- and Academic Hospital at G.) With 18 topographical drawings, 84 ill. Groningen.

4365ᵈ TILBUSSCHER, K. J. zn. J. (1917). "t Sint Anthony Gasthuis of 't Oosterpoortengasthuis te Groningen (1517–1917) (The St. Anthony hospital or the "Oosterpoorten" hospital at G.). *Groningen, 2*, 66–70.

4366 MUNTENDAM, P. (1926). Ziekenhuizen te Groningen in het verleden (Hospitals at G. in the past). *NTG, 70*, I, 987–8 *BGG, VI*, 67–8.
– Review of an article by W. H. Mansholt, entitled: Ziekenhuizen te Groningen in het verleden, het heden en de toekomst, In: *Het Ziekenhuis* (Febr. 1926).

4367 SCHULTE, J. E. (1953). Het jubileum van het Academisch Ziekenhuis te Groningen (The jubilee of the Academic Hospital at G.) *R.K. Artsenbl., 32,* 319–22.

4367ᵃ TONCKENS, N. (1954, 1955). Een eeuw ziekenhuis aan de Munnikeholm (Hundred years of the history of the hospital on the —). I. Een en ander uit het bestaan van het Nosocomium Academicum 1803–1852 (Something from the existence of the — —). *Gron. Volksalm.,* 16–64; II. Het Algemeen Provinciaal, Stads- en Academisch Ziekenhuis (The General Provincial, Municipal and Academic Hospital). *Gron. Volksalm.* (1955), 149–59.

4368 [   ] [1953]. *Gedenkboek van het Algemeen Provinciaal-, Stads-, en Academisch Ziekenhuis te Groningen, 1903–1953* (Memorial Volume of the General Provincial-, Municipal-, and Academic Hospital at G.). 234 pp. Noordhoff, Groningen.

See also 5026, 5482a, 5483

Den Haag (The Hague)

4369 BROES VAN HEEKEREN, W. (1903). Het Sint Antonius gesticht te 's-Gravenhage (The St. Antonius Hospital at The Hague). *Die Haghe, 62,* 62.

4370 MOLL, W. (1925). *Een eeuw Ziekenhuis-geschiedenis. Het Haagsch Gemeenteziekenhuis 1823–1923* (A century of hospital history. The Hague municipal Hospital). Overzicht van den tegenwoordigen toestand der Gemeente-Ziekenhuizen (E. A. Koch). (Survey of the present state of the municpal hospitals). 170 pp., ill., port. Mouton, 's-Gravenhage.
– Reviewed by P. Muntendam: *NTG, 70* (1926), I, 47–8; *BGG, VI,* 21–2.

See also 5028a

Haarlem, Heerlen, 's-Hertogenbosch (Bois-le-Duc).

4371 KERSBERGEN, L. C. (1931). *Geschiedenis van het St. Elisabeth's of Groote Gasthuis te Haarlem* (History of the St. Elisabeth's or Great Hospital at H.). 486 pp., ports. Enschedé & Zn., Haarlem.
– Published on the occasion of the 350th anniversary. Contributions of B. J. Kouwer and other specialists. Reviewed by F. M. G. de Feyfer: *NTG, 75* (1931), IV, 4565–6; *BGG, XI,* 257–8.

4371ᵃ KURTZ, G. H. (1937). Het leven in het oude St. Elisabeth's Gasthuis

(The life in the old St. Elisabeth's Hospital [Haarlem]). *Jbk. Haerlem*, 60–83.

4372 DIJKSTRA, O. H. (1971). Het Gasthuis voor besmettelijke ziekten te Haarlem 1857–1876 (The Hospital for contagious diseases at H.) *Jbk. Haerlem*, 154–63.   *See also* 4633.15

4372ª GILSE, P. H. van (1952). Haarlem, bakermat van het gipsverband, de uitvinding van dr. Anthonius Matthijsen in 1852 (H., birthplace of the Paris bandage, the invention of — — in 1852). *Jbk. Haerlem*, 38–40, ill.

4372ᵇ BLOEMSMA, A. D. (1961). Vrouwe- en Anthony Gasthuis (Women's and Anthony Hospital). *Jbk. Haerlem*, 144–50, ill.
– at Haarlem.

4372ᶜ Os, H. W. M. van (1962). Hoe de broeders van St. Johannes de Deo zich in Haarlem vestigden en daar een ziekenhuis stichtten (How the brothers of — — established themselves at H. and founded a hospital there). *Jbk. Haerlem*, 73–88.

4373 DIETEREN, Remigius (ed.) (1954). *In dienst der zieken; Het St. Joseph Ziekenhuis te Heerlen 1904–1954* (At the service of the sick; The St. Joseph Hospital at H.). 318 pp., ill. Brand, Bussum. 8°.

4374 COOPMANS, J. P. A. (1964). *De rechtstoestand van de Godshuizen te 's-Hertogenbosch vóór 1629* (The legal status of the Charitable Institutions at Bois-le-Duc before —). VIII + 213 pp. Serie: Standen en Landen, no XXXI. Nauwelaerts, Leuven – Béatrice Nauwelaerts, Paris.

4374ª HALLEMA, A. (1933). Het Grootziekengasthuis te 's-Hertogenbosch in den loop der eeuwen (The "Great Hospital" at Bois-le-Duc in the course of the centuries). *Ziekenhuiswezen*, 5, 240.

4374ᵇ ROOY, H. J. M. van (1963). *Het oud archief van het Grootziekengasthuis te 's-Hertogenbosch* (The old archive of the "Great Hospital" at Bois-le-Duc). 3 vols. Godshuizen, 's-Hertogenbosch.

4374ᶜ SPEK, L. A. M. van der (1932). Het Grootziekengasthuis te 's-Hertogenbosch (The "Great Hospital" at Bois-le-Duc). *Ziekenhuiswezen*, 5, 8.

4374ᵈ — and J. A. W. VRIJMAN (1932). *Het Grootziekengasthuis te 's-Hertogenbosch* (The "Great Hospital" at Bois-le-Duc). Godshuizen, 's-Hertogenbosch.

4374^e RUITER, K. de (1974). Enkele grepen uit de historie van het Groot
Ziekengasthuis te 's-Hertogenbosch (Analecta from the history of the
Great Hospital at Bois-le-Duc). *NTG*, *118*, 733–9.

Leiden

4375   VEIT, J. (1899). *Zur Erinnerung an das hundertjährige Bestehen der Lei-
dener Universitäts-Frauenklinik*. 32 pp., port. (of M. S. du Pui). E. J.
Brill, Leiden.
– Address, delivered January 23, 1899.

4376   BARNARD, L. (1959). Een waardige bestemming voor het St. Caecilia
Gasthuis? (A worthy destination for the St. Caecilia Hospital?) [at
Leyden]. *NTG*, *103*, II, 2183–4.

4377   JONGSMA, M. W. (1963). *325 jaar Academisch Ziekenhuis te Leiden*
(325 years Academic Hospital at L.). 37 pp., ill. De Tijdstroom,
Lochem.

4378   DONGEN, M. A. van (1961). Het Sinte Elisabetten Gasthuis te Leiden
(The Saint Elisabeth Hospital at L.). *Ciba-Symp.*, *9*, 74–8, 7 ill.

4378^a LUYENDIJK-ELSHOUT, A. M. (1974). The Caecilia Hospital in Leiden
(1600–1972). In: *Proc. XXIII Int. Congress of the Hist. of Med. London 2–9 Sept. 1972*, Vol. I, 312–7. Wellcome Institute of the History of
Medicine, London.

Middelburg, Nijmegen, Roermond

4379   SCHOUTE, D. (1916). De levensloop van een ziekenhuis. Geschiedenis
van het Gasthuis te Middelburg (The course of life of a hospital. History of the Hospital at M.). *Archief Zeeuwsch Gen. Wetensch.*, 137–285.
– also as a monograph. 149 pp. Altorffer, Middelburg.

4380   — (1917). De levensloop van een ziekenhuis (The course of life of a
hospital). *NTG*, *61*, II, 3–64. [Middelburg].

4381   GELDEREN, D. N. van (1926). De inrichting voor Ziekenverpleging te
Middelburg van 1859–1879 (The Institution for nursing at M.). *NTG*,
70, II, 1084–1103; *BGG*, *VI*, 213–32.

4382   LAMMERTS VAN BUEREN, A. [no d.] *Het Oud-Burgeren Gasthuis te Nijmegen* (The Old-Citizen Hospital at N.). Nijmegen.

4383 LUISSEN, J. (1969). De beide oudste gasthuizen van Roermond (The two oldest hospitals of R.). *De Maasgouw*, *88*, 11–8.

Rotterdam

4383ª SCHREVE, F. H. (1944). Uit de geschiedenis van het Stedelijk Ziekenhuis (From the history of the municipal hospital). *Rott. Jbk.*, 5de reeks, *1*, 109–50, 17 tables, 1 ill.
– At Rotterdam.

4384 SCHAAR, P. J. van der (1951). Het Honderdjarig bestaan van het Gemeentelijke Ziekenhuis aan de Coolsingel te Rotterdam (The 100th anniversary of the Municipal Hospital on the — at R.). *NTG*, *95*, IV, 3303–8, 1 ill.

4385 — and H. J. VALK (1951). *De geschiedenis van een Rotterdams Ziekenhuis: 100 jaar Ziekenhuis Coolsingel 1851–1951* (History of a Rotterdam Hospital: 100 years Coolsingel Hospital). Gemeente Drukkerij, Rotterdam.

4386 KOUWENAAR, W. (1951). Het ziekenhuis aan de Coolsingel te Rotterdam (The Hospital on the — at R.). *NTG*, *95*, IV, 3302.

4387 HERMANS, Hyacinth (1942). *Ons Sint Franciscus Gasthuis 50 jaar* (Our St. Franciscus Hospital 50 years). ill. no pl.

4388 WAALWIJK, H. J. (1965). *Het werk gaat door; 75 jaar Eudokia* (Work is going on; 75 years Eudokia). Paardekoper, Amsterdam.
– with illustrations by Otto Dicke.

4389 LEEDEN, C. B. van der [no d.]. *De ontwikkeling van Diakoniehuis tot Gemeentelijk tehuis voor ouden van dagen te Rotterdam* (Development from Almshouse to Municipal Home for the aged at R.). no pl.

Tilburg

4390 [   ] (1954). *Gedenkboek uitgegeven ter gelegenheid van het 125-jarig bestaan der stichting en het 25-jarig bestaan van het huidige ziekenhuis, 29 November 1954.* (Memorial volume published on the occasion of the 125th anniversary of the foundation and the 25th anniversary of the present hospital). 193 pp., 28 ill. Tilburg. 4°.
– Edited by: Stichting het R.K. Gasthuis St Elisabeth-Ziekenhuis Tilburg.

Utrecht

4391   BRONDGEEST, P. Q. (1901). *Bijdragen tot de geschiedenis van het Gast-huis, het Klooster en de Balije van St. Catharina der Johanniter-ridders en van het Driekoningen-gasthuis te Utrecht* (Contributions to the history of the Hospital, the Cloister and the Bailiwick of St. Catharina of the knights of St. John and of the Epiphany hospital at U.). 128 pp., ill. Hilversum. 8°.

4391ª   ROMBACH, K. A. (1944). Een en ander uit de geschiedenis van de Utrecht-se gast- en ziekenhuizen (Something from the history of the Utrecht hospitals). *Jbk. Oud-Utrecht*, 73–91, ill.

4392   PEKELHARING, C. A. and S. MULLER Fzn. (1921, 1923). *Geschiedenis van de Vereenigde Gods- en Gasthuizen te Utrecht van 1817–1917.* I: (Pe-kelharing). Geschiedenis van het algemeen ziekenhuis, 226 pp. II: (Muller). Geschiedenis van het algemeen gasthuis en van de overige stichtingen, 105 pp. (History of the united charitable Institutions and hospitals at U.). Oosthoek, Utrecht.
       – 2 vols in one binding. Reviewed by A. J. van der Weijde: Vol. I: *NTG, 65* (1921), II, 720–3; *BGG, I*, 332–5. Vol. II: *NTG, 67* (1923), II, 58–60; *BGG, III*, 166–8.

4393   [   ] (1939). Feestnummer ter gelegenheid van het Zilveren jubi-leum van het Homoeopatisch Ziekenhuis 1914 – 18 Maart – 1939 (Memorial issue on the occasion of the silver jubilee of the Homoeo-pathic hospital [Oudenrijn]). Bijblad van het *Homoeopatisch Mbl.*, Maart 1939, 38 pp.

4394   KOUWER, B. J. and H. J. LAMÉRIS (1908). *Iets uit de geschiedenis der klinieken voor Heel- en Verloskunde der Rijksuniversiteit te Utrecht. Met een beschrijving der nieuwe inrichting* (Something from the history of the clinics for surgery and obstetrics of the University of —. With a description of the new institution). 144 pp., ill., ports. Stads Boek en Courant Drukkerij, Kampen.

Venlo, Weert, Zaandistrict, Zaltbommel, Zutphen

4395   PHILIPS, J. F. R. *et al.* (1961). *Een eeuw armen- en ziekenzorg in Venlo. R.K. St. Joseph ziekenhuis 1861–1961* (A century of poor relief and nursing at V. R.C. St. Joseph Hospital). 104 pp., ill., ports. H. C. van Grinsven, Venlo.

4396   [   ] (1969). *St Jans-Gasthuis Weert 1869–1969* (St John's Hospital at W.). 31 pp., ill. Leiter-Nypels, Maastricht.

4397 KUMMER, A. (1965). De Zaanse ziekenhuizen en de Zaanse specialis-ten (The Zaan Hospitals and the Zaan specialists). *Noord-Holland, 10,* 78–83.

4398 AQUOY, J. G. R. (1899). Geschiedenis van het gasthuis te Zaltbommel (History of the hospital at Z.). *Arch. Ned. Kerkgesch.,* 7, 362.

4399 GRAAF, J. de (1917). Stichtingsbrief van het oude en nieuwe gasthuis te Zutphen (A charter of foundation of the old and new hospital at Z.). *Gelre, XX,* 247.

4400 MEINSMA, K. O. *et al.* [1925]. Het oude en nieuwe gasthuis te Zutphen 1625–1925 (The old and new hospital at Z.). no pl.
– Reviewed by D. Schoute: *NTG, 70* (1926), I, 1410–4; *BGG, VI,* 79–83.

4401 GRAAF, J. de (1917). Een tweetal stadsziekentroosters en krankenbe-zoekers te Zutphen en hunne verhouding tot het oude-nieuwe gasthuis aldaar (Two municipal visitors of the sick at Z. and their relation to the old-new hospital). *Gelre, XX,* 209.

See also 4633.–4633.13

C. Leper Houses

General

4402 SCHEVICHAVEN, H. D. J. van (1907). Leprozen en Leprozenhuizen (Lepers en Leper Houses). *Oud-Holland, XXV,* 97.

4403 LINT, J. G. de (1921). Leproserieën (Leper houses). *NTG, 65,* I, 53–62; *BGG, I,* 3–12, 4 ill.

4404 GUYONNET, G. (1957). Lépreux et Léproseries d'autrefois. *Hist. Méd.,* 7, no 6, 9–55, 17 ill.
– also on the Amsterdam leper house.

See also 4850

Local

4405 BROUWER ANCHER, A. J. M. (1899). De Amsterdamsche leprozen-huizen en hun verpleegden (The Amsterdam leper houses and their inmates). *NTG, 35,* II, 1287–96.
– Reviewed by E. Pergens: *Janus, V* (1900), 201–2.

4406   LINT, J. G. de (1921). Les léproseries d'Amsterdam. *Bull. Soc. franç. Hist. Méd.*, *XV*, no 3–4, 107–14.

4407   ROEKEL, G. van (1940). Uit de geschiedenis van een leprozenhuis (From the history of a leper house). [Huissen]. *NTG*, *84*, II, 1323; *BGG*, *XX*, 70.   *See also* 1421, 5034

D. Plague Houses

4407[a]   BRUGMANS, H. (1929). Amsterdamse pesthuizen (Amsterdam plague-houses). *Amstelodamum*, *16*, 16–7.

4407[b]   KOUWENAAR, D. (1937). Het pesthuis (The Plague-house). *Amstelodamum*, *24*, 53–5, ill.

4407[c]   NIJMAN, H. W. (1937). 't Oude pesthuis (The old plague-house). *Amstelodamum*, *24*, 84–7.

4408   HELLINGA, G. (1928). De Amsterdamsche pesthuizen (The Amsterdam plague-houses). *NTG*, *72*, II, 5912–38; *BGG*, *VIII*, 357–83.

4409   — (1929). Het Pesthuis na den brand (1732 tot ongeveer 1839) (The Plague-house after the fire). *NTG*, *73*, I, 35–62; *BGG*, *IX*, 1–28, 6 ill.

4410   EMCK, W. F. (1929). De voormalige pesthuizen te Gorinchem (The former plague-houses at G.). *NTG*, *73*, II, 3751–4; *BGG*, *IX*, 183–6.

4411   PENNING, C. P. J. (1929). Het vroegere pesthuis te Harderwijk (The former plague-house at H.). *NTG*, *73*, II, 3569–71; *BGG*, *IX*, 181–3.

4412   LEEN, J. van der [1934]. *Geschiedenis van het Pest- en Dolhuis der gemeente Rotterdam* (History of the plague-house and lunatic asylum at R.). 48 pp., 13 ill. no. pl. 8°.
– on the occasion of the 25th anniversary of the municipal lunatic asylum "Maasoord"; reviewed by M. A. van Andel: *NTG*, *79* (1935), I, 58–9; *BGG*, *XV*, 17–8.

E. Lunatic Asylums

General

4413   JELGERSMA, G. (1899). Sanatoria voor zenuwzieken (Sanatoria for mental patients). *Alers et al.*, 150.

4414 ANDEL, A. H. van (1899). Over de krankzinnigengestichten in Nederland (On the lunatic asylums in the Netherlands). *Alers et al.*, 21–6.

4415 SCHUURMANS STEKHOVEN, J. H. (1922). *Ontwikkeling van het krankzinnigenwezen in Nederland 1813–1914.* Verzameling van archiefstukken, statistische tabellen, platen, kaarten enz. den minister van Binnenlandsche Zaken aangeboden (Development of lunatic care in the Netherlands. A collection of documents, statistical tables, plates, maps etc., offered to the minister of Home Affairs). 's-Gravenhage. 4°.

4416 HALLEMA, A. (1941). *Gestichtstypen uit den ouden tijd. Centralisatie en decentralisatie in ons vaderlandsch gestichtswezen tijdens de Republiek.* Maatschappelijk hulpbetoon en krankzinnigenverpleging vastgekoppeld aan het gevangeniswezen in de 17de en 18de eeuw (Types of asylums from old times. Centralisation and decentralisation in our national system of institutions during the Republic. Social assistance and mental nursing linked together with the prison-system in the 17th and 18th century). 86 pp. De Tijdstroom, Lochem.

4417 SCHUT, J. (1970). *Van dolhuys tot psychiatrisch centrum. Ontwikkeling en functie* (From lunatic asylum to psychiatric centre. Development and function). 133 pp. De Toorts, Haarlem.

Local

4418 HELLINGA, G. (1932). Het Amsterdamsche dol- of krankzinnigenhuis (The Amsterdam lunatic or madman asylum). *NTG, 76*, II, 1603–20; *BGG, XII*, 61–78.

4418ª SANDER, C. A. L. (1958). Het Dulhuis of Dolhuis aan de Vesten of Kloveniersburgwal (The lunatic asylum on the "Vesten" or —). *Amstelodamum, 45*, 229–238, ill.
– at Amsterdam.

4419 WIERINGA, W. J. et al. (1960). *Een halve eeuw arbeid op psychiatrisch-neurologisch terrein 1910–1960* (Half a century of work in the psychiatric-neurological field). 228 pp., ill., ports. Zomer en Keuning, Wageningen.
– Memorial volume on the occasion of the 50th anniversary of the "Valerius Clinic" at Amsterdam.

4420 DRUYVESTEYN, C. (1897). *Het Provinciaal Geneeskundig Gesticht voor Krankzinnigen "Meerenberg" te Bloemendaal; historisch overzicht* (The

Provincial Medical Institution for lunatics — at B.; historical survey). Tjeenk Willink, Haarlem. *See also* 2282.

4421 [ ] (1949). *Een eeuw Krankzinnigen verpleging 1849–1949*. Gedenkboek ter gelegenheid van het honderdjarig bestaan van het Provinciaal Ziekenhuis nabij Santpoort (voorheen Meerenberg) (A century of mental nursing. Memorial volume on the occasion of the 100th anniversary of the Provincial Hospital near S. (formerly —)). 303 pp., ill., ports. Santpoort.

4422 BOURICIUS, L. G. N. (1927). *Geschiedenis van het geneeskundig gesticht voor krankzinnigen. Het St. Joris Gasthuis en het daarmede verbonden geweest zijnde "Tuchthuis binnen Delft". Uitgegeven ter gelegenheid van het 250-jarig zelfstandig bestaan (1677–1927)* (History of the Medical Institution for mental patients. The St. Joris Hospital and the associated House of Correction at D. Edited on the occasion of the 250th anniversary of independent existence). 155 pp. Delft.

See also 1421

4423 HEEMSTRA, M. J. Barones van (1951). *Honderdjarig bestaan van de Psychiatrische Inrichting te Franeker (1851–1951). Een tehuis voor zenuwzieken in Friesland* (The hundredth anniversary of the Psychiatric Hospital at F. A home for neurotics in Fr.). Leeuwarden.

4424 KLATTER, J. (1973). *Groot Bronswijk 1873–1973*. 472 pp., ill., ports. Buijten & Schipperheijn, Amsterdam.

– "Groot Bronswijk" is a Protestant lunatic asylum at Wagenborgen (Groningen).

4425 DONINCK, A. van (1929). Verblijf der krankzinnigen in het gemeentelijk gasthuis te Gheel, 1680–1860 (Stay of the lunatics in the municipal hospital at G.). *NTG, 73*, II, 3157–67; *BGG, IX*, 157–67.

4426 — (1931). Verplegingsoord van geesteszieken te Gheel: de ziekenkamer (Lunatic asylum at G.: the sick-room). *NTG, 75*, IV, 5498–5506; *BGG, XI*, 293–301.

4427 KOYEN, M. H. (1968). Inventaris van het archief van het gasthuis te Geel (Inventory of the archive of the hospital at G.). *Jbk. Vrijh. Land Geel, 7*, 5–130.

4428 — (1969). *Geschiedenis van het gasthuis te Geel, 1286–1969* (History of the hospital at G.). 139 pp., ill. Geschiedkundig genootschap Geel, Tongerlo.

4429 EYNIKEL, H. (1971). Geel, bakermat van de gezinsverpleging (G., birthplace of boarding out). *Ann. Soc. belge Hist. Hôp.*, *9*, 113–27.

4429ᵃ KOYEN, M. H. (1973). *De gezinsverpleging van Geesteszieken te Geel tot het einde van de 18e eeuw* (Boarding out of mental patients at G. till the end of the 18th century). Geels Geschiedkundig Genootschap, Tongerlo.

4429ᵇ — (1974). Krankzinnigenzorg St Dimpna en Geel (Mental care St D. and G.). *Spiegel Historiael*, *9*, 515–21, 10 ill.

See also 4300–05

4430 SCHADE, H. (1922). De geschiedenis van het krankzinnigengesticht "Reynier van Arkel" (History of the lunatic asylum — —). *NTG*, *66*, I, 1803–20; *BGG*, *II*, 101–18, 9 ill.
– a short report: *BGG, II*, 62.

4431 — (1923). De feestmaaltijden in het geneeskundig gesticht voor krankzinnigen "Reinier van Arckel" te 's-Hertogenbosch (The banquets in the lunatic asylum — — at Bois-le-Duc). *NTG*, *67*, II, 2291–2; *BGG, III*, 349–50.

4432 SCHOUTEN, J. (1966). Een zeventiende-eeuwse dolcel te Gouda (A 17th century madman cell at G.). *Arts en Auto*, *32*, 974–87.

4433 CAHN, L. A. (1970). *Medemblik, een episode in de Nederlandse psychiatrie 1884–1967* (M., an episode of Dutch psychiatry). 95 pp., ill. Wormerveer.

4434 [Anonym] (1965). *Rond de Koepel van St. Bavo 1914–1964. Gedenkboek ter gelegenheid van het gouden jubileum van de psychiatrische inrichting Sint Bavo te Noordwijkerhout van de Broeders van Liefde* (Around the Dome of St Bavo. Memorial volume on the occasion of the golden jubilee of the psychiatric institution at N. of the Brethern of Love). 152 pp., ill. Dekker & Van de Vegt, Nijmegen.

4435 BEEKUM, J. van (1965). Zij zijn van ons geslacht (They belong to our family). *Overijssel*, *1*, 98–103, ill.
– on lunatic asylums in Overijssel. The first asylum in O. was opened in 1835 at Deventer.

4436 LITH, J. van der (1863). *Geschiedenis van het Krankzinnigengesticht te Utrecht, gedurende deszelfs 400-jarig bestaan* (History of the lunatic institution at U. during its 400th anniversary).

4437 HUT, L. J., A. POSLAVSKY, H. LOOIS *et al.* [1961]. *De Willem Arntz Stichting 1461–1961* (The Willem Arntz Foundation). XIV + 568 pp., ill. Oosthoek, Utrecht. 4°.

4438 KORTHALS ALTES, A. P. (1961). *De Willem Arntz Stichting 1461– 1961.* 99 pp. no pl.
      – Memorial address on the occasion of the 500th anniversary of –– at U., January 26, 1961.

4439 [   ] (1971). *Bij ons in Dennenoord. De psychiatrische inrichting in Zuidlaren is 75 jaar* (The psychiatric Institution "Dennenoord at Z., 75 years). J. H. Kok, Kampen.

4440 DIEPSTRATEN, Ph. H. J. *et al.* (1972). *Vijf jaar Prof. Pompekliniek*; lustrumverslag van de Prof. Mr W. P. J. Pompekliniek 1966–1971 (Five years Prof. Pompe clinic; lustrum report). Nijmegen.

                              See also 4283–4305 (mental nursing).

F. Sanatoria

4441 HALLEMA, A. (1935). Het Friesch Volkssanatorium te Appelscha 1910 – 5 September – 1935 (The Frisian Sanatorium at A.). *Ziekenhuiswezen, 8* no 6, 10 pp.
      – On the occasion of the 25th anniversary.

4442 [   ] [no. d.] *Het vijftigjarig bestaan van het R.K. Sanatorium "Dekkerswald"* te Groesbeek (The 50th anniversary of the R. C. Sanatorium — at G.). no pl.

4443 [   ] (1963). R. K. Sanatorium bestaat vijftig jaar (R. C. Sanatorium exists fifty years) [Dekkerswald]. *MC, 18,* 767–8, ill.

4444 [   ] (1968). Sanatorium Sonnevanck 1908–1968. *Tegen de Tuberculose, 64,* 156–7, ill.
      – at Harderwijk.

4445 FRANCKEN, Joh. C. F. (1973). Sonnevancks omschakeling (The changing of —). *Centr. Wbl.,* 19 mei, p. 7, 3 ill.
      – On Sanatorium "Sonnevanck" at Harderwijk, founded 1908. In 1973, on the occasion of the 65th anniversary, the sanatorium was changed into a hospital and it adopted a village in Mali (Africa) for the fight against tuberculosis.

4446 BOELE, H. W. and H. WERKMAN (1902). *Het sanatorium te Hellendoorn.* Erven Tijl, Zwolle.

4447 LOGHEM, J. J. van (1952). Het gouden feest van Hellendoorn (The 50th anniversary of the sanatorium at H.). *NTG*, *96*, II, 1314–5.

4448 PHILIPS, J. F. R. (1971). *Vijftig jaar Sanatorium Hornerheide. Historische beschouwingen over de medische zorg in Limburg* (Fifty years Sanatorium —. Historical observations on medical care in L.). 167 pp., ill. Assen.
– Stud. Sociaal-economische geschiedenis van Limburg XVI; also publ. in: *Jbk. Soc. Hist. Centr. Limburg*, *16*, 1–135.

4449 GEUNS, H. A. van (1967). Davos 100 Jahr Kurort. *Tegen de Tuberculose*, *63*, 18–23; 49–57.

G. Maternity Homes and obstetric Education

4450 VROESOM DE HAAN, J. (1899). De kraaminrichtingen in Nederland gedurende de tweede helft dezer eeuw (The maternity-homes in the Netherlands during the second half of this century). *Alers et al.*, 30–4.

4451 SIEVERTSEN BUVIG, S. (1921). *Geschiedenis van de Rijks-kweekschool voor vroedvrouwen te Amsterdam van 1861–1921* (History of the State's training college for midwives at A.). no pl.

4452 HUITEMA, W. (1962). De kweekschool voor vroedvrouwen te Amsterdam (The training college for midwives at A.). *NTG*, *106*, I, 543–5; *BGG*, *XLII*, 18–20.

4452ᵃ ELAUT, L. (1954). De "Vroedkundige Oeffenschool" van Jan Bernard Jacobs en de kraambedkoorts op het einde van de achttiende eeuw (The "School for teaching midwives" of — — and puerperal fever at the end of the 18th century). *Wetensch. Tijdingen*, *14*, col. 335–42.

See also 3630–35 (Training midwives)

H. Various hospitals and Clinics

Children's hospitals

4453 WELY, D. L. van (1899). De kinderziekenhuizen en herstellingsoorden voor zieke kinderen (The children's hospitals and convalescent homes for sick children). *Alers et al.*, 35–9.

4454   [A.V.B.] (1915). Het vijftigjarig bestaan van het Emma kinderzieken-
       huis te Amsterdam 1865 – 6 Mei – 1915 (The 50th anniversary of the
       Emma Children's hospital at A.). *Eigen Haard, XLI,* 349.

4455   [   ] (1965). *Een eeuw Emma Kinderziekenhuis 1865 Amsterdam 1965*
       (A century Emma Children's Hospital). 36 pp. Arbeiderspers, Amster-
       dam.

4456   [   ] (1951). *Vijftig jaren Johanna Stichting. Gedenkboek 1900–
       1950* (50 years Johanna Foundation. Memorial Volume). 112 pp.
       Arnhem.
       – The "Johanna Foundation" is a home for defective children.

4457   WEVE, H. J. M. (ed.). (1933). *Driekwart eeuw Nederlandsch gasthuis
       voor behoeftige en minvermogende ooglijders te Utrecht 1858–1933.*
       Gedenkschrift ter gelegenheid van het 75-jarig bestaan van het gasthuis
       (Three-quarter of a century Dutch Hospital for indigent and poor
       eye-patients at U. Memorial volume on the occasion of the 75th anni-
       versary of the hospital). 238 pp., ill., ports. De Liefde, Utrecht. 8°.

4458   DOESSCHATE, G. ten (1959). De Stichting van het Nederlandse Gast-
       huis voor Ooglijders te Utrecht (The Foundation of the Ophthalmic
       hospital at U.). *GeWiNa,* no 5, 11.   See also 659

4459   BOSSCHAERT, D. and J. G. van CITTERT-EYMERS (1965). *Kliniek tot
       herkenning en genezing van tand-, oor-, huid-, keel-, en kinderziekten te
       Utrecht 1865–1929* (Clinic for diagnosis and treatment of dental-,
       ear-, skin-, throat-, and children's diseases). 60 pp. Utrechts Univer-
       siteitsmuseum, Utrecht.
       – portrait of H. Snellen.

4460   EIBRINK, G. J. (1915). *Het Doofstommen-Instituut te Groningen 1790 –
       14 April – 1915* (The Institution for the deaf and dumb).

I. Foreign hospitals

4461   KUIJJER, P. J. (1957). Het Hôtel-Dieu te Beaune, een middeleeuws
       ziekenhuis (The Hôtel-Dieu at B., a mediaeval hospital). *NTG, 101,*
       1659–64; *BGG, XXXVII,* 26–31, 2 ill.

4462   THEUNISZ, Joh. (1933). Ziekenhuizen te Napels aan het einde der 17e
       eeuw (Hospitals at Naples at the end of the 17th century). *NTG, 77,*
       II, 2067–8; *BGG, XIII,* 131–2.

4463 HALLEMA, A. (1932). Het Ziekenhuis en de ziekenhuisverpleging aan Kaap de Goede Hoop (±1650 – ±1800) (The Hospital and the nursing at Cape Good Hope). *Ziekenhuiswezen*, *5*, no 2 and 3, 21 pp.

4464 — (1932). Wat op het stuk van Ziekenhuiswezen in onze Westindische Koloniën tot stand is gebracht en ten bate der zieke kolonisten is gedaan (What has been accomplished and what has been done for sick colonists in our West-Indian colonies). *Ziekenhuiswezen*, *5*, no 7, 13 pp., 3 ill.

J. Orphanages

4465 HERDER, T. den (1959). De ziekte van de weeskinderen in 1566 (The disease of the orphans). *Amstelodamum*, *46*, 163–4; 235–6.

4466 KANNEGIETER, J. Z. (1959). De weeshuisziekte van 1566 (The disease in the orphanage). *Amstelodamum*, *46*, 112–7.

4467 ROEKEL, G. van (1940). De "Weeskinderziekte" in 1566 (The disease of the orphans in 1566). *NTG*, *84*, III, 2564; *BGG*, *XX*, 20.

4468 QUERIDO, A. (1958). *Storm in het weeshuis. De beroering onder de Amsterdamse burgerwezen in 1566* (Storm in the orphanage. The turmoil among the Amsterdam city-orphans). 38 pp. Em. Querido's Uitg. Mij., Amsterdam.

4469 — (1959). De beroering onder de wezen in 1566 (The agitation among the orphans). *Amstelodamum*, *46*, 212–3.

4470 HALLEMA, A. (1958). Geneeskundige behandeling in een weeshuis aan het einde van de 17de eeuw (Medical treatment in an orphanage at the end of the 17th century). *NTG*, *102*, II, 1756–7; *BGG*, *XXXVIII*, 20–1.
– The orphanage in question is the "Weeshuis der Gereformeerden binnen Delft" (Orphanage of the Reformed at D.).

4471 — (1964). *Geschiedenis van het Weeshuis der Gereformeerden binnen Delft te Delft* (History of the Orphanage of the Reformed at D.). XV + 544 pp., ill., facs. Delft.
– from *ca* 1575–1964.

4472 BEERNINK, G. (1909). Het weeshuis te Nijkerk in de 17e eeuw (The orphanage at N. in the 17th century). *Gelre*, *12*, 59 pp., 2 ill.

4473 KUNST, A. J. M. (1956). *Van Sint Elisabeths-gasthuis tot Gereformeerd Burgerweeshuis 1485–1814* (From St-Elisabeth Hospital to Calvinistic Orphanage). 333 pp. Van Gorcum, Assen.
– at Utrecht; also published as a thesis (University of Utrecht).

See also 4309

K. Houses of correction (mental treatment in —)

4474 HALLEMA, A. (1950). De medische behandeling van patiënten in de voormalige Nederlandse tuchthuizen (Medical treatment of patients in the former houses of correction in the Netherlands). *NTG, 94*, IV, 3560–5; *BGG, XXX*, 48–53.

4475 — (1951). Nog enkele documenten betreffende de medische behandeling van patienten in het voormalige tuchthuis te Arnhem (Some more documents regarding the medical treatment of patients in the former house of correction at A.). *NTG, 95*, I, 216–21; *BGG, XXXI*, 1–6.

4476 — (1959). Medische behandeling, kontrole en adviezen in de tuchthuizen van Arnhem en Antwerpen in de 17de en 18de eeuw (Medical treatment, supervision and advices in the houses of correction of A. and Antwerp in the 17th and 18th century). *Sci. Hist., I*, 134–48.

Chapter XVIII

Medical Profession

In this chapter entries concerning the various aspects of the professional life of physicians and surgeons have been gathered.

From the late Middle Ages till the French revolution the surgeons were organized in a guild, in the beginning together with craftsmen. Later on they had their own guild that held its meetings in the guild's room where the note-books and some surgical works were kept and where the examinations took place. The local colleges of doctors date from a later period.

Also in medical professional life there is nothing new under the sun: in the past there were also doctor's bills judged to be too high and there occurred serious quarrels between colleagues. Sometimes the municipality had to give sentences or ordinances on doctor's fees. Before a major operation a notarial contract on the fee might be signed and after a spectacular successful operation a report was sometimes drawn up by a notary.

In the eighteenth century several learned societies were founded, some of them had a provincial, others a local character (Hollandsche Maatschappij van Wetenschappen at Haarlem (1752), Zeeuwsch Genootschap der Wetenschappen (1769), Bataafsch Genootschap at Rotterdam).

The Dutch association of physicians dates from 1847; it was called "Nederlandsche Maatschappij ter bevordering van de geneeskunst" (Netherlands Society for the advancement of medicine). The epitheton "Royal" was added to the name of the Association in 1949. It has regional departments of which several have already been in existence for 75 or 100 years.

Associations of specialists date from our century.

A. General

4477 NIJHOFF, G. C. (1923). Hoe zijn wij gekomen aan de "titel van arts"? (How did we get the title "Arts"?). *NTG*, *67*, II, 1610–1; *BGG*, *III*, 264–5.

4478 — (1930). De arts naar zijn afkomst (The physician and his origin). *NTG, 74*, III, 3600–12.
- Address delivered for the Dutch Association of Physicians Leeuwarden, July 7, 1930.

4479 KUIPER, K. (1914). Eenige opmerkingen over de verhouding van den geschoolden arts tot den vrijen genezer in Oud-Hellas (Some remarks on the relation between the trained physician and the free healer in Ancient Hellas). *NTG, 58*, I, 1898–1901.

4480 BECK, J. W. (1914). Iets over artsen en de uitoefening der geneeskunde in de Romeinse wereld (Something on physicians practising medicine in the Roman world). *NTG, 58*, I, 1902–6.

4481 BAUMANN, E. D. (1915). *De dokter en de geneeskunde. I: Maatschappelijk leven.* II: *De wetenschap* (The doctor and medicine. I: Social life, 128 pp. II: Science, 141 pp., ill. Meulenhoff, Amsterdam. 4°.

4482 BRUÏNE PLOOS VAN AMSTEL, P. J. de (1923). Worden doctoren gewaardeerd? (Are physicians appreciated?). *Med. Wbl., 29*, 553; 565; 577.

4483 PUTTO, J. A. (1937). De "Arts" (The physician). *GG, 15*, 450–1.

4484 EERENBEEMT, H. F. J. M. van den (1969). Arts en sociaal besef in Nederland in historisch perspectief (Physician and social consciousness in the Netherlands in historical perspective). *MC, 24*, 1161–4.

4484[a] RENTERGHEM, A. W. van (1910). *De rehabilitatie van den huisarts door verbetering in de opvoeding van den geneesheer* (Rehabilitation of the family doctor by improving the education of the physician). 40 pp. F. van Rossen, Amsterdam.

4485 DANIËLS, C. E. (1900). Docteurs et malades. *Janus, V*, 20–6; 80–6 and 105–12, ill.

4486 PUTTO, J. A. (1936). De dokter bij den zieke in vroeger jaren (The physician with the patient in former years). *GG, 14*, 262–3.

4487 KULSDOM, M. E. (1947). "Doctores consultissimi experientissimi" *NTG, 91*, III, 2534–7; *BGG, XXVII*, 50–3.
- on ceremonious forms of address of physicians.

4488 WEIJDE, A. J. van der (1924). Een vervallen verklaring als lid der maatschappij (An exclusion as a member of the society (of medicine)). *NTG, 68*, I, 37–8; *BGG, IV*, 3–4.

4489 ANDEL, M. A. van (1914). Vrije uitoefening der geneeskunde in de 17de eeuw (Free practice of medicine in the 17th century). *NTG*, *58*, I, 1907–14.

4490 — (1918/19). Spectatoriale vertoogen over de geneeskundige practijk in het laatst der 18de eeuw (Spectatorial representations on the medical practice at the end of the 18th century). *Med. Wbl. 25*, 481; 497; 513.

4491 WEIJDE, A. J. van der (1924). De uitoefening der geneeskunde omstreeks 1860 (Practising medicine about 1860). *NTG*, *68*, I, 36–7; *BGG*, *IV*, 1–2.

4492 BRUINSMA, G. W. (1907). De geneeskundigen in Nederland en hun practijk een halve eeuw geleden (Physicians in the Netherlands and their practice half a century ago). *NTG*, *51*, I, 59–73.

4493 ARTELT, W. (1957). Cito—tuto—iucunde? Arts, rijwiel en auto omstreeks 1900 (Doctor, bicycle and car about 1900). *Ciba-Symp.*, *5* (6), 6–17, ill., port.

4494 BURGER, J. F. (1954). Reclame ten tijde van de Bataafse Republiek (Advertising in the time of the Batavian Republic). *NTG*, *98*, II, 1472.

4495 VRIES, Ph. de (1949). *Geschiedenis van het verzet der artsen in Nederland, 1941–1945* (History of the resistance of the physicians in the Netherlands,). 385 pp., Tjeenk Willink & Zn, Haarlem.
– Written by order of the "Nederlandse Maatschappij ... Geneeskunst".

4496 BORST, J. G. G. (1947). Occupied Holland. Resistance by the Medical Profession. *Brit. med. J. Suppl*, *I*, 57.
– Reprinted in: *Neth. J. Med.*, *16* (1973), 35–8.

4497 KLEIWEG DE ZWAAN, J. P. (1915/16). Het werk der vrouw in de geneeskunde, historische beschouwingen (The work of the woman in medicine, historical reflections). *Med. Wbl.*, *22*, 262; 275; 285; 299; 310; 322 and 334.

4498 VIEYRA, D. (1932). Een practiseerende doktersweduwe uit 1705 (A practising widow of a physician, 1705). *NTG*, *76*, I, 75; *BGG*, *XII*, 16.

4499 ROEKEL, G. van (1940). Een vrouwelijke arts omstreeks 1600 (A female physician about 1600). *NTG*, *84*, I, 841; *BGG*, *XX*, 56.

4500 LEERSUM, E. C. van (1919). Een vrouwelijke collega (?) uit de 17de

eeuw (A female colleague (?) from the 17th century). *NTG, 63,* I,
790–2.

–On Johanna Letocardia van Oostrijck at Leiden who cured several wounds in
arms, hands, fingers etc.

See also 2509–10, 2563, 3480

B. Jewish medicine

4501   Esso, Izaak van (1940). Het aandeel der Joden in de natuurwetenschappen in de Nederlanden (The part of the Jews in the natural sciences in
the Netherlands). In: Brugman & Frank. *Geschiedenis der Joden in
Nederland,* vol. I., 643–79. Van Holkema & Warendorf, Amsterdam.

4502   — (1959). Survey on Jewish physicians in the Netherlands. [Hebrew].
Koroth, 2 (5–6), 201–8.

4502ª VISSER, C. (1927). Vondel en de "de Joodsche docter" (V. and the "Jewish physician"). *Amstelodamum, 14,* 33–4.

4503   COHEN, D. E. (1927). De vroegere Amsterdamsche Joodsche doctoren
(The former Amsterdam Jewish physicians). *NTG, 71,* II, 1385–1401;
BGG, VII, 625–41.

4504   — (1930). De Amsterdamsche Joodsche chirurgijns (The Amsterdam
Jewish surgeons). *NTG, 74,* I, 2234–59; *BGG, X,* 113–35. 3 ill., 1 port.

4505   — (1931). De vroegere Amsterdamsche joodsche apothekers (The
former Jewish chemists at A.). *Ph. W., 68,* 1215-24.

4506   — (1934). De Joodsche geneeskundigen in de noordelijke Nederlanden vóór 1600 (The Jewish physicians in the Northern Netherlands
before 1600). *NTG, 78,* I, 533–43; *BGG, XIV,* 33–43.

4507   RODRIGUES PEREIRA, E. A. (5684 = 1923). Een drietal op de voorgrond
tredende Joodsche geneeskundigen uit het begin der 19de eeuw (Three
prominent Jewish physicians from the beginning of the 19th century).
De Vrijdagavond, I, 244a.

4508   STEPHAN, B. H. (1904). Sterfte en ziekten bij joden en niet-joden (Mortality and diseases with Jews and non-Jews). *NTG, 40,* II, 1631–54;

4508ª SANDERS, J. (1918). *Ziekte en sterfte bij Joden en niet-Joden te Amsterdam* (Disease and death with Jews and non-Jews at A.). Thesis. 128
pp. Van Hengel, Rotterdam.

– also as a monograph.

4509 LEYDESDORFF, Julius (1919). *Bijdrage tot de speciale psychologie van het Joodsche volk* (Contribution to the special psychology of the Jewish people). Thesis University Groningen.

4510 PINKHOF, H. (1914). Een klacht uit de zeventiende eeuw (A complaint from the 17th century), *NTG, 58*, I, 2026–8.
- The complaint on quacks is expressed in the book *Ma'asch Tobiah* (Work of Tobias), Venice 1706, reprinted Krakau 1908. Tobias is Tobias Katz, son of a rabbin at Metz.

4511 — (1934). De clinische urognostiek van een dokter uit de 17de eeuw (Clinical urognostics of a 17th century physician). *NTG, 78*, I, 1029–31; *BGG, XIV*, 54–6.
- The signs to be derived from the urine as expounded in the book *Ma'asch Tobiah*, Venice 1706.

4512 VIEYRA, D. (1935). Geneeskundige Archivalia (From medical records). I. Toestand van den geneeskundigen dienst bij de beide Israelitische gemeenten te Amsterdam omstreeks 1813 (Situation of the medical service of both the Israelian parishes at A. about —). *NTG, 79*, I, 60–1; *BGG, XV*, 19–20.

4513 MENDELS, I. (1926). Onhygiënische toestanden in het begin van de 19e eeuw (Unhygienic situations in the beginning of the 19th century). *NTG, 70*, I, 551–3; *BGG, VI*, 46–8.
- a report on the ritual baths of Jewish women after menstruation.

4514 VRIES, S. P. de (1968). *Joodse riten en symbolen* (Jewish rites and symbols). Amsterdam.

4515 LEIBOWITZ, J. O. (1971). An 18th century manuscript poem by I. Belinfante honouring a medical graduate. *Koroth, 5*, 427–34.
- I.B. *d.*, 1781.

See also 2344, 3714, 4991

C. Professional matters

Conflicts

4516 COHEN, Hk. (1929). Godsvrede tusschen doctoren en apothekers (Political truce between physicians and chemists). *NTG, 73*, II, 3168–74; *BGG, IX*, 168–74.

4517   NUYENS, B. W. Th. (1937). Krakeelende dokters in de 17e en 18e eeuw
(Quarreling physicians in the 17th and 18th century). *NTG, 81*, IV,
5441–2; *BGG, XVII*, 192–3.
– included in a report of a meeting of the "Genootschap".

4518   BRAAT, P. (1938). Artsen als vechtersbazen (Pysicians as fighters).
NTG, 82, II, 2836; *BGG, XVIII*, 113.
– on a scuffle between two surgeons at Roosendaal, December 22, 1673.

4519   KULSDOM, M. E. (1951). Een ouderwets conflict (An old-fashioned
conflict). *NTG, 95*, III, 2195–2200; *BGG, XXXI*, 34–9.
– Letter to the editor (same title) by A. G. J. Hermans: *NTG, 95*, IV, 3893; *BGG,
XXXI*, 102.

Bills

4520   HALLEMA, A. (1954). Dorps- en armenrekeningen als bronnen voor
de geschiedenis der geneeskunde (Villages' and poor' bills as sources
of the history of medicine). *NTG, 98*, IV, 3588–9; *BGG, XXXIV*, 77–8.

4521   GILS, J. B. F. van (1926). Afrekening met gesloten beurzen (Settlement
with closed purses). *NTG, 70*, I, 550; *BGG, VI*, 45.
– in 1566.

4522   EVERDINGEN, Th. J. G. van (1903). Barbier-chirurgijnsrekening uit
het laatst der zestiende eeuw (Barber-surgeon's bill from the end of the
16th century). *Gelre, VI*, 283–4.

4523   KEUNE, W. T. P. J. M. (1968). Een rekening uit het jaar 1586 van
Mr Henrick Rammelman, gesworen chyrurgus van Deventer (A bill
from the year 1586 of —. a sworn surgeon of D.). *NTG, 112*, 1261–3.

4524   POT, J. (1931). Een doktersrekening uit de 16e eeuw (A doctor's bill
from the 16th century). *NTG, 75*, I, 1128–52; *BGG, XI*, 57–81.

4525   BEYERMAN, J. J. (1934). Een overeenkomst op medisch gebied in 1680
(A medical agreement in —). *NTG, 78*, I, 73–4; *BGG, XIV*, 27–8.

4526   DITMAR, J. van (1937). Rekening van een arts in de 17e eeuw (A doctor's bill in the 17th century). *NTG, 81*, III, 4275; *BGG, XVII*, 167.

4527   VIEYRA, D. (1933). Gespecificeerde honoraria van Hollandsche geneeskundigen in Ned.-West-Indië. Anno 1713 (Specified fees of Dutch
physicians in the Dutch West Indies). *NTG, 77*, II, 2066; *BGG, XIII*,
130.

4528 PUTTO, J. A. (1936). Eene "meesters" rekening uit het begin der achttiende eeuw (A "master's" bill from the beginning of the 18th century).
GG, 14, 579–80.

4529 WEIJDE, A. J. van der (1923). Een doktersrekening van 1764 (A doctor's bill from —). *NTG, 67,* II, 904; *BGG, III,* 219.
– on a doctor's bill that was judged to be too high by the Utrecht Collegium Medicum.

4530 FLAMENT, (1907). Rekening van een chirurgijn uit 1769 (A surgeon's
bill from —). *De Maasgouw,* 87.

4531 COHEN, Hk. (1941). Collegiale behandeling (Fraternal treatment).
NTG, 85, II, 1485–7; *BGG, XXI,* 50–2.
– Notary protocol for C. van Wieringen, surgeon at Sommelsdijk, 1776.

Contracts, Instructions

4532 WEIJDE, A. J. van der (1925). Notarieele acte voor het aannemen van
een lijfarts (Notarial act for the appointment of a physician in ordinary). *NTG, 69,* I, 609–10; *BGG, V,* 50–1.

4533 KATE, W. ten (1936). Geneeskundige Archivalia: Verzoek van een
chirurgijn tot vermindering van het officiegeld. Krankzinnigenverpleging in de 18e eeuw (Medical Records: Request of a surgeon for a de-
crease of the registration fee. Mental nursing in the 18th century).
NTG, 80, III, 3564–5; *BGG, XVI,* 124–5.

4534 ANDEL, M. A. van (1921). Verkoop van een practijk in de 17de eeuw
(Sale of a practice in the 17th century). *NTG, 65,* II, 1203; *BGG, I,* 370.

4535 HOEVEN, J. van der (1939). Verzoek om te worden aangesteld als plat-
telandsgeneesheer (Request to be appointed as a country-physician).
NTG, 83, II, 1496; *BGG, XIX,* 72.

4536 DOESSCHATE, A. ten (1937). Verzoekschrift van een geneesheer te
Ootmarsum in 1778 om in voorkomende gevallen sectio caesarea of
symphysiotomie te mogen verrichten (Request of a physician at O.
in 1778 to be allowed to perform caesarean section or symphysiotomy
in occurring cases). *NTG, 81,* II, 2660–1; *BGG, XVII,* 119–20.

4537 GEYL, A. (1911). Arbeidscontracten voor chirurgen en andere ge-
neeskunstoefenaren (Labour-contracts for surgeons and other students
of medicine). *NTG, 55,* II, 1235–9·

4538 ZUIDEN, D. S. van (1917). Een contract tusschen twee doktoren (A contract between two physicians). *NTG, 61*, II, 724–5.

4539 — (1940). Een merkwaardig contract over de genezing van een been (A remarkable contract on the healing of a leg). *NTG, 84*, I, 841; *BGG, XX*, 56.

4540 — (1918). Op welke voorwaarden de hofschoenmaker van den Koning van Denemarken zijn breuk liet opereren (On the conditions on which the court shoemaker of the King of Denmark consented in the operation for his hernia). *NTG, 62*, I, 1535.
  – on a contract for the fee of an operation for hernia to be performed by Mr Rochus van Dijck, town-surgeon of The Hague.

4541 PINKHOF, S. (1924). Uit het Gemeentearchief van Amsterdam. I. Toelating als chirurgijn. II. Toezicht op operaties. III. Verstrekking van orthopaedische hulpmiddelen. IV. Verzoek om anatomisch "materiaal" (From the municipal Record-office of A. I. Conditions of admission as a surgeon. II, Supervision of operations. III. Providing of orthopaedical aids. IV. Request for anatomical "material".). *NTG, 68*, II, 2248–50; *BGG, IV*, 285–7.

4542 RHIJN, N. van (1924). Een oude instructie voor chirurgijns (An old instruction for surgeons). *NTG, 68*, I, 1542–4; *BGG, IV*, 94–6.

4543 SCHELTEMA, W. P. (1940). Instructie voor den chirurgijn en vroedmeester op de Vrije Heerlijkheid Ameland in 1780 (Instruction for the surgeon and accoucheur on the Free Manor Ameland in —). *NTG, 84*, IV, 4823–4; *BGG, XX*, 198–9.

4544 ROEKEL, G. van (1940). Auteurs van wetenschappelijke werken door de overheid gehonoreerd (Authors of scientific works paid by the government). *NTG, 84*, IV, 4824–5; *BGG, XX*, 199–200.

4545 BRAAT, P. (1937). Instructie voor Adr. van Ghert als 's lands doctoor van de Baronie van Breda, gearresteerd den 29en October 1756 (Instruction for A van G. as country physician of the Barony of Breda, confirmed — —). *NTG, 81*, IV, 5834–6; *BGG, XVII*, 220–2.

Ordinances, Sentences

4546 BROUWER ANCHER, A. J. M. (1899). Oude ordonnantiën betreffende Genees-, Heel-, en Verloskundigen, Apothekers, kwakzalvers, enz.

(Old ordinances concerning physicians, surgeons, obstetricians, chemists, quacks, etc.). *NTG, 35,* (2de reeks), I, 1173–97.

– o.a. prescriptions for "gravel-water" and remedies for "flerecijn" (podagra).

4547 DONINCK, A. van (1929). Sprokkels uit oude archivalia. Ordonantie tot uitoefenen der geneeskunde 1540 (Gleanings from old records. Ordinance for practising medicine). *NTG, 73,* I, 68–70; *BGG, IX,* 34–6.

4548 HALLEMA, A. (1956). Dokters en apothekers te Utrecht in de 17e eeuw. Twee merkwaardige ordonnanties van 1655 betreffende doktershonoraria (Physicians and chemists at U. in the 17th century. Two curious ordinances from — concerning doctor's fees). *NTG, 100,* IV, 2914–9; *BGG, XXXVI,* 58–63.

4549 — (1952). Twee vonnissen wegens het onbevoegd uitoefenen der geneeskunst, gewezen te Amsterdam in het jaar 1548 (Two sentences for practising medicine without being registered passed at A.). *NTG, 96,* II, 825–7; *BGG, XXXII,* 10–2.

See also Surgeons general (3460–93)

D. Collegia Medica

4550 BRANS, P. H. (1957). Les Collèges Médicaux dans les Pays-Bas méridionaux. *Janus, XLVI,* 25–40.

4551 GEYL, A. (1907). Bladen uit Archieven der Collegia Medicum, chirurgicum et ad res obstetricias Amstelodamensia en mededeelingen van andere schrijvers (Leaves from the records of the — — — — and communications of other writers). *Gen. Crt.,* 9 February

4552 HAVER DROEZE, J. J. (1921). *Het Collegium Medicum Amstelodamense (1637–1798).* 263 + XXXVI pp., ill. Haarlem. 8°.

4553 WITTOP KONING, D. A. (1947). De voorgeschiedenis van het Collegium Medicum te Amsterdam (The previous history of the — — at A.). *Jbk. Amstelodamum, 41,* 51–66.

4553ª — (1948). Uit de voorgeschiedenis van het Collegium Medicum (From the previous history of the — —). *Amstelodamum, 35,* 72.

4554 NAPJUS, J. W. (1924). Het Collegium Medicum te Groningen. *NTG, 68,* I, 57–8; *BGG, IV,* 23–4.

4555 WILDEMAN, M. G. (1899). In en om Haarlem's Collegium Medico-pharmaceuticum (In and around the — — —). *Haarlemsch Advertentieblad.*   *See also* 2883

4556 BRANS, P. H. (1956). De collegia medica in de zuidelijke Nederlanden (The — — in the Southern Netherlands). *Ph. T. België, 33*, 121–4; *Bull. Pharm*, no 14.

4557 KRUL, R. (1890). De Hage-doctoren (Collegium medicum Hagae Batavorum 1594–1799) (The "the Hague-doctors"). *Tijdspiegel, II*, 292–305.

4558 KULSDOM, M. E. (1951). Het Collegium medicum te Leeuwarden 1686–1774. *NTG, 95*, IV, 3039–49; *BGG, XXXI*, 42–51.

4559 WEIJDE, A. J. van der (1922). Collegium medicum Ultrajectinum. *NTG, 66*, II, 2600–8; *BGG, II*, 343–51.

4560 — (1923). Rapport, uitgebracht door het Utrechtsch collegium medicum (Report delivered by the — — —). *NTG, 67*, II, 466; *BGG, III*, 177–9.

4561 — (1925). Wapenbord van de voorzitters van het Utrechtsche Collegium Medicum (Escutcheon of the chairmen of the — — —) *NTG, 69*, II, 59–74; *BGG, V*, 149–64, 1 ill., 5 ports.

4562 BERGER, J. A. (1931). Een "collegium medicum te Vlissingen". *NTG, 75*, IV, 5510–6; *BGG, XI*, 305–11.

4563 SIMONS, R. D. G. Ph. (1949). Een collegium medicum van 1781 in Suriname (A — — in Surinam). *NTG, 93*, I, 340–2; *BGG, XXIX*, 17–9.

E. Quackery

General

4564 WIELEN, P. van der (1905). De kwakzalver (The quack). *Eigen Haard, 31*, 711, 730 and 749.

4565 THEYS, Constant (1962). Kwakzalvers in de 18e eeuw (18th century quacks). *Eigen Schoon en de Brabander, 45*, 165–6.

4566 — (1966). Kwakzalvers in de 18de eeuw (18th century quacks). *Eigen Schoon en de Brabander, 49*, 326–7.

4567 DROOGLEEVER FORTUYN, H. J. W. (1940). *Kwakzalverij, bijgeloof en geneeskunst* (Quackery, superstition and medicine). 100 pp., Arbeiderspers, Amsterdam.
– 2nd edition: 164 pp., Stafleu, Leiden (1949).

4568 DROGENDIJK, A. C. (1957). De kwakzalverij voorheen en thans (Quackery past and present). *Ziekenfondsgids 11*, 220–4; 250–7.

4569 ELAUT, L. (1958). Ongehoord meer dan tweehonderdjarig sukses van een kwakzalversboekje (Success unheard of and lasting more than 200 years of a little quack's book). *Het Vlaamsche Kruis, 31*, 97–106.

4570 MOULIN, D. de [1972]. Boekaniers, chirurgijns en de "Piratenonderlinge van 1667" (Buccaneers, surgeons and the "Society" of pirates of —). *Organorama, 9*, 15–21, ill.

4571 VADER, J. (1965). Walcherse tovenaars en wonderdokters (Walcheren magicians and quacks). *Neerlands Volksleven, 15*, 114–21.

4572 COHEN, Hk. (1941). Een dominee beschuldigd van kwakzalverij (A vicar accused of quackery). *NTG, 85*, III, 3630–1; *BGG, XXI*, 122–3.
See also 870, 2002–8 (Quacks), 5318, 5374, 5378.

Announcements, measures, prizes, etc.

4573 ANDEL, M. A. van (1928). Kwakzalversbiljetten (Posters of quacks). *NRC*, 9 September.

4574 — (1912). Kwakzalvers-reclames in vroeger eeuwen (Advertising of quacks in former centuries). *NTG, 52*, II, 297–310.

4575 — (1932). Kwakzalversadvertenties in oude couranten (Advertisements of quacks in old journals). *NTG, 76*, III, 3853–65; *BGG, XII*, 141–53.

4576 COHEN, Hk (1941). Kwakzalversprijzen in de 17e eeuw (Fees of quacks in the 17th century). *NTG, 85*, II, 1912; *BGG, XXI*, 66.
– notarial protocol.

4577 ZUIDEN, D. S. van (1919). Een kwakzalverstestament (Will of a quack). *NTG, 63*, I, 688.

4578 WEIJDE, A. J. van der (1923). Maatregelen tegen kwakzalvers in 1548 (Measures against quacks in —). *NTG, 67*, II, 905; *BGG, III*, 220.
– Order of the Utrecht town council.

4579   PUTTO, J. A. (1963). Straffen voor kwakzalvers in de 17e eeuw (Punish-
       ments for quacks in the 17th century). *GG, 41,* 525.

4580   GORTER, C. N. (1906). De Vereeniging tegen de kwakzalverij (Associa-
       tion against Qnackery) *Boons Magazijn, 1,* 109.

Drugs

4581   ABRAHAMS, E. J. (ed.) (1916). *De kwakzalversmiddelen. Hunne inhoud
       en de gevaren die bij het gebruik dreigen* (Quack's remedies. Their con-
       tents and the dangers involved). 137 + XVII pp. Dordrechtsche Druk-
       kerij – Uitg. Mij, Dordrecht.
       – According to analyses made during 35 years by the "Vereeniging tegen de Kwak-
       zalverij".

4582   COHEN, Ernst (1912). Zur Geschichte der chemischen Quacksalberei.
       In: *Feestbundel ... Hector Treub,* 667–75, 1 ill. S. C. van Doesburgh,
       Leiden.

F. Guilds

General

4583   EEGHEN, I. H. van (1965). *De Gilden. Theorie en practijk* (The Guilds.
       Theory and practice). 150 pp., 30 ill. Van Dishoeck, Bussum.
       – On the guilds in general, with a chapter on the Amsterdam surgeons' guild (72–
       100).

4584   ANDEL, M. A. van (1917). Uit de laatste jaren der chirurgijnsgilden
       (From the last years of the surgeons' guilds). *NTG, 61,* II, 1778–84.

4585   BRANS, P. H. (1955). Chirurgijns en Chirurgijnsgilden in de Zuidelijke
       Nederlanden (Surgeons and surgeons' guilds in the Southern Nether-
       lands). *Jbk. Dodonaea, 23,* 327–47.   *See also* 3465, 5222

Local

4586   BRUINVIS, C. W. (1906). Gildebrief der Chirurgijns te Alkmaar (Charter
       of the Surgeons at A.). *Navorscher, 55,* 345.

4587   DOOREN, L. (1938). Een Geldersch melaatschengilde (1554) (A Leper
       Guild in Guelders). *NTG, 82,* II, 2295–6; *BGG,* XVIII, 96–7.

4588 — (1936). Gildebrieff van 't Cherurgijnsgilde te Arnhem (Charter of the surgeons' guild at A.). *NTG, 80*, I, 991–2; *BGG, XVI*, 43–4.

4589 HUNGER, F. W. T. (1930). Over een gildebrief van de stad Bolsward voor de medicijn-meester, chirurgijns en apothekers uit het jaar 1662 met twee supplementen van 1665 en 1675 (On a charter of the town B. for the physicians, surgeons and chemists from the year —, with two supplements from — and —) *De Vrije Fries, XXX* (reprint).

4590 HOEVEN, J. van der (1934). Het chirurgijnsgilde te Deventer (The surgeons' guild at D.). *NTG, 78*, II, 1547–59; *BGG, XIV*, 57–69.

4591 JONKMAN, J. J. (1913). De chirurgijns-gildekamer te Enkhuizen (The room of the surgeons' guild at E.). *PhW, 50*, 390–4.

4592 BROUWER, D. (1924). Het chirurgijns-gilde te Enkhuizen (The surgeons' guild at E.). *NTG, 68*, II, 2256–7; *BGG, IV*, 293–4.

4593 WOERDEN, J. van (1951). Heropening der "chirurgy's camer" te Gouda (Re-opening of the surgeons' guild-room at G.). *NTG, 95*, III, 2201–2; *BGG, XXXI*, 40–1.

4594 FEITH, H. O. L. (1838). *De Gildis Groninganis*. Dissertatio Historica-Juridica inauguralis. Groningen.

4595 LEUFTINK, A. E. (1951). De voorgeschiedenis van het chirurgijnsgilde te Groningen (The previous history of the surgeons' guild at G.) *NTG, 95*, IV, 3881–6; *BGG, XXXI*, 90–5.

4596 BOERMA, N. J. A. F. (1916). Liber legum collegy chirurgiae Groningensis. *NTG, 60*, II, 1593–6.

4597 KRUL, R. (1887). "De Hage-docenten, 1637–1837, en het Haagsche chirurgijnsgilde, 1591–1806 ("The Hague-teachers", and the surgeons' guild of The Hague). *NTG, 23*, II, 412–25.

4598 DOORNINCK, J. I. van and J. NANNINGA UITTERDIJK (1875). Het St. Lucasgilde te Kampen (The St. Luke guild at K.). *Bijdr. Gesch. Overijssel*, 2de deel, 47–57.

4599 STRAAT, H. L. (1932). Het Chirurgijnsgilde te Leeuwarden (The surgeons' guild at L.). *De Vrije Fries, XXXII*, 40 pp.
– Charters from 1550 and the inventory from 1565 and 1585 a.o.

4600 BIJL, W. F. Th. van der (1933). Uit de geschiedenis der chirurgijnsgilden in Zeeland (From the history of the surgeons' guilds in Z.). *NTG, 77*, II, 2046–64; *BGG, XIII*, 110–28.

4601   FOKKER, A. A. (1877). Losse bladen uit de geschiedenis van het chirurgijnsgilde te Middelburg (Loose leaves from the history of the surgeons' guild at M.). *NTG, 21*, II, 333.

4602   MAN, M. G. A. de (1912). Een onbeschreven penning van het chirurgyns- of Cosmas en Damianusgilde te Middelburg (An undescribed medal of the surgeons' or Cosmas and Damianus guild at M.). *T. Kon. Ned. Gen. Munt- en Penningk.*, XX, 121.

4603   SCHOUTE, D. [1913]. *Schets van het Middelburgsche chirurgijnsgilde* (Sketch from the Middelburg surgeons' guild). 55 pp., ill. no pl. pr. pr.

4604   — (1941). Uit boeken die verloren gingen (From books that got lost). *NTG, 85*, III, 3620–9; *BGG, XXI*, 112–21.
    – on books of the surgeons' guild at Middelburg (written by Adolphus van Lare, deacon of the guild), that got lost during World War II (May 17, 1940).

4605   HILTE, A. J. M. (1973). Over het chirurgijnsgilde te Nijmegen (On the surgeons' guild at N.). *Numaga, XX*, no 1, 17–36, 2 ill.

4606   [Anonym]. (1910). Een en ander uit het Rotterdamsche gildewezen. Het chirurgijnsbedrijf (Something on the system of guilds at R. The surgeons' business). *Wbl. Winkeliers- en Handelsbelangen, V*, no 9, Donderdag 2 Juni.

4607   LOON, L. van (1939). Het Rotterdamsche chirurgijnsgilde "S. Cosmas et Damianus" van 1467–1798 (The Rotterdam surgeons' guild — — from — —). I: *NTG, 83*, III, 1485–92; 3911–8; *BGG, XIX*, 61–8; 193–201.

4608   BRUYN, J. A. de (1931). Brief van Schout en Schepenen der stad Schoonhoven, waarbij het chirurgijnsgilde gesticht werd (Letter from the Bailiff and Aldermen of the town of S. founding the surgeon's guild). *NTG, 75*, I, 646–7; *BGG, XI*, 53–4.

4609   WILDEMAN, M. G. (1918). Voorzitters van het doktersgilde te Utrecht in de laatste helft der 18e eeuw (Chairmen of the surgeons' guild at U. in the last half of the 18th century). *NTG, 62*, I, 906–7.

4610   GILS, J. B. F. van (1923). Een merkwaardig overblijfsel van een chirurgijnsgilde (A remarkable remnant of a surgeons' guild). *NTG, 67*, II, 1654–8; *BGG, III*, 308–12.
    – on the biers of the surgeons' guild at Workum.
                See also 1726–9 (A. Titsingh), 4893–6 (Pharmacy), 5028a, 5235.

Examinations

4611 GEYL, A. (1911). Over half voldoende examens en voorwaardelijke be-
voegdheid in vroeger dagen (On half satisfying examinations and conditional competence in former days). *NTG, 55,* I, 642–7.

4612 BIJLSMA, R. (1906). Examen Chirurgicum te Rotterdam de Anno
MDLXXXXV (Surgeon's examination at R. — —). *GenCrt.* 9 en 16
Juni.

4613 ANDEL, M. A. van (1916). Een Examen Chirurgicum in 1636. *NTG, 60,*
II, 346–58.

4614 WEIJDE, A. J. van der (1923). Een examen voor chirugijns in 1766
(A surgeons' examination in 1766). *NTG, 67,* II, 904; *BGG, III,* 219.
– a short note.

4615 STRAAT, H. L. (1923). De kosten van het Barbiersexamen te Leeuwarden (The fees of the barber's examination at L.). *NTG, 77,* II, 1637–8;
BGG, III, 291–2.

4616 — (1924). Iets over de examens van het Leeuwarder en Groninger chirurgijnsgilde (Something on the examinations of the surgeons' guilds
at L. and at G.). *NTG, 68,* I, 48–9; *BGG, IV,* 14–5.

4617 HOEVEN, J. van der (1937). Een en ander over de examens bij de chirurgijnsgilden en over het "vroedkundig examen". (Something on the
examinations of the surgeons' guilds and on the "obstetrical examination"). *NTG, 81,* III, 3142–7; *BGG, XVII,* 121–6.

4618 BOESMAN, Theodoor (1942). *De examens in de chirurgijnsgilden* (The
examinations in the surgeons' guilds). Thesis University Utrecht (Supervisor: G. Remijnse). 143 pp., ill. Keemink & Zn, Utrecht.

See also 1456

4619 GILS, J. B. F. van (1929). Une relique d'une corporation de chirurgiens
et pharmaciens. *VIme Congrès Int. d'Hist. Méd. Leyde-Amsterdam,
1927,* 296–9, 1 ill. Anvers.

Certificates

4620 DOORMAN, G. (1939). Octrooien, verleend aan medici in de 16e en 17e
eeuw (Patents granted to physicians in the 16th and 17th century).
NTG, 83, III, 4328–9; *BGG, XIX,* 219–20.

4621   ZUIDEN, D. S. van (1914). Een merkwaardige acte uit het jaar 1660
       A remarkable act, 1660). *NTG, 58*, II, 1106.

4622   — (1916). Een verklaring over een afdrijvend middel dat gegeven zou
       zijn door den lijfarts van prins Maurits van Nassau (A declaration on
       a laxative that would have been prescribed by the court physician of
       Prince — —). *NTG, 60*, I, 1977–8.

4622ª — (1917). Een verklaring over een bloedstelpend middel (A declara-
       tion on a styptic remedy). *NTG, 61*, I, 1752–3.

4623   — (1917). Een verklaring in plaats van een doctorsbul (A declaration
       instead of a doctor's diploma). *NTG, 61*, II, 809–10.

4624   — (1917). Een verklaring van Dr Helvetius (A declaration of Dr H.).
       NTG, 61, II, 2145.

4625   — (1917). Een notarieele verklaring ten nadele van den chirurgijn Corn.
       S a s b o u t (1600) (A notarial act to the detriment of the surgeon — —).
       NTG, 61, II, 2208–9.   *See also* 1963

4626   — (1936). Notaris en geneesheer (Notary and physician). *NTG, 80*,
       III, 3570–2; *BGG, XVI*, 130–2.

4627   PRINSEN, J. Lzn, J. (1912). Uit het notarisprotocol van Salomon Le-
       naertzn van der Waert. Medische Zaken (From the notarial protocol
       of — —. Medical cases). *Oud-Holland, XXX*, 96.

4628   PINKHOF, H. (1914). Een klacht uit de 17de eeuw (A complaint from the
       17th century). *NTG, 60*, I, 2026.

4629   LEERSUM, E. C. van (1919). Een notarieele geneeskundige verklaring uit de
       18de eeuw (A notarial medical certificate from the 18th century).
       NTG, 63, II, 272–3.

4630   VAZ DIAS, A. M. (1937). Gezondheidsattest (Uit oud Notarieel
       Archief) (Certificate of health. (From the old Notarial Archives)).
       NTG, 81, II, 1462; *BGG, XVII*, 83.

4631   HAKKENBERG VAN GAASBEEK, A. (1972). De dokter en zijn wapen
       (The physician and his coat of arms). *Arts en Auto, 38*, 508–9, 5 ill.
       – on guilds' coats of arms.

4632   BRUINSMA, G. W. (1912). Een rapport uit de oude doos (An antiquated
       report). *NTG, 56*, II, 2011–5.
       – on a report of the military medical service in the Dutch East Indies, 1828.

4632ª EEGHEN, I. H. van (1968). Gezondbrief in tijden van pest (Health certificate in periods of plague). *Amstelodamum, 55, 212.*

G. Archivalia

4633 WIJNDELTS, J. W. (1918–23). Sprokkels uit oude archieven (Gleanings from old records).

4633.1 I. [A Zutphen certificate on a surgeon, 1576]. *NTG, 62,* I, 829.

4633.2 II. Een vroedvrouwen-eed in de 16de eeuw (A midwife's oath in the 16th century). *NTG, 62,* I, 1260.

4633.3 III. Eenige gevallen van doodschouw in Zutphen in vorige eeuwen (Some post-mortems at Z. in former centuries). *NTG, 62,* I, 1647–8.

4633.4 IV. Een geneeskundig attest uit het laatst der 17de eeuw (A medical certificate from the last part of the 17th century). *NTG, 62,* II, 591–2.

4633.5 V. Eenige gevallen van doodschouw te Zutphen in vorige eeuwen (2). (Some inquests at Z. in former centuries). *NTG, 62,* II, 1500.

4633.6 VI. Idem (3). *NTG, 63* (1919), I, 203.

4633.7 VII. Hoe men krankzinnigen behandelde in het midden de 16de eeuw (On treatment of lunatics in the middle of the 16th century). *NTG, 63,* I, 1513.

4633.8 VIII. no title. *NTG, 63,* II, 136.

4633.9 IX. Een belangwekkend geval van doodschouw (An interesting inquest). *NTG, 63,* II, 763.

4633.10 X. Voorbereiding tot een studiereis van een aankomend chirurg in de 17de eeuw (Preparation to a study-tour of a prospective surgeon in the 17th century). *NTG, 63,* II, 1472.

4633.11 XI. no title. [On Zutphen]. *NTG, 64,* (1920), I, 752–3.

4633.12 XII. Rekening van een chirurgijn in het midden der 18de eeuw

(A surgeon's bill in the middle of the 18th century). *NTG, 64,* I, 2309–10.

4633.13 XIII.   Aanstelling van een gemeente-geneesheer in de 15de eeuw, voorkomende in het Protocol van Kentenissen der Stad Zutphen (Appointment of a municipal physician in the 15th century from the Protocol of Minutes of the town of Z.). *NTG, 64,* II, 335–6.

4633.14 XIV.   Attest afgegeven door een tweetal chirurgijns en anderen ter verkrijging van maatschappelijken steun voor een hunner patienten, die tengevolge zijner verwonding hulpbehoevend was geworden (Certificate issued by two surgeons and others to obtain social support for one of their patients who has become invalid in consequence of injuries). *NTG, 64,* II, 1032–3.

4633.15 XV.   [Acte uit het Archief Haarlem, over een vroedvrouw] (certificate from the Archives of H. on a midwife). *NTG, 64,* II, 1931–3.

4633.16 XVI.   Relaas eener ontijdige bevalling (Account of a premature delivery). *NTG, 65,* (1921), I, 686–7; *BGG, I,* 100–1.

4633.17 XVII.   [Notariële acte Hoorn] (Notarial act). *NTG, 65,* I, 2581; *BGG, I,* 239.

4633.18 XVIII.   De dienstbodenplaag in het begin der 18de eeuw (The maidservants' plague in the beginning of the 18th century). *NTG, 65,* II, 727–8; *BGG, I,* 339–40.

4633.19 XIX.   De gevolgen van een gevecht tegen Turksche zeerovers (The results of a fight against Turkish pirates). *NTG, 66* (1922), II, 1098–9; *BGG, II,* 229–30.

4633.20 XX.   [Notariële acte Hoorn] (Notarial act H.). *NTG, 67* (1923), I, 56–7; *BGG, III,* 23–4.

4633.21 XXI.   Hoe men vroeger chirurg werd (How one did become a surgeon in former times). *NTG, 67,* I, 1889–90; *BGG, III,* 122–3.

4633.22 XXII.   [Notariële acte Alkmaar] (Notarial act —). *NTG, 67,* I, 2408–9; *BGG, III,* 142–4.

4633.23 XXIII.   Een vrouwelijke arts in het laatst der 16de eeuw (A female

physician in the last part of the 16th century). *NTG*, *67*, II, 488–9, *BGG*, *III*, 199–200.
Correction to no XXIII: *NTG*, *67*, II, *909*; *BGG*, *III*, 224.

4634 VIEYRA, D. (1935–36). Geneeskundige Archivalia. Een Amsterdamsche medicus wijst in 1817 op den slechten staat van den gezondheidsdienst (Medical Records. An Amsterdam physician [G. d'Ancona] points to the bad condition of the public health service). *NTG*, *79*, I, 474–5; *BGG*, *XV*, 40–1.

4634.1 Request van een wegens hardnekkig bedwateren weggejaagden verpleegde uit het Aalmoezeniers-weeshuis te Amsterdam (Request of a patient turned out of the Almshouse at A. because of bed-wetting). *NTG*, *79*, II, 1611–3; *BGG*, *XV*, 98–100.

4634.2 Een "Garnalen-quaestie" uit 1821 (A "shrimps-question"). *NTG*, *79*, II, 2666–8; *BGG*, *XV*, 138–40.

4634.3 Een Fransche stalknecht met een levenden kikvorsch in zijn maag (A French stableman with a living frog in his stomach). *NTG*, *79*, III, 3313–5; *BGG*, *XV*, 158–60.

4634.4 Request door een zekere dochter, welke men voor een manspersoon wilde doen (door)gaan, aan den Koning (van Frankrijk) overgeleverd Maart 1693 (Request of a certain daughter passed off as a man, delivered up to the King (of France), March —). *NTG*, *79*, III, 4284–6; *BGG*, *XV*, 197–9.

4634.5 Een aan het ongelooflijke grenzende redding van een drenkeling op Woensdag 19 April 1758 (en enkele andere notities) (An almost unbelievable rescue of a drowned person on Wednesday — (and some other notes)). *NTG*, *79*, IV, 4656–8; *BGG*, *XV*, 209–11.

4634.6 De aanstelling van een praelector in de scheepsgeneeskunde te Amsterdam in het jaar 1796 (The appointment of a praelector of naval medicine at A., 1796). *NTG*, *79*, IV, 5661–4; *BGG*, *XV*, 247–50.

4634.7 Isaac Souman junior, chirurgijn, zijn cautie ten behoeve vant Collegium Medicum, Anno 1733, den 25 Maart. – Een apothekersbediende, die geen Latijn kent, etc. – De stedelijke overheid van Amsterdam brengt den apotheker tot rede ... (— —, surgeon, his caution on behalf of the — —, March 25, 1733. – A chemist's assistant who does not know Latin, etc. – The municipal government of A. brings the chemist to reason..) *NTG*, *80*, (1936), I, 56–7; *BGG*, *XVI*, 19–20.

4635   VAZ DIAS, A. M. (1932, 1933, 1934). Sprokkels uit het Oud-Notarieel Archief te Amsterdam (Gleanings from the Old-Notarial Archives at A.).

4635.1   I: *NTG, 76*, IV, 5584–6; *BGG, XII*, 262–4.

4635.2   II: *NTG, 77* (1933), I, 75; *BGG, XIII*, 26.

4635.3   III–IV: *NTG, 77*, I, 1035–8; *BGG, XIII*, 81–4 (a.o. Dr Nic. v. Wassenaer).

4635.4   V–VI: *NTG, 77*, II, 2067–8; *BGG, XIII*, 131–2.

4635.5   VII–IX: *NTG, 78* (1934), II, 1990–1; *BGG, XIV*, 98–9.

4635.6   X: *NTG, 78*, II, 2502; *BGG, XIV*, 117.

4635.7   XI–XV: *NTG, 78*, III, 3162–4; *BGG, XIV*, 145–7.

4635.8   XVI: *NTG, 78*, IV, 4563–4; *BGG, XIV*, 201–2.

4636   DITMAR, J. van (1937). Uit oude boeken (From old books).

4636.1   I.   Huismiddel dat zeer excellent is tegen het graveel. Huismiddel van de Groot-Hertoginne van Toscane, dat aanstonds de pijn in de maag wegneemt. Syroop voor zieltogende. Syroop des levens. Huismiddel tegen pijn in de lendenen. Urine als oogwater. (Domestic remedy being very excellent against gravel. Another of the Grand-Duchess of T. allaying stomach-ache immediately. Syrup for the dying. Syrup of life. Domestic remedy against lumbar pain. Urine as eye-water). *NTG, 81*, III 4275–6; *BGG, XVII*, 167–8.

4636.2   II.   Epidemie te Leiden (Sept. 1669). "Gezwel aan de hals". Griep in 1504. Ordre op de heete ziekte der pest (10 April 1655). (Epidemic at L. "Swelling in the neck". Flu in 1504. Ordinance on the hot disease of plague). *NTG, 81*, IV, 4700; *BGG, XVII*, 179.

4636.3   III.   Ziektegevallen. "Larcke-swam" als middel tegen tering. Dood van Condé. Na de dood van Karel II (Cases of illness. "Larcke-swam" as a remedy against phthisis). Death of —. After the death of Charles II). *NTG, 81*, IV, 5836–7; *BGG, XVII*, 222–3.

4637   JONG, H. W. M. de (1956). Uit de Archives Royales de Mari (From the Archives —). *NTG, 100*, IV, 2922; *BGG, XXXVI*, 66.

H. Societies and Associations

General

4638 LEERSUM, E. C. van (1913). La société historique Néerlandaise des sciences médicales, exactes et naturelles. *Janus, XVIII,* 652–3.

4639 KLEIWEG DE ZWAAN, J. P. (1913). An international federation for the study of the history of medicine and natural sciences. *Janus, XVIII,* 462.

4640 HERINGA, G. C. (1940). *150 jaar Natuurwetenschap* (150 years of Natural Science). 31 pp., 6 ports. no pl.

– Address delivered, 13th November 1940, on the occasion of the 150th anniversary of the "Society for the promotion of physics, medicine and surgery" at Amsterdam.

4641 DELPRAT, C. C. (1915). *De wording en de geschiedenis van het Genootschap van Natuur-, Genees- Heelkunde te Amsterdam, 1790–1915* (The genesis and history of the Association of Natural Science, Medicine and Surgery at A.). 61 pp. Kruyt, Amsterdam.

4642 — (1916). De wording en de geschiedenis van het Genootschap ter bevordering van Natuur-, Genees- en Heelkunde te Amsterdam. Rede ter herdenking van het 125-jarig bestaan van het genootschap (10 November 1915) (The genesis and history of the Association for the promotion of Natural Science, Medicine and Surgery at A. Address in commemoration of the 125th anniversary of the Association). *NTG, 60,* I, 72–103., ill. (also of medals).

4643 — and A. KUMMER, (1965). *De wording en de geschiedenis van het Genootschap ter bevordering van Natuur-, Genees- en Heelkunde te Amsterdam 1790–1915 door Dr. C. C. Delprat, honorair bestuurder, vervolg 1915–1965, door Prof. Dr A. Kummer* (The genesis and history of the Association for the promotion of Natural Science, Medicine and Surgery at A. by —, honorary director, sequel by —). 77 pp., ill., ports. A. Bonn, no pl.

Learned Societies

4644 COLE, F. J. (Editor) (1938). *Observationes Anatomicae selectiores Amstelodamensium 1667–1673* University of Reading, England.

– Reprint of the *Observationes anatomicae selectiores Collegii privati Amstelodamensis.* Amsterdam 1667, and the "pars altera" of 1673. Introduction XI pp.

4645   [   ] (1930). *De Koninklijke Akademie van Wetenschappen, Universiteiten en Hoogescholen in Nederland en Nederlandsch-Indië* (The Royal Academy of Science, Universities and Academies in the Netherlands and in the Dutch East Indies). 102 pp., ill. Leiden.
– Also published in French and German.

4646   BIERENS DE HAAN, J. A. (1952, ²1970). *De Hollandsche Maatschappij der Wetenschappen 1752-1952* (The Dutch Society of Science). 461 pp., ill. ports. Tjeenk Willink & Zn, Haarlem.
– With English summary.

4647   SCHOUTE, D. (1923). De geschiedenis van het natuurkundig gezelschap te Middelburg (History of the society for physics at M. Reprint from: *Archief Zeeuwsch Gen. Wtsch.*, Middelburg. 34 pp.

4648   WEIJDE, A. J. van der (1920). *Bijdrage tot de geschiedenis der geneeskunde in ons vaderland (1793-1843). Ontleend aan den inhoud der Notulen van het "Utrechtsch Geneeskundig Gezelschap Mathias van Geuns"* (Contribution to the history of medicine in our country. Borrowed from the contents of the minutes of the "Utrecht Medical Society —"). Utrecht.

4649   KOOPMAN, J. (1928). Het Genootschap "Servandis Civibus" (1778–1794) (The Society — —). *NTG*, 72, II, 3811-6; *BGG*, VIII, 215-20.

4650   KAISER, Wolfram und VÖLKER, A. (1972). Niederländische Leopoldina-Mitglieder des 17. und 18. Jahrhunderts und ihre Korrespondenz mit dem Akademiepräsidium. *Janus*, LIX, 249-68.

4651   [   ] (1927). *Feestbundel aangeboden door leden en oud-leden van het Klinisch Genootschap te Rotterdam aan Dr. H. Klinkert, ter gelegenheid van zijn 80ste verjaardag* (Festschrift presented by members and former members of the Clinical Society at R. to — — on the occasion of his 80th birthday). 523 pp., ill. Rotterdam.

Royal Dutch Society for the promotion of Medicine

4652   BURGER, H. (1924). Feestrede, uitgesproken bij de herdenking van het vijf-en-zeventigjarig bestaan der Nederlandsche Maatschappij tot bevordering der geneeskunst, in den Koninklijken Schouwburg te 's-Gravenhage, op 8 Juli 1924 (Address delivered at the commemoration of the 75th anniversary of the Dutch Society for the promotion of medicine, in the Royal Theatre at The Hague). *NTG*, 68, II, 308-21.

Also in: H. Burger. *Uitgezochte opstellen en toespraken...*, 64–81. De Bussy, Amsterdam.

4653 SCHOUTE, D. *et al.* (1924). *Gedenkboek der Nederlandsche Maatschappij ter bevordering der Geneeskunst bij haar vijf-en-zeventigjarig bestaan den leden aangeboden 8 Juli 1924* (Memorial Volume of the Dutch Society for the promotion of medicine on the occasion of the 75th anniversary, presented to the members July 8, 1924). 228 pp., ill., ports. Ellerman Harms & Co Amsterdam.
    – Reviewed by P. Muntendam: *NTG, 68* (1924), II, 1271–3; *BGG, IV,* 234–6.

4654 ERP TAALMAN KIP, L. F. C. van *et al.* (1949). *Gedenkboek der Koninklijke Nederlandsche Maatschappij tot bevordering der geneeskunst ter gelegenheid van haar honderjarig bestaan, 7–8–9 Juli 1949* (Memorial Volume of the Royal Dutch Society for the promotion of medicine, on the occasion of the 100th anniversary). 308 pp., ports. De Bussy, Amsterdam.

4655 FESTEN, H. (1962). Uit de geschiedenis van de Maatschappij (From the history of the Society). *MC, 17,* 149–56; 393–5; 416–9.

4655ᵃ — (1974). Honderdvijfentwintig jaar geneeskunst en Maatschappij (125 years of medicine and the Society [for the promotion of medicine]. *MC, 29,* 1305–20.

4655ᵇ — (1974). *125 jaar Geneeskunst en Maatschappij. Geschiedenis van de Koninklijke Nederlandsche Maatschappij tot bevordering der Geneeskunst* (125 years of medicine and Society. History of the Royal Dutch Society for the promotion of medicine). 591 pp., ill., ports. no pl; pr. pr. [Address Society: Lomanlaan, 103, Utrecht]

4656 BURGER, H. (1923). Toespraak gehouden bij de herdenking van het 75-jarig bestaan van den geneeskundigen kring te Amsterdam op 22 September 1923 (Address delivered at the commemoration of the 75th anniversary of the medical circle at A.). *NTG, 67,* II, 1374; not in *BGG.*

4657 — *et al.* (1923). *Gedenkboek uitgegeven ter gelegenheid van de viering van het 75-jarig bestaan van den geneeskundigen kring te Amsterdam 21 September 1923* (Memorial Volume published on the occasion of the celebration of the 75th anniversary of the medical circle at A.). 182 pp., ill., ports. Amsterdam. 8°.
    – Reviewed by P. Muntendam: *NTG, 67* (1923), II, 2296; *BGG, III,* 354.

4658 WEIJDE, A. J. van der *et al.* (1924). *Gedenkschrift uitgegeven door de afdeeling Utrecht der Nederlandsche Maatschappij tot bevordering der geneeskunst, ter gelegenheid van den 75sten verjaardag der afdeeling op 23 Mei 1924* (Memoir published by the section U. of the Dutch Society for the promotion of medicine, on the occasion of the 75th anniversary of this section). 44 pp., ill port. (of F. C. Donders.) Utrecht.
– Reviewed by P. Muntendam: *NTG, 68* (1924), I, 2631–2; *BGG, IV*, 126–7.

4659 ROMBACH, K. A. (1949). *Honderd jaar Utrechtse geneeskundige kring* (A century Utrecht medical circle). 120 pp., ill., ports. no pl.

4660 DROGENDIJK, A. C. (1949). Honderd jaar Afdelingsleven (A century life of the local circle). *Eeuwfeestnr. Med. bl. Afd. Dordrecht*, 24 November.

4661 BOSMAN, J. F. M. (1935). Afdeeling Zutphen en Omstreken der Nederlandsche Maatschappij der Geneeskunst 1845–1935 (Section Z. and its surroundings of the Dutch Society of Medicine). *NTG, 79*, IV, 5655–60; *BGG, XV*, 241–6.

4662 KLOPPER, S. (1965). Honderd jaar artsenkring in Zaanland (A century circle ·of physicians in Z). *Noord-Holland, 10*, 69–75.

4663 [   ] (1952). *Gedenkboek van de afdeling Zwolle en omstreken der Kon. Ned. Maatschappij tot Bevordering der Geneeskunst 1852–1952* (Memorial Volume of the section Z. and its surroundings of the Royal Dutch Society for the promotion of medicine — —). 66 pp., ill., 1 port. J. J. Tijl, Zwolle.
– Compiled on the occasion of the 100th anniversary of the foundation.
See also 695, 5475–6

Special Associations

4664 FESTEN, H. (1964). De totstandkoming van de afzonderlijke organisatie voor specialisten binnen de Maatschappij (Uit de geschiedenis van de Maatschappij, III) (The realization of a separate organisation for specialists inside the Society (of Medicine) *MC, 19*, 681–3.

4665 DIJKSTRA, O. H. (1961). De Nederlandse Patholoog-Anatomen Vereniging veertig jaar oud (The Dutch Association of Pathologists fourty years old). *NTG, 105*, 1654–6.

4666 WOERDEMAN, M. W. (1964). Iets over de geschiedenis van de Nederlandse Anatomen Vereniging (Something on the history of the Dutch Association of Anatomists). *NTG, 108*, II, 1510–1.

4667   HANEVELD, G. T. (1972). De Vereeniging ter beoefening der Ziekte-
       kundige Ontleedkunde (The Association of pathological anatomy).
       NTG, 116, 415.
       – This Association, founded 1850, never flourished and was incorporated into the
       "Genootschap ter bevordering der Natuur-, Genees- en Heelkunde" in 1853.

4668   KRAMER, P. H. (1940). Bij het honderdjarig bestaan van de Rotter-
       damsche Vereeniging "In sociorum salutem" (At the 100th anniver-
       sary of the Rotterdam Association — —). *NTG, 84*, IV, 3891–8;
       BGG, XX, 148–55.

4669   TONGEREN, F. C. van (1963). Officiële herdenkingsrede (Official me-
       morial address). *NTVerl.. Gyn., 63*, 15–39.
       – On the occasion of the 75th anniversary of the "Nederlandsche Gynaecologische
       Vereeniging" on 16 November 1962. The Dutch Gynaecological Association was
       founded at Amsterdam, 1887.

4670   LINDEBOOM, G. A. (1958). De Nederlandsche Internisten Vereeniging
       25 jaar. Rede gehouden op 11 Mei 1957 in het Academisch Ziekenhuis
       te Leiden (The Dutch Association for Internal Medicine 25 years.
       Address delivered on May 11, 1957 in the Academical Hospital at L.)
       Folia Med. Neerl., 1, 25–33.

4671   [   ] (1933). *Gedenkboek uitgegeven ter gelegenheid van het 40-jarig
       bestaan der Nederlandse Keel- Neus- en Oorartsen Vereeniging* (Me-
       morial Volume published on the occasion of the 40th anniversary
       of the Dutch Association for Otorhinolaryngology). Amsterdam.

4672   [   ] (1968). *Gedenkboek Nederlandse keel, neus-, oorheelkundige
       vereeniging. 75. 1893–1968* (Memorial Volume of the Dutch Associa-
       tion for Otorhinolaryngology). 80 pp., ill., ports. Ellerman en Harms,
       Amsterdam.

4672ᵃ [   ]. (1964). *Nederlands Tandartsenblad*. Jubileumnummer ter ge-
       legenheid van het 50-jarig bestaan van de Nederlandsche Maatschap-
       pij tot Bevordering der tandheelkunde (— —. Jubilee issue on the oc-
       casion of the 50th anniversary of the Dutch Society for the promotion
       of dentistry). 116 pp., ill. Den Haag.
       – with many beautiful pictures from the Kalman Klein Collection, (description
       by F. E. R. de Maar).

4673   DOESSCHATE, G. ten (1963). The Netherlands Ophthalmological So-
       ciety 70 years. *Ophthalmologica* (Basel), *145*, 81–7, ill.

4674   DOESSCHATE, J. ten (1968). 75 jaren Nederlands Oogheelkundig Ge-
       zelschap (75 years Dutch Ophthalmological Society). *NTG, 112*, 1185.

4674ᵃ [   ] (1971). *Nederlandse Vereniging van Dermatologen. 75 jarig bestaan* (Dutch Association of Dermatologists. 75th anniversary). 55 pp. no pl. pr. pr.

– pp. 2–21: J. R. Prakken. Driekwart eeuw Dermatologie in Nederland; 75 jaar geschiedenis van de Nederlandse Vereniging voor Dermatologen (75 years of dermatology in the Netherlands; 75 year history of the Dutch Association of dermatologists).

4675 WINCKEL, Ch. W. F. (1957). De Nederlandse Vereniging voor Tropische geneeskunde, 1907–1957 (The Dutch Association for Tropical Medicine). *NTG, 101*, II, 2395–2402.

, 4676 BOESMAN, Th. (1969). Feestrede wegens het 70-jarig bestaan van de Nederlandse Orthopaedische Vereniging (Address delivered on the occasion of the 70th anniversary of the Dutch Orthopaedic Association). *NTG, 113*, 1005.

4677 JONGKEES, L. B. W. (1963). Het Nederlands Kanker-Instituut 50 jaar (The 50th anniversary of the Cancer Institute). *NTG, 107*, II, 1589–92.

4678 GILS, J. B. F. van (1928). *Gedenkboek, uitgegeven ter gelegenheid van het 25-jarig bestaan van de Nederlandsche Centrale Vereeniging tot bestrijding der tuberculose* (Memorial Volume published on the occasion of the 25th anniversary of the Dutch Association for the fight against tuberculosis). 181 pp., ill., ports. 's-Gravenhage.

4679 DROGENDIJK, A. C. (1960). Herdenkingsrede gehouden ter gelegenheid van het Eerste lustrum van de Prot. Chr. Artsenorganisatie (Commemorative address delivered on the occasion of the first lustrum of the Protestant Christian Physicians' Organisation) *Soteria, 4*, 184–8.

4680 SCHREUDER, P. H., G. J. VOS and D. HERDERSCHÉE (1929). *Gedenkboek omtrent zorg voor en onderwijs aan zwakzinnigen* (Memorial Volume of the care and education of mental defectives). ill., port. 's-Gravenhage. 8°.

– Published by the "Vereeniging van onderwijzers artsen, werkzaam aan inrichtingen voor onderwijs aan achterlijke en zenuwzwakke kinderen". 27 December 1903 – 27 December 1928.

4681 RIEL, J. van (1906). Geschiedkundig overzicht der vereeniging over de jaren 1880–1905. (Historical survey of the Association 1880–1905). In: *Gedenkboek van de Vereeniging tegen de Kwakzalverij, ter gelegenheid van het vijf-en-twintig jarig bestaan*, 165–98. Dordrecht.

See also 3999, 4000

Association "Netherlands Journal of Medicine"

4682 BLINK-ROLDER, J. W. van den (1957). Het honderdjarig bestaan van de Vereeniging "Het Nederlandsch Tijdschrift voor Geneeskunde" (toespraak) (The 100th anniversary of the "Association — — — (Address)). *NTG, 101*, II, 2104; (not in *BGG*).

4683 MAYER, Ch. (1957). Het honderdjarig bestaan der Vereeniging "Nederlandsch Tijdschrift voor Geneeskunde" (The 100th anniversary of the Association — — —). *NTG, 101*, II, 2106; not in *BGG*).
– Address.

4684 CLEGG, H. A. (1957). Honderdjarig bestaan van de Vereeniging "Het Nederlandsch Tijdschrift voor Geneeskunde" (The 100th anniversary of the Association — — —). *NTG, 101*, II, 2105–6; (not in *BGG*).

Dutch Society ... Pharmacy

4685 WITTOP KONING, D. A. (1948). *De Nederlandsche Maatschappij ter Bevordering der Pharmacie 1842–1942* (The Dutch Society for the promotion of Pharmacy). Amsterdam.

4686 — (1962). Uit de eerste jaren van de Maatschappij (From the first years of the Society). *PhW*, *97*, 419–25; *Bull. Pharm*, *30*, (October), 9–14.
– From annual reports of the "(Kon.) Nederlandsche Maatschappij ter bevordering van de Pharmacie", 1842–44.

4687 — (1967). De Koninklijke Nederlandse Maatschappij ter Bevordering der Pharmacie in de afgelopen vijf en twintig jaren (The Royal Dutch Society for the promotion of Pharmacy in the past twenty-five years). *PhW*, *102*, 323–46, 8 ports; 2 ill. (of medals). *Bull. Pharm.*, *38* (September), 1–24, port.

4688 BRANS, P. H. (1954). Les organisations mondiales d'Histoire de la Pharmacie. *Arch. Int. Hist. Sci.*, *8*, 49.

4689 — (1955). 5 jaar Kring voor de Geschiedenis van de Pharmacie in Benelux (Five years Circle for the History of Pharmacy in Benelux). *Bull. Pharm.*, *12*, 8.

Society for the History of Medicine, Physics and Mathematics

4690 FEYFER, F. M. G. de (1938). *Herinneringen uit de eerste jaren van de Vereeniging voor Geschiedenis der Geneeskunde, Natuurkunde en Wiskunde* (Memories of the first years of the Association for the History of Medicine, Physics and Mathematics) De Jager, Geldermalsen.
   – Address.

4691 BURGER, D. (1938). *Overzicht van de eerste 25 jaren (1913–1938) van de Vereeniging voor Geschiedenis der Genees-, Natuur- en Wiskunde, sinds 1928 Genootschap voor Geschiedenis der genees-, natuur-, en wiskunde, gevestigd te Leiden* (Survey of the first 25 years of the Association for the History of medicine, physics and mathematics, since 1928 Society for the History — — —, established at L.). 46 pp. Jac. van Campen, Amsterdam.

4692 — (1939). Genootschap voor Geschiedenis der Geneeskunde, wiskunde en natuurwetenschappen (Society for the History of Medicine, mathematics and natural science). *NTG, 83,* I, 532–3; *BGG, XIX,* 37–8, 1 ill.
   – on the 25th anniversary of the Society.

4693 — (1948). *Gedenkboekje bij het 35-jarig bestaan van het Genootschap voor geschiedenis der geneeskunde, wiskunde en natuurwetenschappen, gevestigd te Leiden* (Memorial booklet on the occasion of the 35th anniversary of the Society for the History of medicine, mathematics and natural science, established at L.). 44 pp., 5 ports. Jacob van Campen, Amsterdam.

4694 SCHULTE, B. P. M. (ed.) (1963). *Vijftig jaren beoefening van de geschiedenis der geneeskunde, wiskunde en natuurwetenschappen in Nederland 1913–1963* (Fifty years of practising history of medicine, mathematics and natural science in the Netherlands). 118 pp., ill. Published by the "Genootschap voor geschiedenis der geneeskunde...".
   – p. 9–23: G. A. Lindeboom. De beoefening van de geschiedenis der geneeskunde (with an extensive bibliography, 19–23).

4695 ANDEL, M. A. (1921). Proceedings of the Dutch Society for the History of Medicine, Physics and Mathematics. *Ann. Med. Hist.,* ser.1, *III,* 199–201.

4696 — (1923). The Proceedings of the Dutch Society for the History of Medicine. *Ann. Med. Hist.,* ser.1, *V,* 82–7.
   – letter to the editor.

4697 *Meetings* (listed in the following table).

Date and Place	Secretary	NTG	BGG	Remarks
16/7–X–1920 Gorinchem	v. Andel	65 (1921, 107–10	I, 57–60	*Janus, XXV*, 45–8
18–XII–1920 Amsterdam	v. Andel	65, 687–8	I, 101–2	*ibid*, 48–50 (v. Andel)
12–III–1921 Den Haag	Kroon	65, 2582–5	I, 240–3	*ibid*, 389 (v. Andel)
14–V–1921 Leiden	v. Andel	65, 60–4	I, 313–6	*ibid*, 282–4 Jenner-commemoration
22/3–X–1921 Gorinchem	v. Andel	65, 2828–31	I, 460–2	
18–XII–1921 's-Hertogenbosch	v. Andel	66 (1922), 502–6	II, 59–63	
21/2–X–1922 Gorinchem	Schoute	66, 1986–7	II, 250	*Janus*, 28, 110–9.
10–XII–1922 Utrecht	Lamers	67 (1923), 481–4	III, 50–3	*ibid*, 420–4
20/1–X–1923 Gorinchem	v. Leersum	67, 1597–1603	III, 251–7	10th anniv.
28/9–IV–1923 Groningen	Lamers	68 (1924) 44–58	IV, 10–24	
20/1–X–1923 Gorinchem	Lamers	68, 944–9	IV, 67–72	
31–V–1924 Enkhuizen	Lamers	68, 2253–61	IV, 290–8	
25/6–X–1924 Gorinchem	Muntendam	68, 2250–2	IV, 287–9	
31–V–1924 Enkhuizen	v. Gils	68, 2253–61	IV, 187–90	
25/6–X–1924 Gorinchem	Lamers	69 (1925) 53–5	V, 25–8	
5–IV–1925 Amersfoort	Lamers	69, 2559–65	V, 130–6	
13/4–VI–1925 Zutphen	Lamers	69, 1584–7	V, 264–7	
16/7–X–1926 Gorinchem	Muntendam	70 (1926) 1879–82	VI, 304–8	
15/6–X–1927 Gorinchem	Sluiter	71 (1927) 1974–5	VII, 676–80	
20/1–X–1928 Gorinchem	v. Andel	72 (1928) 5476	VIII, 351–6	
6/7–IV–1929 Gouda	v. Andel	73 (1929) 2180	IX, 130–6	
19/20–X–1929 Gorinchem	v. Andel	73, 5158–62	IX, 298–302	
18/9–X–1930 Gorinchem	v. Andel	74 (1930) 5398	X, 298–300	
2/3–V–1931 Utrecht	v. Andel	75 (1931) 2988	XI, 181–7	

Date and Place	Secretary	NTG	BGG	Remarks
17/8–X–1931 Gorinchem	v. Andel	75, 5908–12	XI, 328–32	
4/5–VI–1932 Breda	v. Andel	76 (1932) 4237	XII, 175–80	
15/6–X–1932 Gorinchem	v. Andel	76, 5181–4	XII, 241–4	
10/1–VI–1933 Deventer	v. Andel	77 (1933) 3057	XIII, 172–6	
28/9–IV–1934 Leiden	v. Andel	78 (1934) 3165	XIV, 148–54	
20/1–X–1934 Gorinchem	v. Andel	78, 5065–8	XIV, 211–4	
6/7–IV–1935 Haarlem	v. Andel	79 (1935) 2109 –12	XV, 121–4	
19/20–X–1935 Gorinchem	v. Andel	79, 5163–6	XV, 226–9	
28/9–III–1936 Eindhoven	Burger	80 (1936) 2622 –6	XVI, 95–9	
17/8–X–1936 Gorinchem	v. Andel	80, 5043–6	XVI, 193–6	
17/8–IV–1937 Rotterdam	v. Andel	81 (1937) 1966 –8	XVII, 96–8	
23/4–X–1937 Gorinchem	v. Andel	81, 5440–8	XVII, 191–9	
22/3–X–1938 Gorinchem	v. Andel	82 (1938) 5415 –21	XVIII, 297– 303	
29/30–IV–1939 Groningen	v. Andel	83 (1939) 2634 –7	XIX, 168–71	
22/3–X–1939 Leiden	v. Andel	83, 5288–91	XIX, 249–52	
20/1–IV–1940 Delft	v. Andel	84 (1940) 1722 –9	XX, 89–96	
20–X–1940 Leiden	v. Andel	84, 4294–8	XX, 178–82	
11–V–1941 Utrecht	Schoute	85 (1941) 2706 –9	XXI, 77–80	
19–X–1941 Leiden	Burger	85, 4543–7	XXI, 152–6	
31–V–1942 Utrecht	Burger	86 (1942) 1718 –24	XXII, 99–105	
25–X–1942 Leiden	Schierbeek	86, 3082–5	XXII, 160–3	
6–VI–1943 Utrecht	Burger	87 (1943) 1498 –1501	XXIII, 74–7	
24–X–1943 Leiden	Burger	87, 1709–11	XXIII, 92–4	
4–VI–1944 Utrecht	Burger	88 (1944) 727– 8	XXIV, 14–5	
20–I–1946 Leiden	Burger	90 (1946) 383– 4	XXVI, 10–1	

Date and Place	Secretary	NTG	BGG	Remarks
19–V–1946 Leiden	Burger	*90*, 921–3	*XXVI*, 31–3	
27–X–1946 Leiden	Burger	*90*, 1973–5	*XXVI*, 54–6	
31–V–1947 Amsterdam	Burger	*92* (1948) 42–5	*XXVIII*, 1–4	
26–X–1947 Den Haag	Burger	*92*, 505–7	*XXVIII*, 5–7	
22/3–V–1948 Hoorn	Burger	*92*, 3209–11	*XXVIII*, 12–4	
6/7–XI–1948 Haarlem	Burger	*93* (1949) 45–7	*XXIX*, 12–4	
7/9–V–1949 Leiden	Burger	*93*, 3003–5	*XXIX*, 55–7	
29/30–X–1949 Gouda	Burger	*94* (1950) 40–3	*XXX*, 4–7	
20/1–V–1950 Wageningen	Burger	*94*, 2622–4	*XXX*, 31–3	
21/2–X–1950 Gorinchem	Burger	*95* (1951) 221–4	*XXXI*, 7–9	
28/9–IV–1951 Amersfoort	Burger	*95*, 3441–4	*XXXI*, 86–9	
27/8–X–1951 Gorinchem	Burger	*96* (1952) 829–31	*XXXII*, 14–6	
17/8–V–1952 Maastricht	Burger	*96*, 3209–11	*XXXII*, 46–8	
15/6–XI–1952 Utrecht	Burger	*97* (1953) 1149–51	*XXXIII*, 30–2	
6/7–VI–1953 Gorinchem	Burger	*98* (1954) 39–41	*XXXIV*,13–5	
21/2–XI–1953 Enschede	Brans	*98*, 708–10	*XXXIV*, 29–31	
30/1–X–1954 Kampen	Brans	*99* (1955) 1592–3	*XXXV*, 52–3	
21/2–V–1955 Dordrecht	Brans	*99*, 3532–3	*XXXV*, 106–7	
22/3–X–1955 Gorinchem	Brans	*100* (1956) 935–7	*XXXVI*, 28–30	
2/3–VI–1956 Arnhem	Brans	*100*, 2920–2	*XXXVI*, 64–6	
27/8–X–1956 Rotterdam	Brans	*101* (1957) 777–8	*XXXVII*, 10–1	
15–VI–1957 Den Haag	Brans	*101*, 2215–6	*XXXVII*, 40–1	*GeWiNa* (1957), no 2, 4–8
8/9–VI–1963 Gorinchem		—	—	*Physis*, V, 349 50th anniv.

Date and Place	Secretary	*GeWiNa*
26/7–X–1957 Deventer	Wittop Koning	no 3 (1958), 3–6
19/20–IV–1958 Gorinchem	Wittop Koning	no 4 (1958), 4–7
8/9–XI–1958 Utrecht	Wittop Koning	no 5 (1959), 4–6
25/6–IV–1959 Nijmegen	Wittop Koning	no 6 (1959), 4–6
14/15–XI–1959 Delft	Wittop Koning	no 7 (1960), 5–7; 11–8
14/5–V–1960 Amersfoort	Wittop Koning	no 8 (1960), 3–6
5/6–XI–1960 Breda	Van Cittert-Eymers	no 9 (1961), 3–8
13/4–V–1961 Harderwijk	Van Cittert-Eymers	no 10 (1961), 4–9
11/2–XI–1961 Amsterdam	Van Cittert-Eymers	no 11 (1962), 2–9
12/3–V–1962 Amsterdam	Van Cittert-Eymers	no 12 (1962), 2–7
29–IX–1962 St. Niklaas (Belgium)	Van Cittert-Eymers	no 13 (1963), 2–5
8/9–VI–1963 Gorinchem	Van Cittert-Eymers	no 14 (1963), 2–12
9/10–XI–1963 Zutfen	Van Cittert-Eymers	no 15 (1964), 5–9
2/3–V–1964 Gouda	Van Cittert-Eymers	no 16 (1964), 2–7
3/4–X–1964 Leuven		no 17 (1965).
23–X–1965 Hoorn	Brongers	no 19 (1966), 2–4
14–V–1966 Nijmegen	Brongers	no 20 (1966), 2–4
19/20–XI–1966 Utrecht	Brongers	no 21 (1967), 3–7
7/8–V–1967 Zwolle	Brongers	no 22 (1967) 2–4
21/2–X–1967 Maastricht	Brongers	no 23 (1968), 3–4
11/2–V–1968 Zierikzee	Brongers	no 24 (1968), 3–4
26/7–X–1969 Franeker	Brongers	no 25 (1970) 2–3
4/5–IV–1970 Amsterdam	Smeur	no 26 (1970), 1–2
17/8–X–1970 Luxemburg	Smeur	no 27 (1971), 2–3
17/8–IV–1971 Enschede	Smeur	no 28 (1971), 1–2

Date and Place	Secretary	*GeWiNa*
7/8–XI–1971 Haarlem	Smeur	no 29 (1972), 1–3
15/6–IV–1972 Amersfoort	Smeur	no 30 (1972), 1–3
28/9–IV–1973 Gorinchem	Smeur	no 32 (1973), 1–2

4698 ANDEL, M. A. van (1922). Geschiedkundige sectie op de Hundertjahrfeier der Gesellschaft Deutscher Naturforscher und Aerzte (Historical section on the 100th anniversary of the — — —) *NTG*, *66*, II, 2635–6; not in *BGG*.

4699 HALBERTSMA, K. T. A. (1937). *Het eeuwfeest van het Gesellschaft der Aerzte in Wien (1837–1937)* (Centenary of the — — —). 24 pp. Waltman, Delft.

I. Congresses

4700 [Editorial] (1972). Chronologische lijst van vroegere congressen (Chronological list of former congresses of history of medicine). *AP*, no 6, januari, 19.

4701 LINT, J. G. de (1920). Het [eerste] congres voor de geschiedenis der geneeskunde te Antwerpen (The [first] medical-historical congress at Antwerp). *NTG*, *64*, II, 930–3.

4702 ANDEL, M. A. van (1921). The second international medical-historical congress at Paris (1–6 July 1921). *Janus*, *XXV*, 391–6.

4703 GILS, J. B. F. van (1921). Tweede congres voor de geschiedenis der geneeskunde (Second medical-historical congress). *NTG*, *65*, II, 1201–3.

4704 — (1922). Derde congres voor geschiedenis der geneeskunde 17–22 Juli) te Londen (Third medical-historical congress at L.) *NTG*, *66*, II, 1095–8; *BGG*, *II*, 226–9.

4705 ANDEL, M. A. v. (1925). Fünfter Internationaler Kongress für Geschichte der Medizin von 20–25 Juli in Genf. *Janus*, *XXIX*, 259–70.

4706 GILS, J. B. F. van (1925). Het vijfde internationale congres voor de

Geschiedenis der Geneeskunde (The fifth medical-historical congress (20–25 July at Geneva). *NTG, 69*, II, 1581–3; *BGG, V*, 261–3.

4707 RIJNBERK, G. van (1927). Het VIe internationale congres voor de Geschiedenis der Geneeskunde (The 6th international medical-historical congress (18–25 July 1927 at Leiden-Amsterdam). *NTG, 71*, II, 506–7; *BGG, VII*, 517–8.

4708 ANDEL, M. A. van (1927). Het 6e internationale congres voor de Geschiedenis der Geneeskunde (The 6th international medical-historical congress). *NTG, 71*, II, 665–7; *BGG, VII*, 574–6.

4709 TRICOT-ROYER, J. J. G. (1927). Autour du congrès médico-historique de Leyde-Amsterdam (18–23 juillet 1927). *Janus, XXXI*, 423–43.

4710 LAIGNEL-LAVASTINE, M. (1927). VIᵉ congrès international d'histoire de la médecine. Leyde-Amsterdam (18–23 juillet 1927). *Bull. Soc. Fr. Hist. Méd., XXI*, 335–61.

4711 [ ] (1929). *VIᵉ Congrès International d'Histoire de la Medecine. Leyde-Amsterdam 18–23 juillet 1927.* 376 pp., ill. "De Vlijt", Anvers.

4712 ANDEL, M. A. van (1935). The Xth historical medical congress in Madrid and its significance for the propagation of the study of the history of medicine. *Janus, XXXIX*, 203–6.

4713 — (1935). Het 10e Internationaal Historisch-Geneeskundig Congres te Madrid, 22–30 September 1935 (The 10th International historical-medical congress at — —). *NTG, 79*, IV, 5158–62; *BGG, XV*, 221–5.

4714 NUYENS, B. W. Th. (1938). Het XIe internationale congres voor Geschiedenis der Geneeskunde, gehouden te Zagreb, Belgrado en Dubrovnik van 1–14 September 1938. (The XIth international medical-historical congress). *NTG, 82*, IV, 5409–15; *BGG, XVIII*, 291–7.

4715 SCHLICHTING, Th. H. (1955). Het 14e internationale congres voor de geschiedenis der geneeskunde (The 14th international medical-historical congress 13–20 September 1954 at Rome and Salerno). *NTG, 99*, II, 1593–5; *BGG, XXXV*, 53–5.

4716 PANHUYS, L. C. van (1931). Het verhandelde op het gebied van de geschiedenis der geneeskunde op het Amerikanisten congres te Hamburg (The proceedings of the congress of Americanists at H. concerning the history of medicine). *NTG, 75*, II, 2994–9; *BGG, XI*, 187–92.

4717 SYPKENS SMIT, J. H. (1950). Het [zesde] internationaal congres voor de geschiedenis der natuurwetenschappen (The [6th] international congress of the history of the natural sciences). *NTG*, *94*, IV, 2928–31; *BGG, XXI*, 34–7.

4718 BRANS, P. H. (1957). De congressen over geschiedenis der wetenschappen te Florence-Milaan en te Luzern-Bazel (The congresses on the history of science). *NTG*, *101*, I, 778–80; *BGG, XXXVII*, 11–3.

4719 — (1954). Het eerste Beneluxcongres voor de geschiedenis der wetenschappen (The first Benelux-congress for the history of science). *NTG*, *98*, III, 2525–6; *BGG, XXXIV*, 77–8.

4720 — (1954). Le congrès Bénélux d'Histoire des Sciences à Haarlem. *J. Pharm. Belg.*, *9*, 229.

4721 RIJNBERK, G. van (1910). 3e Congrès de la Société Italienne pour l'histoire critique des sciences médicales et naturelles. Tenu à Vénise le 26–28 Septembre 1909. *Janus, XV*, 41–4.

4722 [   ] (1968). *Acta quinti conventus Historiae Scientiae, Medicinae, Matheseos Naturaliumque excolendae. Mosae Traiecti ... MCMLXVII.* 109 pp., 13 ill., 12 figs. E. J. Brill, Leiden.
– reprint from *Janus, LIV* (1967), 161–269.

4723 LINT, J. G. de (1921). Le premier congrès de l'histoire de l'art de guérir. Anvers le 7 au 12 août 1920. *Janus, XXV*, 23–32.

4724 PERGENS, Ed. (1901). Xe Congrès international d'ophthalmologie à Lucerne, du 13 au 17 Septembre 1904. Partie historique. *Janus, VI*, 616–9.

4725 LINT, J. G. de (1931). 6e Internationale congres voor militaire geneeskunde en pharmacie (6th International congress for military medicine and pharmacy). *NTG*, *75*, I, 1163; *BGG, XI*, 92.
– refers to the historical exhibition on military medicine to be held at the forthcoming congress (15–20 June 1931).

Pharmacy

4726 BRANS, P. H. (1955). Congrès International d'Histoire de la Pharmacie à Rome. *Bull. Pharm.*, *XI*, 8.

4727 — (1958). Cercle Benelux d'histoire de la pharmacie. *Arch. int. Hist. Sci.*, *11*, 284–6.

4728 — (1959). Kring voor de Geschiedenis van de Pharmacie in Benelux. Verslag van het congres te Bergen (België) op 10 en 11 mei 1958. (Circle for the history of pharmacy in —. Report of the congress at B. (Belgium). *Bull. Pharm.*, no 18 (June), 12; French translation: *ibid.*, no 19, (August), 20–1.

4729 WITTOP KONING, D. A. (1959). De geschiedenis van de farmacie in het F.I.P. congres te Brussel (The history of pharmacy at the F.I.P. congress at Brussels). *Bull. Pharm.* no 18, 14.

4730 — (1959). *Kring voor de Geschiedenis van de Pharmacie in Benelux.* Programma en historische data ter gelegenheid van de najaarsverga-dering 1959 (gehouden te Maastricht). Overzicht van de Tentoonstel-ling "De oude Apotheek van het Maasland"(Circle for the History of Pharmacy in –. Programme and historical data on the occasion of the autumnal meeting — —. Survey of the exhibition The old chemist's shop in the region of the —). 22 pp. no pl.

4731 BRANS, P. H. (1961). Bij het tweede lustrum van de Kring voor de Geschiedenis van de Pharmacie in Benelux (At the second lustrum of the Circle for the history of Pharmacy in —). *Ph. T. België*, *38*, 96–9.

4732 — (1961). Le deuxième lustre du Cercle Bénélux d'Histoire de la Phar-macie. *J. Pharm. belge*, sept-oct., 345; *Bull. Pharm.*, no 28.

4733 — (1963). Het Internationale Congres voor Geschiedenis der Pharma-cie te Rotterdam (International congress for the history of pharmacy at R.). *PhW.*, *98*, 6 december, 1182–3.

4734 — (1963). Le Congrès International d'Histoire de la Pharmacie. *France Pharmacie*, 1033.

4735 WITTOP KONING, D. A. (1962). Cinquante ans de F[éderation] I[nter-nationale] P[harmaceutique]. 1912–1962. *J. mond. de Pharm.* 141–262.

4736 HUEGEL, Herbert and W. SCHNEIDER (1963). Internationaler Kongress für Geschichte der Pharmazie in Rotterdam 17. bis 21. September 1963. Bericht von Herbert Huegel mit einem Rückblick auf Rotter-dam von W. Schneider. *Dtsch. Apoth. Ztg*, *103*, 1267–76; 1702–4.

                                                        See also 3829a

J. Varia

4737   Vos, T. A. (1972). Arts en wereld in vroeger tijden (Physician and world in former times). I. Over kerken, kloosters en scholen (On churches, cloisters and schools). *Arts en Wereld*, 5, no 4, 11–21, 10 ill. 5. Het Duecento. *Ibid.*, 5, no 10, 7–16, 9 ill. 6. Bevolking en medicus (Population and physician). *Ibid.*, 5, no 11, 31–4, 7 ill.

Chapter XIX

Pharmacy

During the Middle Ages medicinal herbs were cultivated by friars in monastery-gardens. Moreover they were often collected and dispensed by some women ("geneesjoffers"). In the sixteenth century pharmacists made their first appearance. In some towns, such as Leyden, the apothecaries gathered into guilds. The pharmacists' guilds exercised supervision of the chemist's shops and examined apprentices before admitting them into their guild. In Amsterdam the supervision was exercised by the collegium medicum, which drew op a municipal pharmacopoea in 1636 at the proposal of Nic. Tulp.

The training for pharmacist was entirely practical and took four years. The apprentices came into the apothecary at an early age, for example of 14 or 16 years. They had to learn to know the medicinal herbs, preferably in a botanical garden.

The apothecaries had not only to provide all kinds of drugs (also such as theriac) and leeches, but, at least in the seventeenth century, they did administer clysters to the patients at their home. Several apothecaries applied themselves to chemistry, and others studied medicine to practise as a doctor too. The training for pharmacist sometimes was a step to medical education for young men who had not enough money to afford medical study. Frederik Ruysch and Gerard van Swieten qualified first as apothecaries, later on they became physicians.

A. Historical surveys

4738   STOEDER, W. (1891). *Geschiedenis der Pharmacie in Nederland* (History of Pharmacy in the Netherlands). Amsterdam.

– Reviewed by C. E. Daniëls: *NTG*, 27 (1891), II, 414. Reprint 1974, Schie-Pers, Schiedam.

4739   WITTOP KONING, D. A. (1951). Brevi Notizie della Farmacia in Olanda. *Il Farmacista*, 5, 429.

4740 — (1956). Streifzug durch die Geschichte der Pharmazie in Holland. *Zur Gesch. Pharm.*, *8*, 29–30.

4741 WIELEN, P. van der (1914, 1915). *Monumenta pharmaceutica*. 2 vols. 's-Gravenhage. 4°.

4742 KNIJFF, C. (1967). Overzicht over 125 jaar farmacie. Inhoud van een perscommuniqué ter gelegenheid van het 125-jarig bestaan van de K.N.M.P. [Koninklijke Nederlandse Maatschappij ter bevordering der Pharmacie] (Survey of 125 years of pharmacy. Contents of a press-communiqué on the occasion of the 125th anniversary of the Royal Dutch Society for the promotion of pharmacy). *PhW.*, *102*, 419–26.

4743 WITTOP KONING, D. A. (1955, 1956, 1961). Historische tijdschrift-artikelen (Historical articles in periodicals). *Bull. Pharm.* no *IX*, 16–7; no *XIV*, 28–9; no *XXVII*, 15–6.

4744 — (1962). Probleme der Periodisierung in der Pharmaziegeschichte. *Veröff. Int. Gesellsch. Gesch. Pharm.*, *20*, 95–8.

4745 — (1963). De beoefening van de geschiedenis van de farmacie (The study of the history of pharmacy). *Bull. Pharm.*, no 31, 89–95.

4746 LINSTAED, Hugh (1967). Some contributions by Dutch pharmacists to international pharmacy. *PhW*, *102*, 399–404.

4747 WITTOP KONING, D. A. (1953). Uit de geschiedenis van het Pharma-ceutisch studentenleven (From the history of the pharmaceutical students' life). *Lustrumgids A.N.P.S.V.*, 8–11.

4748 — (1960). Hooggeleerden in de pharmacie uit vervlogen jaren (Professors of pharmacy from years past). *De Geuzenpenning*, *10*, 44–5.

4749 — (1967). De farmacie in Nederland in de tijd van Jeroen Bosch (Pharmacy in the Netherlands at the time of — —). *Specimina Specia*, *8*, 25–9.

4750 SCHRIJNEN, D. (1902). Pharmaceutische Folklore (Pharmaceutical Folk-lore). *PhW*, *39*, 833-7.

4751 PINKHOF, H. (1934). Houd uw pharmacognosie bij! (Keep up your pharmacognosy). *NTG*, *78*, II, 1570; *BGG*, *XIV*, 80.
– short note with the advice of the physician Jehoedah Ibn Tibbon (1120 – *ca* 1190).

4752 WITTOP KONING, D. A. (1952). De herkomst van onze Nederlandsche Pharmaceutische Ordonnantiën (The origin of our Dutch Pharmaceutical Ordinances). *Ph. T. België*, *29*, 77–81; *Bull. Pharm.* no *III*, 1–4.

4753   — (1957). De oudste pharmaceutische ordonnantiën van Antwerpen
        (The oldest pharmaceutical ordinances of Antwerp). *Bull. Pharm,*
        no 15, 1–7.

4754   MATTELAER, B. (1972). Twintig jaar farmacie geschiedenis in Benelux
        (Twenty years history of pharmacy in —). *Bull. Pharm.* no 44, 41–61.

4755   WITTOP KONING, D. A. (1955). De rol van Antwerpen in de geschie-
        denis van de pharmacie (The role of Antwerp in the history of pharm-
        acy). *Ph. T. België, 32,* 5; *Bull. Pharm,* no *12,* 1–6.

4756   BRANS, P. H. (1951). Overzicht van de geschiedenis der pharmacie in
        Nederlands-Oost-Indië (Survey of the history of pharmacy in the
        Dutch East Indies). *PhW., 86,* 841–63; 881–99.

4757   LASHLEY, E. A. C. (1940). Gegevens betreffende de geschiedenis van
        de pharmacie in Suriname (Data concerning the history of pharmacy
        in Surinam). *PhW., 77,* 1166 and 1229.

> *See also* 1195, 2547, 2785a–d (Cosmas and Damianus),
> 2746, 3822–6 (naval medicine), 3841, 3934–8 (military med-
> icine), 4230a, 4685–9 (Associations), 4726–9 (Congresses),
> 5416.

B. Foreign Relations

4758   WITTOP KONING, D. A. (1954). Relations pharmaco-historiques entre
        l'Italie et la Hollande. *Vorträge Hauptvers. int. Gesells. Gesch. Pharm.,*
        159–63. Rom.

4759   — (1959). Les relations pharmacologiques entre la France et les Pays-
        Bays. *Les Conférences du Palais de la Découverte,,* Série D, no 64, 22
        pp., ill.

4760   — (1960). De invloed van Frankrijk op de Nederlandse Farmacie
        (The influence of France on Dutch Pharmacy). *Specimina Specia, 2,*
        6–7.

4761   — (1966) Some historical pharmaceutical relations between Great-
        Britain and the Netherlands. *Veröff. Int. Gesells. Gesch. Pharm.,*
        N.F., 28, 305–8, ill.

4762   BRANS, P. H. (1953). Une journée de l'Histoire de la Pharmacie à
        Paris. *J. Pharm. Belg., 8,* 488.

4763 — (1954). Een avond gewijd aan de geschiedenis van de pharmacie te Parijs (An evening dedicated to the history of pharmacy at Paris). *Bull. Pharm.*, no. *VIII*, 15.

4764 — (1963). Mitarbeiter der "Oost-Indische Compagnie" aus deutschen Ländern. *Dtsch. Apoth. Ztg.*, *103*, 905.

4764ª Esso Bzn., I. van (1938). *De pharmaceutische handelsbetrekkingen tusschen Nederland en Rusland in de 17ᵉ en 18ᵉ eeuw. De geschiedenis der Nederlandsche apotheekers en alchemisten in Rusland. De geschiedenis van tinctura Bestuchewii* (The pharmaceutical commercial relations between the Netherlands and Russia in the 17th and 18th century. History of the Dutch chemists and alchemists in Russia. History of the tinctura —). Amsterdam *8°*.

C. Drug trade and Prizes

4765 WITTOP KONING, D. A. (1958, 1959). Bijdragen tot de pharmaceutische prijsgeschiedenis (Contributions to the history of pharmaceutical prices). *Econ. Hist. Jbk.*, *27*, 1–38, 3 pl; *ibid.*, *28* (1959), 259–78.

4766 — (1958). Bijdragen tot de pharmaceutische prijsgeschiedenis (Contributions to the history of pharmaceutical prices). I. Het schuldboek van apotheker Mylius te Kampen (The sold ledger of the chemist — at K.). *Bull. Pharm.*, no 17, 38 pp. II. Het debiteurenboek van Anthonie d'Ailly 1819–20 (The sold ledger of — —). *Bull. Pharm.*, no 17, 11–38. III. Een viertal inventarissen van het pharmaceutische bedrijf van A. d'Ailly uit de jaren 1799–1802 (Four inventories from the pharmaceutical business of —). *Bull. Pharm.*, no 28, 1–20.

4767 GRENDEL, E. (1962). Een prijscourant van farmaceutisch glaswerk uit 1853 (A price-list of pharmaceutical glass-ware from 1853). *PhW.*, *97*, 97–102, ill; *Bull. Pharm.*, no 29, 2 pp.

4768 WITTOP KONING, D. A. (1942). *De handel in geneesmiddelen te Amsterdam tot omstreeks 1637* (The trade in remedies at A. till about 1637). Thesis University Amsterdam (Supervisor: P. van der Wielen). 136 pp. Muusses, Purmerend.
  – Reviewed in *PhW.*, *81* (1946), 577–82.

4769 — (1950). *N.V. Koninklijke Pharmaceutische Fabrieken v/h Brocades-*

Stheeman en Pharmacia 1800–1950 (The Royal Pharmaceutical Factory, — — Ltd. — —). 57 pp., ill. Haarlem.

4770 — (1954). De geschiedenis van de groothandel in geneesmiddelen (History of the wholesale trade in remedies). *Ph. T. België 31*, no 7; *Bull. Pharm.*, no IX, 1–5.

4771 — (1971). Farmaceutisch-historische veiling bij Lempertz in Keulen (Pharmaceutical-historical auction at L. at Cologne). *Bull. Pharm.*, no *43*, 28.

4772 — (1973). Niederländische Einblattdrucke über Heilmittel. *Veröff. int. Ges. Gesch. Pharm.*, *40*, 183–204.

D. Mortars, jars and weights

4773 SALM, Laura (1917, 1920). De vijzels van François en Pierre Hemony (The mortars of François and Pierre —). *Oud-Holland 35*, 93; *Ibid.*, *38*, 63.

4774 WITTOP KONING, D. A. (1953). *Nederlandse vijzels* (Dutch mortars). 114 pp, 45 ill. Deventer.
– legends in English, Dutch, French, German.

4775 — (1969). De vijzels van de gebroeders Hemony (The mortars of the Hemony brothers). *Bull. Museum Boymans-van Beuningen*, *20*, 37–41.

4776 — (1959). Vijzels (Mortars). *Noury Post*, *6*, no 4.

4777 — (1947). Vijzels (Mortars) *Hobby*, *I*, 197–9.

4778 — (1947). De jubileumvijzel van het Departement Amsterdam (The jubilee-mortar of the Department —). *Ph.W*, *82*, 389–91.

4779 — (1941). Persoonsnamen op vijzels (Names of persons on mortars). *Ned. Leeuw*, *59*, Kol. 57–63.

4780 — (1939). Opschriften op vijzels (Inscriptions on mortars). *PhW.*, *76*, 1471–86. Addition: *Ibid.*, *77* (1940), 905–8.

4781 — (1948). Apothekersbenodigdheden (Chemists' requisites). *Hobby*, *2*, 73–7.

4782 WIELEN, P. van der and Hk COHEN (1938). Noord- en Zuid-Nederlandse vijzelgieters (Mortar-casters in the Northern and Southern Netherlands). *PhW.*, *75*, 830–1.

4783 WITTOP KONING, D. A. (1939). Noord- en Zuid-Nederlandse vijzel-gieters (Mortar-casters in the Northern and Southern Netherlands). *PhW.*, *76*, 874–99.

4784 — (1968). De grote vijzel van Wilhelmus Wegenaert (The large mortar of — —). *PhW.*, *103*, 824–6; *Bull. Pharm.*, no *40* november, 9–10.

4785 — (1962). Mechelse vijzels (Mechlin mortars). *Ph. T. België*, *39*, 95–9, ill.

4786 PIT, A. (1905). De apothekerspot van Albarello (The apothecaries' jar of —). *Het Huis, III*, 193.

4787 WITTOP KONING, D. A. (1959). Nederlandse apothekerspotten (Dutch apothecaries' jars). *Noury Post*, *6*, no 7.

4788 — (1964, 1965). Niederländische Apothekengefässe. *Ph. Ztg. 109*, 1751–8, ill; *Bull. Pharm.*, no *33* (1965), febr.; *Österr. Apoth. Ztg, 19*, 189–96.

4789 — (1964). Haarlemse apothekerspotten (Haarlem apothecaries' jars). *Ned. Ceramiek*, no 36 (september), 23–5, 1 ill.

4790 — (1961). Apothekerspotten van Adrianus Kocx (Apothecaries' jars of — —). *Ned. Ceramiek 23*, 1–2.

4791 — (1954). *Delftse Apothekerspotten* (Delft apothecaries' jars). 174 pp. De Yssel, Deventer.

4792 — (1958). De wordingsgeschiedenis van de Delftse apothekerspot (The genesis of the Delft apothecaries' jar). *Ned. Ceramiek*, *2*, 1–2.

4793 — (1964). Gemerkte "Delftse" apothekerspotten (Marked "Delft" apothecaries' jars). *Ned. Ceramiek*, no 34 (maart), 80, 1 ill.

4794 — (1954). *Delft drug-jars*. 174 pp. Yssel Press, Deventer.

4795 — (1966). Singulière série de marques sous les piluliers en Delft. *Rev. d'Hist. Pharm.*, *18*, 39–40, 1 ill.

4796 SCHOUTEN, J. (1970). De pauw op Delftse apothekerspotten (The peacock on Delft apothecaries' jars). *Antiek*, *5*, nr 2, 100–7.

4797 [   ] [   ]. Answers by Prof. Trease, M. E. Collard, and P. H. Brans to a query on the use of Delft pill tiles. *Rev. Hist. Pharm.* (Paris), *44* (151), 465–6.

4798 WITTOP KONING, D. A. (1949). Een 17de-eeuwse Engelse apothekers-pot, geschenk van de Pharmaceutical Society of Great Britain (A 17th century English apothecaries' jar, a gift of the — — —) *PhW.*, *84*, 675–7.

4799 — (1970). Raerener Apothekengefäsze. Die Vorträge der Hauptver-sammlung in Luxemburg. *Veröff. Int. Gesells. Gesch. Pharm.*, *36*, 185–95.

4800 KRET, André (1965). Un vase de pharmacie en Chine de commande. *Soc. d'hist. Pharm.*, *XVII*, no 187 (december), 441–4.

4801 SCHOUTEN, J. (1967). Theriak en theriakpotten (Theriac and theriac-jars). *Antiek*, *1*, no 10, 13–8.

4802 GRENDEL, E. (1972). Farmaceutische zuinigheid (Pharmaceutical economy). *Bull. Pharm.*, no 45, 6–8, ill.

4803 — (1972). Spanen dozen (Chip boxes). *Bull. Pharm.*, no 45, 35–7, ill. – on pill boxes.

4804 STARING, W. C. H. (1885). *Lijst van alle binnen- en buitenlandse maten, gewichten en munten* (List of all home-made and foreign measures, weights and coins). Van Nooten, Schoonhoven.

4805 ZEVENBOOM, K. M. C. and D. A. WITTOP KONING (1953, ²1971). *Ne-derlandse Gewichten, Stelsels, ijkwezen, vormen, makers en merken* (Dutch weights, systems, gauging, forms, makers and marks). 247 pp., ill. Rijksmuseum Geschiedenis Natuurwetenschappen, Leiden. 2nd ed.: Lochem.

4806 WITTOP KONING, D. A. (1949). Een ijkmeesterskistje uit de 18e eeuw (A 18th century box of an inspector of weights and measures). *Hobby*, *3*, 184–5.

4807 — (1951). Muntgewichten (Weights of coins). *Jbk. Munt- en Pennink.*, *38*, 88–93.

4808 — (1950). De ijkletters van het Nederlands troois gewicht (The gauge-letters of the Dutch troy weight). *Jbk. Munt- en Pennink.*, *37*, 123–6.

4809 — (1959). Medicinaal gewicht (Medicinal weight). *Noury Post*, *6*, no. 12.

4810 — (1951). De Amsterdamse balansenmakersfamilie Linderman (The Amsterdam balance-makers family —). *Jbk. Munt- en Penningk.*, *38*, 122–6.

E. Antidotaria, pharmacopoeia's, prescription books

4811 VANDEWIELE, Leo J. (1972). Welke uitgaaf van het Ricettario Fiorentino lag er aan de basis van het Antidotarium van Clusius? (Which
edition of the — — was the basis of the — of —?). *Bull. Pharm., 44,*
41–8, facs.

4812 BERG, W. S. van (1917). *Eene middel-nederlandsche vertaling van het
Antidotarium Nicolai* (MS 15624–15641), Kon. Bibl. te Brussel)) *met
den latijnschen tekst en eerste gedrukte uitgave van het Antidotarium
Nicolai* (A Middle-Dutch translation of the — — (Royal Library,
Brussels), with the Latin text and first printed edition of the — —).
Leiden. 8°.

4813 BRAEKMAN, W. und Gundolf KEIL (1971). Fünf mittelniederländische
Uebersetzungen des "Antidotarium Nicolai". Untersuchungen zu
pharmazeutischen Fachschriften der mittelalterlichen Niederlande.
SA, 55, 257–320.   *See also 2763–65*

4814 LEEUW, P. C. de (1962). *Pharmaceutische encyclopaedie, bevattende alle
gegevens omtrent herkomst, samenstelling en gebruik van de meest voorkomende drogerijen, chemicaliën en geneesmiddelen* (Pharmaceutical
encyclopedia, containing all data concerning origin, composition and
use of the most frequently occurring drugs, chemicals and remedies).
2 nd ed. 484 pp. Enschede.

4815 — (1965). *Pharmaceutische gids bevattende de officiële latijnse namen,
volksnamen en synoniemen voor chemicaliën, drogerijen en geneesmiddelen* (Pharmaceutical guide containing the official Latin names, popular names and synonyms of chemicals, drugs and remedies). 239 pp.
Enschede.
- 4th edition (completed by W. F. de Leeuw).

4816 VANDEWIELE, L. J. and WITTOP KONING, D. A. (1973, 1974). *Opera
Pharmaceutica Rariora.* Vol. I–VIII. De Backer Publ., Ghent (Belgium)
- Vol. III: Carolus Clusius. *Antidotarium, sive de exacta componendorum miscen-
dorumque medicamentorum ratione libri tres* (1561); Vol. V: *Pharmacopoea Hagien-
sis 1659.*

4817 WITTOP KONING, D. A. (1960). De geschiedenis van de Farmacope
(History of Pharmacopoeia). *Noury Post, 7,* no 3.

4818 — (1963). Was ist eine Pharmakopöe? *Veröff. Int. Gesells. Gesch. Pharm.*, *22*, 181–91.
- also in: *Festschrift zum 65. Geburtstage von G. E. Dann*, 181–91 Stuttgart.

4819 — (1963). Die niederländischen Pharmakopöen als Zeugen der europäischen Geschichte. *Veröff. Int. Gesells. Gesch. Pharm.*, *21*, 119–23.

4820 WIELEN, P. van der (1936). De eerste Nederlandsche Pharmacopee. 1636 – 5 Mei – 1936. (The first Dutch Pharmacopoeia). *NTG*, *80*, II, 1917–23; *BGG, XVI*, 57–63.

4821 GRENDEL, E. (1967). Pharmacopoea pauperum – Armen Apotheken. *PhW.*, *102*, 760–9.

4822 WITTOP KONING, D. A. (1938). Uit de geschiedenis van de Pharmacopoea Almeriana Galeno- Chymica (From the history of the — — —). *PhW.*, *75*, 821–30.

4823 — (1938). Een supplement op de Pharmacopoea Almeriana (A supplement to the — —). *PhW.*, *75*, 1200–2.

4824 — (ed.) (1961). *Facsimile of the first Amsterdam Pharmacopoeia 1636* With an introduction by the editor on the precursors of this pharmacopoeia. *Dutch Classics on History of Science*, no 1. 133 pp., port. (of Nic. Tulp). B. de Graaf, Nieuwkoop.
- Reviewed by W. F. Daems: *Sci. Hist.*, *4* (1962), 44–5.

4825 — (1950). De oorsprong van de Amsterdamse Pharmacopee van 1636 (The origin of the Amsterdam Pharmacopoeia). *PhW.*, *85*, 801–3.

4826 — (1953). Der Ursprung der Amsterdamer Pharmacopoea von 1636. *Zur Gesch. Pharm.*, *5*, 19–20.
- also in: *Geschichtsbeil. Dtsch. Apoth. Ztg.*, *93*, 19–20.

4826ᵃ BRUGMANS, H. (1936). De Amsterdamse Pharmacopee (The Amsterdam Pharmacopoeia). *Amstelodamum*, *23*, 89, ill.

See also 828

4827 VANDEWIELE, L. J. (1960). De zeldzame Pharmacopoea Amstelredamensis, editio tertia (The rare — — —). *Ph. T. België*, *37*, 5–6, ill. *Bull. Pharm.*, no 23, (october) 13–5.

4828 KULSDOM, M. E. (1949). Een oude stadspharmacopee (An old city-pharmacopoeia [Leeuwarden]. *NTG*, *93*, III, 2993–3002; *BGG*, *XXIX*, 45–54.

4829 WITTOP KONING, D. A. (1952). De te Zutphen gebruikte Pharmacopee (The pharmacopoeia used at Z.). *PhW.*, *87*, 41–2; *Bull. Pharm.*, no IV, 1–2.

4830 — (1956). Editions Néerlandaises des pharmacopées étrangères. *Actes VIII Congrès int. d'Hist. Sci.*, Florence, 555–60.

4831 VANDEWIELE, L. J. (1963). Die städtischen Pharmakopoën in Nord- und Süd-Niederland. *Dtsch. Apoth. Ztg.*, *103*, 1167–9.

4832 DAEMS, W. F. and L. J. VANDEWIELE (1955). *Noord- en Zuidnederlandse Pharmacopeeën* (Pharmacopoeias of the Southern and Northern Netherlands). 199 pp., 136 ill. Itico N.V. Mortsel- Antwerp-Joppe.
– also published in French: *Pharmacopées communales des Pays-Bas du Nord et du Sud.*

4833 WITTOP KONING, D. A. (1959). De Nederlandse en Belgische uitgaven van buitenlandse pharmacopeeën (Dutch and Belgian editions of foreign pharmacopoeias). *PhW.*, *93* (1958), 977–82; *Bull. Pharm.* no 18, 6–12.

4834 — (1952). De Belgische Pharmacopeeën (The Belgian Pharmacopoeias). *PhW.*, *87*, 144–8; *Bull. Pharm.*, no 2, 1–5.

4835 — (1951). The Belgian Pharmacopoeas during the Union with Austria, 1714–1794. *Vorträge Jubiläums-Hauptvers. Int. Gesells. Gesch. Pharm.*, 117–23. Salzburg.

4836 SCHOOR, O. van (1930). Brève étude sur l'histoire des pharmacopées officielles en général et celles de Belgique et des Pays-Bas en particulier. *El Monitor de la farmacie* (Madrid).
– Reviewed by S.V.G.: *Rev. Hist. Pharm, I*, 182–3.

4837 GRENDEL, E. (1972). Zestig jaar "Pharmacotherapeutisch vademecum" (Sixty years — —). *Bull .Pharm.*, no 45, 1–5.

4838 BRANS, P. H. (1952). Een Nederlands-Indische Pharmacopee (A Dutch-East-Indian Pharmacopoeia). *Bull. Pharm., II*, 19; *PhW.*, *89*, 149.

4839 — (1963). Zur Geschichte der in Niederländisch-Indiën gebrauchten Pharmakopöen. *Veröff. Int. Gesells. Gesch. Pharm.*, N. F. *21*, 9–20, facs.

4840 WITTOP KONING, D. A. (1957). Niederländische Drucke deutscher Pharmakopoeen. *Veröff. Int. Gesells. Gesch. Pharm.*, *10*, 200–8, ill.
– With French summary.

4841 — (1957). Dutch editions of English Pharmacopoeias. *Pharm. J.* 421–2.

4842 GANZINGER, K. (1962). Die österreichische Provinzial-Pharmakopöe (1774–1794) und ihre Bearbeiter. *Zur Gesch. Pharm.*, *14*, 17–24, ports., refs.
– also on Gerard van Swieten.

4843 VREESE, W. L. de (1894). *Middelnederlandsche Geneeskundige Recepten en Tractaten, Zegeningen en Tooverformules* (Middle Dutch medical prescriptions and treatises, blessings and magical formulas). Gent. 8°.

4844 BRAEKMAN, W. L. (1970). *Middelnederlandse Geneeskundige recepten. Een bijdrage tot de geschiedenis van de Vakliteratuur, in de Nederlanden* (Middle Dutch medical prescriptions. A contribution to the history of the special literature in the Netherlands). 499 pp., facs. Gent.

4845 VANDEWIELE, L. J. (1961). Het "Licht der Apothekers" (The "Light of Apothecaries"). *Ph. T. België*, *38*, 1–10; *Bull. Pharm.*, no 27, 1–9.

4846 WITTOP KONING, D. A. (1967). *Quiricus de Augustis Dlicht d'Apothekers 1515.* The prescription-book printed in the Low Countries. Facsimile with an introduction by —. Dutch Classics in History of Science, no XVI., 26 + 144 pp., ill. B. de Graaf, Nieuwkoop.
– Review: *GeWiNa*, no 22, 7.

4847 EEGHEN, W. van (1966). Brusselse Dichters. XXVI, 57. Thomas van der Noot. 52. Dlicht der Apothekers (1516) (Brussels poets. 52. The "Light of Apothecaries"). *Brusselse Post*, *16*, no 6, 2.
– on the Dutch translation of Quirian Augustis' *Lumen Apothecariorum*.

4848 [JACOBS,] [1906]. Een receptenboek uit het Huis van Prins Willem van Oranje (A prescription-book from the House of Prince William of Orange). In: F. J. L. Krämer, E. W. Moes and P. Wagner. *Je Maintiendrai*, vol. II, 61–79. A. W. Sijthoff, Leiden no d. 4°.
– The book belonged to Juliana of Nassau, sister of Prince William the Silent and may have belonged to their mother Juliana of Stolberg.

4848ᵃ EEGHEN, I. H. van (1952). De inhoud van het zalfkastje in het Koninklijk Paleis op de Dam (The contents of the ointment-cabinet in the Royal Palace on the Dam [at Amsterdam]). *Amstelodamum*, *39*, 113–6.

4849 HEEREN, J. J. M. (1964). Een oud Helmonds notitieboekje met recepten (A small old Helmond note-book with prescriptions). *Brabants Heem, 16,* 115-7.

4850 WITTOP KONING, D. A. (1937). Recepten der bekende zalven en dranken van het leprozenhuis (Prescriptions of the well-known unguents and draughts of the leper-house). *PhW., 74,* 1260-6.

4851 — (1949). Het nachtrecept (The prescription in the night). *PhW., 84,* 824.

4851ª EEGHEN, I. H. van (1955). Een Amsterdam receptenboek uit de 18de eeuw (An Amsterdam prescription-book from the 18th century). *Amstelodamum, 42,* 17-21.

4852 MÜLLER, P. L. J. (1936). Medicynboekje, uitgegeven door twee vermaarde doctoren (Prescription-book, published by two famous physicians). *PhW., 73,* 2-19.

4853 RIJKENS, R. G. (1919). De receptuur en de apotheek vóór een halve eeuw (Dispensing and the chemist's shop half a century ago). *NTG, 63,* I, 1203-5.

See also 1961, 2766-71 (Middle Ages)

F. Chemists

4854 ANDEL, M. A. van (1916). Praktizerende apothekers in de 17de en 18de eeuw (Practising chemists in the 17th and 18th century). *NTG, 60,* II, 1330-7.

4855 — (1919). Concurrentie tusschen apothekers en doctoren in den ouden tijd (Competition between chemists and doctors in older times). *Ph. W., 56,* 9-17 and 55-67.

4856 ROEKEL, G. van (1939). De apotheker in vroeger tijd (The chemist in former times). *NTG, 83,* IV, 5673-4; *BGG, XIX,* 271-2.

4857 COHEN, Hk. (1930). Van leerjongen tot meester apotheker (I.). (From apprentice to master chemist). *Ph. W., 67,* 997-1020.

4858 WITTOP KONING, D. A. (1946, 1956, 1968). Uit den goeden ouden tijd. Van leerjongen tot meester apotheker (From the good old days. From apprentice to master chemist).

II. *PhW.*, *81*, 545–9; III. *Ibid.*, *91* (1956), 745–7 (on: Ant. d'Ailly and Arn. van Covent). IV: *Ibid.*, *103* (1968), 1193–1201 (on: H. Prinssen and L. Zijnen). V: (by P. A. Jaspers). *Ibid.*, *104* (1969), 413–7 (on: P. Pirovano (1655–1731), F. Pirovano (*b.* 1694) and Chr. Pirovano (1728–?), chemists at Venlo).

4859   — (1948). *Verschuivingen in het apothekersvak in de loop der eeuwen* (Shiftings in the chemist's profession in the course of the ages). Amsterdam.
  – Public lecture.

4860   — (1971). Hoe vind ik iets over de apotheker? (How can I find something on the chemist?) *Onze Voorouders en hun Werk*, (Amsterdam), 262–70.

4860ª [Anonym] (1941). Request van een Amsterdamse gasthuisapotheker (Request from a Amsterdam hospital chemist). *Amstelodamum*, *28*, 12–3.

4861   JULIEN, Pierre (1973). Le cahier de cours d'histoire naturelle pharmaceutique d'un étudiant de Maestricht (1816). *Rev. Hist. Pharm.*, *21*, no 217, 417–9.

4862   SCHENKEVELD, A. (1967). De strijd tegen de Apothekerskamer (The fight against the apothecaries' chamber.). *PhW.*, *102*, 865–9.

4863   WINTERS, J. H. (1969). Bij het 40-jarig bestaan van de Groep van Ziekenhuisapothekers (At the 40th anniversary of the Group of Hospital pharmacists). *PhW.*, *104*, 1569–70.

4863ª SCHULTE, M. J. (1969). Omzien na veertig jaar (Looking back after fourty years). *PhW.*, *104*, 1571–7.
  – 40th anniversary of the "Association of Hospital pharmacists"

4864   PEETERS, K. C. (1963). De apotheker en de artsenijbereidkunde in het volksleven (The chemist and the pharmaceutics in the life of the people). *Kon. Apoth. Ver. Antwerp*, *125-jarig jubileum*, 39–66.

4865   GRENDEL, E. (1971). Hoe de indeling in de leerboeken over de receptuur voor onze assistenten tot stand kwam (How the classification in the manuals on dispensing for our assistants has been effected). *Bull. Pharm.*, no 43, 16–9.

4866   — (1969, 1971). Knecht, bediende, assistent. Ontwikkelingsgeschiedenis van het pharmaceutisch hulppersoneel (Servant, employee, assistant. Developmental history of pharmaceutic auxiliary personnel). *PhW*, *104*, (1969), 1356–70; *Bull. Pharm.*, no 43 (1971), 1–15, ill.

4867 WHITTET, T. D. (1963). From apothecary to pharmacist: a) study of changes of title; b). Titles used in Holland. *Chem. and Drugg.*, *179*, 584.

4868 LUEDTKE, C. (1963). Niederländer als Reformatoren des Apothekerswesens in Mecklenburg. *Dtsch. Apoth. Ztg.*, *103*, 1169–71.

4869 SCHLICHTING, Th. H. (1956). De invloed van de Engelse apothekers op de medische opleiding (Influence of the English chemists on medical education). *NTG*, *100*, IV, 2919–20; *BGG*, *XXXVI*, 63–4.
  – review of an article by Z. Cope: *Brit. Med. J.* (1956), I, 1.

4870 DOOREN, L. (1939). Een apothekersrekening van 1438 (A chemist's bill from —). *NTG*, *83*, III, 3354; *BGG*, *XIX*, 190.

4871 GIJSBERTI HODENPIJL, A. K. A. (1919). Een apothekers-instructie uit 1680 (A chemist's instruction from —). *NTG*, *63*, I, 535.

4872 GRENDEL, E. (1973). Apothekers diploma uit 1845 (Pharmacist's diploma from —). *PhW.*, *108*, 61–2.

4872ᵃ ANSINGH, E. W. (1973). Een apothekersdiploma uit 1846 (Pharmacist's diploma from —). *Bull. Pharm.*, no 48, 25.

4873 WITTOP KONING, D. A. (1940). Apothekersgraven in de kerken van Nederland (Graves of chemists in the churches in the Netherlands). *PhW*, *77*, 929–34.

4874 ARKEL, C. G. van (1965). De apotheker in de literatuur (The chemist in literature). *PhW*, *100*, 30–44, ill; *Bull. Pharm.*, no 33, 1–14.

4875 [   ] (1964). Dr Pieter Hendrik Brans, Rotterdam 65 Jahre. *Dtsch. Apoth. Ztg*, *104*, 506, port.

4876 BRANS-de GROOT, C. (1967). *Pieter Hendrik Brans. 1917–1967. 50 jaar pharmacie* (— — —. 50 years of pharmacy). 19 pp., port. Rotterdam. pr. pr.
  – In Dutch and French.

4877 [   ] (1971). Dr Phil. Willem F. Daems, 60 Jahre alt am 3. Dezember 1971. *Schweiz. Apoth. Ztg.*, *109*, 952, port.

4878 POSTMA, C. (1960). *Pieter Karel Drossaart, apotheker 1835–1845, burgemeester 1858–1863 te Vlaardingen* (A chemist and burgomaster at V.). 33 pp., ill., table. Vlaardingen.

4879 WITTOP KONING, D. A. (1941). Hercules Kruys. *PhW.*, *78*, 89.

4880 GRENDEL, E. (1959). Hans Martens, koopman, kruidenier, apotheker (—, merchant, grocer, chemist). *Bull. Pharm.*, no 19.

4881 JASPERS, P. A. Th. M. (1966). Het apothekersexamen van Jan Pieter Minckelers (1748–1824) (The chemist examination of — —). *PhW.*, *101*, 141–4, 2 ill; *Bull. Pharm.*, no 36 (juni), 3–6, facs.

4881ª LINDEBOOM, G. A. (1973). David en Nicolaas Stam, apothekers te Leiden (— — —, pharmacists at L.) *PhW*, *108*, 153–60, ill.; also in: *Bull. Pharm.*, no 48, 18–25, ill.

4882 DANN, Georg Edmund (1971). Ein niederländischer Pharmaziehistoriker – Dirk Arnold Wittop Koning. *Beitr. Gesch. Pharm.*, *23*, no 2–3, 9–10, port.

4883 AHLRICHS, E. L. (1972). 3 September 1971. Dr D. A. Wittop Koning 60 jaar. *Bull. Pharm.*, no 44 (febr.), 93.

Chemist's shops

4884 WITTOP KONING, D. A. (1960). De apotheek in de middeleeuwen (The chemist's shop in the Middle Ages). *MKVAW.*, *XXII*, 3–15; *Bull. Pharm.*, no 24, 3–15.

4885 — (1961). Die Ratsapotheke in den Niederlanden. *Pharm. Rundschau*, *3*, 3.

4886 — (1961). Oude apotheken in Nederland (Old chemist's shops in the Netherlands). *Noury Post*, *8*, nr 1.

4887 — (1966). *De oude apotheek* (The old Chemist's shop). 112 pp. 66 ill., 8 col. pl. Fibula-van Dishoeck. Bussum.

4888 SEGERS, E. G. and D. A. WITTOP KONING (1958). *Apothicaireries anciennes en Benelux.* 50 pp., 35 ill. Davo, Deventer.

4889 WITTOP KONING, D. A. (1961). Oude apotheken in België (Old chemist's shops in Belgium). *Noury Post*, *8*, no 2.

4890 BRANS, P. H. (1953). Een voorloper van de "Bataviasche Apotheek" van 1746? (A precursor of the "Batavian Pharmacy"?) *PhW.*, *90*, 420; *Bull. Pharm*, no V, 1.

4891 BRANS-DE GROOT, Cora H. J. (1970). *Een honderdjarige apotheek 1870–1970* (A hundred years old pharmacy). 16 pp. (not numbered), 8 ill. no pl.
– On the chemist's shop of P. H. Brans, Rotterdam.

4892 HARRISON, F. M. (1966). An old Dutch pharmacy. *Chem. Drugg., 185,* 87.

4892ª HUENDER, A. (1935). Een 250-jarige apothekerszaak (A 250 years old pharmacy). *Amstelodamum, 22,* 5–8.
– formerly at the corner Heerengracht/Vijzelstraat, Amsterdam.

Guilds

4893 BRANS, P. H. (1953). De Dordtse confrery en de plaats tussen de andere apothekersgilden (The Dordrecht fraternity and the place among the other apothecaries' guilds). *Ph. W., 88, 358.*

4894 — (1954). Gilden in België, Nederland en Luxemburg, waartoe apothekers hebben behoord (Guilds in Belgium, in the Netherlands and in Luxemburg to which chemists did belong). *Ph. T. België, 31,* no 6, 127–53; *Bull. Pharm.,* no 9, 5–30.

4895 — (1956). Über Apothekerzünfte in den Niederlanden *Vortr. Hauptvers. Int. Gesells. Gesch. Pharm. Rom,* 31.

4896 WITTOP KONING, D. A. (1957). De zilveren penning van het apothekersgilde te Utrecht (The silver medal of the apothecaries' guild at U.). *Jbk. Munt en Penningk., 44,* 60–2.

G. Drugs

General

4897 ECK, P. N. van (1905). Iets over eenige geneesmiddelen uit vroegere eeuwen (Something on some remedies from former centuries). *Natuur, XXV,, 7.*

4898 ITALLIE, L. van (1907). *De vermeerdering onzer kennis omtrent geneesmiddelen in de 19de eeuw* (The increase of our knowledge of remedies in the 19th century). 38 pp. S. C. van Doesburgh, Leiden.
– Inaugural address, 25th September 1907, University Leiden.

4899 BERG, C. van den (1964). Herinneringen aan de wordingsgeschiedenis van de Wet op de Geneesmiddelenvoorziening (Memories of the genesis of the Act on the Supply of drugs) *T. Soc. Geneesk.*, *42*, 12–5.

4900 WIELEN, P. van der (1914). Van de kruiden, die genazen (On healing herbs). *NTG*, *58*, I, 1961–9.

4901 PRAKKEN, J. R. (1972). Mercurialisten en antimercurialisten (Mercurialists and anti-mercurialists). *NTG*, *116*, 30–5.

4902 MOULIN, D. de (1973). Nieuwe middelen tegen oude kwalen. De na-oorlogse ontwikkeling van de natuurwetenschappelijke geneeskunde (New remedies for old ailments. Post-war development of scientific medicine). *Onze jaren 45–70*, no. 97, 3075–9, ill.

4902ᵃ FORBES, R. J. (ed.) (1968). *Het zout der aarde* (The Salt of the earth). 379 pp., 70 ill. Kon. Ned. Zoutindustrie, Hengelo. pr. pr.
– published on the occasion of the 50th anniversary of the "Koninklijke Nederlandsche Zoutindustrie Hengelo"; with chapters on "Het zout in alchemie en chemie" (Salt in alchemy and chemistry), pp. 1–21 by R. J. Forbes; "Zout in de taal en het volksgeloof der Nederlanden (Salt in language and popular belief, pp. 23–50; and "Het zout in de volksgeneeskunde (Salt in folk-medicine), pp. 46–50 by P. J. Meertens.

Bezoar

4903 HALLEMA, A. (1935). Een vonnis uit de 17de eeuw betreffende de vervalsching van het classieke wondermiddel van den bezoarsteen, een eigenaardige vorm van kwakzalverij of volksgeneeskunde in de 17de eeuw (A sentence from the 17th century concerning the falsification of the classical panacea of the bezoarstone, a peculiar form of quackery or folk-medicine in the 17th century). *NTG*, *79*, IV, 5647–54; *BGG*, *XV*, 233–40.

4903ᵃ EERDE, J. C. van (1926). De samenstelling van "Bezoarsteenen" (The composition of "Bezoarstones"). *Bijdr. Taal-Land-Volk. Ned. Indië*, *82*, 306–9.

4904 KREEMER, J. (1934). *Bezoarsteenen, Moestika's en Goeliga's* (Bezoarstones, — and —). 79 pp. Becherer, Leiden.

4904ᵃ RIJCKEVORSEL, J. L. A. A. M. van (1937). De Bezoar en zijn doos (The bezoar and its box). *Historia*, *3*, 142–6.

4904ᵇ WAGENAAR, M. (1939/40). Een en ander over den Bezoarsteen (Something on the bezoarstone). *PhW.*, *77*, 950–6.

4905   WITTOP KONING, D. A. (1949). Bezoarstenen (Bezoarstones). *Hobby*, *3*, 61–3.

4905ᵃ TASSEL, R. van (1970). *Bezoars and the Collection of Henri van Heurck (1838–1909)*. 60 pp., Antwerpen.

4905ᵇ — (1973). Bezoars. *Janus, LX*, 241–59.

See also 4949.7 and 4949.10

4906   KALFF, S. (1921). Indische geneeskrachtige steenen (Indian therapeutic stones). *Natuur, XLI*, 138.

Chemical drugs

4907   WITTOP KONING, D. A. (1951). Calomel. *PhW.*, *86*, 91–2.

4908   FEYFER, F. M. G. de (1907). Soda als geneesmiddel voorheen en thans (Sodium as a remedy past and present). *Med. Rev., VII*, 509.

4909   BRUNSTING, H. (1972). Terra Sigillata. *Westerheem, 21*, 252–68.

4910   PIETERS, J. (1971). Terra sigillata in de farmacie (— — in pharmacy). *Biekorf* (België), *72*, 247. *See also* 4949.11.

4911   WITTOP KONING, D. A. (1966). Suiker in de Farmacie (Sugar in pharmacy). *Suiker, 1*, no 3.

4912   RIJKENS, R. G. (1909). Uit de geschiedenis van de slaapmiddelen (From the history of soporifics.) *Vrag. Dag, XXIV*, 460.

4913   PINKHOF, H. (1929). Sal polychrestum Glaseri. *NTG, 73*, II, 3179–80; *BGG, IX*, 179–80.

4914   WITTOP KONING, D. A. (1957). De apotheek en de wijn (The chemist's shop and wine). *Wijn*, 5–6.

4915   — (1960). Clareit "goet voor coude vrouwen" (Spiced wine good for frigid women). *Wijn*, 12.   See also 120, 2774–76

4916   VANDEWIELE, L. J. (1964). De eerste publicatie in het Nederlands over Alcohol (The first Dutch publication on —). *Ph. T. België, 41*, 65–80.

4917   WIELEN, P. van der (1913). De ontdekking en de ontdekker van het jodium (The discovery and the discoverer of iodine). *NTG. 57*, II, 1668–74.

– on the Frenchman B. Courtois (?–1838) maker of saltpetre cf: *Ann. de Chimie* (1813), 31 december, 304.

4918   — (1914). Een drietal wondermiddelen. "Haarlemmer Olie, Pinkpillen
en Abdijsiroop" (Three panacea's. "Haarlem Oil, Pinkpills and Abbey-
sirup"). *NTG, 58,* I, 2028–35.

4919   WITTOP KONING, D. A. (1972). Beitrag zur Geschichte des Haar-
lemer Öls. *Veröff. Int. Gesells. Gesch. Pharm., 38,* 289–300.

See also 2008

Vegetable drugs

4920   SCHOUTEN, J. (1968). Kwassi en het befaamde kwassihout (Kwasibita)
(Quassia and the famous bitterwood). *Specimina Specia, 9,* no 43,
1–10.

4921   ANDEL, M. A. van (1923). Belladonna. *NRC,* 3 Januari.

4922   LACKEN, George (1946). *De geschiedenis der penicilline* (History of
penicillin). 38 pp., ill. "De Librije", Haarlem.
– translated into Dutch by Jhr P. Elias and P. Kapteyn-Schröder; with a foreword
by Sir A. Fleming.

4923   LAAGE, R. J. C. V. ter (1973). De ontdekking van penicilline – een
dubbeltje op zijn kant (The discovery of penicillin – a mere toss-up).
AP, no 13, 69–77.

4924   WITTOP KONING, D. A. and A. LEROUX (1972). *La chicorée dans l'histoire de la médecine et dans la céramique pharmaceutique.* 30 pp. Soc.
d'Hist. de la Pharmacie, Valenciennes.
– with the collaboration of L. Cotinat and P. Julien.

4925   ANDEL, M. A. van (1927). Tabak als geneesmiddel (Tobacco as a
drug). *Haagsche Post,* 16 Juli. *See also* 3358–64.

4926   PROOSDIJ, C. van (1965). Snuiftabak, "Het voetsel der neuzen" (Snuff,
"the food for noses"). *NTG, 109,* I, 38–40; *BGG, XLV,* 11–3.

Quinine, Guaiac

4927   DROSSAART LULOFS, P. E. (1933). Een en ander uit de geschiedenis
der kina (Something from the history of quinine). *NTG, 77,* III, 3974–
85; *BGG, XIII,* 201–12.

4928   PUTTO, J. A. (1938). Kinine (1638–1938). (Quinine). *GG, 16,* 698.

4929   WINCKEL, Ch. W. F. (1949). Intraveneuze inspuiting van kinine in

1830 (Intravenous injection of quinine). *NTG*, *93*, IV, 3756–7; *BGG*, *XXIX*, 67–8.

4930   DITMAR, J. van (1937). Kina (Quinine). *NTG*, *81*, IV, 4274; *BGG*, XVII, 166.
– a short note.

See also 5414

4931   LINT, J. G. de (1932). Eine der ersten Guajakschriften. *Janus*, *XXXVI*, 384–5.
– Nachschrift: *Janus*, *XXXVII* (1933), 320–2.

Medicinal herbs

4932   PROOYEN, A. M. van [1933]. *Schetsen uit de geschiedenis der drogerijen* (Sketches from the history of drugs). 80 pp. Enschedé.
– with a foreword by N. Schoorl; reviewed by M. A. van Andel: *NTG*, 77, IV, 4591–2; *BGG,XIII*, 237–8. (1933).

4933   — (1937–1973). During many years Van Prooyen published a great many articles on various medicinal herbs in one and the same periodical of which, however, the name was changed twice:
   a) *Pharmaceutisch Tijdschrift* (Ph. T.). XV–XIX (1937–1941)
   b) *Pharmaceutisch Tijdschrift voor Vlaanderen* (Ph. T. Vl.) XX–XXII (1942–1944)
   c) *Pharmaceutisch Tijdschrift voor België* (Ph. T. Belg.) XXIII–L (1946–1973).

4933[1] Summitates Absinthii, *Ph. T.*, *XV* (1937), 2; Aconitum, *XV*, 105; Althaea, *XV*, 209; Anisum – Anisum stellatum, *XVI* (1938), 3; Arnica, *XVI*, 21; Artemisia, *XVI*, 206; Aurantium, *XVII* (1939), 21; Belladonna, *XVII*, 97; Calamus, *XVII*, 181; Cnicus benedictus, *XVII*, 241;

4933[2] Centaurium, *XVIII* (1940), 43; Chamomilla, *XIX* (1941), 8; Aloe, *Ph. T. Vl.*, *XX* (1942), 13; Asa foetida, *XX*, 49; Benzoe-Styrax, *XX*, 77; Carrageen-Lichen islandicus, *XX*, 102; Cinnamomum chinense, *XXI* (1943), 5; Cinnamomum zeylanicum, *XXI*, 25; Camphora, *XXI*, 52; China, *XXI*, 73 and 109; Colchicum, *XXII* (1944), 1;

4933[3] Cacao, *XXII*, 25; Coca, *XXII*, 51; Cannabis, *XXII*, 85; Digitalis, *Ph. T. Belg.*, *XXIII* (1946), 2; Filix mas, *XXIII*, 33; Foeniculum, *XXIII*, 53; Frangula, *XXIII*, 83; Galbanum, *XXIV* (1947), 9; Gentiana, *XXIV*, 41; Granatum, *XXIV*, 70;

4933[4] Helenium *XXIV*, 143; Hyoscyamus, *XXV* (1948), 17; Ipecacuanha, *XXV*, 36; Iris, *XXV*, 78; Jalapa, *XXV*, 101; Juniperus, *XXV*, 131; Lavandula, *XXVI* (1949), 14; Liquiritia, *XXVI*, 33; Lupulus, *XXVI*, 76; Lycopodium, *XXVI*, 105;

4933[5] Majorana, *XXVI*, 141; Mastix, *XXVI*, 176; Mentha, *XXVII* (1950), 11; Myrrha, *XXVII*, 42; Nux moschata, *XXVII*, 79; Nux vomica, *XXVII*, 109; Amygdalae-Oleum amygdalarum, *XXVII*, 145; Malva, *XXVIII* (1951), 9; Melissa, *XXVIII*, 45; Morus, *XXVIII*, 71;

4933[6] Linum-Oleum Lini, *XXVIII*, 119; Oleum Olivarum, *XXVIII*, 139; Laurus-Oleum Lauri, *XXVIII*, 185; Oleum Ricini, *XXIX* (1952), 28; Caryophylli-Oleum Caryophyllorum, *XXIX*, 46; Rheum, *XXIX*, 81; Crocus, *XXIX*, 121; Salvia *XXIX*, 167; Cochlearia, *XXIX*, 210; Sambucus, *XXX* (1953), 7;

4933[7] Sarsaparilla, *XXX*, 60; Saleb, *XXX*, 106; Secale cornutum, *XXX*, 161; Senega-Polygala, *XXX*, 207; Scilla, *XXX*, 263; Sinapis, *XXXI* (1954), 12; Santonicum (cina), *XXXI*, 60; Senna, *XXXI*, 116; Stramonium, *XXXI*, 193; Succinum, *XXXI*, 269;

4933[8] Thymus, *XXXI*, 310; Tragacantha, *XXXII* (1955), 34; Tilia, *XXXII*, 80; Myrtillus-Uva ursi, *XXXII*, 128; Citrus, *XXXII*, 174; Valeriana, *XXXII*, 216; Tanacetum, *XXXII*, 268; Populus, *XXXIII* (1956), 43; Angelica, *XXXIII*, 91; Convallaria, *XXXIII*, 124;

4933[9] Ulmaria, *XXXIII*, 177; Podophyllum, *XXXIII*, 231; Quassia-Simaruba, *XXIV*, (1957), 32; Balsamum copaivae, *XXXIV*, 69; Balsamum peruvianum en B. tolutanum, *XXXIV*, 164; Foenum graecum, *XXXV* (1958), 17; Hippocastanum, *XXXV*, 89; Laurocerasus, *XXXV*, 169; Coriandrum, *XXXVI* (1959), 67; Tamarindus, *XXXVI*, 133;

4933[10] Verbascum, *XXXVII* (1960), 65–70; Capillus veneris, *XXXVII*, 154–8; Cydonia, *XXXVIII* (1961), 14–21; Rosmarinus, *XXXVIII*, 48; Gnaphalium, *XXXVIII*, 106; Lobelia, *XXXVIII*, 132–8; Rhoeas, *XXXVIII*, 143–9; Capsicum, *XXXVIII*, 200–7; Juglans, *XXXIX* (1962), 42–51; Zingiber, *XXXIX*, 99;

4933[11] Vanilla, *XXXIX*, 155; Triticum, *XXXIX*, 211; Elemi, *XL* (1963), 21–8; Euphorbium, *XL*, 42–8; Rubus idaeus, *XL*, 175–81; Gummi arabicum, *XL*, 201–12; Gutti, *XLI* (1964), 29–36; Cola-Coffeinum, 1 and 2, *XLI*, 48–56 and 81; Sabadilla (Veratrinum), *XLI*, 128; Solani amylum, *XLI*, 170;

4933[12] Maydis amylum, *XLI*, 259–69; Tritici amylum, *XLII* (1965), 8–20; Oryzae amylum, *XLII*, 78–88; Calumba, *XLII*, 106–12; Jaborandi, *XLII*, 143–9; Strophantus, *XLII*, 181–9; Terebinthina (veneta), *XLIII* (1966), 12; Manna, *XLIII*, 31–45; Saccharum 1 and 2, *XLIII*, 104–17 and 172–84; Ratanhia (Tormentilla), *XLIII*, 195–208;

4933[13] Condurango, *XLIII*, 243–7; Cousso, *XLIV* (1967). 48; Physostigma (Calabar), *XLIV*, 91–7; Guaiacum, *XLIV*, 110–23; Quillaja (Saponaria), *XLIV*, 176–86; Curcuma (Zedoaria), *XLIV*, 226; Indigo, *XLV* (1968), 27; Lacca musci (Orseille), *XLV*, 117; Petroselinum (Apiol), *XLV*, 162; Gossypium 1 and 2, *XLV*, 225 and 249;

4933[14] Hydrastis, *XLVI* (1969), 178; Opium 1 and 2, *XLVI*, 235 and 253; Gummi plasticum, *XLVII* (1970), 36; Rosa 1 and 2, *XLVII*, 49 and 101; Boldo, *XLVII*, 191; Croton (Crotonis oleum), *XVLII*, 218; Eucalyptus (en Kino), *XLVII*, 258; Oleum Cajuputi and Ol. Niaouli, *XLVIII* (1971), 198–204; Oleum Santali-Lignum Santali, *XLIX* (1972), 31–41; Chrysarobinum, *XLIX*, 191–5; Hamamelis, *L* (1973), 25–30.

See also 2725

Animal drugs

4934 VANDEWIELE, L. J. (1964). Les animaux, leurs parties et leur excréments, dans les pharmacopées communales des Pays-Bas méridionaux. *J. Pharm. Belg.*, *19*, 351–70.

4935 DANIELS, C. E. (1911). Ons oudste Pharmaceutisch wapen. Een en ander over de Theriak (Our oldest pharmaceutical weapon. Something on Theriac). *PhW.*, *48*, 53–67 and 74–86, 5 ill.

4936 — (1911). Notre plus ancienne arme pharmaceutique. Observations sur la thériaque. *Janus*, *XVI*, 371–80, 1 ill.; 457–65, 4 ill.

4937 WITTOP KONING, D. A. (1973). Theriakkapseln. *Betr. Gesch. Pharm.*, *25*, 23–4, ill.

4938 WEIJDE, A. J. van der (1923). Mumia. *NTG*, *67*, I, 2407; *BGG*, *III*, 141.
   – Letter to the editor; in the Utrecht pharmacopoeia (1749) mumia is still mentioned.

4939 HEUVELMANS, Bernard (1957). Ook bij ons leven er nog eenhoorns (Also with us there are still unicorns). *Motorama*, October, 8–11.

See also 2554

4940 GILS, J. B. F. van (1922). Unicornu. *NTG, 66*, I, 1287–8; *BGG, II,* 98–9.

4941 ANDEL, M. A. van (1923). De slangentong of glossopetra (The serpent's tongue or —). *NTG, 67*, II, 1611–4; *BGG, III,* 265–8, 1 ill.

4942 [Anonym] (1959). Tongue Therapy. Revival of a quaint Dutch pharmacy custom. *MD. med. Newsmag., 3,* 50–1, ill.

4943 DORSSEN, J. M. H. van (1900). Et parva utilia! *NTG, 36,* I, 869–71.
– letter to the editor dealing with: the "brijn van Hij": the brains of the shark, used as a remedy for various ailments.

4944 — (1901). Nog eens "Bryn van Hy" (Once again — —). *NTG, 37,* II, 1345.

4945 ANDEL, M. A. van (1924). Het dierlijke bad, een overblijfsel der primitieve geneeskunst (The animal bath, a remainder of primitive medicine). *NRC,* 5 september.

4946 — (1937). Potvisschen (Cachalots). *NRC,* 7 March.

4947 — (1925). Lever als geneesmiddel bij nachtblindheid (Liver as a remedy for night-blindness). *NTG, 69,* I, 599–601; *BGG, V,* 40–2.

4948 SJOLLEMA, B. [1924]. Geschiedenis der levertraan als huis- en geneesmiddel (History of cod-liver oil as a pallative and as a remedy). *Volksvoeding, 2,* no 31.
– Reviewed by E. Sluiter: *NTG, 68* (1924), I, 2633; *BGG, IV,* 128.

Panacea and secret drugs

4949 ANDEL, M. A. van (1921–1928). Klassieke wondermiddelen (Classical panacea).

4949.1   I.   Unicornu. *NTG, 65,* II, 2302–16; *BGG, I,* 405–19.

4949.2   II.   Hippomanes. *NTG, 66* (1922), I, 1280–4; *BGG, II,* 90–4.

4949.3   III.   Adeps hominis. *NTG, 66,* II, 1645–50; *BGG, II,* 231–6.

4949.4   IV.   Mumia. *NTG, 67* (1923), II, 1872–82; *BGG, III,* 105–15.

4949.5   V.   Het balneum. *NTG, 68* (1924), I, 1966–72; *BGG, IV,* 97–103.

4949.6   VI.   Amber. *NTG, 68,* II, 666–73; *BGG, IV,* 202–9, 3 ill., port.

4949.7   VII.   Bezoar. *NTG, 69* (1925), II, 47–58; *BGG, V,* 137–48.

4949.8 VIII. De mandragora, een verdoovingsmiddel der oudheid (Mandrake an anaesthetic from antiquity). *NTG, 70* (1926), II, 1802–9; *BGG, VI*, 105–12.

4949.9 IX. Edelsteenen (Jewels). *NTG, 71* (1927), I, 1164–78; *BGG, VII*, 161–75.

4949.10 XI. Bezoarstenen (Bezoar stones). *NTG, 72* (1928), II, 3793–3802; *BGG, VIII*, 197–206.

4949.11 XII. Terra sigillata. *NTG, 72*, II, 3803–11; *BGG, VIII*, 207–15. See: 4909–10.

4950 — (1928). *Klassieke wondermiddelen* (Classical panacea). J. Noorduyn & Zn, Gorinchem;
– Reviewed by F. M. G. de Feyfer: *NTG, 73* (1929), II, 3175–6; *BGG, IX*, 175–6.

4951 — (1921). L'Hippomanes. Un rémède antiépileptique populaire. *Bull. Soc. franc. Hist. Méd., XV*, 10.

4952 ZUIDEN, D. S. van (1918). Preservator Magnus Vita. *NTG, 62*, II, 766.
– on the selling of a therapeutic powder of Dr Salomon New.

4953 GRENDEL, E. (1964, 1965). Een keizerlijk decreet voor geheime geneesmiddelen (An imperial decree for secret remedies). *Ph. W., 99*, 843–7; *Bull. Pharm.*, no 33 (1965), Febr., 15–9.

4954 HINSBERGEN, Ph. van (1954). Een universeel, maar geheim geneesmiddel (A universal but secret remedy). *NTG, 98*, I, 41–2; *BGG, XXXIV*, 15–6.

See also Folk medicine

H. Pharmacology and Toxicology

4955 GREVENSTUK, A. (1930). *Pharmacologie en Volksgeneeskunde* (Pharmacology and Folk-medicine). 24 pp. Kolff, Weltevreden.
– Inaugural address January 24, 1930.

4956 BIJLSMA, U. G. (1962). Geschiedenis van de farmacologie aan de Universiteit te Utrecht (History of pharmacology at Utrecht University). *GG, 40*, 429–36.

4957 LEERSUM, E. C. van (1907). De dageraad der moderne pharmacologie (The daybreak of modern pharmacology). *NTG, 51*, I, 47–51.

See also 265, 1210, 1211, 1603

4958 GILS, J. B. F. van (1946). Besmetting en vergiftiging op afstand (Infection and poisoning at distance). *NTG, 90*, II, 624–7; *BGG, XXVI*, 16–9.

4959 BOLTEN, G. C. (1923). Geschiedkundige bijzonderheden aangaande morphinisme en cocainisme (Historical details concerning morphinism and cocainism). *NTG, 67*, II, 1670–3; *BGG, III*, 325–8.

4960 ANDEL, M. A. van (1921). Giftplanten als genees- en toovermiddelen (Poisonous plants as remedies and charms). *NTG, 65*, I, 1854; *BGG, I*, 18.

4961 — (1927). Hyoscine of Scopolamine. Vergift, genot-geneesmiddel (Hyoscine or Scopolamin. Poison, luxury or drug). *Haagsche Post*, 30 april.

4962 — (1930). Voorzorgsmaatregelen tegen vergiftiging aan de Middeleeuwsche tafel (Precautionary measures against poisoning at the medieval table). *NRC*, 18 may.

4963 ECK, P. N. van (1922). Vergiftige pijlen (Poisonous arrows). *Natuur, XLII*, 257.

4964 THIEME, P. J. van ELDIK (1905). Giftmengers in de zeventiende eeuw (Poisoners in the 17th century). *Alb. Nat.*, 46.

4965 LEYDEN, W. K. (1936). *Goeie Mie of de Leidsche giftmengster* ("Good Mie" or the Leiden poisoner). Batteljée & Terpstra, Leiden.

4966 ELAUT, L. (1962). Het aandeel van de Nederlanders in de opheldering van de etiologie der loodvergiftiging (The part of the Dutchmen in the enlightenment of the etiology of lead poisoning). *Sci. Hist., 4*, 183–91.

4966ᵃ KUSTERS, E. (1974). Historisch overzicht van de toxicologie van kwik (Historical survey of the toxicology of mercury). *T. Soc. Geneesk., 52*, 443–6.

See also 2535, 2553

I. Various subjects

4967 WITTOP KONING, D. A. (1953). Noordwijk, Schoonhoven en Nordhorn. *Bull. Pharm, VI*, Umschlag.

4968 — (1942). De klokkengieters Segewin en Frans Hatiseren (The bell-founders — and —). *Oud-Holland, 59*, 46–57.

4969 BRANS, P. H. (1962). Dieren in de artsenijbereidkunde (Animals in pharmacy). *Jbk. Dodonaea, 30*, 563–72.

4970 — (1952). De Kaapkolonie, Jan van Riebeeck en de pharmacie (Cape Colony, — — and pharmacy). *Ph. T. België, 29*, 4.

4971 — (1962). Dieren in de Artsenijbereidkunde (Animals in Pharmacy). *Jbk Dodonaea, 30*, 563–72, 5 ill.

4972 ECK, P. N. van (1907). Kleurstoffen uit het dierenrijk afkomstig (Colouring-matters from the animal kingdom). *Natuur, XXVII*, 225.

4973 — (1908). Luxe-artikelen en sieraden uit het dierenrijk afkomstig (Articles of luxury and ornaments from the animal kingdom). *Natuur, XXVIII*, 27 and 40.

4974 — (9107). Reukstoffen uit het dierenrijk afkomstig (Smell materials from the animal kingdom). *Natuur, XXVII*, 3.

J. Pharmacy and Art

4975 WITTOP KONING, D. A. (1950). *De pharmacie en de kunst*. I. (Pharmacy and Art. I.) 13 pp., 10 ill., 42 pl. De Yssel, Deventer.
- Reviewed by M. M. Hilfman: *NTG, 96* (1952), 829; *BGG, XXXII*, 14. Vol. II: A second collection of 42 plates, formerly published on apothecaries' calendars (1958). De Yssel, Deventer.
Vol. III: (1964). 94 pp. De Yssel, Deventer.

4976 — (1958). La Pharmacie et l'Art. *Terre d'Europe*, 24–8.

4977 — (1960). De pharmacie in de beeldende kunst (Pharmacy in Arts of design). *Noury Post, 7*, no 5 and 7.

4978 — (1972). Het Pharmaceutische wapen (The emblem of pharmacy). *PhW., 107*, 598–600, 2 ill. also in: *Bull. Pharm.*, no 48 (1973), 11–3, ill.

4979 KNIJFF, C. (1971). Hobby-ist verzamelde 19e-eeuwse apotheek (A hobbyist collected a 19th century pharmacy). *Bull. Pharm.*, no. 43, augustus, 23–4, ill.

4980 GRENDEL, E. (1959). De ooievaar en de apotheker, of de oudste beeltenis van een apotheker in de Nederlandse literatuur (The stork and the chemist or the oldest picture of an chemist in Dutch literature). *PhW.*, *94*, 97–102.

– The "Dyalogus creaturarum" (1480) has a woodcut representing an apothecary.

4981   WITTOP KONING, D. A. (1958). Nederlandse Pharmaceutische Zinne-beelden (Dutch Pharmaceutical Symbols). *Noury Post*, *7* (1960), no 2; *GeWiNa*, no 4 (1958), 9–10.

4982   — Niederländische pharmazeutische Sinnbilder. *Veröff. Int. Gesells. Gesch. Pharm.*, N.F. *13*, 225–36, ill.

4983   — and W. H. HEIN (1969). Bildkatalog zur Geschichte der Pharmazie. *Veröff. Int. Gesells. Gesch. Pharm.*, *33*, 288 pp.

4984   [   ] (1961). *Kunstenaar en Apotheek* (Artist and chemist's shop). Catalogue of a small exhibition on the occasion of the Congress of the "Kon. Ned. Maatschappij tot bevordering van de Pharmacie" te Arnhem. 84 numbers.

4985   SCHOUTEN, J. (1963). Symboliek in een achttiende-eeuwse klooster-apotheek (Symbolism in an 18th century monastery pharmacy). In: *Album discipulorum J. G. van Gelder*, 137–41. Utrecht.

4986   WITTOP KONING, D. A. (1961). Gapers. *Bull. Pharm.*, no 26, 1 p.

4987   HOFMAN, J. J. (1928). Pharmaceutische Ex-libris in Nederland en België (Pharmaceutical book-plates in the Netherlands and Belgium). *PhW.*, *65*, 427–39.

– French summary: *J. Pharm. Belg.*, *X*, 295.

See also 2267–8, 5424–39 (Medico-pharm. museum Amsterdam), 5501–4.

K. Periodicals

4988   ARKEL, C. G. van (1965). Pharmaceutisch Weekblad 1864–1964. (Pharmaceutical Weekly — —). *PhW.*, *100*, 6–15.

4989   PINXTEREN, J. A. (1965). L'hebdomadaire *Pharmaceutisch Weekblad* a cent ans. *PhW.*, *100*, 1–6.

Chapter xx

Local Medicine and Local Pharmacy

Several physicians and pharmacists, dabbling in medical history, have devoted their spare time to the past of the town where they were living. From their efforts many contributions providing valuable information have resulted. Needless to say that an endless field of study is still lying unused in the local or provincial archives.

For the sake of convenience of those interested in the medical past of some Dutch towns, it has been thought advisable to insert the data on local pharmacy in a separate section of this chapter.

As in both sections the items are listed alphabetically according to the name of the towns, it will be easy for the reader interested in a special town or district to check if anything has been written on the subject in question.

The entries on botanical gardens that were closely related to the exercise of pharmacy and medicine have already found a place in chapter VI under the heading Botany (*botanical gardens*). Likewise the entries on local hospitals have been included in chapter XVII. Entries on local epidemics have been included in chapter VII under the heading of the disease (leprosy, plague).

A. Local medicine

General

4990 BLAEU, Joan (1649, 1966) *Tooneel der steden van de Vereenighde Nederlanden met hare Beschrijvingen.* Uitgegeven By —. Holland en West-Vriesland. (Theatre of the towns of the "United Netherlands" and their descriptions. Edited by —. Holland and West-Vriesland). 112 pp., facs. Lamanne, Sequoia – Elsevier, Amsterdam-Brussel.

See also 2168a

Amsterdam

4991 BRUGMANS, H. (1928). Anatomie te Amsterdam (Anatomy at A.). *Amstelodamum, 15,* 78–9.

4992 KANNEGIETER, J. Z. (1972). Hevige sterfte te Amsterdam in 1727 (High mortality at A. in 1727). *Amstelodamum, 59,* 49–56, 2 ill.

4993 DANIËLS, C. E. (1910). Lues-behandeling te Amsterdam in 1685 (Treatment of syphilis at A. in 1685). *NTG, 54,* II, 1844.

4993ª RINGOIR, P. H. (1974). Amsterdamse chirurgijns in 1742 (Amsterdam surgeons in 1742). *AP,* no 16/17, 77–94.

4993ᵇ BRUGMANS, H. (1928). De kraamzaal (The lying-in room). *Amstelodamum, 15,* 16.

4993ᶜ Esso Bzn, I. van (1939). Het eerste dokterskoetsje in Amsterdam (The first doctor's brougham at A.). *Amstelodamum, 26,* 138.

4994 SCHILTMEIJER, J. R. [no d.]. *Amsterdam in 17e eeuwse prent* (A. in 17th century pictures). 192 pp., 110 ill. Minerva, Zandvoort aan Zee.
    – with informations on old hospitals.

> See also 1517–21 (Sarphati), 1726–9 (A. Titsingh). 1747–52
> (N. Tulp), 2876–78, 3107, 3146, 3212a, 3231a, 3256a, 3782–
> 83, 4019, 4039a, 4322–57 (hospitals), 4404–09, 4418–9,
> 4451–52, 4454–55, 4465–69, 4503–5, 4508a, 4551–3 (Coll.
> Medica), 4633–7 (Archivalia).

Antwerp

4995 SCHEVENSTEEN, A. F. C. (1927). De Hygiënische maatregelen van het magistraat van Antwerpen in de 15e eeuw (Hygienic measures of the magistrature of Antwerp in the 15th century). *NTG, 71,* I, 2479–92; *BGG, VII,* 329–42.

4996 — (1932). Naamlijsten van Antwerpsche Geneesheeren, chirurgijns, enz. opgemaakt uit de voornaamste fondsen van het Stadtarchief (List of names of the Antwerp physicians, surgeons, etc., drawn up from the principal funds of the municipal Archives). *Antwerpsch Archievenblad,* 7, 122–60.   *See also* 972, 3116, 4476

Arnhem

4997 VEEN, J. S. van (1924). Behandeling van pokken te Arnhem in 1599 (Treatment of smallpox at —). *NTG, 68,* II, 1757–8; *BGG, IV,* 265–6.

4998 RIBBIUS, P. (1927). Medici en medische toestanden te Arnhem door alle tijden (Physicians and medical situations at A. through the times). *NTG, 71*, II, 623–48; *BGG, VII*, 532–57.

4999 DOOREN, L. (1936). De oudste Arnhemsche Stadsgeneesheeren (The oldest town-physicians at A.) *GG, 14*, 501–4.

5000 — (1937). Croniek van Arnhem, betreffende geneeskundige toestanden en personalia van 1426–1662 (Chronicle of A., regarding medical situations and personalia). *NTG, 81*, I, 604–6; *BGG, XVII*, 38–40.

5001 — (1938). Beoefening van de Anatomie in de 16e eeuw te Arnhem (Practice of anatomy in the 16th century at A.). *NTG, 82*, I, 665; *BGG, XVIII*, 36.

See also 888, 3140, 4057a, 4086, 4358, 4456, 4475–6, 4588

Baambrugge

5002 MUNTENDAM, P. (1924). Geneeskundige hulp op het platteland in de 17de en 18de eeuw (Medical care in the country in the 17th and 18th century). *NTG, 68*, I, 1536–9; *BGG, IV*, 88–91.
– Review of an article (with the same title) of J. G. Th. Grevenstuk in *Jaarboekje van het Oudheidkundige Genootschap "Niftarlake"*, 1923. (From the minutes of the church council at Baambrugge).

Bergen op Zoom

5003 LEVELT, H. (1924). Een heelmeester en operatie te Bergen op Zoom in de 15de eeuw (Juli 1471) (A surgeon and an operation at — in the 15th century). *NTG, 68*, I, 1979; *BGG, IV*, 110.

5004 — (1924). Een chirurgisch attest te Bergen op Zoom in 1568 (A surgical certificate at —). *NTG, 68*, II, 1275; *BGG, IV*, 238.

5005 — (1925). Waarheen zond in de 15de en 16de eeuw Bergen op Zoom zijn "lepralijders" ten schouw? (To what place did Bergen op Zoom send its lepers for examination?). *NTG, 69*, II, 1147–8; *BGG, V*, 234–5.

5006 — (1925). Bergen op Zoomsche "Lepralijders" naar Haarlem ten schouw gezonden (17de eeuw) (The lepers of — sent to H. for examination). *NTG, 69*, II, 2122–3; *BGG, V*, 291–2.

5007 — (1926). Bordeelen prostitutie binnen Bergen op Zoom in de 15de en 16de eeuw (Brothel prostitution at — in the 15th and 16th century). *NTG, 70*, I, 1422–3; *BGG, VI*, 91–2.

5008   ENSINK, H. J. (1940). *Moederschapszorg in het Markiezaat van Bergen op Zoom* (Maternity welfare in the Marquisate of —). 215 pp., Thesis Amsterdam. Bergen op Zoom.   *See also* 3165–6

Breda

5009   LINT, J. G. de (1919–20). Besmettelijke ziekten tijdens het beleg van Breda in 1625 (Contagious diseases during the siege of B.). *Med. Wbl.*, *26*, 313–9 and 325–31.

5010   BRAAT, P. (1938). Aanstelling van vroedvrouwen in de Baronie Breda (Appointment of midwives in the Barony of Breda). *NTG, 82*, III, 3868–9; *BGG, XVIII*, 141–2.

5011   HALLEMA, A. (1962). Specialistenhulp voor Bredase zieken in de 16e eeuw elders dan ter plaatse (Medical assistance of sick people by specialists at B. in the 16th century elsewhere than in that town). *NTG, 106*, I, 32; *BGG, XLII*, 5.   *See also* 408, 3477, 4359

Broek in Waterland

5012   BAKKER, C. (1924). Aanteekeningen over de vroedvrouwen te Broek in Waterland in de 17de en 18de eeuw, uit de Resolutieboeken dier Gemeente overgenomen (Notices on the midwives at — in the 17th and 18th century, borrowed from the Resolution-books of that municipality). *NTG, 68*, I, 1973–7; *BGG, IV*, 104–8.
                    See also 2438–42

Brummen

5013   DOOREN, L. (1938). Verloskundige hulp in het ambt Brummen (Obstetrical assistance in the region —). *NTG, 82*, II, 1608; *BGG, XVIII*, 79.

Dordrecht

5014   DROGENDIJK, A. C. (1935). *De verloskundige voorziening in Dordrecht van 1500 tot heden* (Obstetrical provision at D. from 1500 till present). Thesis University Amsterdam (Supervisor: van Rooy. IX + 350 pp., 7 ill. 8°, H. J. Paris, Amsterdam.

5015   — (1953). Verloskundige schetsen uit het verleden der Merwestad. De

15e en 16e eeuw (Obstetrical sketches from the past of the "Merwe-town" [Dordrecht]. The 15th and 16th century). *Med. blad, Afd. Dordrecht*, 25 juni.

5016 — (1956). De verloskundige voorziening te Dordrecht in de eerste helft van de 17e eeuw (Obstetrical provision at D. in the first half of the 17th century). *NTG, 100*, 928–35; *BGG, XXXVI*, 21–8.

5017 — (1954). Verloskundige schetsen uit het verleden der Merwestad. De 18e eeuw (Obstetrical sketches from the past of the "Merwe-town". The 18th century). *Med. bl. Afd. Dordrecht*, 28 January, 25 February and 25 March.

5018 — (1954). — De Franse tijd (The French period). *Ibid.*, 22 April, 26 May, 24 June and 29 July.

5019 — (1954). — De periode van 1840–65 (The period of 1840–65). *Ibid.* 25 November and 23 December.

5020 — (1955). — De periode van 1865–±1930 (The period of 1865–±1930). *Ibid.* 24 March, 28 April, 26 May and 23 June.

5021 PUTTO, J. A. (1961). Een "Instructie voor den Stadtsvroedmeester" van Dordrecht van 1792 (An "Instruction for the town-accoucheur" at D.); *GG, 39*, 229–30.

See also 3148, 3167, 3628–9, 4363–5

Gorinchem

5022 ANDEL, M. A. van (1913). Public Hygiene in a mediaeval Dutch town [Gorinchem]. *Janus, XVIII*, 626–34.

See also 699, 3150, 3168, 3200

Gouda

5023 BIK, J. G. W. F. (1955). *Vijf eeuwen medisch leven in een Hollandse stad* (Five centuries of medical life in a Dutch town [Gouda]). Thesis University Groningen (Supervisor: A. Querido). 634 pp., 45 ill., Van Gorcum, Assen.

5024 — (1964). Welke invloed had het vroegere stadsbestuur van Gouda op de gezondheidszorg? (What influence did the former municipality of G. have on public health?). *GeWiNa, 16*, 14–6.

See also 3149, 4432, 4593

Groningen

5025 ALI COHEN, L. (1860). Bijdrage tot de geschiedenis van de prostitutie
      en hare regeling in de stad Groningen van 1425 tot heden (Contribu-
      tion to the history of the prostitution and its regulation in the town of
      G. from 1425 up to the present). *NTG, 5, 533.*

5026 SCHOUTE, D. (1939). De stad Groningen en de geschiedenis onzer oude
      ziekenhuizen (The town of Groningen and the history of our old hos-
      pitals). *NTG, 83,* III, 3336-43; *BGG, XIX,* 172-9.

5027 TRIP, H. J. (1867). *Geschiedenis der ziekten die in de 17e, 18e en het
      begin der 19e eeuw algemeen geheerscht hebben te Groningen* (History
      of diseases having prevailed at G. in the 17th, 18th and in the beginning
      of the 19th century). Groningen. 8°.

      See also 3667, 4460, 4554, 4594-6

5027ª [M] (1896). Misverstand ontstaan door onbekendheid met de platte-
      lands Groninger taal (Misunderstanding from unfamiliarity with the
      Gronings country language). *Gron. Volksalm.,* 115-9.

's-Gravenhage (The Hague)

5028 KRUL, R. (1891). *Haagsche Doctoren, chirurgen en apothekers in den
      ouden tijd* (Doctors, surgeons and apothecaries from The Hague in
      olden times). 220 pp. Van Stockum & Zn, Den Haag.

5028ª PABON, N. J. (1936). Bijdragen over het godsdienstig, zedelijk en maat-
      schappelijk leven in Den Haag tot het einde der 16de eeuw (Contribu-
      tions to the religious, moral and social life at The Hague till the end of
      the 16th century). *Die Haghe,* 36-258.
      – with chapters on Poor relief, Hospitals (p. 83-109), Education, Guilds (p. 141-56).

5029 HALLEMA, A. (1934). Onderscheiding van overheidswege aan de Haag-
      sche doctoren, die deel genomen hadden aan de cholera-bestrijding in
      1832 (Governmental honours to the The Hague doctors, who had taken
      part in the fight against cholera). *NTG, 78,* I, 75-7; *BGG, XIV,* 29-31.

5030 ENDTZ, L. J. (with the cooperation of H. M. Mensonides and M.
      van Hasselt (1972). *De Hage-Professoren. Geschiedenis van een chirur-
      gische school* (The "Hague-Professors". History of a surgical school).
      171 pp., portrs. and ill., Specia, Amstelveen.
      – With a foreword by G. A. Lindeboom. Reviewed by J. R. Prakken: *NTG, 117*
      (1973), 1060.

      See also 2880, 2944, 4365a-4368 (hospitals)

Haarlem

5031 OVERMEER, W. P. J. (1905). De geneesheeren, chirurgijns, advocaten, procureurs en notarissen te Haarlem in de 18de eeuw (The physicians, surgeons, lawyers, solicitors and notaries at H. in the 18th century). *Alg. Ned. Familiebl., XVII,* 17.

5032 BITTER, H. (1915). *Vroedvrouwen en leerling-vroedvrouwen te Haarlem in de zeventiende en achttiende eeuw* (Midwives and aspirant midwives at H. in de seventeenth and eighteenth century). Haarlem.

See also 3475, 3494, 4371–72c (hospitals), 4555

Harderwijk

5033 [Anonym] (1923). Dokter en ziekenoppasseres te Harderwijk omstreeks 1500 (Physician and nurse at H.). *NTG, 67,* II, 2300–1; *BGG, III,* 358–
–9. See also 4444–5

Hunsingo

5034 FOLMER, [   ] (1883). Voormalige en hedendaagsche schedelvorm in Hunsingo (Former and present shape of the skull in Hunsingo). *NTG, 19,* 325–35.

Huissen

5035 [Anonym] (1923). Instructie voor de bewaerders van het leprozenhuis te Huissen (Instruction for the caretakers of the leper house at H.) *NTG, 67,* II, 2301–2; *BGG, III,* 359–60.

See also 4407

Jisp

5036 HANEVELD, G. T. (1965). Jisp. *Arts en Auto* (Kerstnummer, 1392–3.
– On the "bone-setters at Jisp" in particular Mr. Cornelis (Ploeg).

Kampen

5037 NANNINGA UITERDIJK, J. (1877). Stadsdoctoren te Kampen (Town physicians at Kampen). *Bijdr. Gesch. Overijssel, IV,* 26–60.

5038   — (1880). De chirurgijns te Kampen (The surgeons at K.). *Bijdr. Gesch. Overijssel, VI*, 1–47.   *See also* 3152, 4598

Leiden

5039   RHIJN Jr., W. P. van (1919–20). Spaansche griep te Leiden (Spanish flu at L.) *Med. Wbl.*, 26, 119.

5040   NAPJUS, J. W. (1930). Twee posten uit de thesauriersrekening van Leiden in 1643 (Two items from the treasurer's bill from —). *NTG, 74*, II, 3452–4; *BGG, X*, 206–8.
    – The items refer to the providing of obstetrical care. In addition an order against too copious maternity meals; and the bill for the embalming of princess Anne, widow of the prince of Orange, Willem IV, (1759).
                                                        See also 1966, 4375–78a

Middelburg

5041   SCHOUTE, D. (1942). Uit het jongste verleden der geneeskunde binnen de Middelburgsche samenleving (From the recent past of medicine in the M. society). *Archief*, 1–14.
                                                See also 921, 2452, 3114, 4379–81

Nijmegen

5042   BAUMANN, E. D. (1925). De dysenterie te Nijmegen in 1736 (Dysentery at N.) *NTG, 69*, II, 605–19; *BGG, V*, 169–83.

5043   PENNING, C. P. J. (1927). Eenige gevallen van simulatie te Nijmegen in 1750 en de bestraffing (Some cases of simulation at N. in — and the punishment). *NTG, 71*, II, 2383–5; *BGG, VII*, 714–6.

5044   ROGIER, L. J. (1960). Uit de geschiedenis van de beoefening der geneeskunde inzonderheid te Nijmegen (From the history of the practice of medicine, particularly at N.) *Numaga, 7*, 134–200.
    – a.o. on Michael (*d*. 1636), Emanuël (*d*, 1661) en Gualtherus de Mandeville.

5045   MEYER, Fieke (1960). De hygiënische toestanden in Nijmegen 1850–1880 (Hygienic situations at N.). *Numaga, 7*, 69–122, ill.

5046   VELDE, G. C. J. van der (1967). Gezondheidszorg te Nijmegen in de periode 1816–1865. De werkzaamheden van de "Plaatselijke Commissie van Geneeskundig Toevoorzigt" (Public health at N. in the period

— —. The activities of the "Local Committee of Medical Supervision").
Numaga, 14, 5–39.   *See also* 966, 1144, 4382, 4440

Rotterdam

5047 ELIAS, J. Ph. (1911). Een en ander over het geneeskundig Rotterdam
der zestiende en zeventiende eeuw (Something on medical R. in the
16th and 17th century). *NTG, 55,* II, 117–23.

5048 — (1912). *Overzicht van de geschiedenis der geneeskunde in Rotterdam*
(Survey of the history of medicine in R.) 88 pp. Nijgh & van Ditmar,
Rotterdam, 8°.

5048ª KRAMER, P. H. (1948). Rumor in casa in de Rotterdamse medische
wereld van 1730 (Rumor in casa in the Rotterdam medical world in
1730). *Rott. Jbk.,* 5de reeks, *6,* 188–200.
– with some data on W. Vink, C. Nieuwaart, J. Alphen, A. van Deutekom, P.
Garneau, J. van Wijk.

5049 MELLES, J. (1961). Rotterdamse chirurgijns in vroeger eeuwen (Rotterdam surgeons in former centuries). *NRC* (Weekly suppl.) 18 November.
                              See also 1205, 1286, 3156, 3157, 3207, 3299, 4022, 4383a–89,
                              4412

Tilburg

5050 ROUKENS, C. D. (1959). Zuigelingensterfte en -zorg te Tilburg op het
einde der 19e en in het begin van deze eeuw (Infant mortality and care
at T. at the end of the 19th and in the beginning of the 20th century).
Brabantia, 8, 184–92.   *See also* 4390

Utrecht

5051 BOSSCHAERT, D. (1969). *De stad Utrecht als medisch ontwikkelingsge-
bied* (Proceeding Medical Care for the underprivileged in Utrecht town
during the Nineteenth Century), 441 pp., ill., portrs. Thesis Utrecht
(Supervisor: R. Hornstra) Bronder-Offset, N.V. Rotterdam.
– With English summary; reviewed by L. Elaut: *Sci. Hist., 11* (1969), 187–8.

5052 WEYDE, A. J. van der (1923). Over lepra te Utrecht in de Middeleeuwen (On leprosy at U. in the Middle Ages). *NTG, 67,* II, 1604–9;
BGG, III, 258–63.

5053   — (1924). Over lepra te Utrecht in de middeleeuwen (On leprosy at U. in the Middle Ages). *NTG, 68*, I, 947–8; *BGG, IV*, 70–1.

5054   — (1926). Iets over het toezicht op de volksgezondheid te Utrecht in vroeger tijd (Something on the supervision of public health at U. in former times). *NTG, 70*, II, 669–75; *BGG, VI*, 199–205.

5055   — (1926). De uitoefening der geneeskunde in vroeger tijd te Utrecht (The practice of medicine at U. in former times). *Jbk. "Oud-Utrecht"*, 45–75.

5056   — (1927). Bijdrage tot de geschiedenis der pest te Utrecht (Contribution to the history of the plague at U.). *NTG, 71*, I, 3119–39; *BGG, VII*, 384–404, ill.

5057   BERGH, A. J. van den (1945) *Utrechtsche hygiënische vraagstukken. Historisch beschouwd.* (Hygienic problems at U. Historical review). Kemink, Utrecht.
– posthumously published thesis.

5058   HALLEMA, A. (1955). Archiefsprokkels (Gleanings from records) *NTG, 99*, III, 2228–31; *BGG, 35*, 71–4.
– Data from the resolutions of the council and the corporation of the town of Utrecht 1548–1638.

5059   HOOGLAND, Sr. R. A. (1968). De Utrechtse Schouboecken (The Utrecht books of autopsy). *NTG, 112*, 2164.

5060   SCHRETLEN, E. D. A. M. (1969). De evolutie in de benadering van het begrip ziekte met op de achtergrond enkele facetten uit de medische historie van de stad Utrecht (Evolution in the approach to the concept of disease with, in the background, some facets from the medical past of the town of Utrecht). *Med. afd. Utrecht Kon. Med. Mij. t.b.d. Geneesk., no. 225*, (23 Mei).

5060ᵃ GRAADT van ROGGEN, W. van (1953). De Utrechtse jaarmarktkermis (The Utrecht annual fair). *Jbk. Oud-Utrecht*, 159–77.
– pp. 173–7 on medicine and surgeons, etc.
                    See also 1383, 3158, 3170–1, 3201, 3205, 4391–4, 4436–8,
                    4457–9, 4473, 4559–61

Veere

5061   BIJL, W. F. Th. van der (1932). Benoemingsbesluit van een gemeente-geneeskundige te Veere in het jaar 1486 (Resolution of appointment of a municipal physician at V. in the year 1486). *NTG*, *76*, III, 3306–7; *BGG*, *XII*, 138–9.   See also 3487

Zaltbommel

5062 EPKEMA, E. (1903). Eenige instructies van Zaltbommel in de 18e eeuw (Some instructions of Zaltbommel in the 18th century). *Gelre*, *VI*, 285–97.

5063 — (1909). Beoefenaars der genees- en heelkunde te Zaltbommel in de zeventiende en achttiende eeuw (Some medical and surgical practitioners at Z. in the 17th and 18th century). *Gelre*, *XII*, 163–208.

5064 DOOREN, L. (1939). Sollicitatie naar het chirurgijnsambt te Zaltbommel (Application for the surgeoncy at Z.). *NTG*, *83*, I, 529–30; *BGG*, *XIX*, 34–5.   See also 4398

Zwolle

5065 DOESSCHATE, A. ten (1928). Geneeskunde in Oud-Zwolle (Medicine in Old-Zwolle). *Versl. Med. Ver. tot beoef. Overijsselsch regt en Gesch.*, 45ste stuk, 2de reeks, 21ste stuk, 1–89.

5066 — (1928). Overzicht van de geschiedenis der geneeskunde te Zwolle (Survey of the history of medicine at Zwolle). *NTG*, *72*, I, 1680–95; *BGG*, *VIII*, 81–96.
  –cf: letter to the editor by A. C. A. Hoffman. *NTG*, *72*, I, 2225; *BGG*, *VIII*, 148, referring to the previous item, with remarks on Hahnemann's view on the infectiousness of cholera.

5067 [K.]. (1859). Groote sterfte te Zwolle in 1636–37 (High mortality at Z. in 1636–37). *Navorscher*, *9*, 331–2.

5068 HASSELT, W. J. C. van (1860). Groote sterfte te Zwolle (High mortality at Z.) *Navorscher*, *10*, 79.

Provinces and districts

5069 ENKLAAR, D. Th. (1925). Twee oorkonden betreffende de geneeskundige verzorging in Noord-Nederlandsche steden in de latere middeleeuwen (Two charters regarding the medical care in Northern Netherlands towns in the later Middle Ages). *NTG*, *69*, II, 1146–7; *BGG*, *V*, 233–4.

5070   MULDER, R. D. (1960). Volksgezondheid en medici in het oude Drente (Public health and physicians in old —). *Nwe Drentse Volksalmanak*, *78*, 50–74.

5070[a]   — (1952). *Drenthe's strijd tegen epidemieën* (D's. fight against epidemics). 40 pp. pr. pr.
- Published on the occasion of the 100th anniversary of the Department Assen and Surroundings of the Royal Dutch Society for the promotion of medicine. Also published in: *Nwe Drentsche Volksalm.* (1952), 19–54.

                 See also 567a, 2354a

5070[b]   WENTZEL, G. (1974). Veluwse Geneeskunde (Veluwe medicine). *Ned. Historiën*, *8*, no 2, 71–4, 1 ill.

5071   SNUIF, C. J. (1928). De geneeskundige toestand in Twente (1663–1698). De chirurgijn Adolph de Meyer te Goor (The medical situation in — —. The surgeon — — at G.). *Versl. Med. Ver. Overijsselsch regt en gesch.*, 45ste stuk, 2de reeks, 21ste stuk, 92–126.

5072   RINGELING, J. H. A. (1962–63). Het aandeel van de familie Van Kleef in de geneeskundige zorg op Schokland (1800–1832) (The part of the family — in medical care on — —) *Kamper Almanak*, 199–232.

5073   STARMANS, J. H. (1930). *Verloskunde en kindersterfte in Limburg. Folklore, Geschiedenis, Heden* (Obstetrics and infant mortality in —. Folklore, History, Present). Thesis. 451 pp. Gebr. van Aalst, Maastricht
- reviewed by M. A. van Andel: *NTG*, *74* (1930), 3911–2; *BGG*, X, 229–30.

                 See also 920

5073[a]   AERTS, M. C. M. *et al.* (1974). *Ziek zijn, vroeger* (Being ill in former times). 60 pp., ill. Stichting "Brabantse Dag", Heeze, pr. pr.

5074   DOELEMAN, [   ] (1958). "Zeeuwse koortsen" (Zealand fevers). *MC*, *13*, 768.

5075   FEIBEL, Robert N. (1968). What happened at Walcheren: the primary medical sources. *BHM*, *42*, 62–79.
- on the diseases in the English Army that occupied Walcheren in 1809.

5076   GEIST-HOFMAN, A. M. (1969). Wat gebeurde op Walcheren in 1809 (What happened at Walcheren in 1809?). *NTG*, *113*, I, 32.
- referring to the previous item.

5077   LOO, [   ] (1910). *Les fièvres zélandaises et leur influence sur l'expédition anglaise en 1809*. G. B. van Goor, Gouda.

5078   McGUFFIE (1947). "The Walcheren expedition and the Walcheren fever". *Eng. Hist. Rev.*, *62*, 191–202.

5078ª CROWE, K. E. (1973). The Walcheren expedition and the new Army Medical Board: a reconsideration. *Engl. Hist. Rev.*, *88*, 770–85.

5079 FOLMER, H. R. (1927). Volksgebruiken in Zeeland bij geboorte en kraambed (Popular customs in Z. at birth and childbed). *NTG*, *71*, I, 3112–18; *BGG*, *VII*, 377–83.

See also 4571, 4600

5080 BERGER, J. A. (1930). De geneeskundige verzorging der Salzburgers in Staats-Vlaanderen (The medical care of the Salzburg people in States' Flanders). *NTG*, *74*, II, 3899–3907; *BGG*, *X*, 217–25. (*see also*: 2446a, 3117, 3172).

See also leprosy (3114–21); plague (3146–50); cholera (3199–3209); 3636–43 (midwives); 4321–4401 (hospitals), 4405–07 (leper houses), 4408–12 (plague houses), 4418–40 (lunatic asylums); 4441–76 (other hospitals); 4586–4610 (guilds).

B. Local Pharmacy

Alkmaar

5081 WITTOP KONING, D. A. (1969). Alkmaar en de farmacie. *Alkmaars Jbk.*, *5*, 79–91.

Amersfoort

5082 — (1971). Amersfoort en de pharmacie. *Flehite*, *4*, 33–41, ill. Also in: *Bull. Pharm.*, no 45, 26–34; *PhW.*, *107*, Suppl. M. 317–21, 329. (1972).

Amsterdam

5083 BREEN, J. C. (1915). De Hoogduitsche Apotheek, Prinsengracht 578 (The "High German" Pharmacy, Amsterdam). *Jbk. Amstelodamum*, *XII*, 181.

5084 KRUIZINGA, J. H. (1965). Amsterdamse verzamelaars. III. In het domein van de apotheker. Dr Wittop Koning verzamelt apothekers-benodigdheden (Amsterdam collectors. III. In the domain of the chemist. — — collects apothecaries' requisites). *Ons Amsterdam*, *17*, 34–42, ill.

5085   WITTOP KONING, D. A. (1967). 125 jaar Departement Amsterdam van
       de K.N.M.P. (125 years of the Department Amsterdam of the —).
       PhW., *102*, 650–7.
       – on the Royal Dutch Society for the promotion of pharmacy; address.

5085ª WIELEN, P. vander (1932). Amsterdam en de Pharmacie (— and Phar-
       macy). *PhW.*, *69*, 793–808.

                                    See also 4768, 4778, 4810, 4824–7

Antwerp

5086   WITTOP KONING, D. A. (1955). De rol van Antwerpen in de geschie-
       denis van de pharmacie (The role of Antwerp in the history of pharma-
       cy). *Ph. T. België*, *32*, 5; *Bull. Pharm.*, no 12, 1–6.

5087   — (1956, 1957). De oudste pharmaceutische ordonnantiën van Ant-
       werpen (The oldest pharmaceutical ordinances of Antwerp). *Ph. T.
       België*, *33*, 249–55; *Bull. Pharm.*, no 15 (1957), 1–7.

5088   VANDEWIELE, L. J. (1963). Enkele losse bladzijden uit de geschiedenis
       van de farmacie te Antwerpen (Some loose pages from the history of
       pharmacy at Antwerp). *Kon. Apoth. Ver. Antwerp, 125-jarig jubileum*,
       19–37.

Breda

5089   WITTOP, KONING, D. A. (1953). Breda en de Pharmacie. *PhW*, *88*,
       349–54; *Bull. Pharm.*, no 5, 2–7.

5090   REHM, G. J. (1959, 1960, 1961). De Bredase apotheken van de 15ᵉ tot
       het begin der 19ᵉ eeuw (The chemist's shops at B. from the 15th till the
       beginning of the 19th century). *De Brabantse Leeuw*, *8*, 53–8; 68–72;
       90–5; 109–12; 113–7; 129–34; 145–9; 173–81; *Ibid.*, *9*, 1–6; 17–22;
       33–9; 49–54; 65–8; 81–4; 97–100; 113–7; 129–34; 161–7; 177–83.
       Ibid., *10*, 1–7; 17–21; 33–4; Also in: *Bull. Pharm.*, no 22 (1960), 24
       pp.; *Ibid.*, no 25 (1961), 24 pp., port.; *Ibid.*, no 26 (1961). 22 pp., ill.,
       port.

Brielle

5091   WITTOP KONING, D. A. (1951). Brielle en de pharmacie. *PhW.*, *86*, 75–
       81.

Delft

5092 WIELEN, P. van der (1918). Schets voor een pharmaceutische geschiedenis van Delft (Sketch for a pharmaceutical history of D.) *PhW*, *55*, 852–64.

5093 — (1960). De simpliciakast van het Collegium Medico Pharmaceuticum te Delft (The cupboard of simplicia of the — — at D.). *Bull. Rijksmuseum*, *8*, 69–82.

5094 SNELDERS, H. A. M. (1970). De Delftse apotheker en chemicus Petrus Johannes Kipp (1808–1864). The Delft pharmacist and chemist — —). *Sci. Hist.*, *12*, 79–92, ill.

See also 4791–6 (jars)

Deventer

5095 GELDER, J. B. van, E. GRENDEL and D. A. WITTOP KONING (1966–1967). Deventer en de farmacie. *PhW.*, *101*, 940–52; *Bull. Pharm*, no. 37 (mei 1967), 6–18, ill.

Eindhoven

5096 BERG, M. J. van den (1959). Uit Eindhoven's historie (From the history of E.). *Bull. Pharm.*, no 20 (oct.). inside of the cover, 12 pp.
– some data on the chemist's shops at E. in the 19th century.

Goes, Gouda

5097 SMIT, A. de (1962). Goes in de farmacie in de zeventiende eeuw (G. in pharmacy in the 17th century). *PhW.*, *97*, 33–6; *Bull. Pharm.*, no 30, 1–3.

5098 GRENDEL, E. (1955). *De ontwikkeling van de artsenijbereidkunde in Gouda tot 1865* (The development of pharmacy in — —). Thesis University Amsterdam (Supervisor: R. J. Forbes). 590 pp., ill. Koch en Knuttel, Gouda.

The Hague

5099 SCHIM, H. (1901). "Op de Nieuwe Haegsche Apotheek" ("On the New Hague Pharmacy"). *Die Haghe*, *60*, 266.

5100 WITTOP KONING, D. A. (1947). De simpliciekast van het Haagsche Collegium Pharmaceuticum (The cupboard of simplicia of the — — of The Hague). *PhW.*, *82*, 185–8.

5101 — (1949). 's-Gravenhage en de Pharmacie. *PhW.*, *84*, 710–6; *Med. Bur. Statistiek en Voorl.*, 207–11; *Die Haghe*, *126*, 49–65.

Haarlem

5102 BITTER, H. (1915). Haarlemsche apothekers in de 17de en 18de eeuw (Haarlem chemists in the 17th and 18th century). *PhW.*, *52*, no 34, 1161 –78.   See also 2883, 4789

Harderwijk, Kampen

5103 WITTOP KONING, D. A. (1941). Apothekers te Harderwijk (Chemists at H.). *PhW.*, *78*, 1046–7.

5104 NANNINGA UITTERDIJK, J. (1883). Apothekers te Kampen (Chemists at K.). *Bijdr. Gesch. Overijssel*, *VII*, 330–70.
                                                                 See also 4766

Maastricht, Roermond

5105 WIELEN, P. van der and E. C. J. M. HOLLMAN (1921). Bijdrage tot de geschiedenis der pharmacie in Maastricht (Contribution to the history of pharmacy at M.). *PhW.*, *58*, 758.

5106 KRUYTZER, E. M. (1959, 1960). Les pharmaciens de Maestricht du 19ᵉ siècle et les sciences naturelles. *Natuurhist. Mbl.*, *48*, 138–41; *Bull. Pharm.*, no 21 (1960), febr., 4 pp.   See also 4861

5107 WITTOP KONING, D. A. (1954). De geschiedenis van de pharmacie te Roermond en Venlo (History of pharmacy at R. and at V.). *PhW.*, *89*, 641–7; *Bull. Pharm.*, no 10, 12–6.

Rotterdam

5108 COHEN, Hk (1928). De apotheek van een Rotterdamsch geneesheer in 1603 (The chemist's shop of a physician at R.). *NTG*, *72*, II, 3308–14; *BGG*, *VIII*, 179–84.

5109 — (1928). Een apotheekhoudend Geneesheer te Rotterdam in de zestiende eeuw (A chemist-physician at R. in the 16th century). *PhW.*, *65*, 401–13.

5110 BRANS, P. H. (1954). Uit het pharmaceutisch verleden van Rotterdam (From the pharmaceutical past of R.). *PhW.*, *91*, 361; *Bull. Pharm.*, no 10, 23.

5111 — (1963). Streiflichter auf Rotterdam und die Pharmazie. *Dtsch. Apoth. Ztg,. 103*, 905–10.

5111ᵃ KONING, J. C. de (1971). Apothekers en Apotheken te Rotterdam gedurende de laatste 125 jaar (Chemists and chemist's shops at R. during the last 125 years). *Rott. Jbk.*, 7de reeks, *9*, 207–24.

See also 4875–6, 4891

Tiel

5112 BRANS, P. H. (1954). Tiel en de Pharmacie. *PhW.*, *91*, 648; *Bull. Pharm.*, no 10, 5.

Utrecht, Vianen

5113 WITTOP KONING, D. A. (1957). Utrecht en de Farmacie. *Jbk Oud-Utrecht*, [35], 58–72.

5114 GRENDEL, E. (1962, 1963). Vianen en de farmacie. *PhW.*, *97*, 197–208; *Bull. Pharm.*, no 31 (1963), 1–11; 12–23.

Zierikzee

5115 WITTOP KONING, D. A. (1954). Zierikzee en de Pharmacie. *PhW.*, *89*, 164–7; *Bull. Pharm.*, no 10, 1–4.

5116 BARTENS, J. (1965). Een Zierikzeese apotheker die Jezuietenbroeder werd (A Zierikzee apothecary, who became a Jesuit friar). *Arch. Gesch· Kath. Kerk Zeeland*, *7*, 116–28.

– Engelbert Capwel (1642–1733), author of *Enchiridium Medicum oft Medicijn Boecksken*, Antwerp, 1734 (several times reprinted).

Zwolle

5117 MEULEMEESTER, P. J. A. J. (1928). Kort overzicht van de geschiedenis van een Zwolsche apotheek 15-1-1728—15-1-1928 (Short survey of the history of a chemist's shop at Z.). *Ph. W.*, *65*, 84–7.

Provinces and regions

5118   WITTOP KONING, D. A. (1960). Gelderland en de farmacie (Guelders and pharmacy). *PhW.*, *95*, 245–54.

5119   JASPERS, P. A. Th. M. (1966). *De ontwikkeling van de pharmacie in Limburg gedurende de Franse tijd (1794–1814)* (The development of pharmacy in L. during the French period). Thesis University Amsterdam. 126 pp., 12 ill., facs. Dagblad voor Noord-Limburg, Venlo.

5120   HEGGEN, M. H. M. (1971). *Oude pharmaceutische boeken bijeengebracht in het Land van Herle*. Ter gelegenheid van de voorjaarsvergadering van de Kring voor de Geschiedenis van de Pharmacie in Benelux ... te Heerlen op 17 en 18 april 1971) (Old books on pharmacy collected in the region of Herle. On the occasion of the meeting of the Circle for History of Pharmacy in the Benelux). Heerlen.

See also 4830–36

Chapter XXI

Other Countries

From its very beginning Leiden University and its Medical Faculty received very many foreign students, especially Englishmen, from which resulted many relations with other countries, Great-Britain in the first place. The relations with England culminated in the first half of the eighteenth century when Boerhaave flourished. Though several German scholars were appointed professor in Dutch universities, the relations with Germany in the field of medicine were decidedly less close than with England. Connections with Austria were established in the second half of the eighteenth century as a result of Gerard van Swieten's appointment as physician in ordinary of the Empress Maria Theresa.

From Sweden, for a long time, many students came to Holland only to take their degree, mostly at Harderwijk.

Oversea trade and the possession of colonies such as Ceylon and the Dutch East Indies involved experience in tropical medicine and from the factory at Deshima, the small artificial island of Nagasaki, Western medicine was introduced into Japan through the intermediary of Dutch doctors and Dutch medical books.

The Dutch medical officer Pompe van Meerdervoort trained the first Japanese students after the pattern of Western Medicine. – In this chapter are also included entries of Dutch medical historians concerning medicine in other countries.

A. Benelux

5121 LINDEBOOM, G. A. (1958). Medisch-wetenschappelijke betrekkingen tussen Noord- en Zuid-Nederland in vroeger dagen (15e tot 17e eeuw). (Medical-scientific relations between the Northern and the Southern Netherlands in former days (15th – 17th century)). *NTG*, *102*, II,

1753–5; *BGG, XXXVIII*, 17–9. Also in: *Le Scalpel, III*, 498–504; *Yperman, 5*, no 6, 7 pp.

5122   BRANS, P. H. (1960). Coopération scientifique au sein du Bénelux. *Janus, XLIX*, 137–41.

5122ᵃ BOEYNAEMS, P. (1974). Irish doctors in the Southern Netherlands. In: *Proc. XXIII Int. Congr. Hist. Med. London 2–9 Sept. 1972*, Vol. I, 730–2. Wellcome Institute of the History of Medicine, London.

5122ᵇ ELAUT, L. (1974). Waarheen ging de afgestudeerde arts uit Zuid-Nederland (België) voor post-universitaire scholing tijdens de negentiende en twintigste eeuw? Een onderzoek naar de beweegredenen van zijn keus (Where did the certificated physician from the Southern Netherlands (Belgium) go for post-graduate training during the 19th and 20th century? An investigation into the motives of his choice). In: *Circa Tiliam*, 107–21.

See also 1029, 1596, 2258, 4236–8, 4888–9, 4894

B. England

5123   LEVERE, T. H. (1970). Relations and rivalry: interactions between Britain and the Netherlands in eighteenth century science and technology. *Hist. Sci., 9*, 42–53.

5124   LINDEBOOM, G. A. (1973). *Boerhaave and Great Britain*. Three lectures on Boerhaave with particular reference to his relations with Great Britain. *Analecta Boerhaaviana, VII.*, 75 pp., 16 ill. E. J. Brill, Leiden.

See also 1238, 1535, 4105, 4158–60, 4761

C. Scotland

5125   GUTHRIE, D. (1957). Leyden and Edinburgh. *Brit. med. J.*, (ii), 223.
         – abstract of an address.

5126   — (1957, 1959). The influence of the Leyden School upon Scottish medicine. *Scot. Soc. Hist. Med. Proc.*, 9–14; *Med. Hist., III* (1959), 108–22.
         – Paper read at a meeting of the Scottish Society of the History of Medicine in October, 1957.

5127 MOULIN, D. de (1966). Honderd jaar geleden in Glasgow (Hundred years ago at G.). *NTG*, *110*, 906–7.

5128 WALLACE, A. B. (1965). The Hippocratic tradition in the Netherlands and Scotland. *Brit. J. Pract. Surg.*, *18*, 233–7.

See also 344, 345

D. France

5129 ZEEMAN, D. H. (1878). *Bijdrage tot de geschiedenis der Chirurgie in Frankrijk* (Contribution to the history of surgery in France). Thesis Leiden. 8°.

5130 NOYON, I. (1941). Een medische studiereis in de "Franse tijd" (A medical study-tour in the "French time"). *NTG*, *85*, III, 3615–9, *BGG*, *XXI*, 107–11.

5131 SERGESCU, P. (1956). Savants français en Hollande. *Rev. d'Hist. des Sci.*, *VIII*, 74–8.

5132 LEEMANS, W. F. (1966). Nederlanders aan de Universiteit van Dôle Bourgondië (Dutchmen at the University of Dôle in Burgundy). *Ned. Leeuw.*, *83*, 4–8.

5133 KNEGTEL, A. P. C. H. (1964). Médecins Néerlandais à Paris en 1818–1823–1842. *Hist. de la Méd.*, *13*, Mai, 3–11, 5 ill., 8 ports.
– Notes of C. B. Tilanus, C. J. Broers and P. J. I. de Frémery on their stay at Paris.
See also 894–5

5134 GOMOIU, V. (1963). Les relations de l'Ecole de Montpellier avec les institutions médicales des diverses nations au cours des siècles. *Scalpel*, *116*, 489–98.

5134ᵃ BRUNET, P. (1926). *Les physiciens hollandais et la méthode expérimentale en France au 18e siècle*. Paris.

See also 3521, 3748a, 4196, 4239, 4759–60, 4762–3 (Pharmacy).

E. Italy

5135 CASTIGLIONI, A. (1929). Les étudiants en médecine flamands à l'Université de Padoue. *VIme Congrès Int. d'Hist. de la Méd. Leyde- Amsterdam, 1927*, 313–7, Anvers.

5136   BOEYNAEMS, P. (1955). De invloed van Salerno op de Nederlanden vóór de stichting der Leuvense Universiteit (The influence of Salerno on the Netherlands before the foundation of the University of Louvain). *Belg. T. Geneesk.*, nr. 20, 988–98.

5137   — (1960). Influences Salernitaines aux Pays Bas avant la fondation de l'Université de Louvain (1425). *Atti del XIV Congresso Internaz. di storia della Medizina Roma – Salerno 13–20 Settembre 1954*, Vol. II, 9 pp. Roma.

5138   DONADI, G. C. (1969). L'Olanda nella Storia della medicina con particolare riguardo alle relazioni culturali mediche italo-olandesi. *Pag. Storia Med. 13* (4), 78–90.

See also 331, 358, 1567, 1567a, 4242, 4758

F. Austria

5139   HALBERTSMA, K. T. A. (1936). *De beteekenis van de Weensche school voor de ontwikkeling der geneeskunde gedurende de laatste 150 jaar* (The significance of the Vienna school for the development of medicine during the last 150 years). 46 pp., D. Prooper, Delft.

     – Address, delivered at a meeting of the Association: "Nederland en Oostenrijk", december 18, 1935. Rev. by M. A. van Andel: *NTG, 80* (1936), II, 1931; *BGG, XVI*, 71.

5140   — (1948). *De geneeskundige betrekkingen tussen Nederland en Oostenrijk uit historisch oogpunt* (The medical relations between the Netherlands and Austria from an historical point of view). 46 pp., portr., "Humanitas", 's-Gravenhage, 8°.

5141   MICHOLITSCH, A. (1966). Nederlandse studenten aan de Universiteit van Weenen 1365–1659 (Dutch students at the University of Vienna). *Ned. Leeuw, 83*, 220–32.

5142   LINDEBOOM, G. A. (1950). Gerard van Swieten als hervormer der Weense medische faculteit (— as a reformer of the medical faculty at Vienna). *NTG, 94*, II, 1277–85; *BGG, XXX*, 12–20.

5143   PROBST, Chr. (1972). *Der Weg des ärztlichen Erkennens am Krankenbett.* Herman Boerhaave und die ältere Wiener medizinische Schule. Band I (1701–1787). *SA*, Beiheft *15*, 235 pp., Steiner Verlag, Wiesbabaden.

See also 351–55 (Boerhaave), 880–82 (A. de Haen), 1670–78
(G. v. Swieten), 1883a, 1889, 4134.

G. Poland

5143ᵃ KLEY, J. J. van der (1936). De Polen en de geneeskunde (The Poles and medicine). *NTG, 80*, II, 1488-9; *BGG, XVI*, 55-6.

– on the polish physicians L. Neugebauer (1821-90); Raciborski (1809-71); Balinski (1827-1902); Jan Mierzejefski (1839-1908), and others.

See also 4247b

H. Germany

5144 SNELDERS, H. A. M. (1973). *De invloed van Kant, de Romantiek en de "Naturphilosophie" op de anorganische natuurwetenschappen in Duitsland* (The influence of —, Romanticism, and "Natur-Philosophie" on the inorganic natural sciences in Germany). Thesis Utrecht (Supervisor: R. Hooykaas). 243 pp., no pl., pr. pr.

See also 346-50, 3746b, 4106, 4161, 4170-1, 4241, 4251, 4650

I. Sweden and Iceland

5145 RIJNBERK, G. van (1938). De geschiedenis der wetenschappen in Zweden (The history of science in Sweden). *NTG, 82*, II, 2828-30; *BGG, XVIII*, 105-7.

5146 JÓNSSON, Vilmundur (1949). Laekningar – curationes – séra Thorkels Arngrímsonar (Icelandic), Reykjavik.

– Thorkell (Torchillus) Arngrímson (1629-77), son of the well-known clergyman and Latin author Arngrímur Jónsson (sometimes using the family name Vídalín or Vidalinus) studied medicine at Leyden 1651-52. Later he became a clergyman in his native country (Iceland), practising his medical knowledge along with his clerical duties. See also: Lárus, H. Blöndal og Vilumundur Jónsson: *Leaknar á Islandi* (sec. edition), Reykjavík, 1970, I, p. 13-4, see also pp., 20, 25, 26) – Arngrímsson is the only Icelander who has studied medicine at Leyden.

5147 WRANGEL, E. (1901). *De betrekkingen tusschen Zweden en de Nederlanden op het gebied van letteren en wetenschap, voornamelijk gedurende de zeventiende eeuw* (The relations between Sweden and the Netherlands in the field of letters and science, particularly during the 17th century). 420 pp., E. J. Brill, Leiden.

– Translated from Swedish into Dutch by Mrs. Beets-Damsté; a.o. on Joh. Wullen (Wullenius).

See also 989-92a, 1165, 3492

J. Switzerland

5148   SNAPPER, I. (1924). *Bericht über die dritte Studienreise holländischer Aerzte in der Schweiz.* (23. August bis 6. September 1924). Purmerend, 8°.

K. Portugal

5149   SILVA CARVALHO, A. da (1929). Sur quelques médecins portugais qui ont étudié ou exercé en Hollande. *VIme Congrès Int. d'Hist. de la Méd. Leyde – Amsterdam, 1927,* 346–7, Anvers.

L. Russia

5150   ESSO BZN., I. van (1938). Hollandsche vroedvrouwen in Rusland i n de 18de eeuw (Dutch midwives in Russia in the 18th century). *NTG, 82,* II, *2831–3; BGG, XVIII,* 108–10.

5151   BUWALDA, J. (1938). Hollandsche vroedvrouwen in Rusland (Dutch midwives in Russia). *NTG, 82,* III, *3353; BGG, XVIII,* 128.

5152   ESSO BZN., I. van (1938). Vreemde artsen in Russiche staatsdienst, in Holland gestudeerd hebbende (Foreign physicians having studied in Holland, in Russian public service). *NTG, 82,* IV, *5399–409; BGG, XVIII,* 281–91.

5153   HANS, N. (1957). [Article on Russian students at Leyden in the 18th century]. *Slav. east. Europ. Rev.,* 35, 551–62.

5154   ESSO BZN., I. van (1938). Hollandsche artsen in Russischen hof- en staatsdienst in de 16de, 17de en 18de eeuw (Dutch physicians in public and court service in Russia in the 16th, 17th and 18th century). *NTG, 82,* II, *1582–92; BGG, XVIII,* 40–50.

5155   LINDEBOOM, G. A. (1957). *Medische indrukken uit Rusland* (Medical impressions from Russia). 123 pp., ill., Bohn, Haarlem.

5156   RICHTER, Wilhelm Michaël (1813, 1815, 1817, 1965). *Geschichte der*

Medizin in Russland, 3 vols.: Vol. I. XXIII + 457 pp., Vol. II, XXXII + 440 + Beil. 170 pp., [Russian] + 8 pp.; Vol. III. XXXII + 629 pp. N. S. Wsewolojsky, Moskwa.

– Reprographical reprint: Zentral Antiquariat der D.D.R., Leipzig 1965. In these vols. several Dutch physicians are dealt with.

See also 357, 973, 1502–07 (F. Ruysch), 1511, 4764a

M. South Africa

5157 PENNING, C. P. J. (1946). Een reis met hindernissen naar Transvaal in 1882 (A voyage with obstacles to the Transvaal in 1882). *NTG, 90,* III, 787–8; *BGG, XXVI,* 29–30.
– a case of smallpox on board ship and quarantine measures.

5158 MENKO, H. S. N. (1954). *Contributions of the Netherlands to the development of South African medicine (1652–1902)*. Thesis University of Amsterdam (Supervisor: W. Kouwenaar)., 152 pp., ill., portr. (Jan van Riebeeck). De Bussy, Amsterdam-Capetown-Pretoria.

5159 BURROWS, E. H. (1956). The Leyden tradition in South African medicine (S. African students educated at L.) *S. Afr. med. J., 30,* 257–8.

5160 PRICE, C. H. (1962). Medicine and pharmacy at the Cape of Good Hope. 1652–1807. *Med. Hist., 6,* 169–70.

5161 PIJPER, C. (1919). *De Volksgeneeskunst in Transvaal* (Folkmedicine in the Transvaal), Thesis University of Leyden (Supervisor: E. C. van Leersum), 71 pp. J. J. Groen & Zn., Leiden.

See also 970, 1440–43 (J. van Riebeeck), 1959, 3970a, 4463

N. Dutch East Indies, Dutch New Guinea

5162 BROCKELMANN, C. H. J. (1962). Deutsche Ärzte in Niederländisch-Indien. *Med. Welt,* 1527–31.

5163 MCLEAN, J. (1972). Enige gegevens over verzamelaars van voorwerpen van natuurlijke historie in het voormalig Nederlandsch Indië (Some data on collectors of objects of natural history in the former Dutch Indies). *Sci. Hist., 14,* 51–60.

5163ª BIERDRAGER, J. (1960). Geschiedenis en ontwikkeling van de gezondheidszorg in Nederlands Nieuw Guinea (History and development of
public health care in Dutch New Guinea). *MC*, *15*, 133–6 and 143–5.

O. Surinam

5164 OUDSCHANS DENTZ, F. (1917). Huldiging van een Schotsch geneesheer
in Suriname in 1816 (Honouring of a Scotch physician) *Navorscher*,
LXVI, 126 and 225.

5165 WIERSMA, P. (1902, 1973). *Verslag eener zending naar Britsch-Indië,
ter bestudeering van het emigratie-wezen aldaar, voor zoover betreft de
werving, het in depots onder dak brengen en het afschepen van Britsch-
Indische emigranten naar Suriname* (Report of a mission to British
India, for studying emigration, concerning the recruitment, accommo-
dating in depots and shipping of the British-Indian emigrants to Surinam). 88 pp. Eldorado, Paramaribo.

– With a foreword by L. S. F. Lutchman. This report was found as a carbon copy
at an Amsterdam antiquarian. It was compiled in 1902 by –. It gives also a description of public health and medical care in Surinam.

See also 81, 501, 967, 1444a, 1454, 4055a, 4464, 4527, 4563, 4764

P. America

5166 COURTNEY, J. W. (1929). The versatility of Dutch pioneers in American medicine. *VIme Congres Int. d'Hist. de la Méd. Leyde-Amsterdam,
18–23 juillet 1927*, 191–4, Anvers.

5167 STRUIK, D. J. (1964). De wetenschappelijke betrekkingen tussen Amerika en de Nederlanden in de Koloniale Periode (The scientific relations between America and the Netherlands in the Colonial Period).
Post Iucundam Iuventutem, no. 42, 1–5.

5168 GUTHRIE, Douglas (1958). The contribution of Holland and Scotland
to the evolution of Medical Education in America. In: F. Marti-
lbanez (ed.). *History of American Medicine*, 165–7. MD. Publ. New
York. *See also 4090*

See also 360, 697, 4105

5169 NIEUWENHUIS, A. W. (1924). Principles of Indian Medicine in American ethnology and their psychological significance. *Janus, XXVIII*, 304–56.

5170   — (1932, 1933). Urformen des Naturwissenschaftlichen Denkens der Naturauffassung auf dem Amerikanischen Festlande. *Janus, XXXVI*, 27–42; 49–58; 93–113; 146–68; 190–201; 228–34; 251–64; 283–96; 318–26. *Janus, XXXVII*, 84–96; 122–8 and 153–60.

5171   BALEN, W. J. van (1930). De geneeskunde der oude Incas (Medicine with the ancient Inca's). *NTG, 74*, II, 3913–7; *BGG, X*, 231–5.

5172   MELCHIOR, A. (1954). De geneeskunde in het Amazonegebied (Medicine in the region of the Amazone). *NTG, 98*, IV, 3250–4; 3327–30; 3424–8; 3501–4; 3607–10; 3684–7; 3745–8. 20 ill.

5173   FERIZ, H. (1965). Een Indiaanse mythe over het ontstaan der geslachten (An Indian myth on the genesis of the sexes). *Organorama, II*, no. 5, 18–21.   *See also* 2416

Q. Japan

5174   ESSO Bzn., I. van (1941). Die medizinischen Beziehungen zwischen Japan und Holland im 17., 18. und 19. Jahrhundert. *Janus, XLV*, 114–36.

5175   HALBERTSMA, K. T. A. (1941–42). De betekenis van de Hollandse geneeskunde voor Japan in haar historische ontwikkeling (The significance of Dutch medicine to Japan in historical development).
I. *NTG, 85*, IV, 4196–200; *BGG, XXI*, 145–9.
II. Engelbert Kaempfer (1651–1716), *NTG, 86* (1942), 326–30; *BGG, XXII*, 20–4.
III. Carl Peter Thunberg (1743–1828). *NTG, 86*, I, 564–7; *BGG, XXII*, 28–31.
IV. Philipp Franz von Siebold (1796–1866). *NTG, 86*, II, 834–8; *BGG, XXII*, 44–8.
V. Jhr. Dr. J. L. C. Pompe van Meerdervoort (1829–1908). *NTG, 86*, II, 1088–92; *BGG, XXII*, 61–5.
VI. A. F. Bauduin (1829–1890). G. C. van Mansvelt (1832–1912). W. K. Gratama (1831–1888). A. J. C. Geerts (1843–1883). *NTG, 86*, III, 1956–60; *BGG, XXII*, 106–10, 4 ports.

5176   — (1941). *De beteekenis van de westersche geneeskunde met name de*

Hollandsche voor Japan in hare historische ontwikkeling (The significance of western medicine, particularly Dutch medicine to Japan in
historical development). 56 pp., 4 ill. Drukkerij Waltman, Delft.

5177 MA, Eiko (1959). Japan's encounter with western medical Science:
"The beginning of Dutch study", being the memoirs of a 18th century
doctor. *BHM, 33*, 315–29.

5178 — (1961). The impact of Western medicine on Japan. Memoirs of a
pioneer. Sugita Gempaku, 1733–1877. *Arch. int. Hist. Sci., 14*, 65–84.
– Western medicine penetrated into Japan by the translation of Dutch works.
Gempaku wrote his memoirs under the title: *The beginning of Dutch Studies*
(Rangaku Kotohajime).

5178ª ACHIWA, G. (1973). The change-over from Dutch to German for the
learnings of western medicine in the local parts of Japan in the early
Meiji period. *Nihon Ishigaku Zasshi, 19*, 1–18 [Japanese with English
abstract].

5178ᵇ — (1974). On the Westernization of Japanese Medicine: with emphasis
on the influence of Herman Boerhaave. In: *Circa Tiliam*, 49–60. Brill,
Leiden.

5179 PAS, P. W. van der (1964). The earliest microscopical observations
in Japan. *Arch. int. Hist. Sciences, 17*, 223–38, 8 ill.
– Some of the illustrations of Murishina Churyo's book *Komo Zatsuwa* (Edo, 1787),
are plates from J. Swammerdam's work *Historia generalis ofte Algemeene Verhandeling der bloedeloose Dierkens* (Utrecht, 1669).

5180 WAGENSEIL, F. (1959). Die drei ersten unter europäischem (holländischen) Einflusz entstandenen japanischen Anatomiebücher. *SA, 43*,
61–85, 7 ill.
– refers to translations into Japanese of the book of Justus Danckers *Ontleding des
menschelijke Lichaems*, Amsterdam, 1634, 1635, 1667) and of the Leyden physician
Gerard Dicten *Anatomische Tabellen*, Amsterdam 1734.

5181 ACHIWA, Goro (1963). A list of Dutch original medical books (the
HANAURA or KAHO medic. school's library: 1876–1878). [Japanese].
Studium Historiae Medicae (published by Collegium ad stud. Hist.
Med. Osaka University, medical school. Kitaku, Osaka (Japan).

5182 — (1966). The list of Foreign books belonging to HANAURA (KAHO)
Hospital. *Reports Ass. Hist. Eng. Language*, no. 57.

5183 OHYA, Zensetsu (ed.) (1973). *Geneesku(n)dig Nederlandsch-Japansch*

Woordenboek (Dutch-Japanese Medical Dictionary). 227 pp. Kane-hara's Uitgevers-Maatschappij. Tokyo-Kyoto.
– With a preface (in Dutch) by G. A. Lindeboom.

5184 ACHIWA, Goro (1965). Gottlieb Salomon: *Handleiding tot de verlos-kunde*, 2de druk, Amsterdam (1826), translated by YADABE KYOUN into Japanese (1845). [Japanese]. *Japanese Medical Journal*, 18 Nov., 1965 no. 2166.
– This book introduced the caesarian section into the Japanese medical world. Salomon was doctor medicinae and lecturer on obstetrics at Leyden. The first edition dates from 1817.

5184ª OTAKI, T. (1973). "Seisetsu-naika-senjo", the first translated book of internal medicine. *Nihon Ishigaku Zasshi*, *19*, 19–28, 165–73; 333–42. [Japanese with English abstract].
– also on Joh. de Gorter (1689–1762).

5184ᵇ KOUSBROEK, Rudy (1974). Als een wit paard. De ontleedkundige ta-felen 200 jaar geleden in het japans vertaald (As a white horse. The anatomical tables translated in Japanese 200 years ago). *NRCHandels-bl.*, 8 june, Cult. Suppl., no 191, 1.

5185 RIPKA, B. K. (1968). Die Japanische Ausgabe des Werkes für die Oftal-mologie von J. J. Plenck. *Communic. de Historia Artis Medicinae* (Boedapest), no. 45, 135–42, ill.
– The Japanese translation of Plenck's *De morbis oculorum* (Kyoto, 1815) was made after the Dutch translation of M. Pruys (Rotterdam, 1787). J. J. E. Plenck (1733–1807) wrote textbooks on all branches of medicine (*Doctrina de morbis oculorum*, Vienna, 1777).

5186 [Anonym] (1963). Koan Ogata (1810–1863); promotor van Neder-landse geneeskunst in Japan (Koan Ogata (1810–1863): promotor of Dutch medicine in Japan). *M.C.*, *18*, 564, portr.

5187 AOKI, J. (1969). On S. Tuboi, a pupil of Ogata's school of Dutch Learn-ing. *Nihon Ishigaku Zasshi*, *15*, 209–13.
– Japanese with English abstract.

5188 DROOGLEEVER FORTUYN, A. B. (1926). Takano Nagahide. *NTG*, *70*, I, 983–7; *BGG*, *VI*, 63–7.

5189 ITAKURA, K. and R. ITAKURA (1962). Studies of trajectory before the days of Dutch learning. Reprinted from: *Japanese studies in the his-tory of science*, n. 1, 83–93, ill., 8° Firenze.

5190 [   ] (1971). *Rangaku in Japanese culture*. Proceedings of the Symposium on the Historical Relations between the Netherlands and Japan, Leyden, September 7–13, 1969 (Japanese with English summaries), 405 pp., Tokio.

– Rangaku is Dutch learning; with an important chapter (IV) on Dutch-Japanese relations in Medicine in the 17th century; with a.o. contributions on Boerhaave's influence, on Willem ten Rhijne and on Pompe van Meerdervoort. Chapter V deals with Dutch learning in local communities (Okayama, Osaka, Niigata).

5190[a] LUYENDIJK-ELSHOUT, A. M. (1974). Vesalius en Rangaku. De introductie van westerse anatomie in Japanse tekstboeken (V. and Rangaku. Introduction of western anatomy into Japanese textbooks). *NTG, 118,* 988.

– short report of a paper. (Vesalius is not mentioned).

5190[b] LUYENDIJK-ELSHOUT, A. M. (1973). "Anatomia reformata". The Dutch handbook of anatomy from the Baroque period. *Nihon Ishigaku Zasshi, 19,* 377–83 [Japanese].

– on Dutch anatomical works (a.o. of Kulmus) translated into Japanese.

5191 BOWERS, John Z. (1965). *Medical Education in Japan.* From Chinese medicine to Western. 174 pp., ill. Harper & Row, New York, Evanston and London.

– provides much information on the influence of Dutch medicine in Japan: On Pompe van Meerdervoort: 27–32, 143.

5192 ACHIEE ACHIWA, Goro (1965). The influence of European medicine on Japanese surgery [Japanese]. *Nihon Ishigaku Zasshi (J. Japanese Soc. Med. Hist., 11,* 1–27.

5193 OFFNER, C. B. and H. VAN STRAELEN (1963). *Modern Japanese religions with special emphasis upon their doctrines of healing.* Brill, Leiden.

5194 SUGITA, Genpaku (1969). *Dawn of Western Science in Japan. Rangaku Kotohajime.* XXX + 74 pp., 11 ill. The Hokuseido Press, Tokyo.

5195 MACLEAN, J. (1973). Natural Science in Japan I. Before 1830. *Ann. Sci., 30,* 257–98.

5196 KLEIWEG DE ZWAAN, J. P. (1918). *Oude betrekkingen tusschen Nederland en Japan* (Old relations between the Netherlands and Japan). Amsterdam, 8°.

– Published by Jap. Comm. of the "Ver. tot verbreiding van kennis over Nederland in den Vreemde", no. 2. Also in: *Kolon. T. VII,* no 5 and 6.

5197 SAKAGUCHI, Masao (1968). On the pharmaceutical reference books used by the author Udagawa Yôan of the Seimi-Kaisô [Japanese]. *Kagakushi Kenkyu,* 7, 49–56.

– The sources for this pharmaceutical work were chiefly Dutch versions of works by J. B. Trommsdorff, Karl Gotfried Hagen, H. J. van Houte and J. A. van Water. *See also* 363–5 (Boerhaave), 1411–3 (Pompe v. Meerdervoort), 1435–9, 1552, 1730.

R. China

5198 KLEIWEG DE ZWAAN, J. P. (1917). *Völkerkundliches und Geschichtliches über die Heilkunde der Chinesen und Japaner mit besonderer Berücksichtigung der holländischen Einflüsse.* Nat. Verh. Holl. Mij Wetenschap. 3e Verz., VII, Haarlem, 4°.

5199 SNAPPER, I. (1941). *Chinese lessons to Western medicine* (A contribution to geographical medicine from the clinics of Peking Union Medical College), New York-London.
– 2nd edition [1965?].

5200 KAN, L. B. (1965). Introduction to Chinese medical literature. *Bull. Med. Libr. Ass.*, *53*, 60–70.

5201 DUNNING, A. J. (1972). Prikken tegen pijn. Acupunctuur (Pricking against pain. Acupuncture). *Elsevier's Magazine*, *28*, no. 42, 14 Okt., 105–13.

5202 KOSTER, S. (1921). Iets over de geneeskunde in China en Japan, speciaal wat betreft de verzorging van krankzinnigen (Something on medicine in China and Japan, especially concerning the care of lunatics). *NTG*, *65*, I, 3100–13; *BGG*, *I*, 267–80, 2 ill.

5202[a] KOOPMAN, J. (1921). Over Chineesche letters in verband met de geneeskunde (On Chinese letters in connection with medicine). *NTG*, *65*, I, 1913–4.

5202[b] [Anonym] (1962). De Chinese en westerse invloed op de geneeskunde in Japan (Chinese and western influence on medicine in Japan). *Periodiek*, *17*, 195–202.
– also on the influence of Dutch medicine.

Chapter XXII

Medicine and Art

Art has served medicine by illustrating medical works and drawing title-prints.

On the other side artists have made portraits of doctors, or have pictured them at their work as an anatomist, physicians visiting their patients, etc. Patients suffering from various diseases as well as surgical procedures have often been pictured.

Literature has often dealt with physicians and their professional behaviour in an admiring or a satyrical way. The doctor has often been introduced into poetry, stage and opera. Some authors have made medical-musical historical studies.

The entries in the section museums are alphabetically arranged according to the towns.

In this chapter sections are also inserted referring to exhibitions, philately etc.

A. Painting, drawing and plastic art

General

5203 [   ] (1895–1933). *Atlas van Stolk*, Katalogus der historie-, spot- en zinneprenten, betrekkelijk de geschiedenis van Nederland (Atlas of Stolk, Catalogue of historical and emblematical prints and caricatures related to the history of the Netherlands), 10 vols., register, no pl.

5204 LEERSUM, E. C. van and W. MARTIN (1910). [116] *Miniaturen der lateinischen Galenos-Handschrift der königlichen oeffentlichen Bibliothek in Dresden. Db. 92–93 in phototypischer Reproduktion.* Leiden, f°.

5205 WALSUM, G. C. van (1930). Een vergeten medicus-schilder (A forgotten physician-painter). *NTG, 74,* I, 529–30; *BGG, X,* 51–2.
– on S. H. W. van Trigt (Dordrecht).

5206 DONGEN, J. A. van (1962). The Role of the Netherlands in the Evolution of Medicine. Illustrated with Dutch Pictorial Art. *J. Int. Coll. Surgeons*, *38*, 377–88, 3 ill.

5207 SETERS, W. H. van (1963). Lyonet's Kunstboek. (Lyonet's Art-book). *Med. and biol. Ill.*, *13*, 255–64, ill. *See also* 1208

5208 LINT, J. G. de (1921). Afbeeldingen van enkele geneesheren uit de oudheid (Pictures of some physicians from antiquity). *NTG*, *65*, I, 1262–72; *BGG*, *I*, 113–22, 4 ill.

5209 SCHOUTEN, J. (1967). "De antieke geneeskunst" ("Ancient medicine"). *Imago*, calendar of Nederlands Klassiek Verbond.

5210 RIJNBERK, G. van (1935). Over portretten en portretalbums naar aanleiding van een geschenk door de familie *Tilanus* (On portraits and photograph-albums with reference to a gift from the family —). *NTG*, *79*, 3296–9; *BGG*, *XV*, 141–4.

5211 LAMERS, A. J. M. (1923). L'importance de quelques drapelets de pélerinage flamands pour l'histoire de la médecine. *Janus*, *XXVII*, 8–14, ill.

5212 CORTEJOSO VILLANUEVA, L. (1962). La pintura holandesa del siglo XVII y su visión de la enfermedad. *Bol. Cult. Cons. Col. méd. Esp. 25* (161), 65–71, ill.

5213 NUYENS, B. W. Th. (1923). Van een Hollandschen goudsmid, die Galenus voorstelt (On a Dutch goldsmith, representing Galenus). *NTG*, *67*, II, 1625–9; *BGG*, *III*, 279–83, 2 portrs.

5214 [   ] (1918–1927). Geneeskundige kunstkalender voor het jaar 1927 (Medical art-calendar for the year 1927). J. Philip Kruseman, Den Haag.
– Nine volumes, with each *ca* 26 ill.

5215 WELCKER, A. (1951). Aesculapius en Hygieia. Onbekende aesculaapvoorstellingen uit het cinquecento naar aanleiding van een tekening toegeschreven aan Jan Stephen van Calcar (Aesculapius and Hygieia. Unknown aesculapius-pictures from the cinquecento with reference to a drawing attributed to Jan Stephen van Calcar). *NTG*, *95*, 1373–6; *BGG*, *XXXI*, 15–8, 2 ill.

5216 PROPER, R. (1959). Jan Stephan van Calcar-Portraits of the Artist. *J. Hist. Med.*, *14*, 519–22, portr.

5217 — (1959). Jan Stephan van Calcar: a little-known self-portrait. *BHM.* *33*, 466–9, portr.

5218 Gils, J. B. F. van (1925–1926, 1936). Hippocrates' bezoek bij Democritus (Hippocrates on a visit to Democritus). *NTG, 69*, II, 1132–40; *BGG, V,* 219–27. *NTG, 70,* (1926), I, 542–5; *BGG, VI,* 37–40, 2 ill. *NTG, 80,* (1936), 3171; *BGG, XVI,* 115.

5219 Hofstede de Groot, C. (1925). Hippocrates op bezoek bij Democritus (Hippocrates on a visit to Democritus). *NTG, 69*, I, 30–5; *BGG, V,* 1–6.

5220 Kroon, B. L. (1925). Hippocrates op bezoek bij Democritus (Hippocrates on a visit to Democritus). *NTG, 69,* I, 597–9; *BGG, V,* 38–40.

5221 Phillipovich, E. von (1959). De arts in de ogen van de patient (The doctor in the eyes of the patient). *Ciba-Symposium, 7,* 77–9 4, ill.
 – on 4 paintings attributed to Werner van den Valckert (*ca* 1620) and representing the physician as Christ, as an angel, as a man and as a devil. The representation is borrowed from etchings of Hendrik Goltzius.

5222 Haak, B. (1972). Regenten en regentessen, overlieden en chirurgijns (Amsterdamse groepsportretten van 1600 tot 1835) (Governors and ladys governors, members of the board, surgeons. (Amsterdam group portraits from — till —)). *Antiek, 7,* 81–116, 47 ill.; 287–302, 20 ill.; also as a monograph.

5222ª Vos, T. A. (1974). Wandelingen (III). Museumwandeling. Oog in magie en kunst (Walks (III). Museum-walk. Eye in magic and art). *Arts en Wereld, 7* no 4, 29–43, 5 ill.

Anatomy

5223 Krivatsky, Peter (1968). Le Blon's Anatomical Color Engravings. *J. Hist. Med., 23,* 153–8, col. pl.
 – refers to a colour plate of the shoulder published by Arent Cant (1695–1723) as a sheet.

5224 Chastel, A. (1966). L'anatomie artistique et le sentiment de la mort. *Méd. France,* no 175, 17–32.
 – with pictures of Y. Diemerbroeck, F. Ruysch and G. Bidloo.

5225 Bynum, William F. (1968). "Anatomy lecture on the brain". Pen and ink drawing by an unknown 17th century Dutch master. *J. Hist. Med., 23,* 196, 1 ill.

5226 LINT, J. G. de (1923). Een skeletprent van Peter de Wale (A picture of a skeleton from — —). *NTG, 67*, II, 1618–21; *BGG, III*, 272–5.

5227 ANDEL, M. A. van (1940). Twee anatomische beeldjes (Two anatomical statuettes). *NTG, 84*, IV, 3899–3901; *BGG, XX*, 156–8.

5228 COCKX-INDESTEGE, Elly (1971). Twee anatomische planodrukken met beweegbare onderdelen, uitgegeven bij Silvester van Parijs te Antwerpen, ca 1540–1550 (Two anatomical broadsides with movable parts, printed in Antwerp by — —, ca — —). *Sci. Hist., 13*, 91–102, 4 ill.
– The male figure has six, the female seven superimposed flaps.

5229 LEFANU, William (1960). Anatomical drawings by Jacobus Schijnvoet. *Oud-Holland, 75*, 54–8, ill.
– A part of an illustration of William Cheselden's *Osteographia* (1723) is made by the Dutch engraver Jac. Schijnvoet (1685– after 1733).

5230 WEERSMA, P. (1940). Bij eenige teekeningen van Leonardo da Vinci (To some drawings of — —). *NTG, 84*, III, 2555–60; *BGG, XX*, 111–6, ill.

5231 LEERSUM, E. C. van (1913). Leonardo da Vinci and the acupuncture of the heart. *Janus, XVIII*, 351–6, 3 ill.

5232 SCHOUTEN, J. (1972). Hartsymboliek (Heart-symbolism). *Antiek, 7*, no 7, 520–6.

5232ª HANEVELD, G. T. (1974). De plotselinge (hart)dood op oude afbeeldingen (Sudden (heart)death on old pictures). *Arts en Wereld, 7*, no 3, 33–6, 2 ill.

Anatomy Lessons

5233 LINDEBOOM, G. A. (1960). L'anatomie dans l'art des Pays-Bas septentrionaux. *Janus, XLIX*, 182–6.

5234 FINLAY, J. F. (1958). Anatomy lessons by the 17th and 18th century Dutch artists. *Dent. Mag.* (London), *75*, 9–15, ill.

5235 NUYENS, B. W. Th. (1928). *Het ontleedkundig onderwijs en de geschilderde Anatomische lessen van het Chirurgijnsgilde te Amsterdam in de jaren 1550 tot 1798* (Anatomical teaching and the painted anatomical lessons of the surgeons' guild at A. in the years 1550 till 1798). *Jaarversl. Kon. Oudheidk. Gen.* (1928).
– Also separately: 50 pp., ill. P. N. van Kampen en Zn., Amsterdam. 4°.

5236   CETTO, Anna Maria (1961). Ontleedkundige afbeeldingen. VIII. Een
       portret van een onbekend anatoom (Anatomical pictures. VIII. A
       portrait of an unknown anatomist). *Ciba-Symposium*, *9*, 23–5. ill,
       – design of an anatomy lesson. The anatomist may be J. J. Rau (1668–1719),
       professor at Leyden.

5237   — (1961). Ontleedkundige afbeeldingen. IX. Groep portret en voor-
       studie (Anatomical pictures. IX. Portrait of a group and preparatory
       study). *Ciba-Symposium*, *9*, 70–3, 6 ill.
       – on the Anatomy of Dr. Willem Roëll, painted by Cornelis Troost (1697–1750),
       and the drawing made for it.

5238   GEYL, A. (1906). Kleine bijdragen tot de geschiedenis van de schilde-
       rijen van 't Amsterdamsch chirurgijnsgild, o.a. van de anatomische
       les van Rembrandt (Small contributions to the history of the pictures
       of the Amsterdam surgeons' guild, o.a. of the Anatomy Lesson of —).
       Oud-Holland, XXIV, 38.

5239   SIX, J. (1905). De ligging van het lijk in Rembrandts Anatomische les
       van Dr. Deyman (The position of the corpse in Rembrandt's Anatomy
       lesson of —). *Oud-Holland, XXIII*, 37.

5240   CETTO, Anna Maria (1958). "L'Anatomie du docteur Deyman" de
       Rembrandt. *Ciba-Symp.*, *6*, 122–5, ill.

5241   — (1958). Rembrandts Anatomische les van Dr. Deyman (Rembrandt's
       Anatomy of Dr. —). *Ciba-Symp.*, *6*, 112–5, ill.

5241ª EEGHEN, I. H. van (1948). De anatomische lessen van Rembrandt
       (The anatomy lessons of —). *Amstelodamum*, *35*, 34–6, ill.

5242   HECKSCHER, W. S. (1958). *Rembrandt's Anatomy of Dr. Nicolaas Tulp.
       An Iconological Study.* X + 283 pp., 85 ill. N.Y. Univ. Press, Washing-
       ton.
       – reviewed by W. J. Cathey: *BHM, XXXV* (1961), 183–5.

5242ª — (1974). Petites perceptions: an account of sortes Warburgianae. 8.
       A baroque palimpsest. [Rembrandt's "Anatomy of Dr Nicolaas Tulp"].
       J. mediev. Renaiss. Stud., *4*, 120–2.

5243   QUERIDO, A. (1967). De anatomie van de Anatomische Les (The ana-
       tomy of the Anatomy Lesson). *Oud-Holland, 82*, 128–36, 5 ill.
       – on Rembrandt's Anatomy of Dr Tulp.

5244   FRIIS, H. (1962). Rembrandts ungdomsvaerk: Dr. Tulp anatomifore-
       laesning. *Medicinisk Forum* (Copenhague), *15*, 124–8, ill.

5245 SCHOUTEN, J. (1970). Een onbekende Anatomische Les van Dr. Nicolaas Tulp door Christiaan Coevershoff (An unknown Anatomy Lesson of N.T. by —). *Opstellen voor H. van de Waal*, 174–84, Amsterdam-
Leiden.

5246 EEGHEN, I. H. van (1971). De anatomische les van Christaen Coeuers-
hof of Op zoek naar een notoir misdadiger (Anatomy Lesson of — or
looking for a notorious criminal). *Jbk. Centr. Bur. Geneal.*, 181–97, ill.
See also 5413

5247 HELLINGA, G. (1929). [No title.] *NTG*, *73*, II, 4172; *BGG, IX*, 232.
- A satyrical poem on the Anatomical theatre at Amsterdam.

Physicians, pathology

5248 DONGEN, J. A. van (1967). *De zieke mens in de beeldende kunst*
(The sick in pictorial art). 274 pp., 200 ill., 8°. Mycofarm, Delft.

5249 [ ] (1958). La thèse de Tony Torrilhon – Brueghel était-il médecin? *Connaissance des Arts* (Paris), Oct., no 80, 68–76, 21 ill.
- on the unpublished medical thesis of – : *La pathologie chez Bruegel* (Paris 1958,
Supervisor: Prof. Alajouanine).

5249ᵃ TORRILHON, T. M. (1973). La pathologie chez Bruegel. *Orvostört.
Közl.*, *69/70*, 15–55, ill. refs.

5250 JOWELL, F. (1965). The paintings of Hieronymus Bosch. *Proc. Roy.
Soc. Med.*, *58*, 131–6.

5251 LUCAS, A. R. (1968). The imagery of Hieronymus Bosch. *Amer.
J. Psychiat.*, *124*, 1515–25.

5252 FROMM, E. (1969). The manifest and the latent content of two paintings
by Hieronymus Bosch: a contribution to the study of creativity.
Amer. Imago, *26*, 145–66.

5253 KRAMER, M. K. (1970). A study of the paintings of Vermeer of Delft.
Psychoanal. Quart., *39*, 389–426.

5254 CARSTENSEN, R. and M. PUTSCHER [ ]. Ein Bild von Vermeer in
medizin-historischer Sicht. *Dtsch. Ärztebl. ärzt. Mitt.*, *68*, 3460–2, ill.

5255 BONNEURE, Fernand (1960). Ziekte en dood in de schilderkunst (Disease and death in the art of painting). *West-Vlaanderen*, *9*, 393–403, ill.

5256 MILLER, P. W. (1965–'66). Provenience of the death symbolism in
Van Gogh's cornscapes. *Psychoanal. Rev. 52*, 60–6
See also 2053

5257 RIJNBERK, G. van (1920–1923). De geneesheer en geneeskunst in Nederlandsche prentverbeeldingen (Physician and medicine in Dutch pictures).
1. Inleiding (Introduction), *NTG*, *64*, (1920), 9–42, 35 ill.;
2. Phantastische Heelkunde (Fantastic Surgery). Het snijden van de kei (Cutting for the stone), *NTG*, *64*, II, 1555–63, 6 ill.;
3. De lagere heelkunst (Lower surgery). *NTG*, *65* (1921), I, 82–97, 14 ill.; *BGG*, *I*, 32–47;
4. De kiezentrekker (The tooth-drawer). *NTG*, *65* (1921), 1878–84; *BGG*, *I*, 165–75, 9 ill.;
5. Militaire chirurgie (Military surgery). *NTG*, *66* (1922)., I, 59–70; *BGG*, *II*, 1–12, 11 ill.;
6. Het aderlaten (Blood-letting). *NTG*, *66* (1922), II, 75–9; *BGG*, *II*, 169–73, 5 ill.;
7. De melaatschen en de lazarusklep (The lepers and the leper's clapper). *NTG*, *67* (1923), I, 34–41; *BGG*, *III*, 1–8, 8 ill.

5258 — (1929). De geneesheer en de geneeskunst in Nederlandsche prentverbeeldingen (Physician and medicine in Dutch pictures). V [8]. Het steensnijden (Cutting for the stone). *NTG*, *73*, I, 1113–23; *BGG*, *IX*, 73–83, 8 ill., 2 portrs.

5259 MEIGE, Henry (1896–97). Les arracheurs de "Pierres de tête" *Janus*, *I*, 393–6; 497–502, ill.

5260 LIÉTARD, (1897–'98). (Un arracheur de pierres de tête). *Janus*, *II*, 375, ill.
   – Letter to the editor. With a drawing after D. Teniers.

5261 GILS, J. B. F. van (1940). Het snijden van de kei (Cutting for the stone). *NTG*, *84*, II, 1310–8; *BGG*, *XX*, 57–65, 4 ill.

5262 MENDEN, J. F. (1969). Operation for stones in the head. An engraving by Nicolaes Weydmans. New Haven, Yale Medical Library, Clements C. Fry Collection. *J. Hist. Med.*, *24*, 211.

5262[a] GROOT, I. M. de and D. de MOULIN (1974). De keisnijding. Een gravure van Johannes Theodoor de Bry (Cutting for the stone. An engraving by — —). *Organorama*, *11*, no 2, 28–30, 3 ill.

Leprosy

5263 ANDEL, M. A. van (1918). Afbeeldingen van leprozen op Nederland-sche kunstwerken (Pictures of lepers on Dutch works of art). *NTG*, 72, II, 1210–4.

5264 GOLDMAN, L. (1968). Favus mistaken for leprosy by artists of the Re-naissance. *Arch. Derm.* (Chicago), *98*, 660–1.

5265 ANDEL, M. A. van (1919). Quelques figures de lépreux dans l'art clas-sique des Pays-Bas. *Janus, XXIV*, 135–45, ill.

5266 — (1937). De leproos in de plastische kunst (The leper in plastic art). *NTG, 81*, 3848–54; *BGG, XVII*, 145–51.

5267 LINDEBOOM, G. A. (1968). Leprosy in the Art of the Low Countries. *Verh. XX. Intern. Kongress Gesch. Medizin, Berlin, 22.–27. August 1966*, G. Olms, Hildesheim, 521.

5268 — (1967). Die Leprösen in der alten Kunst der Niederlande. *Grünen-thal Waage, 6*, 90–4, ill.

5269 KOENEN, J. (1929). Over drie teekeningen van Hans Burgkmair (On three drawings by Hans Burgkmair). *NTG, 73*, 1107–12; *BGG, IX*, 67–72, 3 ill.
– H. Burgkmair (1473–ca. 1531) German painter and engraver. One picture re-presents the royal touch, another lepers.

Various topics

5270 MEIGE, Henry (1906). Un barbier-chirurgien de Gérard Dow. (Coll. Léopold Favre, à Genève). *Nouv. iconogr. de la Salpêtrière, XIX*, 3. Mai-Juin, 293–6, ill.

5271 MANUELIDES, Laura K. (1967). Kopster. An etching by Cornelis Dusart (1660–1704). New Haven Yale Med. Library. Clements C. Fry Collection. *J. Hist. Med.*, 22, 82, ill.

5272 HOFMEIER, H. (1961). Zur Abbildung einer Mamma-amputation bei Romeyn de Hooghe aus dem Jahre 1688. German, English and French summaries. *Münch. med. Wschr., 103*, 1162–4, ill.

5272ᵃ MOULIN, D. de and I. M. de GROOT (1974). De kankeroperatie door Romeyn de Hooghe (The cancer operation by — —). *Organorama, 11*, no 5, 22–3.

5273 COHEN, M. H. (1922). Een Middeleeuwsch Ziekenhuis (A Hospital in the Middle Ages). *NTG, 66*, II, 2621–2; *BGG, II*, 365–6, ill.

5273ª HANEVELD, G. T. (1974). Mensen met hoorns (Men with horns). *Arts en Wereld, 7*, no 1, 19–22, 4 ill.

5274 WEYDE, A. J. van der (1925). Vergrooting van de schildklier op oude schilderijen (Enlargement of the thyroid gland on old paintings). *NTG, 69*, II, 1149; *BGG, V*, 236.

5275 TRICOT-ROYER J. J. G. (1926). Les giants macabres de Boussu, Bruxelles, Vilvorde, Strasbourg, Beaune, Troyes, Enkhuyzen. *Bull. Soc. Fr. Hist. Méd. 20*, 84–90, ill.; 199–205.

5276 ANDEL, M. A. van (1938). Het portret van Heer *Henric van Naeldwijc*, een pathologisch document uit de Middeleeuwen (The portrait of Mr. —, a pathological document from the Middle Ages). *NTG, 82*, 1099–1102; *BGG, XVIII*, 37–40.
– The portrait shows a classical rhinophyma.

5277 REUTER, H. (1965). Holländischer Meister: Bildnis eines Unbekannten mit Rhinophym. *Berlin Med., 16*, 479.

5278 POSTMA, J. U. (1972). Leed Pejeron aan een paralyse van Erb-Duchenne? (Did — suffer from Erb-Duchenne paralysis?). *NTG, 116*, 1129–31.

5279 HOFMEIER, H. (1960). Das Podagra bei Jan Luyken und Abraham a Santa Clara (Zum Gedenken an den 250 jährigen Todestag des P. Abrahams). *Neue Ztschr. ärzt. Fortbild., 49*, 625–9, ill.

5280 SMALBRAAK, Jan (1957). *Trophoblastic growths. A clinical, hormonal and histo-pathologic study of hydatidiform mole and chorionepithelioma.* Thesis Utrecht, XII + 342 pp., ill. Planeta, Haarlem.
– with a picture of the wooden tablet in the church of Loosduinen, relating the story of the birth, in 1276, of the 365 "children" (all baptized!) of the Countess of Henneberg.

5281 HOEVEN, J. van der (1932). Een teruggevonden onbekende teekening van "stiers wreedheid" (Unknown picture of bull's cruelty). *NTG, 76*, 5579–82; *BGG, XII*, 257–60.
– on a "caesarean section" by a furious bull in 1647 at Zaandam.

5282 MEIGE, Henry (1901). Une extraction de la filaire vers la fin du XVIIe siècle. *Janus, VI*, 95–6, ill.
– on a drawing of Jan Luyken; on the removing of a round-worm from a knee.

5283 ENSELME, J. (1965). Le mirage des urines au XVIIe siècle, d'après la peinture hollandaise. *Rev. Lyon Med., 14*, 851–68.
– Essai d'iconographie médicinale.

5284 HOEVEN, J. van der (1929). Visioenen van een koortslijder (Visions of a fever patient). *NTG, 73*, I, 2173–4; *BGG, IX*, 123–4, 1 ill.
– Drawing of visions of a fever patient (J. E. Heemskerk, 1821).

5285 BERNET KEMPERS, A. J. (1936). Oogheelkunde in een Indisch reliëf (Ophthalmology in an Indian perspective). *NTG, 80*, III, 4030–2; *BGG, XVI*, 140–2.

5286 WEVE, E. (1931). De bril en de kunst (Spectacles and art). *NTG, 75*, 2991–2; *BGG, XI*, 184–5.
– included in the report of a meeting of the "Genootschap".

5287 — (1927). Over brillenafbeeldingen in de plastische kunst (On pictures of spectacles in plastic art). *NTG, 71*, II, 649–61; *BGG, VII*, 558–70, ill.

5288 NATER, J. P. (1972). Dermatologie en Schilderkunst I (Dermatology and art of painting). *Arts en Wereld, 5*, no. 5, 12–3; 4 ill.
See also 3748a

5289 CONE, T. E. J. (1964). Pediatrics in Art; home life of children in the sixteenth century. *Amer. J. Dis. Child., 107*, 147–8.

5290 H[OWARD], J. B. (1963). The dentist. An engraving by Lucas van Leyden (1494–1533). New Haven Yale Medical Library, Clements C. Fry Coll. *J. Hist. Med. 18*, 378, 1 pl.

5291 EBERT, G. (1958). David Teniers: der Alchemist. *Neue Ztschr. ärztl. Fortb. 47*, 528, ill., portr.

5292 BRINKMAN, A. A. A. M. (1967). The influence of Brueghel's print "The Alchemist". *Janus, LIV*, 141–5, 4 ill.
See also 2795

5293 TRICOT-ROYER, J. J. G. (1925). Tabatières Hollandaises à gravures médicales. *Bull. Soc. Fr. Hist. Méd. XIX*, 125–8.

5294 GRENDEL, E. (1964). Kupferstiche von Philipp Galle nach den Bildern des Stradanus. *Zur Gesch. Pharm., 16*, 14–5, ill.
– J. or H. Stradanus (van der Straat), a painter ,born at Brussels 1530, died at Florence 1605.

5295 ZIELONKA, J. S. (1972). "The circumcision". Copperplate engraving (1549) by Heinrich Goltzius (1558–1617). *J. Hist. Med., 27*, 80, 1 pl.
– In the New Haven. Yale Med. Library, Clements C. Fry Collection
See also 2978, 2980a (thoracopagus)

Rembrandt

5296 LINT, J. G. de (1930). *Rembrandt.* 113 pp. J. Ph. Kruseman, den Haag, 64 ill.
- Reviewed by G. van Rijnberk: *NTG, 74*, II, 5942; *BGG, X*, 321-2. Series: *Great Painters and their works as seen by a doctor*, Vol. I. (Series not continued).

5297 EMDE BOAS, C. van (1971). Rembrandt als erotischer Künstler. *Z. Psycho-som. Med., 17*, 187–93.

5298 [Anonym] (1958). Shadow and soul. The artistic insight of Rembrandt. *M.D. med. Newsmag., 2* (8), 77–81, ill.

5299 JARCHO, S. (1969). Rembrandt's "Eye-operation". *Bull. N.Y. Acad. Med., 45*, 1396–8.

5300 GRABMAN, James P. (1973). Tobit recovering his sight. Engraving by A. de Marcenay after Rembrandt. *J. Hist. Med.*, XXVIII, 45.
- Antoine de Marcenay de Ghuy (1724-1811), painter, sculptor, engraver and essayist.

5301 SCHMIDT-DEGENER, R. (1922). Rembrandt und Vondel. F. Saxl (ed.). *Studien der Bibl. Warburg*, nr. IX.

5302 SCHOUTEN, J. (1969). Rembrandt en de geneeskunde (R. and medicine). *Specimina Specia*, september, 1–9.

5303 GRECO, T. (1970). Rembrandt e il cancro della mammella. *Osped. Ital. Chir., 22*, 141–4.

5303ª EEGHEN, I. H. van (1969). Rembrandt en de mensenvilders (— and the human skinners). *Amstelodamum, 56*, 1–11, 3 ill.
See also 1959a, 2080–3; 5239–45 (Anatomy Lessons)

Jan Steen

5304 JULIEN, P. (1970). Un empirique de Jan Steen. *Rev. Hist. Pharm.* (Paris), *20*, 163–4, ill.

5305 GILS, J. B. F. van (1920, 1921). Een detail op de doktersschilderijen van Jan Steen (A detail in the doctor's paintings of —). *Oud-Holland XXXVIII* (1920), 200; *NTG, 65*, I, 2561; *BGG, I*, 219.

5306 — (1921). Het vuurtje op Jan Steen's schilderijen (The little fire in the paintings of —). *NTG, 65*, I, 2868; not in *BGG*.

5307 — (1934). Jan Steen en de dokters (Jan Steen and the physicians).
NTG, *78*, 3168–9; *BGG*, *XIV*, 151–2.
– Short report of a lecture, communicated by Van Andel.

5308 EBSTEIN, E. (1931). Jan Steen, der Maler des Krankenzimmers. *Ther. Ber. 8*, 113–6, 5 ill.

5309 VRIES, J. de (1903). De zieke dame van Jan Steen (The ill lady of —). *Eigen Haard*, 648.

5310 VERHOEFF, A. (1921). Een detail op de doktersschilderijen van Jan Steen (A detail on the paintings of a physician by —). *NTG*, *65*, I, 2733.

5311 MEIGE, Henry (1900). Les médecins de Jan Steen. *Janus*, *V*, 187–90; 217–28, ill.

5312 — (1899). Les peintres de la médecine (école hollandaise) Le vieillard malade de Jan Steen. *N. Iconogr. Salpêtrière*, *12*, 497–500.

5313 CHURCHMAN, J. W. (1907). The physician in the paintings of Jan Steen. *Bull. Johns Hopkins Hosp.*, *18*, 480–3.

See also 5499

Frans Hals

5314 REGNAULT, Félix (1929). Frans Hals vu par un médecin. Un portrait de paralyse faciale. Ivrognerie de sa vieillesse due à la misère comme pour Rembrandt. *Bull. Soc. Fr. Hist. Méd. XXIII*, 28–31.

5315 VINKEN, P. J. and E. DE JONGH (1963). De Boosaardigheid van Hals' Regenten en Regentessen (The malice of Hals' Governors and Lady Governors). *Oud-Holland*, *78*, 1–26.

Popular prints, caricatures, varia

5316 LINT, J. G. de (1918). *Geneeskundige volksprenten in de Nederlanden* (Medical popular prints in the Netherlands). Thesis Leiden, 122 pp., ill. Gorinchem, 8°.
– also as a monograph.

5317 — (1919). Volkstümliche Bilder auf dem Gebiete der Medizin in den Niederlanden. *Janus*, *XXIV*, 253–302, ill.

5318 RIJNBERK, G. van (1914). De kwakzalver in de Nederlandsche prent-kunst (The quack in pictorial art in the Netherlands). *NTG*, *56*, I, 1924–8, 3 ill.

5319   VETH, Cornelis [1927]. *De arts in de caricatuur* (The physician in caricature). ill. Van Munster, Amsterdam no d.

– With an introduction by G. van Rijnberk. Reviewed by J. G. de Lint: *BGG*, *VII* (1927), 410–1.

5320   — (1927). *Der Arzt in der Karikatur*. Stollberg, Berlin.

5321   HOEVEN, J. van der (1930). Inleiding tot een demonstratie van eenige caricaturen en prenten betreffende Gall en diens leer (Introduction to a demonstration of some caricatures and pictures with regard to Gall and his doctrine). *NTG*, *74*, 5922–7, 2 ill.; *BGG*, *X*, 301–6.

5322   ANDEL, M. A. van (1940). Een ivoren spierbeeldje en zijn maagschap (An ivory muscle-statuette and its relationship). *NTG*, *84*, 2942–8; *BGG*, *XX*, 121–7.

5323   THIENEN, Trithjof van (1930). *Das Kostüm der Blütezeit Hollands.* 180 pp., 72 pp., 8°. (Kunstwissenschaftliche Studien, Bd 4). Deutscher Kunst Verlag, Berlin.

5324   VINKEN, P. J. (1960). H. L. Spiegel's Antrum Platonicum. A Contribution to the Iconology of the Heart. *Oud-Holland, LXXV*, 125–42.

5325   LUBBERS-VAN DER BRUGGE, C. J. M. (1957). Het schilderij "Na de Promotie" van N. van der Waay (The painting "after the Graduation" by —). *Jbk. Amstelodamum, 49*, 129–45, 11 ill.

Emblems

5326   SCHOUTEN, J. (1963). *De slangestaf van Asklepios als symbool van de geneeskunde* (The serpent staff of Asklepios as a symbol of medicine). Thesis Leiden (Supervisor: H. van de Waal), 214 pp., 61 ill., Schotanus & Jens, Utrecht.

– also as a monograph, with a foreword by G. A. Lindeboom. Brocades-Stheeman, Amsterdam-Meppel, 2nd ed. (no d.); contains also descriptions of many medals, coins, etc.

5327   — (1967). *The Rod and Serpent of Asklepios Symbol of Medicine*. 260 pp., ill., Amsterdam-London-New York.

5328   — (1968). *The pentagram as a medical symbol*. 78 pp., 41 ill., De Graaf, Nieuwkoop, 8°.

– reviewed by F. R. Forbes: *J. Hist. Med.*, *24* (1969), 363 and by: Cathey, W.J.: *BHM, XLIV* (1970), 489.

5329 — [no d.]. *Het pentagram als medisch teken* (The pentagram as a medical symbol). 79 pp., Den Haag.

5330 ASSIES, W. J. (1951). Het medische embleem zoals wij het voeren (Our nowadays medical emblem). *MC, 6,* 158–66, 1 ill.

5331 GILS, J. B. F. van (1921). Emblemata met geneeskundige voorstelling (Emblems with medical representations). *NTG, 65,* I, 661–70; *BGG, I,* 75–84, 8 ill.

5332 ANDEL, M. A. van (1928). Vroedvrouwenbordjes (Signboards of the midwives). *NTG, 72,* 2665–9; *BGG, VIII,* 149–53.

5333 HOFMEIER, H. K. (1972). Die emblematische Bedeutung des Falhutes in der niederländischen Literatur. Beitrag zur niederländischen Emblematik. *Med. Welt* (Stuttgart), *23,* 1614–5, ill.

5334 BOO, J. A. de (1971). Medische emblemen in de heraldiek (Medical heraldic emblems). *Spiegel Historiael, 6,* 226–33, 41 ill.

5335 HANEVELD, G. T. (1973). Het blazoen van de Colleoni's. Beeld van een zeldzame aandoening (The blazon of the — Picture of a rare affection). *Arts en Wereld, 6,* n° 12, 18–9, 3 ill.
– The rare affection is triorchism (three testicles).

5336 VINKEN, P. J. (1959). The modern Advertisement as an Emblem. *Gazette, 5,* 234–43.

Stone-tablets, Epitaphs, etc.

5337 ANDEL, M. A. van (1934). De gevelsteen en de geneeskunst (The stone-tablet and medicine). I. *NTG, 78,* III, 3575–9; *BGG, XIV,* 155–9, 10 ill.; II. *NTG, 78,* IV, 4558–63; *BGG, XIV,* 196–201. 10 ill.

5338 BOERMA, N. J. A. F. (1932). Grafschrift op het kerkhof te Bedum (Epitaph in the cemetery at B.) *NTG, 76,* IV, 5586; *BGG, XII,* 264.

5339 — (1939). Grafschrift te Vierhuizen (Epitaph at V.) *NTG, 83,* IV, 4868; *BGG, XIX,* 232.

5340 GILS, J. B. F. van (1920). Overblijfsel van een chirurgijnsgilde (Rest of a surgeons' guild). *NTG, 64,* I, 445.
– On the pictorial bier of the surgeons' guild at Workum; included in a report of a meeting of the "Genootschap".

5340ᵃ DIJKSTRA, O. H. (1973). De Gasthuispoort aan het Groot Heiligland te Haarlem (The Hospital gate on — — at H.). *Jbk. Haerlem*, 100–12, 5 ill.

Title-pages

5341 COHEN, Hk (1929). Les titres-planches de quelques anciens herbiers et pharmacopées édités en Hollande. *VIᵐᵉ Congrès Int. d'Hist. Méd. Leyde-Amsterdam 1927*, p. 112–3. Anvers.

5342 ANDEL, M. A. van (1933–34). De geneeskundige practijk der 17e eeuw naar titelprenten (The medical praxis of the 17th century with regard to title-pages). I. *NTG*, 77, 4991–5; *BGG*, *XIII*, 241–5, 7 ill.; II. *NTG*, 77, 5402–5; *BGG*, *XIII*, 270–3, 6 ill.; III. *NTG*, 78, 69–73; *BGG*, *XIV*, 23–6, 6 ill.

5343 HOFMEIER, H. K. (1961). Die von François van Bleiswijck zur Zeit Boerhaaves gestochenen Titelseiten der Leidener medizinischer Doktorsdissertationen. *Ärztl. Mitt.* (Köln), 46, 2504–6, ill.

5344 — (1962). Schöne Titelseiten medizinischer Doktorsdissertationen aus Leiden zur Zeit Boerhaaves. *Ärztl. Mitt.*, (Köln), 47, 1098–1102, ill.

5344ᵃ LINT, J. G. de (1930). Titelprenten met geneeskundige voorstellingen van Jan Luyken (Title-pages with medical images by —). *Oude Kunst*, 7, no. 8, 229–41.

See also 333–42 (Boerhaave), 1830–8 (Vesalius), 2409, 2511 4975–86 (Pharmacy and Art).

B. Literary Art

Prose

5345 BURGER, D. (1949). Geneeskundige toekomstvisioenen in de literatuur van vijf eeuwen (Medical visions of the future in the literature of five centuries). *NTG*, 93, 3752–6; *BGG*, *XXIX*, 63–7.

5346 VISSER, Ab (ed.) (1965). *Hippocrates en Hermandad*. 243 pp. Kon. Ned. Gist- en Spiritus fabriek, Delft.
– An Anthology of murder-stories with some medical aspect. (Conan Doyle et al).

5347 LODATO, Gaetano (1971). Virgilius gezien door een medicus (— seen by a physician). *Hermèneus, 43*, no. 1, 1–11.
– On the veterinary aspects of Virgilius' *Georgia.* translated from the Italian by C. Ypes.

5348 TORREN, J. van der (1942). Daniël Defoe's *Robinson Crusoe* en de aanvangskoorts bij malaria (Defoe's *Robinson Crusoe* and the initial malarial fever). *NTG, 86*, III, 3085–6; *BGG, XXII*, 163–4.

5349 SCHLICHTING, Th. H. (1939). Thomas More over neigingen tot zelfmoord (— and suicidal thoughts). *NTG, 83*, II, 1492–6; *BGG, XIX*, 68–72.

5350 ERNSTING, W. (1962). Menno ter Braak en de psychoanalyse (— and psychoanalysis). *NTG, 106*, I, 83–4.

5351 THOMASSEN, M. H. J. P. (1905). Cervantes et la médecine. *Janus, X*, 543.

5352 PENNING, C. P. J. (1935). Het ongehoorde wonder (The wonder unheard of). *NTG, 79*, IV, 5167–9; *BGG, XV*, 230–2.
– on a novel by H. Zschokke (1771–1848).

5353 GILS, J. B. F. van (1946). De slaap (Sleep). *NTG, 90*, I, 627–32; *BGG, XXVI*, 19–24.

5354 VINKEN, P. J. (1958). Some Observations on the Symbolism of the Broken Pot in Art and Literature. *American Imago, 15*, 149–74.

5355 HERMANS, Eduard H. (1961, 1962) *Humor in de geneeskunde* (Humour in medicine). 2 vols. I: 153 pp., ill. II: 154 pp., ill. Kon. Ned. Gist- en Spiritusfabriek, Delft.

See also 701–3 (F. v. Eeden), 974–8 (J. P. Heye).

Poetry

5356 ANDEL, M. A. van (1937). Geneeskundige poëzie uit het begin der 19de eeuw (Medical poetry from the beginning of the 19th century). *NTG, 81*, IV, 4261–2; *BGG, XVII*, 153–4.

5357 WALSEM, G. C. van (1928). Een vergeten medicus-dichter (A forgotten physician-poet). *NTG, 72*, II, 5474–6; *BGG, VIII*, 349–51.
– on Nicolaas Jansz. van Wassenaer (Haarlem).

5358 — (1930). *Med. Dr. Nicolaas van Wassenaer. Harlemias, het beleg der stad Haarlem in een Griecksch gedicht verhaald*, en opnieuw uitgegeven

door — (M.D. — —, the siege of the city of H. told in a Greek poem and edited again by —). Sijthoff, Leiden.
  – Reviewed by G. van Rijnberk: *NTG*, *74* (1930), IV, 5937–8; *BGG*, *X*, 316–7.

5359 THEUNISZ, Joh. (1934). "Demokriets en Herakliets pelgrimasie" (The pilgrimage of — and —). *NTG*, *78*, III, 3584–6; *BGG*, *XIV*, 164–6.

5360 BOSHOUWERS, H. (1910/1911). Dante en de geneeskunde (— and medicine). *Med. Wbl.*, *17*, 25.

5361 GREWEL, F. (1949). A cent diables la vérolle. *NTG*, *93*, III, 3006; *BGG*, *XXIX*, 58.
  – on a poem on lues; cf: letters to the editor (with same title) by W. C. A. H. Essed: *NTG*, *93*, IV, 3757–8; *BGG*, *XXIX*, 68–9 and by A. G. J. Hermans: *NTG*, *93*, IV, 3758–9; *BGG*, *XXIX*, 69–70.

5361ᵃ STOPPELAAR, F. de (1974). De eerste dichtende medicus in de lage landen was een hekeldichter (The first poet-physician in the Low Countries was a satirist). *Specimina Specia*, *15*, dec., 10–12, ill.
  – On Jan de Weert (?–1362) who published in 1351 his "Nieuwe Doctrinael", a didactic work.

5362 DONINCK, A. van (1931). Bilderdijk en de geneeskunde: "De ziekte der geleerden" (— and medicine: "The illness of learned men"). *NTG*, *75*, II, 2361–70; *BGG*, *XI*, 137–46.

5363 GILS, J. B. F. van (1943). Kopper(tjes)maandag. Een geestig misverstand van Bilderdijk (Printers' Monday. A witty misunderstanding of —). *NTG*, *87*, III, 1492–5; *BGG*, *XXIII*, 68–71.

5364 VISSER, R. P. W. (1972). De dichter Bilderdijk en de plantenanatomie (The poet — and plant-anatomy). *Sci. Hist.*, *14*, 17–28.
  – with English summary.

5365 ANDEL, M. A. van (1927). De geneeskunst in de werken van Jacob Cats (Medicine in the works of — —). *NTG*, *71*, II, 2350–63; *BGG*, *VII*, 68–94.

5366 GILS, J. B. F. van (1943). Vader Cats en anderen over wanlusten (Father — and others on extravagant appetite). *NTG*, *87*, I, 485–62; *BGG*, *XXIII*, 21–5.

5367 HOFMEIER, H. (1967). Zwei Gedichte des niederländischen Schriftstellers Jakob Cats (1577–1660) über das Zahnziehen. *Zahnärtzt. Mitt.*, *57*, Heft 12, ill.

5368 BISSELING, G. H. (1921). Tanden en tandheelkunst in de dichtkunst der eeuwen (Teeth and dentistry in poetry through the centuries). *T. Tandh.*, *XXVIII*, 969.

5369 [   ] (1925). Bladvulling (Stop-gap). *NTG*, *69*, I, 1139; *BGG*, *V*, 72.
- A small poem of the Dutch poet Tollens for patients with cholera and their families, 1853).

5370 LINT, J. G. de (1918). Een gedicht van den dichter-geneesheer J. Ant. van der Goes (A poem of the physician-poet — —). *NTG*, *62*, I, 1408.

5371 PINKHOF, H. (1927). De Muzen en de Koepokken (The Muses and cowpox) *NTG*, *71*, II, 112; *BGG*, *VII*, 516.

5372 KOOPMAN, J. (1928). Een gedicht over de inenting (A poem on vaccination). *NTG*, *72*, II, 4986; *BGG*, *VIII*, 323–4.

5373 FRANCIS, W. W. (1957). On the Death of Harvey. A premature threnody by Nikolaas van Assendelft. *J. Hist. Med.*, *XII*, 254–5.

The Stage

5374 WINKEL, J. te (1915). De kwakzalver op ons tooneel in de 16de eeuw (The quack on our stage in the 16th century). *NTG*, *59*, I, 1915–23.

5375 GILS, J. B. F. van (1917). *De dokter in de oude Nederlandsche tooneel literatuur* (The physician in the old Dutch stage-literature). Thesis University Leiden (Supervisor: E. C. van Leersum). Haarlem. 8°.

5376 — (1917). *Der Arzt in der alten niederländischen Bühnenliteratur*; Leiden.
- Reviewed by F. M. G. de Feyfer: *Janus*, *XXII* (1917), 414–5.

5377 ANDEL, M. A. van (1917/'18) De dokter in het Oud-Hollandsche blijspel (The physician in the Old Dutch comedy). *Med. Wbl.*, *24*, 385; 404.

5378 — (1917/'18). De kwakzalver in het Oud-Hollandsche blijspel (The quack in the Old Dutch comedy). *Med. Wbl.*, *24*, 577; 593.

5379 — (1918/'19). De dokters van Molière op het Hollandsch tooneel (The physicians of — on the Dutch stage). *Med. Wbl.*, *25*, 209; 227; 241.

5380 — (1922). Les médecins de Molière au théatre classique des Pays-Bas. *Cptes Rend. 2me Congrès Int. d'Hist. Méd., Paris, Juillet 1921*. Evreux.

5381 GILS, J. B. F. van (1922). Molière's Zwanenzang (M. 's Swan-song) *NTG*, *66*, I, 322; not in *BGG*.

5382 — (1924). Psychiatrie op het tooneel (Psychiatry on the stage), *NTG*, *68*, II, 2255–6; *BGG*, *IV*, 292–3.

5383 — (1929). De inenting tegen de pokken op het tooneel (Vaccination against small-pox on the stage). *NTG*, *73*, II, 4660–2; *BGG*, *IX*, 261–3.

5384 DRIEL, B. M. van (1919). Een tooneelstuk met Pasteur als hoofdpersoon (A stage-play with — as principal character). *NTG*, *63*, I, 1971.

5385 GILS, J. B. F. van (1919). Narrenspiegel des Lebens. *NTG*, *63*, I, 2289.
 - Drama in five acts by K. Schönherr (1867–1943) an Austrian dramatist.

5386 — (1943). Het drama van den dood in het kraambed (The drama of death in childbed). *NTG*, *87*, I, 657–61; *BGG*, *XXIII*, 35–9.

C. Musicians, music, opera

5387 KOOPMAN, J. (1925). Mozart en zijn geneeskundigen (— and his physicians). *NTG*, *69*, I, 35–43; *BGG*, *V*, 7–15. (I).

5388 — (1925–1932). Geneeskundige-Muziekhistorische Studiën (Medical-music-historical studies. II. Franz Schubert. *NTG*, *69*, II, 1567–73; *BGG*, *V*, 247–53. III: Beethoven (not published in this journal; publication as a monograph was planned). IV: Glück. *NTG*, *73* (1929), II 5752–6; *BGG*, *IX*, 336–40 V: Drie krankzinnige toonkunstenaars (Three mad musicians). *NTG*, *74* (1930), I, 2918–26; *BGG*, *X*, 176–84. VI: Smetana. *NTG*, *75* (1931), IV, 4066–71; *BGG*, *XI*, 247–52. VII. Johann Sebastiaan Bach *NTG*, *76* (1932), II, 2235–8; *BGG*, *XII*, 101–4.

5389 — (1932). Arzt und Heilkunde in der Oper. *Med. Mitt.* (Schering-Kahlbaum), *4*, 106–11.

5390 COUL, P. G. Op de (1932). Naar aanleiding "Geneeskundig-muziekhistorische studies" VII. (With reference to "Medical-music-historical studies" VII). *NTG*, *76*, II, 2819; *BGG*, *XII*, 124.

5391 GRIMBERT, Charles (1924). La mélothérapie dans l'antiquité et son application à la mélancholie du peintre Hugo van der Goes (1420–1482). *Bull. Soc. Franc. Hist. Méd.*, *XVIII*, 149–52.

5392 KLEIWEG DE ZWAAN, J. P. (1913/'14). De muziek in de geschiedenis der geneeskunde (Music in the history of medicine). *Med. Wbl.*, *20*, 493.

5392ᵃ OLOF, Theo (1974). Medici & muziek (Physicians and music). *Organorama*, *11*, no 5, 17–20.

5393 KOOPMAN, J. (1927–1932). De geneesheer (dokter) op het operatooneel (The physician on the opera-stage).

5393.1 I. *NTG*, *71* (1927), I, 763–7; *BGG*, *VII*, 156–60
Doktor und Apotheker (Text: Stefani Jr. composer C. Ditters von Dittersdorf); Lo Speziale (opera buffa), J. Haydn): Der Waffenschmied (G. A. Lörtzing); Crispino e la comare (Le docteur Crispin), L. and F Ricci; Die toten Augen (text: H. H. Evers and M. Henry, composer: d'Albert).

5393.2 II. *NTG*, *71*, II, 1405–8; *BGG*, *VII*, 645–8
Der neue krumme Teufel (text: J. Kurz, composer J. Haydn). Guten Morgen, Herr Fischer (text: W. Friedrich, composer E. Stiegmann); Der Dorfbarbier (text: J. Weidemann Schenk, composer Joh. Schenk); Der Arzt der Sobeide (text: Zoref, composer Hans Gal); Isabelle et Pantalon (text: Mac Jacob, composer R. Manuel).

5393.3 III. *NTG*, *72* (1928), I, 1704–7; *BGG*, *VIII*, 105–8.
Der Augenarzt (text: Em. Veith, composer Adalbert Gyrowetz); Don Pasquale (text: and composer: G. Donizetti; L'elisire d'amore (text: Romani, composer G. Donizetti), the same text as used in the opera Le Philtre (composer: Auber); Hoffmann's Erzählungen (text: Barbier, composer J. Offenbach).

5393.4 IV. *NTG*, *72*, II, 3822–4; *BGG*, *VIII*, 226–8
Cosi fan tutte (text: Lorenzo da Ponte, composer W. A. Mozart) Chirurgie (text and composer: P. O. Ferroud).

5393.5 V. *NTG*, *73* (1929), II, 5162–4; *BGG*, *IX*, 302–4
Le médecin turc (text: Villiers and Gouffé, composer Isouard); La médecine sans médecin (text: Scribe and Bayard, composer Ferd. Hérold); Doktor Peschke oder Kleine Herren (text: D. Kalisch, composer A. Conradi); Le docteur Ox (text: Gille and Mortier, composer J. Offenbach); Apothécaire et perruquier (text: Frebault, composer J. Offenbach).

5393.6 VI. *NTG*, *74* (1930), I, 526–8; *BGG*, *X*, 48–50.
Unknown text-writer and composer. The name of the opera is also

unknown. The following announcement occurs: Bekant-Machungh
von der Baron B ... Kaiserliche Hoffracht und Leib-Medicus von Ade-
lichen Geblühte, aus dem althen hause N.: Professor Medicinae, Anatomiae, Chimiae & Philosophiae, etc. (perhaps Doktor Eisenbart,).
Le docteur Isambart (text: Kelm, composer "Vicomte de Flaross").
L'amore ammalato (Die Krackende Leibe) or: Antiochus und Strato-
nice (text: B. Feind, composer C. Graupner)

5393.7 VII. *NTG, 74*, I, 1782–5; *BGG, X*, 109–12.
Noel (text: Ferrier, composer Fr. D. Erlanger); Hannele's Himmel-
fahrt (text: Georg Graener, composer P. Graener); La Forza del Des-
tino (text: Piave, composer G. Verdi); Wozzeck (text: G. Buchner,
composer Alban Berg); "Arlecchino", ein theatralisches Capriccio
(text and music: Ferruccio Busoni); Mirjam or "das Maifest" (text:
Ganghoeffer, composer R. Heuberger); Der arme Heinrich (text:
and music Hans Pfitzner).

5393.8 VIII. *NTG, 74*, II, 4451–4; *BGG, X*, 257–60
Christelflein (text and music: Hans Pfitzner; Der Ferne Klang (text
and music: Franz Schreker); Der Barbier von Bagdad (text and music:
Peter Cornelius); Doktor Eisenbart (text: Falckenberg, composer
Hermann Zilcher).

5393.9 IX. *NTG, 75* (1931), II, 1810–13; *BGG, XI*, 133–6
"Das Mädchen von Pskoff" (text: Mesch, composer Rimsky-Kor-
sakoff); Die Leipziger Messe (text and music Sperontes); Le docteur
Magnus (text: Cormon and Carré, composer E. Boulanger); Der Dieb
des Glücks (text: Richard Schuster, composer Bernard Schuster);
Mandragola (text: Paul Eger, composer Ign. Waghalter).

5393.10 X. *NTG, 75*, IV, 5019–21; *BGG, XI*, 282–4
Die Apotheke (text: Engel, composer G. C. Neefe); Lukas der
Arzt (text: Math. von Kralik, composer Richard von Kralik); Die
Herzenskrankheit (text and music: Fritz Kaufman); Le docteur Blanc
(text: Catulle Mendès, composer Gabriel Pierné); Der schwarze Dok-
tor (text and music: Sepp Rosegger); Ein Damenkaffee oder der junge
Doktor (text and music: Alex. Dorn).

5393.11 XI. *NTG, 76* (1932), I, 77–9; *BGG, XII*, 18–20
Der Fidele Bauer (text: Victor Leon, composer Leo Fall); Friederike
(text: Herzer and Lohner, composer F. Léhar); Der Vogelhändler
(text: West and Held, composer Zeller); Hin und Zurück (text:

Schiffer, composer P. Hindemith); Gianni Schicchi (text and music: Puccini); Der Schatzgräber (text and music: Schreker); Turandot (text and music: Busoni).

See also 1952

D. Medals

5394 REYS, J. H. O. (1936). Medici op penningen (Physicians on medals). *NTG, 80,* III, 4044–5; *BGG, XVI,* 154–5, 14 ill.

5395 WEIJDE, A. J. van der (1929). Nederlandsche penningen, uitgereikt in verband met het inenten tegen pokken (Dutch medals presented in connection with vaccination). *NTG, 73,* II, 5149–55; *BGG, IX,* 289–95, 4 ill.

5396 — (1930). Nog een vaccinatiepenning (Again a vaccination-medal). *NTG, 74,* I, 61; *BGG, X,* 24.

5397 Esso Bzn, I. van (1937). Over een gouden medaille uitgereikt aan Dr J. van Renesse, te 's-Gravenhage in het jaar 1840 (On a gold medal presented to — — at The Hague in —). *NTG, 81,* II, 1462–3; *BGG, XVII,* 83–4, 3 ill.

5398 [Editorial] (1943). Winkler-medaille. *Psych. neurol. Bl., 46,* 208. – cf: *NTG, 99* (1955), II, 1134.

5399 [   ] (1966). De "Snellen-penning" door Prof. Dr J. ten Doesschate uitgereikt aan Mevrouw Dr. J. Schappert-Kimmijser (The presentation of the "Snellen-medal" to — —). *NTG, 110,* II, 1677. – included in a report of a meeting of the Dutch Society for Ophthalmology, 11 December 1965).

5400 GEMMIL, Ch. L. (1973). Medical Numismatic notes XI: Commemorative medals issued at the international physiological congresses. *Bull. N.Y. Acad. Med., 49,* 556–66, 6 ill. – with a picture of a medal of F. C. Donders (Groningen, 1913) and one of A. Vesalius (Brussels, 1956).

5401 WITTOP KONING, D. A. (1952). De nieuwe erepenning van de K.N.M.P. (= Koninklijke Nederlandse Maatschappij ter bevordering der Pharmacie) (The new medal of honour of the Royal Dutch Society for the promotion of Pharmacy). *PhW, 87,* 848-9, *Bull. Pharm.,* no IV.

5402 — (1972). *Pharmazeutische Münzen und Medaillen.* 48 pp. Govi–Verlag, Frankfurt a.M.

5402ª   ZWIERINGA, W. H. F. (1927). Gasthuis-Penningen (Hospital-badges). *Amstelodomum, 14,* 9.

> *See also* 31, 342, 394, 499, 500, 866, 1135, 1605, 2878, 3203, 4301, 4687, 4896, 5326.

E. Philately, emergency Money

Philately.

5403   WERSCH, L. van and W. H. WOLFF (1936). Artsen en postzegels (Physicians and stamps). *NTG, 80,* I, 400–1; *BGG, XVI,* 30–1, ill.

5404   GALLAS, Th. (1939). Medische philatelie (Medical philately). *NTG, 83,* III, 3921–3; *BGG, XIX,* 203–5.

5405   SCHMEINK, C. J. (1965–1967). Artsen op postzegels (Physicians on stamps). I. *NTG, 109,* II, 1253–60; *BGG, XLV,* 17–24; II, *NTG, 110* (1966), 26; III, *NTG, 111* (1967), 33.

5406   BOSMAN-JELGERSMA, H. A. (1973). Postzegels als venster op de geneeskunde (Stamps as a window to medicine). *Organorama, 10,* no 2, 11–4, ill.

5407   [   ] (1961). Philatelic personalities; Herman Boerhaave 1668–1738. *Brit. J. clin. Pract., 15* (1), 22.

5408   [   ] (1957). Illustration of a Pieter Camper postage stamp issued in the Netherlands in 1940. *Brit. J. clin. Pract., 11,* 397, ill.

5409   [   ] (1961). Medical stamps. Camilo de Castelo Branco (1825–1890) and Frans Cornelis Donders (1818–1889). *Wiss. med. J., 60,* 338.

5410   [   ] (1961). Philatelic personalities: Jean-Baptiste van Helmont 1577–1644. *Brit. J. clin. Pract., 15,* 877, ill.
  – A Belgian stamp, 1942

5411   [   ] (1961). Philatelic personalities: Gerhard Freiherr van Swieten 1700–1772. *Brit. J. clin. Pract., 15,* 596, ill.
  – An Austrian stamp, 1937

5412   [   ] (1961). Medical Stamps. Antonio Grossich (1849–1928) and Sape Talma (1847–1918). *Wiss. med. J., 60,* 306, ill.

5413   MAY, D. (1971). Stamps. "The Anatomy Lesson of Dr Tulp" on a Cameroon stamp. *Med. News-Trib., 3,* 18 October, 13, ill.

5414 SMITS, J. W. (1972–1973). Medische filatelie (Medical Philately) Red Cross 1972: *GG*, *3*, 361, ill.; Wereldgezondheidsmaand van het Hart (April 1972) (The World Health month of the Heart) *GG*, *3*, 421, ill.; Kinine (Quinine) *GG*, *3*, 479, ill.; Insulin (Three stamps: Switzerland (with a portrait of Banting); Canada (with an illustration of laboratory tools); Belgium (5 test-tubes, filled with the liquid of Fehling – blue to orange) *GG*, *3*, 518, ill. Cholera. *GG*, *4* (1973), 19, ill; Auto-inoculatie (Auto-inoculation), *GG*, *4*, 73, ill.; Longtuberculose bij historische personen (Lungtuberculosis with historical persons). *GG*, *4*, 251, 1 ill.; Gehandicapten (Handicapped persons). *GG*, *4*, 296; Gewonden (Wounded persons). *GG*, *4*, 146; 189; Phtisis pulmonum bij historische personen (Phtisis pulmonum with historical persons). *GG*, *5* (1974), no 4, 10, ill.

5415 MAY, D. (1973). Stamps (Red Cross, Netherlands). *Med. News*, april 30, 13, ill.

5416 FENECK, F. F. (1965). De geschiedenis van tuberculose, weergegeven aan de hand van postzegels (History of tuberculosis rendered with the help of stamps). *Tegen Tuberculose*, *61*, 14–9, ill.

5417 BRANS, P. H. (1952). Een pharmaceutische postzegel (A pharmaceutical stamp). *Bull. Pharm.*, no II, 29. See also 4204

Money

5418 HARTOG, C. den (1936). Medische voorstellingen op Duitsch noodgeld (inflatiegeld) (Medical pictures on German emergency money (inflation-money). *NTG*, *80*, II, 1485–9; *BGG*, *XVI*, 52–6, 6 ill.
– cf: letters to the editor (with same titles) by Th. Gallas: *NTG*, *80*, II, 2626–7; *BGG*, *XVI*, 99–100 and by J. L. H. Mendels: *NTG*, *80*, II, 2627; *BGG*, XVI, *100*.

F. Museums

5419 ROOSEBOOM, M. (1958). The history of science and the Dutch collections. *The Museum Journal*, *58*, 10 pp.

5420 WITTOP KONING, D. A. (1937). Nederlandsche openbare en particuliere pharmaceutische verzamelingen. Pharmaceutica in het Stedelijk museum te Alkmaar (Dutch public and private pharmaceutical collections. Pharmaceutica in the Municipal Museum at —). *Ph. W.*, *74*, 1585–9.

5421   STOKVIS, B. J. (1891). Het Koloniaal-Geneeskundig Museum te Amsterdam (The Colonial-medical Museum at A.). *NTG*, *27*, II, 245–52.

5422   DANIËLS, C. E. (1903). Het Koloniaal-Geneeskundig Museum te Amsterdam. Een ziektegeschiedenis (The Colonial-medical Museum at —. A case history). *NTG*, *39*, II, 1354.

5423   VEDER, W. R. (1911). Het St. Anthonius poorthuis te Amsterdam (The St. Anthonius gate-house at A.). *Eigen Haard*, *XXXVII*, 218; 270; 292; 358; 461; 565 and 764.

5423ª [V.] (1902). Het geschiedkundig medisch-pharmaceutisch Museum (The Historical medico-pharmaceutical museum). *Vox Med.*, *2*, no 23, 181.

5424   PIJNAPPEL, M. W. (1902). Een geschiedkundig medisch-pharmaceutisch museum (A historical medico-pharmaceutical museum). *Eigen Haard*, *XXVIII*, 727.

5425   [Editorial] (1912) Zu Anlass der Ausbreitung des Medischpharmazeutischen Museums in Amsterdam. *Janus*, *XVII*, 62–3.

5426   VALK, J. W. van der (1912). De Boerhaave-zaal in het Geschiedkundig medisch-pharmaceutisch museum (The Boerhaave-room in the historical medico-pharmaceutical museum). *Eigen Haard*, *XXXVIII*, 84.

5427   DANIËLS, C. E. (1902/03). Het geschiedkundig medisch-pharmaceutisch museum te Amsterdam (The historical medico-pharmaceutical museum at A.). *Bull. Ned. Oudh. Bond*, *IX*, 89.

5428   — (1905). *Gids voor de bezoekers van het Geschiedkundig Medisch-Pharmaceutisch Museum te Amsterdam* (Guide for the visitors of the Historical Medico-pharmaceutical Museum at A.) ill, Amsterdam. 8°.

5429   — (1907). De oude krankzinnigenzaal van het Geschiedkundig Medisch-pharmaceutisch Museum, in het Stedelijk Museum te Amsterdam (The old insane ward of the Historical Medico-pharmaceutical Museum, in the Municipal Museum at A.). *Eigen Haard*, *XXXIII*, 518.

5430   — (1907). *De Oud-Hollandsche krankzinnigenzaal van het Geschiedkundig Medisch-Pharmaceutisch Museum in het Stedelijk Museum*

(The Old Dutch insane ward of the Historical Medico-Pharmaceutical Museum in the Municipal Museum [at Amsterdam]. Amsterdam.
– on the occasion of the International Congress for psychiatry, neurology, etc.

5431 WITTOP KONING, D. A. (1953). Het Medisch Pharmaceutisch Museum (The Medical Pharmaceutical Museum). *PhW.*, *88*, 354–7; *Bull. Pharm.*, no. *V*, 7–10.

5432 — (1953). De Delftse apothekerspotten van het Medisch Pharmaceutisch Museum te Amsterdam (The Delft apothecary jars of the Medico-Pharmaceutical Museum at A.). *PhW.*, *88*, 710–7; *Bull. Pharm.*, *VI*, 14–21.

5433 — (1954). The Amsterdam Historical Medical-Pharmaceutical Museum. *Endeavour*, *13*, 128–33, portr., ill.

5434 — (1957). Das medizinisch-pharmazeutische Museum in Amsterdam. *Dtsch. Apoth. -Ztg.*, (Geschichtsbeilage), *9*, 24–5, ill. Also in: *Zur Gesch. der Pharmazie*, *9*, 24–5.

5435 — (1959). Het medisch-pharmaceutisch museum te Amsterdam, de medische afdeling (The medico-pharmaceutical museum at A., the medical section). *Noury Post*, *6*, nr. 10.

5436 DONGEN, J. A. van (1955). Het historisch Medisch-pharmaceutisch Museum in de Koestraat bij de Nieuwmarkt te Amsterdam (The historical Medico-pharmaceutical Museum in the — near the — at A.). *NTG*, *99*, I, 971–3; *NGG*, *XXXV*, 33–5.

5437 — (1961). Een portrettengalerij van medici uit de vorige eeuw; aanwinst van het geschiedkundig, Medisch-Pharmaceutisch Museum te Amsterdam (A gallery of portraits of physicians from the last century; an acquisition to the historical Medico-Pharmaceutical Museum at A.). *NTG*, *105*, I, 39; *BGG*, *XLI*, 7.

5438 WITTOP KONING, D. A. (1962). Het Nederlands Historisch Medisch Pharmaceutisch Museum (The Netherlands Historical Medico-pharmaceutical Museum). *Ons Amsterdam*, *14*, 24–7, ill.

5439 LINT, J. G. de (1922). Een blijvend monument voor de geschiedenis der geneeskunde (A lasting monument to the history of medicine). *NTG*, *66*, I, 1467; *BGG*, *II*, 122.
– on a collection in Belgium that was planned to be bought for the Medico-pharmaceutical Museum at Amsterdam.

5440 JONKMAN, J. (1913). De chirurgijnskamer te Enkhuizen (The surgeons' room at E.). *PhW*, *50*, 390. Also in: *Telegraaf*, 9 april 1913.

588   MEDICINE AND ART

5441 WESTRA VAN HOLTHE, J. (1930). *Catalogus van de voorwerpen in het
Waagmuseum en de Chirurgijnskamer te Enkhuizen* (Catalogue of the
subjects in the Waag Museum and the "Surgeons' Room" at E.).
no pl.
– Reviewed by M. A. van Andel: *NTG, 74* (1930), II, 4919; *BGG, X,* 279.

5442 SCHOUTEN, J. [no d.]. *De chirurgijnskamer in het Catharina-Gasthuis
te Gouda* (The surgeons' room in the Catharina-hospital at G.).
52 pp., 24 ill., Stedelijke Musea, Gouda. Imperator, Lisse.

5443 HOFMEIER, H. K. (1962). Die Chirurgenkammer im "Gasthaus" zu
Gouda. *Mat. med. Nordmark, 14,* 741–9, ill., refs.

5444 BOERMA, N. J. A. F. (1903). *Catalogus van de geschiedkundige verzameling verloskundige instrumenten der Universiteits-Vrouwenkliniek te
Groningen* (Catalogue of the historical collection of obstetrical instruments in the University Women's clinic at G.).

5445 BIERENS DE HAAN, J. A. (1941). *De Geschiedenis van een verdwenen
Haarlemsch Museum van Natuurlijke Historie 1759–1856* (History of
a vanished Haarlem Museum of Natural History). Bohn, Haarlem.

5446 [   ] (1967). *Natuurkundig Kabinet van Teylers Museum.* Beknopte
rondleiding langs een aantal belangrijke natuurkundige objecten in
het Natuurkundig Kabinet (Physical Cabinet of Teylers Museum.
Short guide to a number of important objects in the Physical Cabinet).
30 pp., ill., Haarlem.

5447 CROMMELIN, C. A. (1931). *Het Nederlandsch historisch natuurwetenschappelijk museum* (The National Museum for the History of Science).
Leiden, 4°, ill.

5448 LINT, J. G. de (1934). Openingsrede voor de geneeskundige afdeeling
van het Natuurwetenschappelijk Museum te Leiden op 28 April 1934
(Inaugural address for the medical section of the Museum for the
History of Science). *NTG, 78,* II, 2503–7; *BGG, XIV,* 118–22, ill.
– a.o. on the instruments of Solingen.

5449 ROOSEBOOM, Maria (1938). De geneeskundige afdeeling van het
Nederlands Historisch Natuurwetenschappelijk Museum te Leiden
(The medical section of the Dutch Museum for the History of Science).
NTG, 82, III, 4348–52; *BGG, XVIII,* 168–72, 3 ill.

5450 — (1959). Rijksmuseum voor de Geschiedenis der Natuurwetenschappen. Verslag van de directrice over het jaar 1957. (The National Mu-

seum for the history of Science. Report of the director on the year 1957). *Verslagen der Rijksverzamelingen over Geschiedenis en Kunst*, *79*, 131–41.

5451 — (1959). The National Museum for the History of Sciences at Leyden (Russian). *Voprosy Istorii Estetvosnaniia i Tekhniké*, 7, 113–20.

5452 — (1964). Rijksmuseum voor de Geschiedenis der Natuurwetenschappen. Verslag van de Directrice over het jaar 1962 (National Museum for the History of Science. Annual report 1962). *Versl. Rijksverz. Gesch. en Kunst*, *84*, 155–64.

5453 — (1965). Rijksmuseum voor de Geschiedenis der Natuurwetenschappen. Verslag van de Directrice over het jaar 1963 (National Museum for the History of Science. Annual report (1963). *Versl. Rijksverz. Gesch. en Kunst*, *85*, 225–38, ill.

5454 — (1966). Rijksmuseum voor de Geschiedenis der Natuurwetenschappen. Verslag van de Directrice over het jaar 1964 (National Museum for the History of Science. Annual report (1964). *Versl. Rijksverz. Gesch. en Kunst*, *86*, 203–17.

5455 — (1967). Rijksmuseum voor de Geschiedenis der Natuurwetenschappen. Verslag van de Directrice over het jaar 1965 (National Museum for the History of Science. Annual report 1965). *Versl. Rijksverz. Gesch. en Kunst*, *87*, 224–36.

– following reports have appeared in the succeeding yearbooks of which the name was changed into *Nederlandse Rijksmusea* in 1971 (report of 1972 appeared in 1974).

5456 LIGNAC, G. O. E. (1948). Het ontstaan en de ontwikkeling van het Pathologisch-Anatomisch Museum te Leiden (Origin and development of the Pathology Museum at L.). *NTG*, *92*, IV, 3700–1.

5457 ELSHOUT, A. M. (1950). De restauratie der praeparatenverzameling uit de 18e eeuw, van het anatomische Laboratorium te Leiden (The restauration of the collection of preparations of the Anatomical Laboratory at L. from the 18th century). *NTG*, *94*, I, 205–7.

5457ᵃ [Anonym] (1974). *Gids voor het museum van het anatomisch laboratorium van de rijks universiteit te Leiden* (Guide to the museum of the anatomical laboratory of Leiden University). 10 pp., pr. pr. Luctor et Emergo, Leiden.

5458 KRUYTZER, E. M. (1961). Le Musée d'Histoire naturelle de Maastricht. *Janus, L,* 62–5.

5459 VISSER CASIMIR, K. (1941). *Van de heksenwaag te Oudewater en andere weinig bekende zaken* (From the witches' weighhouse at Oudewater and other little known cases). 118 pp., ill. De Tijdstroom, Lochem.

5460 BOS, H. J. M. (1968). *Mechanical instruments in the Utrecht University Museum. Descriptive catalogue.* 70 pp., 40 ill., Utrecht.

5461 LAVEN, W. J. and J. C. VAN CITTERT-EYMERS (1967). *Electrostatical instruments in the Utrecht University Museum. Descriptive Catalogue.* 78 pp., 49 ill., Utrecht.

5462 CITTERT, P. H. van (1934). *Descriptive Catalogue of the Collection of Microscopes in charge of the Utrecht University Museum.* With an introductory historical survey of the Resolving power of the Microscope. 110 pp., ill., Groningen.
– Reviewed by M. A. van Andel: *NTG, 79* (1935), I, 906–7; *BGG, XV,* 68–9.

5463 VREEDENBURGH Jr, C. (1913). Een merkwaardig museum (A remarkable museum). *Natuur, XXXIII,* 289–95
– Museum of Typography at Haarlem, founded by Ch. Enschedé; Its library contains some old books by Dutch physicians.

5463ᵃ HANEVELD, G. T. (1974). The Schroeder van der Kolk museum collection. In: *Proc. XXIII Int. Congr. Hist. Med. London 2–9 Sept. 1972,* Vol. I, 733. The Wellcome Institute of the History of Medicine, London.

Foreign musea

5464 FRISON, E. (1966). *Henri van Heurck Museum. Geillustreerde inventaris van de historische microscopen onderdelen en uitrusting* (Illustrated inventory of the historical microscopes parts and outfit). Kon. Mij v. Dierkunde en Min. Nat. Opvoeding en Cultuur, Antwerpen.
– Text in Flemish, French, German and English. *See also* 4905a

See also 972

5465 ANDEL, M. A. van (1914). Een bezoek aan het Wellcome historical-medical museum te Londen (Visit to the Wellcome historical-medical museum at L.). *NTG, 58,* II, 1545–50.

5466 DONGEN, J. A. van (1959). Hall of Fame. De Nederlandse afdeling van de Hall of Fame van het International College of Surgeons te Chicago

(The Dutch section of the Hall of Fame of the International College of Surgeons at C.). *NTG, 103*, I, 40–2.   See also 5512a

5467   MAC LEAN, J. (1972). Enige gegevens over verzamelaars van voorwerpen van natuurlijke historie in het voormalige Nederlandsch Indië (Some details on collectors of objects of natural history in the former Dutch Indies). *Sci. Hist., 14*, 51–60.   See also 1865a

G. Exhibitions

5468   ANDEL, M. A. van (1921). Een historisch-hygiënische tentoonstelling (A historical exhibition on hygiene). *NRC*, 7 augustus.

5469   RIJNBERK, G. van (1961). Een geschiedkundige hygiënische tentoonstelling (A historical exhibition on Hygiene). *NTG, 65*, II, 32–3; *BGG, I*, 285–6.
        – On the historical section of the great exhibition on hygiene. (Amsterdam, october 1921); cf: letter to the editor (same title) by M. A. van Andel: *NTG, 65*, II, 758; not in *BGG*.

5470   NUYENS, B. W. Th. (1929). Exposition Médico-Historique à Amsterdam. *VIme Congrès Int. d'Hist. de la Méd. Leyde-Amsterdam 1927*, 200–3, Anvers.

5471   [   ] (1932). *Catalogus van de Tentoonstelling t.g.v. 3de eeuwfeest instelling Hooger Onderwijs (1632–1932)* (Catalogue of the Exhibition on the occasion of the 3rd centenary of the foundation of Higher Education). *XV* + 175 pp., 46 facs., 1081 nrs. Stedelijk Museum, Amsterdam.

5472   WITTOP KONING, D. A. (1953). Amsterdam: it houses one of Europe's finest scientific exhibits. *The Laboratory, 23*, 56–7.

5473   [   ] (1899). *Catalogus van de Historisch-Geneeskundige Tentoonstelling 1849–1899, ... te Arnhem, ter gelegenheid van het vijftigjarig bestaan der Nederlandsche Maatschappij ter bevordering der Geneeskunst* (Catalogue of the Historical-Medical Exhibition ... at A., on the occasion of the 50th anniversary of the Dutch Society for the Promotion of Medicine), III pp., G. J. Thieme, Arnhem.
        – Contains also a list of the exposed objects and a list of portraits of well-known Dutch physicians.

5474   [   ] (1949). *Catalogus van de schilderijen, tekeningen, grafiek, sculpturen, penningen, boeken en handschriften, oude instrumenten en curiosa op de Medisch-Historische Tentoonstelling ter gelegenheid van het eeuwfeest der Nederlandsche Maatschappij tot bevordering der geneeskunst in de Waag te Amsterdam, 7 Juli – 31 Augustus 1949* (Catalogue of paintings, drawings, graphic art, coins, books and manuscripts, old instruments and curiosa on the Medico-Historical Exhibition on the occasion of the centenary of the Dutch Society for the Promotion of Medicine, in the Weigh-house). 195 pp., ill. Ellerman Harms, Amsterdam.

5475   SLUITER, E. (1949). De medisch-historische tentoonstelling ter gelegenheid van het eeuwfeest der Kon. Ned. Maatschappij tot bevordering der geneeskunst (The medico-historical exhibition on the occasion of the 100th anniversary of the Dutch Society for the Promotion of Medicine). *NTG, 93*, III, 3021–3. (not in *BGG*).

5475ᵃ   HANEVELD, G. T. en A. M. LUYENDIJK-ELSHOUT (1974). *Arts & diagnose*. Tentoonstelling ter gelegenheid van het 125-jarig bestaan van de koninklijke nederlandsche maatschappij tot bevordering der geneeskunst (Physician and diagnosis. Exhibition on the occasion of the 125th anniversary of the Royal Dutch Society for the promotion of medicine). [30 pp.], ill. Drukkerij De Brink, Leiden.

5475ᵇ   [Anonym] (1974). Medische Tentoonstelling in Gouda. Over huisbezoek, artsen, diagnosen en artsenijbereiders (Medical Exhibition at G. On visitation, physicians, diagnoses and pharmacists). *Reform. Dagbl.*, Vrijdag 13 Sept.

5476   DONGEN, J. A. van (1949). Medisch-historische tentoonstelling (Medico-historical exhibition). *NTG, 93*, III, 2371–2; *Med. Cont., 4*, 409–10.

    – On the exhibition in the Weigh-house at Amsterdam, (a.o. manuscripts, old books and portraits).

5477   [   ] (1950). *Vroedmeester, pillendraaier en liefhebber der Natuur. Catalogus van de oude schilderijen, tekeningen, … instrumenten, kraamkamer, oude apotheek etc.* Op de historische tentoonstelling op verloskundig, pharmaceutisch en biologisch gebied, genaamd —) (1 Juli – 30 September 1950. In de Waag, Nieuwmarkt te Amsterdam) (Accoucheur, pill-roller and lover of nature. Catalogue of the pictures, drawings, … instruments, lying-in room, old pharmacy, etc. On the historical exhibition on obstetrics, pharmacy and biology, named —) [No pl.]

– Review by E. Sluiter *NTG* (1950), *94*, III, 2126–8 (not in *BGG*) and D. A. Wittop Koning, J. A. van Dongen and H. Engel: *Ons Amsterdam 2* (1950), 184–8 and by J. A. van Dongen: *MC*, *5* (1950) 520; *Elsevier's Wbl.*, 12 Augustus 1950.

5478 DONGEN, J. A. van (1960). De tentoonstelling over fertiliteit en steriliteit bij mens en dier in historie en kunst (The exhibition on fertility and sterility in man and animal, in history and art). *NTG*, *104*, I, 183–5; *BGG, XL*, 1–3.
– Amsterdam, 6–14 June 1959.

5479 [   ] (1973). *Catalogue Exhibition. Reinier de Graaf Tercentenary Symposium* Wednesday 8 – Saturday 11 August 1973 "de Leeuwenhorst", Noordwijkerhout. 13 pp. pr. pr.
– Symposium organised by the Society of Obstetrics and Gynecology of the Netherlands.

5480 GOGELEIN, A. J. F. (et al.) (1973). *Leven en werk van Antoni van Leeuwenhoek 1632–1723. Tentoonstelling ingericht ter gelegenheid van de officiële opening van het Antoni van Leeuwenhoek-Ziekenhuis 28 oktober – 27 november 1973* (Life and work of —. Exhibition held on the occasion of the official opening of the A. v. L. Hospital). 20 pp., ill. no pl.

5481 [   ] (1972). *Van Medicijnman tot medicus.* Panorama van meer dan twintig eeuwen medisch kunnen; van de kenners, de ziekten en de zieken; van de wereld er omheen. Catalogus van de Tentoonstelling 5 april – 3 juli 1972, in het Frans Hals museum te Haarlem (From Medicine-man to physician. Panorama of more than twenty centuries of medical knowledge; from the scientists, the diseases and the patients; and the world around them. Catalogue of the exhibition in the Frans Hals Museum at H.)

5482 [   ] (1939). *Catalogus van de tentoonstelling ter herdenking van den 150sten sterfdag van Petrus Camper, 1722–1789, gehouden te Groningen van 30 april tot 7 mei 1939* (Catalogue of the exhibition in commemoration of the 150th dying-day of Petrus Camper, held at G.). 50 pp., 5 ill. Groningen.

5482ᵃ [   ] (1953). *Gulden Strijd. 1903–1953. Catalogus medisch-historische herdenkingstentoonstelling ter gelegenheid van het 50-jarig bestaan der tegenwoordige vestiging van het Algemeen provinciaal stads- en academisch ziekenhuis van Groningen ... 1953.* (Golden fight. Catalogue of the medico-historical commemorative exhibition on the occasion of the 50th anniversary of the present establishment of the General provincial, municipal and academic hospital at G.). 32 pp. Ill. P. Noord-hoff Groningen.

5483 SCHLICHTING, Th. H. (1954). De tentoonstelling bij het 50-jarig bestaan van het Stads-, provinciaal- en academisch Ziekenhuis te Groningen (The exhibition on the occasion of the 50-years existence of the Muni-cipal provincial and academical Hospital at G.). *NTG*, *98*, I, 35–9; *BGG*, *XXXIV*, 9–13.

5484 STRENGERS, Th. (1907). De historische tentoonstelling op het aanstaan-de Natuur- en Geneeskundig Congres (The historical exhibition at the coming Congress of natural sciences and medicine). *Chem. Wbl.*, *IV*, 34.

5485 LEERSUM, E. C. van (1907). Mededeelingen over de tentoonstelling (Information on the exhibition). *Hand. 11e Ned. Nat. Gen. Congres* (April). *See* 5486.

5486 —, F. M. G. DE FEYFER and P. C. MOLHUYSEN (1907). *Catalogus van de geschiedkundige Tentoonstelling van Natuur- en Geneeskunde, te houden te Leiden 27 Maart – 10 April 1907 ter gelegenheid van het XIe Neder-landsche Natuur- en Geneeskundig Congres* (Catalogue of the historical exhibition of Natural Science and Medicine, to be held at L., on the occasion of the XIth Dutch Congress of Natural Science and Medicine). Ill., Leiden, 8°.

5487 — (1907). Exposition historique des sciences naturelles et de la mé-decine (27 Mars – 10 Avril 1907). Discours prononcé à l'occasion de l'ouverture du onzième congrès de Sciences naturelles et de médecine le 4 avril 1907 à Leyde. *Janus*, *XII*, 319–31.

5488 FEYFER, F. M. G. de (1907, 1908). Die historische Ausstellung der Na-tur- und Heilkunde in Leiden, 27 März – 10 April 1907. *Janus*, *XII*, 605–15 and 694–700; *XIII* (1908), 88–103, ill.

5489 MYNLIEFF, C. J. (1907). Het reddingswezen in de 18e en eerste helft der 19e eeuw (The life-saving service in the 18th and in the first half of the 19th century). *Catalogus van de Geschiedk. Tentoonst. van Natuur- en Geneesk. te Leiden*, 214.

5490 [   ] (1973). *History of the treatment of Bladder Stones and Cystos-copy. From Lichtleiter to fibre optics.* An Exhibition on the occasion of the XVth Congress of the International Society for Urology. 26 pp. Rijksmuseum voor de Geschiedenis der Natuurwetenschappen, Leiden Mededeling nr. 139.

5491 HUNGER, F. W. T. (1917). *Catalogus van de tentoonstelling gehouden te Leiden 29 Juni 1917, ter gelegenheid van den 400sten geboortedag van Rembertus Dodonaeus* (Catalogue of the exhibition held at Leyden 29 June 1917, on the occasion of the 400th anniversary of the birthday of —), Portr. Leiden, 8°.

5492 KROON, J. E. (1918). *Catalogus van de tentoonstelling te Leiden 30 Dec. 1918 – 31 Jan. 1919 ter gelegenheid van den 250en geboortedag van Herman Boerhaave* (Catalogue of the exhibition at L., on the occasion of the 250th anniversary of the birthday of —). Leiden, 8°.

5493 — (1919). Boerhaave-tentoonstelling (Boerhaave-exhibition). *NTG, 63*, I, 205.

5494 — (1919). De Boerhaave-tentoonstelling te Leiden (The Boerhaave exhibition at Leyden). *Bibliotheekleven, IV*, 33.

5495 LINT, J. G. de (1914). *Catalogus van de tentoonstelling over oude anatomie gehouden te Leiden, Jan. 1915, ter gelegenheid van de herdenking van den geboortedag van Andreas Vesalius, met een bijdrage van J. Boeke* (Catalogue of the exhibition on ancient anatomy held at L., on the occasion of the commemoration of the birthday of —, with a contribution by —), 1 ill., Gorinchem 8°maj.

5496 — (1934). De tentoonstelling en het portret van Volcher Coiter te Leiden (The exhibition and the portrait of — at L.). *NTG, 78*, II, 2486–7; *BGG, XIV*, 101–2.

5497 [   ] (1925). *Catalogus van de tentoonstelling ter herdenking van het driehonderdvijftig-jarig bestaan der Leidsche Universiteit* (Catalogue of the exhibition in commemoration of the 350th anniversary of Leyden University), 32 pp. 7 ill. Museum "De Lakenhal", Leiden, February MCMXXV, A. W. Sijthoff, Leiden.

5498 KRET, A. (1968). Rekonstruktion eines alchemistischen Laboratoriums des 16. Jahrhunderts im Museum für die Geschichte der Naturwissenschaften in Leiden. *Zur Gesch. Pharm., 20*, 1–3.

5499 GILS, J. B. F. van (1926). Naar aanleiding van de Jan Steen-tentoonstelling (With reference to the exhibition of —). [Lakenhal Leiden]. *NTG, 70*, II, 680–2; *BGG, VI*, 210–2.

5500 MUNTENDAM, P. (1925). Tentoonstelling te Alkmaar (Exhibition at Alkmaar). 17 Sept. – 1 Oct. 1925. *NTG, 69*, II, 1149; *BGG, V*, 236.
  – On the occasion of the 50th anniversary of the Noord-Holland Association "Het Witte Kruis". Paintings (several mentioned), drawings, plates, books etc.

5501 WITTOP KONING, D. A. (1949). *De oude Apotheek, tentoonstelling ter gelegenheid van het 200-jarig bestaan van de Gemeenteapotheek te 's-Gravenhage* (The old chemist's shop, exhibition on the occasion of the 200th anniversary of the Municipal pharmacy at The Hague), 's-Gravenhage.

5502 BRANS, P. H. (1959). Tentoonstelling "Schoonheid in de Pharmacie" en de najaarsvergadering van de kring voor de Geschiedenis van de Pharmacie in Benelux te Gouda, 22 en 23 november 1958 (Exhibition "Beauty in Pharmacy" and the autumnal meeting of the Circle for the History of Pharmacy in Benelux at —). *Bull. Pharm.*, no. *18* (June), 12–4.

5503 MOULIN, D. de and E. van der KLEYN (1972). *De artsenijbereidkunde vroeger en vandaag.* Tentoonstelling ter gelegenheid van de officiële opening van het opname gebouw van het Sint Radboud Ziekenhuis. 4 november – 3 december 1972 (Pharmacy in past and present). Exhibition on the occasion of the official opening of the admission building of the Radboud Hospital [Nijmegen]). 32 pp., 20 ill., Bur. Pers en Voorlichting Sint Radboud Zhs., Nijmegen.

5504 BERNET KEMPERS, A. J. (1971). "Bitter in de mond", een nieuwe tentoonstelling in het kruidentuinhuisje ("Bitter in the mouth", a new exhibition of bitter herbs in the botanical garden-house). *Ned. Openluchtmuseum. Bijdragen en mededelingen, 34*, no 1, 19–31.
      – description of the bitter herbs, exposed in the botanical garden house of the Museum at Arnhem.

5505 COBBEN, J. J. (1957). De tentoonstelling "Magie" te Antwerpen in de Stedelijke Feestzaal, Meir; 27 juli tot 15 september 1957 (The exhibition "Magics" at A. in the Municipal Festive Hall, Meir). *NTG, 101*, II, 2216; *BGG, XXXVII,* 41.

5506 WITTOP KONING, D. A. (1971). "Bezeten bezit" in het historisch Museum te Rotterdam ("Possessed possession" in the historical museum at Rotterdam). (Exhibition). *Bull. Pharm.*, no. *43*, augustus, 26–8, ill.

5507 CITTERT, P. H. van (1928). Historische tentoonstelling van antieke natuurkundige instrumenten te Utrecht (Historical exhibition of ancient physical instruments at U.). *NTG, 72*, I, 2224–5; *BGG, VIII,* 147–8.

5508 UNGER, W. S. (1926). Tentoonstelling betreffende de geschiedenis der genees- en natuurkunde in Zeeland (Exhibition concerning the history of medicine and physics in Zealand). *NTG, 70*, II, 661–9; *BGG, VI*, 191–9, portrs., 2 ill.

5509   [   ] (1960). *Oude drukken uit de Nederlanden.* Boeken uit de Collectie Arenberg, thans in de verzameling Lessing J. Rosenwald. Tentoonstelling Den Haag. Museum Meermanno-Westreenianum 29 augustus tot 9 october 1960. – Brussel Albert I-Bibliotheek 21 oktober tot 31 december 1960 (Old editions in the Netherlands. Books from the Collection Lessing J. Rosenwald. Exhibition at The Hague. – Brussels Albert I-Library). VIII + 158 pp., 19 fig., M. Nijhoff,

– See also French edition: *Livres anciens des Pays Bas. La collection Lessing J. Rosenwald provenant de la Bibliothèque d'Arenberg.* Bruxelles, 1960.

See also 2280

5509ᵃ   [   ] (1913). *Tentoonstelling "De Vrouw" 1813–1913* (Exhibition "The Woman" — —). 526 pp., Concordia, Amsterdam.

– Catalogue of the exhibition, held from May–October 1913 in "Meerhuizen", Amsterdam. With chapters on Hygiene, Education, Nursing etc.

See also 4975–87 (Pharmacy and Art)

Exhibitions in Foreign musea

5510   LEERSUM, E. C. van (1906). Ausstellung der Geschichte der Medizin in Kunst und Kunsthandwerk. 1 Mars au Avril 1906. *Janus, XI*, 196–200.

5511   KLEIWEG DE ZWAAN, J. P. (1906). De historisch-geneeskundige tentoonstelling te Berlijn (The historical-medical exhibition at Berlin). *Nosokomos, VI*, 244 and 263.

5512   — (1913). De geschiedkundige tentoonstelling te Londen (The historical exhibition at London). *NTG, 67*, II, 1326.

5512ᵃ   ROOSEBOOM, M. and J. A. van DONGEN (ed.) (1958). *Catalogue of the Netherlands Room* [Hall of Fame, Chicago], 59 pp. pr. pr. [Rijks Museum voor Geschiedenis Natuurwetenschappen, Leiden].

See also 5466

Indexes

Index of Authors

The references are to entry numbers, no page numbers are used in the index.

In case a reference mentions more than one author, only the name of the first author is included. The names of reviewers are not entered.

Likewise the names of secretaries of meeting reports and those of supervisors ("promotores") are not inserted in this index.

Double-barrelled names are to be looked for at the first name.

Index of (historical) Persons

This Index contains the names mentioned in the titles of the entries, the authors' names have been listed in a separate index.

References are to entry numbers. No page numbers are used in the index.

Index of Places

List of Sources

Abbrevations

Arch.	Archief, Archiv, Archive
Congr.	Congress
Gen.	Genootschap (Society)
Genootschap	Genootschap voor geschiedenis der geneeskunde, wiskunde, natuurwetenschappen en techniek (Society for the history of medicine, mathematics, natural sciences and techniques).
Jbk	Jaarboek (Yearbook)
Jrg	Jaargang (Volume)
Mbl.	Maandblad (Monthly)
Med.	Medical, medicine
N.R.	Nieuwe reeks (New series)
Nwe	Nieuwe (New)
Pr. pr.	Privately printed
Wbl.	Weekblad (Weekly)

Some Dutch periodicals, of which the complete title is given in the text, are not inserted in this index.

Abbottempo	Tijdschrift samengesteld door Abbott Universal Ltd. In Nederland: Abbott N.V. Amsterdam.
Acad. Med. N.J. Bull.	Academy of medicine of New Jersey Bulletin. New Jersey.
Acad. Rev.	Academy Review of the California Academy of Periodontology.
Acta allerg.	Acta allergologica. Kopenhagen.
Acta Belg. medic. et pharmac. milit.	Acta Belgica de arte medicinali et pharmaceutica militari. Brussel.
Acta Endocr.	Acta Endocrinologica. Copenhagen.
Acta Med. Hist. patav.	Acta Mediae Historiae patavina. Padova.
Acta méd. Tenerife	Acta médica de Tenerife. Santa Crux de Tenerife.
Acta Physiol. Pharmacol. Neerl.	Acta Physiologica et Pharmacologica Neerlandica North-Holland Publishing Company, Amsterdam.
Acta psychol.	Acta psychologica. Amsterdam.

Acta septimi	*Acta Septimi Conventus Historiae Scientiae Medicinae Mathesos Na-*
conventus	*turaliumque excolendae.* Amsterdam, 1974
Acta Univ. palack.	Acta Universitatis palackianae olomucensis Facultas medica. Tsjecho-
olomuc. Fac. med.	Slowakaije.
Adler	Zeitschrift für Geneaologie und Heraldik. Wien.
Ärztl. Mitt.	Ärztliche Mitteilungen. Köln.
Ärztl. Praxis	Ärztliche Praxis. München.
Ärztl. Viertel-	Ärztliche Vierteljahresrundschau.
jahresrundschau	
Afrika	Afrika, Maandblad van het Afrika Instituut. Den Haag (The Hague).
Alb. Nat.	Album der Natuur. Haarlem.
Alers et al.	Alers et al. (1899). *De ziekenverpleging en de zorg voor de openbare*
	gezondheid in de laatste 50 jaren. Ned. Tijdschrift voor Geneeskunde.
	Van Rossen, Amsterdam. 8°. These were previously published in the
	Catalogus der Historisch-Geneeskundige Tentoonstelling te Arnhem,
	Juli 1899.
Alg. Ned.	Algemeen Nederlandsch Familieblad, Tijdschrift voor Geschiedenis,
Familiebl.	Geslacht- en wapen- en zegelkunde, etc. 's-Gravenhage.
Alg. T. Wijsbeg.	Algemeen Nederlands Tijdschrift voor Wijsbegeerte en Psychologie.
Psych.	Van Gorcum, Assen.
Alkmaars Jbk.	Alkmaars Jaarboekje. Alkmaar.
Allg. Ztschr. f.	Allgemeine Zeitschrift für Psychiatrie und Psychische gerichtliche
Psychiatrie und	Medizin. Berlin.
Psychische gerichtli-	
che Medizin	
Ambix	Ambix. The Journal of the Society for the Study of Alchemy and Early
	Chemistry. W. Heffer, Cambridge.
Am. Heart J.	American Heart Journal. St.-Louis, USA.
Amer. J. Cardiol.	American Journal of Cardiology. New York.
Amer. J. Dis.	American Journal of Diseases of Children. Chicago.
Child.	
Am. J. Psychiatr.	The American Journal of Psychiatry. Baltimore, USA.
American Imago	American Imago. New York.
Amstelodamum	Amstelodamum. Maandblad voor de kennis van Amsterdam. Orgaan
	van het Genootschap Amstelodamum (see Jbk. Amstelodamum). De
	Bussy Ellerman Harms BV, Amsterdam.
Anaesthesiology	Anaesthesiology. Philadelphia.
Angéiologie	Angéiologie, organe officiel de la Société française d'angéiologie et
	d'histopathologie et du Collège international d'angéiologie. Paris.
Ann. Belg. Ver.	Annalen van de Belgische Vereniging voor Hospitaal Geschiedenis.
Hosp. Gesch.	Bruxelles,
Ann. Démog. hist.	Annales de Démographie historique. Paris.
Ann. Gesch. Oudhk.	Annalen der Geschiedenis van de Oudheidkundige Kring Ronse.
Kring Ronse	België.
Ann. Int. Med.	Annals of Internal Medicine. Philadelphia.
Ann. Méd. psychol.	Annales Medico-Psychologiques. Paris.
Ann. R.K. stud. Ned.	Annuarium der Roomsch-Katholieke Studenten in Nederland. Leiden.
Ann. Sci.	Annals of Science, includes Bulletin of the British Society for the His-
	tory of Science. Taylor & Francis, London. (Quarterly.)
Ann. Soc. belge	Annales des Sociétés belges d'Histoire des Hospitaux. Bruxelles.
Hist. Hosp.	
Ann. Soc. belges	Annales des Sociétés belges de Médecine tropicale, de Parasitologie et
Méd. trop.	de Mycologie. Anvers.

Ann. Soc. Méd.	Annales de la Société de médecine d'Anvers. Anvers.
Ann. Soc. Méd. Chir.	Annales de la Société Médico-chirurgicale de Liège. Liège.
Antiek	*Antiek*, Tijdschrift voor liefhebbers en kenners van oude kunst en kunstnijverheid. De Tijdstroom, Lochem.
Antonie van Leeuwenhoek	later: *Tijdschrift voor Hygiene en microbiologie en serologie.* Amsterdam.
Antwerps Arch. Bl.	Antwerpsch Archievenblad. Antwerpen.
AP	Aere Perennius. Verslagen en Mededelingen uit het Medisch-Encyclopaedisch Instituut der Vrije Universiteit Amsterdam. Amsterdam. (restricted circulation).
Archeion	Archivio di Storia della Scienza. Later: *Archives Internationales d'Histoire des Sciences.* Académie Internationale d'Histoire des Sciences, Paris.
Archeologia	Archeologia, Revue mensuelle. Paris-Bruxelles-Berne.
Arch. chir. neerl.	Archivum chirurgicum Neerlandicum. H. Veenman & Zn., Wageningen.
Arch. Dem.	Archives of Dermatology. Chicago.
Arch. Gesch. Med.	Archiv für Geschichte der Medizin (Leipzig). In 1929 continued as: *Sudhoffs Archiv.* F. Steiner Verlag, Wiesbaden.
Arch. Int. d'Hist. Sci.	Archives Internationales d'Histoire des Sciences. Paris.
Arch. Int. Med.	Archives of Internal Medicine. Chicago.
Arch. Int. Sci.	Archives Internationales des Sciences.
Archief (Arch. Zeeuws. Gen.).	Mededelingen van het Koninklijk Zeeuwsch Genootschap der Wetenschappen. Middelburg.
Archimedes	Archimedes, publication of the Foundation for Education, Science and Technology. South Africa.
Arch. Ned. Kerkgesch.	Archief voor Nederlandsche Kerkgeschiedenis. Den Haag.
Arch. néerl. Physiol. de l'homme et des animaux	Archives Néerlandais de la Physiologie de l'homme et des animaux. La Haye.
Arch. néerl. scienc. et nat.	Archives Néerlandaises des Sciences exactes et naturelles. La Haye. (Série III B = Sciences naturelles).
Arch. Ortop.	Archivio di Ortopedia. Milano.
Arch. Psicol. Neurol. Psichiat.	Archivio di Psicologica, Neurologica e Psichiatria. Milano.
Arch. Stenogr.	[Archiv für Stenographie]. (German).
Arch. di Storia della Scienza	Archivio di Storia della Scienza. Milano.
Arch. Zeeuws Gen.	See: *Archief.*
Arkh. Anat. Gistol. Embriol.	Arkhiv Anatomii Gistologii i Embriologii. Moskou.
Ars medici	Ars medici, Revue internationale pour le médecin praticien. Gand.
Art Digest	Art Digest. USA.
Art. méd.	L'Art médical. Nice.
Arts en Wereld	Arts en Wereld. Medisch pharmaceutisch tijdschrift. Medische Uitgeversmaatschappij "Arts en Wereld", Den Haag. (Monthly.)
Arthr. and Rheum.	Arthritis and Rheumatism. New York.
Arq. Anat. Antrop.	Arquivos de Anatomia y Antropologia. Lisboa.
Arq. bras. Natr.	Arquivos brasileiros de Nutriçao. Rio de Janeiro.
Atti del reale Ist. Veneto Sci lett. e Arti	Atti del reale Istituto Veneto di Scienze lettere ed Arti. Venetië.

Atti e Mem. Accad.   Atti e Memorie dell'Accademia di Storia dell'Arte Sanitaria (issued
Stor. Arte Sanit.   with *Rassegna di Clinica, Terapia e Scienze affini*). Roma.

BDHM Hyderabad   Bulletin of the Department of History of Medicine Hyderabad. Hyderabad.

Beaken   It Beaken. Tydskrift utjown fan de Fryske Akademy (Journal of the
Frisian Academy). Assen.

Beaufortia   Beaufortia. Series of miscellaneous publications of the Zoological
Museum of the University of Amsterdam. Amsterdam.

Been's Hist. Frag-   Been's Historische Fragmenten, C. Bredée. The Hague. Only a few
menten   issues have appeared. (1911–1913?).

Beitr. Gesch. Dort-   Beiträge zur Geschichte Dortmunds und der Grafschaft Mark. Dort-
munds u.d. Grafschaft   mund.
Mark

Beitr. Gesch. Pharm.   Beiträge zur Geschichte der Pharmazie und ihrer Nachbargebiete.
Berlin.

Ber. ROB   Berichten van de Rijksdienst voor het Oudheidkundig Bodemonder-
zoek in Nederland. Amersfoort.

Berl. Med.   Berliner Medizin, Organ für die gesamte praktische und theoretische
Medizin. Berlin.

BGG   Bijdragen tot de Geschiedenis der Geneeskunde Uitgave van het
Nederlands Tijdschrift voor Geneeskunde. Amsterdam; Bohn, Haarlem.

BHM   Bulletin of the History of Medicine. Organ of the American Association of the History of Medicine and of the Johns Hopkins Institute of
the History of Medicine. The Johns Hopkins Press, Baltimore.

Bibliotheekleven   Bibliotheekleven. Orgaan der Centrale Vereniging voor Openbare lees-
zalen en bibliotheken en van de Nederlandse Vereniging van Biblio-
thecarissen en bibliotheekambtenaren. Amsterdam.

Bibliothèque d'Huma-   Bibliothèque d'Humanisme et Renaissance. Genève.
nisme et Renaissance

Biblos   Biblos. Oesterreichische Zeitschrift fuer Buch- und Bibliothekswesen.
Dokumentation Bibliographie und Bibliophilie. Wien.

Biekorf   Biekorf. Dat is een leer- en leesblad voor alle verstandige Vlamingen.
Brugge.

Bijdr. Dierk.   Bijdragen tot de Dierkunde. Leiden.

Bijdr. Gesch.   Bijdragen voor de Geschiedenis der Nederlanden. Den Haag (The Hague).

Bijdr. Gesch.   Bijdragen voor de Geschiedenis van het Bisdom Haarlem. Haarlem.
Bisdom Haarlem

Bijdr. Gesch.   Bijdragen tot de Geschiedenis van Overijssel. Zwolle.
Overijssel

Bijdr. Gesch. Prov.   Bijdragen van de Geschiedenis van de Provincie der Minderbroeders
Minderbroeders in de   in de Nederlanden. Rotterdam.
Nederl.

Bijdr. Med./   Bijdragen en mededelingen van het Historisch Genootschap. Gronin-
Hist. Gen.   gen.

Bijdr. Med. Rijks-   Bijdragen en Mededeelingen van het Rijksmuseum voor Volkenkunde.
museum Volkenk.   Leiden.

Bijdr. Taal-, land-,   Bijdragen tot de taal-, land-, en volkenkunde van Nederlandsch-Indië.
Volkenkunde Ned.
Indië

Biogr. Mem. Fellows   Biographical Memoirs of Fellows of the Royal Society. London.
Roy. Soc.

Biol. in der Schule	Biologie in der Schule.
Bio-Lex.	*Biographisches Lexikon der hervorragenden Ärzte aller Zeiten und Völker.* 8 Vols. 3rd unchanged edition. Urban & Schwarzenberg, München-Berlin. (1962).
Bol. Cult. Cons. Col. méd. Esp.	Boletin Cultural e Informativo Consejo general de Colegios médicos de Espana. Madrid.
Bol. Inst. Stor. ital. arte San.	Bollettino dell'Istituto Storico Italiano dell'arte Sanitaria. Rome.
Boll. della R. Accad. medica di Roma	Bollettino e Atti della R. Accademia medica di Roma. Rome.
Boll. Soc. Ital. Farm. osped.	Bollettino della Società italiana di Farmacia ospedaliera.
Book Collector	Book Collector. London.
Boon's Magazijn	Boon's geïllustreerd Magazijn, continued as: *Morks Magazijn.* Amsterdam.
Bouwers van Indië	Bouwers van Indië. Een serie levensbeschrijvingen, uitgegeven in opdracht van het Koloniaal Instituut. Deventer.
Brabantia	Brabantia. Tweemaandelijks Tijdschrift van het Provinciaal Genootschap van Kunsten, Wetenschappen in Noord-Brabant en de Stichting Brabantia Nostra. 's-Hertogenbosch (Bois-le-Duc).
Brabants Heem	Brabants Heem. Tweemaandelijks Tijdschrift voor Brabantse Heem- en Oudheidkunde. Oisterwijk.
De Brabantse Leeuw	De Brabantse Leeuw. published by: Provinciaal Genootschap van Kunsten en Wetenschappen in Noord-Brabant, Genealogisch-Heraldische Sectie. Rotterdam.
Brit. dent. J.	British Dental Journal. London.
Brit. J. Addict.	British Journal of Addiction. London.
Brit. J. clin. Pract.	The British Journal of Clinical Practice. London.
Brit. J. Derm.	British Journal of Dermatology. London.
Brit. J. Hist. Sci.	The British Journal for the History of Science. London.
Brit. J. med. hypn.	British Journal of medical hypnotism. Kingsway, Sussex.
Brit. J. Plast. Surg.	British Journal of Plastic Surgery. Edinburgh.
Brusselse Post	Maandblad voor Brusselse Vlamingen. Brussel.
Brüsseler Ztg.	Brüsseler Zeitung.
Buiten	Buiten. Geïllustreerd Weekblad; (later "Het Landhuis") Amsterdam. 4°.
Bull. Cleveland med. Libr.	Bulletin of the Cleveland medical Library. Cleveland.
Bull. Hosp. Jt. Dis.	Bulletin of the Hospital for Joint Diseases. New York.
Bull. int. Soc. Secur. Ass.	Bulletin of the International Social Security Association. Genève.
Bull. Johns Hopkins Hosp.	Bulletin of the Johns Hopkins Hospital. Baltimore, USA.
Bull. Kol. Inst. Amsterdam	Bulletin van het Koloniaal Instituut te Amsterdam. Amsterdam.
Bull. Med. Libr. Ass.	Bulletin of the Medical Library Association. Chicago.
Bull. Mém. Soc. Int. d'hist. Méd.	Bulletin et Mémoires de la Société Internationale d'histoire de la Médecine. Ed.: F. A. Sondervorst Le Scalpel, Bruxelles.
Bull. Boymans	Bulletin van het Museum Boymans-Van Beuningen. Rotterdam.
Bull. Ned. Oudh. Bond	Bulletin van den Nederlandsen Oudheidkundigen Bond. Amsterdam.
Bull. N.Y. Acad. Med.	Bulletin of the New York Academy of Medicine. New-York.
Bull. Pharm.	Bulletin van de Kring voor de Geschiedenis van de Pharmacie in Bene-

lux. Cercle Bénelux d'histoire de la Pharmacie. Bruges & Amsterdam. (Irregular.)

Bull. Rijksmuseum Bulletin van het Rijksmuseum Amsterdam. Staatsuitgeverij, Den Haag (The Hague).

Bull. Séances Acad. royal. Sci. d'Outre Mer Bulletin des Séances de l'Académie Royale des Sciences d'Outre-Mer. Bruxelles.

Bull. signal. Hist. Sci. Techn. Bulletin signaletique Histoire des Sciences et des Techniques. Revue trimestrielle. Paris.

Bull. Soc. belge d'Ophthalm. Bulletin de la Société belge d'Ophthalmologie. Bruxelles.

Bull. Soc. fr. hist. Méd. Bulletin de la Société française d'histoire de la Médecine. Paris.

Bull. Soc. Roy. Bot. Belg. Bulletin de la Socétié Royale de Botanique de Belgique. Bruxelles.

Canad. med. J. Canadian medical Association Journal. Toronto.

Canad. psychiat. Ass. J. Canadian Psychiatric Association Journal. Ottawa.

Castalia Castalia. Rivista di Storia della Medicina. Milano, (Quarterly.)

Centaurus Centaurus. International Magazine of the History of Mathematics, Science and Technology. Munksgaard, Copenhagen.

Centr. Wbl. Centraal Weekblad voor de Gereformeerde kerken in Nederland. Drukkerij Libertas, Utrecht.

Cereb. Palsy Bull. Cerebral Palsy Bulletin. London.

Chem. Drugg. Chemist and Druggist. London.

Chemie en Techniek Chemie en Techniek Revue. Periodiek voor Procesindustrie en Laboratorium. Leiden.

Chem. Wbl. Chemisch Weekblad. Orgaan van de Koninklijke Nederlandse Chemische Vereniging. Den Haag (The Hague).

Chron. Botan. Chronica Botanica. International Plant Science Publications Society. Massachusetts, USA.

Chron. Univ. Liège Chronique de l'Université de Liège. Liège.

Ciba-Symposium Ciba-Aktiengesellschaft. Basel. (Bi-monthly.)

Ciba-Ztschr. Ciba-Zeitschrift. Ciba Aktiengesellschaft. Basel.

Circa Tiliam *Circa Tiliam. Studia Historiae Medicinae Gerrit Arie Lindeboom Septuagenario oblata.* E. J. Brill, Leiden, 1974.

Circulation Res. Circulation research. New York.

Clio Med. Clio Medica, Acta Academiae Internationalis Historiae Medicinae. Pergamon Press Ltd. Oxford-New York. From 1971: B. M. Israël, Amsterdam. (Quarterly.)

Clin. Orthop. Clinical Orthopaedics; continued as: *Clinical Orthopaedics and related research.* Toronto.

Cobouw Cobouw. Centraal Orgaan voor de Bouwwereld. Den Haag (The Hague).

Comm. biohist. Ultraj. Communicationes Biohistoricae Ultrajectinae. Utrecht (stencilled edition, Biohistorical Institute, Utrecht).

Compt. Rend. hebd. Séances acad. Sci. Comptes Rendus hebdomadaires des Séances de l'Académie des Sciences. Paris.

Curr. Problems in Hist. Med. Aktuelle Probleme aus der Geschichte der Medizin. Current Problems in History of Medicine. Proceedings XIXth International Congress for the History of Medicine (Basel, 7–11 September 1964) S. Karger. Basel-New York 1966.

Current Works in the An international bibliography. The Wellcome Historical Medical
History of Medicine Library. London. Quarterly.

Dej. Ved. Techn.	Dejiny Ved a Techniky. Academy of Science, Prague.
Dent. Mag.	Dental Magazine and Oral Topics. London.
Deutsch. med. J.	Deutsches medizinisches Journal. Berlin.
Dietsche Warande &	Dietsche Warande & Belfort. Antwerpen.
Belfort	
DMW	Deutsche Medizinische Wochenschrift. Stuttgart.
Doc. bl. (Werkgr.)	Documentatieblad Werkgroep 18e eeuw. Witsenburgselaan 35, Nij-
18e eeuw	megen.
Doc. Geigy	Documenta Geigy. Basel.
Dtsch. Apoth. Ztg.	Deutsche Apotheker-Zeitung. Stuttgart.
Dtsch. Ärztebl.	Deutsches Ärzteblatt; ärztliche Mitteilungen. Köln.
ärztl. Mitt.	
Duisburger Forschun-	Duisburger Forschungen. Schriftenreihe für Geschichte und Heimat-
gen	kunde Duisburgs. Duisburg.
Dymphna	Dymphna. Tijdschrift voor verplegenden van zenuw- en zielsziekten. Roermond.

Econ. Hist. Jbk.	Economisch Historisch Jaarboek. Later: *Economisch en sociaal histo-risch jaarboek*. Den Haag (The Hague).
Edinb. med. J.	Edinburgh Medical Journal. Edinburgh.
Eigen Haard	Eigen Haard. Wekelijksch Tijdschrift voor het Gezin. Haarlem.
Endeavour	Endeavour. Quarterly of the Imperial chemical Industries. London.
Engl. Hist. Rev.	English Historical Review. London.
Engl. Studies	English Studies, ed. by G. H. Goethart, P. I. H. O. Schut and R. W. Zandvoort. Amsterdam.
Epilepsia	Epilepsia. Journal of the International League against Epilepsy. Amsterdam.
Epistème	Epistème. Rivista critica di Storia delle scienze mediche e biologiche. Via M. Picco 31, Milano Quarterly.
Essays in Biohist.	P. Smit & R. J. Ch. V. ter Laage (eds.) (1970). *Essays in Biohistory and other contributions .. presented to Frans Verdoorn on the occasion of his 60th birthday*. 426 pp., ill., ports. A. Oosthoek, Utrecht (Series: *Regnum Vegetabile*, Vol. 71).
Europ. orthodont.	European orthodontic Society Transactions. Newcastle upon Tyne,
Soc. Rep.	England.
Ewiges Volk	Ewiges Volk, edited by the "Verband deutscher Sippenforscher in den Niederlanden". Soest (Holland). [appeared during the German occupation of Holland].

Il Farmacista	Bollettino della Federazione degli ordini dei farmacisti d'Italia. Biella.
Feestbundel Klinkert	Feestbundel aangeboden door leden en oudleden van het Klinisch
(1927)	Genootschap te Rotterdam aan hunnen voorzitter Dr. H. Klinkert ter gelegenheid van zijn tachtigste verjaardag op 3 September 1927. 520 pp. Brusse, Rotterdam.
Flehite	Flehite. Tijdschrift van Verleden en Heden van Oost-Utrecht. Amersfoort.
Fol. med. neerl.	Folia medica neerlandica. Bohn, Haarlem Afterwards De Bussy-Ellerman Harms, Amsterdam.
Fol. Psych. Neurol.	Folia Psychiatrica, Neurologica et Neurochirurgica Neerlandica.
Neurochir.	Amsterdam.

Fortschr. Med.	Fortschritte der Medizin. Halle.
Fracastoro	Fracastoro. Bollettino degli Istituti ospitalieri di Verona. Verona.
France Pharm.	France-Pharmacie. Paris.
Gamma	Gamma. Tijdschrift van de Nederlandse Vereniging van Radiologische Laboranten. Utrecht.
Gazette	Gazette (French).
Geldersche Volks-almanak	Geldersche Volksalmanak. Arnhem. *1* (1835) – *71* (1947) Vol. 71 = N.R. Vol. 1.
Gelre	Bijdragen en mededelingen van Gelre. Vereniging tot beoefening van de Geldersche Geschiedenis, oudheidkunde en recht. Arnhem.
Gen. Crt.	Geneeskundige Courant voor het Koninkrijk der Nederlanden. Tiel. Published from 1847–1912.
Gen. T. Ned. Indië	Geneeskundig Tijdschrift voor Nederlandsch-Indië. Batavia.
Geneesk. T. Zeemagt	Geneeskundig Tijdschrift voor de Zeemagt.
Geront. clin.	Gerontologia Clinica. S. Karger, Basel.
Gesnerus	Gesnerus. Vierteljahrschrift herausgegeben von der Schweizerischen Gesellschaft für Geschichte der Medizin und der Naturwissenschaften. H. R. Sauerländer & Co., Aarau.
Geuzenpenning	De Geuzenpenning. Munt- en Penningkundig Nieuws. Amsterdam.
GG	*Geneeskundige Gids*, magazine voor medici. Misset-Fonorama, Amersfoort. (Monthly).
G&W	Geloof en Wetenschap, orgaan van de Christelijke Vereniging van Natuur- en geneeskundigen in Nederland. Loosduinen. Not continued after 1971.
GeWiNa	Mededelingen van het Genootschap voor Geschiedenis der geneeskunde, wiskunde en natuurwetenschappen. Utrecht. (stencilled periodical with restricted circulation).
Gezondheidszorg	Gezondheidszorg. Maandblad van het Groene Kruis. Formerly: *Het Groene en Witte Kruis.* Utrecht.
Gids (De)	De Gids. Algemeen Cultureel Maandblad. Amsterdam.
Giorn. crit. d. Fil. Ital.	Giornale critico della Filosofia Italiana.
Groningen	Groningen. Tijdschrift voor de Volkstaal, Geschiedenis, Volksleven, etc. van de provincie Groningen. J. C. Mehel, Winssum.
Groninger Univ. bl.	Groninger Universiteitsblad. Groningen.
Groninger Volksalmanak	Groninger Volksalmanak. Jaarboekje voor Geschiedenis, taal- en letterkunde der provincie Groningen. Groningen.
Groot Nederland	Letterkundig Maandschrift voor den Nederlandschen Stam. Amsterdam.
Grünenthal Waage	Die Grünenthal Waage. Medizin-wissenschaftliche Abteilung der Chemie Grünenthal. continued as: *Die Waage* Stolberg im Rheinland.
GTNI	Geneeskundig Tijdschrift voor Nederlandsch-Indië. Batavia.
Gulden Passer.	De Gulden Passer. Driemaandelijksch Bulletin van de Vereniging der Antwerpsche Bibliophilen. Antwerpen.
Gut	Gut. The Journal of the British Society of Gastroenterology. British Medical Association London.
Gynaek. Rundschau	Gynaekologische Rundschau. Basel.
Haagsch Jbk.	Haagsch Jaarboekje. Den Haag (The Hague).
Haagsch Mbl.	Haagsch Maandblad. Den Haag (The Hague).
Haagsche Post	Haagsche Post. Den Haag (The Hague) (Weekly).
Haarlemsch Advert. bl.	Haarlemsch Advertentieblad. Haarlem.
Haghe, Die	Die Haghe. Bijdragen en mededelingen van de Vereniging "Die Haghe". Den Haag (The Hague).

Harofe Haivri	The Hebrew medical Journal. New York. (Semi-annual).
Hart-Bulletin	Hart-Bulletin. Driemaandelijkse uitgave van de Nederlandse Hartstichting. Kruyt NV, Bussum. (Quarterly).
Hautarzt	Hautarzt, Zeitschrift für Dermatologie, Venerologie und verwandte Gebiete. Springer-Verlag, Berlin.
Heb. med. J.	Hebrew medical Journal (Harofe Haivri). New York.
Hermèneus	Hermèneus. Tijdschrift voor de antieke cultuur. Tjeenk Willink-Noorduyn, Culemborg.
Herv. Durgerdam	Hervormd Durgerdam. Uitgave der Hervormde Kerk te Durgerdam.
Hippokrates	Hippokrates. Hippokrates Verlag. Stuttgart.
Hist. Méd.	Histoire de la Médecine, organe officiel de la Société Française d'Histoire de la Médecine Paris. Discontinued as from 1-1-1974.
Hist. Sci.	History of Science. An annual Review of Literature, Research and Teaching. Cambridge.
Hist. Sci. méd.	Histoire des Sciences médicales. Colombes.
Historia	Historia. Maandschrift voor Geschiedenis en Kunstgeschiedenis.
Hobby	Hobby. Tijdschrift voor Verzamelaars. Rotterdam.
Horizon	Horizon. Gereformeerd Apologetisch Tijdschrift. Delft. (not continued).
Il Giardino di Esculapio	Il Giardino di Esculapio. Ediz. trimestrale. Milano.
Illustr. med. Ital.	L'Illustrazione medica Italiana. Genua.
Image	Image Roche. Published in English, German, French, Greek, Dutch, Portuguese and Spanish. F. Hoffmann – La Roche & Co, Basel.
Imprensa Médica	Imprensa Médica. Lisboa.
Ind. Gids	Indische Gids, Staatkundig, Economisch en Letterkundig Tijdschrift. Amsterdam.
Int. Kirchl. Ztschr.	Internationale Kirchliche Zeitschrift. Bern.
Invest. Urol.	Investigative Urology. Baltimore.
Isis	Isis. International Review devoted to the History of Science and its Cultural Influences, is the official quarterly journal of the History of Science Society, Inc. Baltimore, Maryland.
Israel Ann. Psychiat.	Israel annals of Psychiatry and Related Disciplines. Jerusalem.
Itan	Itan. Journal of the Kansai Branch of the Japanese Society of Medical History. Osaka.
JAMA	Journal of the American Medical Association. Chicago.
Janus	Janus. Revue internationale d'histoire des sciences, de la médecine, de la pharmacie et de la technique. Blikman, Laporte & Dosse, Amsterdam.
	Janus appeared from 1896–1941 (Vol. *I–XLV*); from 1957 (Vol. *XLVI* –); [1961–3 one vol.: *L.*].
Jbk. Amstelodamum	Jaarboek van het Genootschap Amstelodamum. De Bussy Ellerman Harms BV, Amsterdam.
Jbk. Breda "De Oranjeboom"	Jaarboek en registers van de geschied- en oudheidkundige kring van stad en land van Breda "De Oranjeboom". Breda.
Jbk. Centr. Bur. Geneal.	Jaarboek van het Centraal Bureau Genealogie. Den Haag (The Hague).
Jbk. Dodonaea	Biologisch Jaarboek Dodonaea, published by the "Koninklijk Natuurwetenschappelijk Genootschap Dodonaea" at Ghent. De Sikkel, Antwerp, afterwards Ghent.
Jbk. Haarlem	Jaarboekje voor de stad Haarlem. Haarlem.
Jbk Mij. Ned. Letterk.	Jaarboek van de Maatschappij der Nederlandse Letterkunde te Leiden. E. J. Brill, Leiden.

Jbk Munt- en   Jaarboek Munt- en Penningkunde. Amsterdam.
Pennink.
Jbk. Ned. Bot. Ver. Jaarboek Nederlandse Botanische Vereniging. H. Veenman & Zn.,
                      Wageningen.
Jbk. Oudhk. Gen.   Jaarboekje van het Oudheidkundig Genootschap "Niftarlake". Utrecht.
"Niftarlake"
Jbk. Oudhk. Kring   Jaarboek Oudheidkundige Kring "De Ghulden Roos" (Roosendaal).
"De Ghulden Roos" Roosendaal.
Jbk. Oud-Utrecht   Jaarboek van de Vereniging tot beoefening en tot verspreiding van de
                      kennis der geschiedenis van de stad en de provincie Utrecht. Utrecht.
                      (1 = 1923).
Jbk. R.U. Groningen Jaarboek der Rijksuniversiteit te Groningen. J. B. Wolters, Groningen.
Jbk. Soc. Hist.   Jaarboek Sociaal Historisch Centrum voor Limburg. Maastricht.
Centrum Limburg
Jbk Vrijh. Land Geel. Jaarboek van de Vrijheid en het Land van Geel. Geel (Belgium).
J. Am. dent. Ass.   Journal of the American Dental Association. Chicago.
J. Amer. diet. Ass. Journal of the American dietetic Association. Chicago.
J. Amer. Optom. Ass. Journal of the American Optometric Association. St. Louis.
J. belge Radiol.   Journal belge de Radiologie. Bruxelles.
J. Hist. behav. Sci. Journal of the History of the behavioral Sciences. Brandon/Vermont
                      USA.
J. Hist. Biol.   Journal of the History of Biology. Cambridge/ Massachussetts.
J. Hist. Med.   Journal of the History of Medicine and allied Sciences. Quarterly of
                      the Department of the History of Medicine, Yale University. New Ha-
                      ven, Connecticut.
J. Inst. Brewing   Journal of the Institute of Brewing, containing the Transactions of the
                      various sections records of the Research scheme communications to-
                      gether with abstracts of papers published in other journals. London.
J. Int. Coll.   Journal of the International College of Surgeons. Chicago.
Surg.(eons)
J. Jap. Soc.   Journal of the Japanese Society of Medical History. Tokyo.
Med. Hist.
J. Nutr.   Journal of Nutrition. Philadelphia.
J. med. Education   The Journal of Medical Education. New York.
J. mediev.   Journal of Medieval and Renaissance Studies. Duke University Press.
Renaiss. stud.   Durham, North Carolina.
J. ment. Sci.   Journal of Mental Science. London.
J. mond. Pharm.   Journal mondial de Pharmacie. Den Haag (The Hague).
J. Obst. Gyn.   The Journal of Obstetrics and Gynecology of the British Common-
                      wealth. London.
J. Path.   The Journal of Pathology. formerly: *The Journal of Pathology and
                      Bacteriology.* Leeds.
J. Path. Bact.   Journal of Pathology and Bacteriology. later: Journal of Pathology.
                      London.
J. Pediatr. Surg.   Journal of Pediatric Surgery. New York.
J. Pharm. Belg.   Journal de Pharmacie de Belgique. Bruxelles.
J. Psychiat. Nurs. Journal of Psychiatric Nursing and mental health services. Philadel-
                      phia.
J. Soc. Bibliogr.   Journal of the Society for the Bibliography of Natural History. Lon-
Nat. Hist.   don.
J. South-Afr. Bot. Journal of South African Botany. Parow (South Africa).

Kagakushi Kenkyu	Kagakushi Kenkyu. Japan.
Kamper Almanak	Kamper Almanak. Kampen.
K.(Kath.) Artsenbl.	Katholiek Artsenblad, Blad voor metamedische vraagstukken van de Katholieke Artsenvereniging. After 1969 continued as *Metamedica* Utrecht. (Monthly).
Khirurgiia	Khirurgiia. Moskou.
Klin. Med.	Klinicheskaia Meditsina. Moskou.
Klin. Montsbl. Augenheilk.	Klinisches Monatsblatt Augenheilkunde. Stuttgart.
Klin. Oczna	Klinika Oczna. Acta Ophthalmologica Polonica. Warszawa.
Klin. Wschr.	Klinische Wochenschrift. Berlin.
Kolon. T.	Koloniaal Tijdschrift, uitgegeven door de Vereniging van ambtenaren bij het binnenlandsch bestuur in Nederlandsch-Indië. Den Haag (The Hague). 4°.
Koroth	Koroth. Quarterly Journal of the Israel Society for the History of Medicine and Sciences. Jerusalem – Tel Aviv.
Korresp. bl. Zahnärzte	Korrespondenzblatt für Zahnärzte. Berlin.
Kwart. Hist. Nauki Techn.	Kwartalnik Historii Nauki i Techniki. Warszawa.
Laboratory, The	The Laboratory. Published by Fisher Scientific Co. Pittsburgh P. A.
Lancet, The	The Lancet. London.
Landarzt, Der	Der Landarzt. Stuttgart.
Landbouwk. T.	Landbouwkundig Tijdschrift voor Nederlands Indië. Buitenzorg.
Leids(ch) Jbk.	Jaarboek voor Geschiedenis en Oudheden van Leiden en Rijnland. Leiden.
Leuvense Bijdr.	Leuvense Bijdragen. Tijdschrift voor Germaanse Filologie. Leuven.
Levende Natuur	Levende Natuur. Nederlands Tijdschrift voor Veldbiologie. Amsterdam.
Limburg	Limburg. Maandelijks Tijdschrift voor Limburgse geschiedenis, Oudheidkunde, Kunst en Folklore. Maaseik.
Lucerna	Lucerna. Gereformeerd interfacultair Tijdschrift. Voorburg.
Lychnos	Lychnos. Annual of the Swedish History of Science Society. Stockholm
Maasgouw	De Maasgouw. Orgaan voor Limburgsche Geschiedenis, Taal- en letterkunde. Maastricht.
Mannheimer Gesch. bl.	Mannheimer Geschichtsblätter.
Marquette med. Rev.	Marquette medical Review. Milwaukee.
Mat. med. Nordmark	Materia medica Nordmark. Hamburg.
Mbl. Ver. bestrijding Kwakz.	Maandblad der Vereniging tot bestrijding der kwakzalverij. Leeuwarden.
MC	Medisch Contact, weekblad van de Koninklijke Nederlandsche Maatschappij tot bevordering der Geneeskunst. Reflex, Rotterdam.
MD	MD of Canada, medical newsmagazine. MD Publication, Westmount, Canada. (monthly).
Med. Bild	Medizinisches Bild; Illustrierte Zeitschrift für die gesamte Medizin und ihre Grenzgebiete. Jena.
Med. biol. Engng.	Medical and biological Engineering. Continuation of: Medical Electronics and Biological Engineering. Oxford.
Med. Biol. Ill.	Medical and Biological Illustration. London.
Med. Bur. Statistiek en Voorl.	Mededelingen van het Bureau Statistiek en Voorlichting te 's-Gravenhage. Den Haag (The Hague).

Méd. et Hyg.	Médecine et Hygiène, Journal d'informations médicales. Genève.
Méd. Europ.	Médecine de l'Europe [?].
Méd. France	Médecine de France. Olivier Perrin, Paris.
Med. Hist.	Medical History, a quarterly journal devoted to the History and bibliography of Medicine and the Related Sciences. Dawson & Sons, London.
Med. Hist. J.	Medizin Historisches Journal. Georg Olms, Hildesheim.
Med. J. and Record	Medical Journal and Record. New York. (Continued as *Medical Record*. A National Review of Medicine and Surgery).
Med. Landbouw-hogesch. Wageningen	Mededelingen van de Landbouwhogeschool te Wageningen. Wageningen.
Med. Life	Medical Life: incorporating the: Missisippi Valley Medical Journal; Medico-historical Bulletin. American Journal of Urology Nashville J. of Medicine and surgery Detroit medical J.; Medical Quip 20–45 (1920–38) New York. (No more published.)
Med. Monschr.	Medizinische Monatschrift. Stuttgart.
Med. Ned. Hist. Inst. Rome	Mededelingen Nederlands Historisch Instituut Rome. Ministerie CRM, Den Haag (The Hague).
Med. nei Sec.	Medicina nei Secoli. Official Bulletin of the Institute for the History of medicine at the University of Rome. E. Cossidente, Rome.
Med. News Trib.	Medical News-Tribune; continuation of: Medical News. Alperton.
Med. Revue	Medische Revue. Maandelijks overzicht der binnen- en buitenlandsche literatuur voor den practiseerenden geneesheer. Published from 1901–1913.
Med. Sci. Law	Medicine Science and the Law. The official Journal of the Britsh Academy of Forensic Sciences. Sweet & Maxwell, London.
Med. Techn. Radiol.	Medizinisch-Technische Radiologie. Fachzeitschrift für Röntgen Assistentinnen und Assistenten. Ermer K. G. Homburg-Saar. W-Deutschland.
Med. Wbl.	Medisch Weekblad voor Noord- en Zuid Nederland, gewijd aan de practische genees- heel- en verloskunde. Orgaan voor Praktizeerende geneeskundigen. Scheltema & Holkema, Amsterdam. (published from 1894–1925).
Med. Welt	Medizinische Welt. F. K. Schattauer Verlag. Stuttgart-New York.
Medica mundi	Medica mundi.
Mensch en Maatschappij	Mensch en Maatschappij. Tweemaandelijks Tijdschrift voor Sociale Wetenschappen. P. Noordhoff, Groningen.
Metamedica	Metamedica. Formerly Katholiek Artsenblad. Herenstraat 35, Utrecht. (Monthly).
MGT	Militair Geneeskundig Tijdschrift. Den Haag (The Hague).
Midwives Chron.	Midwives Chronicle and Nursing Notes. London.
Mikrobiologiia	Mikrobiologiia. Moskou.
Mil. Spectator	De Militaire Spectator, Tijdschrift voor het Nederlandsche Leger en dat in de overzeesche bezittingen. V. Loosjes, Haarlem.
Minerva Med.	Minerva Medica. Gazzetta Bisettimanale per il medico pratico. Torino.
Minn. med.	Minnesota medicine. St. Paul.
Mitt. Gesch. Med. Naturwiss.	Mitteilungen zur Geschichte der Medizin und der Naturwissenschaften. Hamburg-Leipzig.
Mitt. Österr. Sanitätsverw.	Mitteilungen Österreichische Sanitätsverwaltung. Wien.
MKNAW	Mededelingen Koninklijke Nederlandse Akademie van Wetenschappen. Noord-Hollandse Uitgevers Maatschappij, Amsterdam.

MKVAW	Mededelingen van de Koninklijke Vlaamse Academie van Wetenschappen, letteren en schoone kunsten van België, Bruxelles.
Mndschr. Kindergeneesk.	Maandschrift voor Kindergeneeskunde. H. E. Stenfert Kroese, Leiden.
Mndschr. locale Gezondhz.	Maandschrift voor locale Gezondheidszorg ten dienste van de autonome gebiedsdelen in de provincie Oost-Java. Soerabaia.
Monsp. Hippocrates	Monspeliensis Hippocrates. Revue de la Société Montpelliéraine d'Histoire de la Médecine. Montpellier. (Quarterly).
Motorama	Motorama.
Mt Sinai J. med.	Mount Sinai Journal of Medicine. New York.
Münch. med. Wschr.	Münchener medizinische Wochenschrift. München.
Nachr. Dtschen. Gesell. Med.	Nachrichten der Deutschen Gesellschaft der Medizin.
Natura Docet	Natura Docet. Orgaan van de Stichting Nederlandse Bond voor Natuurgeneeswijze en natuurkundige inrichtingen. Amsterdam. (Monthly)
Nature	Nature. Mac Millan Journals Ltd. London.
Natuur	De Natuur. Populair geïllustreerd Maandblad gewijd aan de Natuurkundige Wetenschappen en hare toepassingen. Utrecht.
Natuurhist. Mbl.	Natuurhistorisch Maandblad; published by: Natuurhistorisch Genootschap in Limburg. Maastricht.
Natuurwtsch. T.	Natuurwetenschappelijk Tijdschrift. In opdracht van de Natuur- en Geneeskundige vennootschap V.Z.W. uitgegeven. Gent.
Navorscher	De Navorscher. Een middel tot gedachtenwisseling en letterkundig verkeer tusschen allen die iets weten, iets te vragen hebben of iets kunnen oplossen; since 1950 including: Nederlands Archief voor Genealogie en Heraldiek. Amsterdam.
NBW	Nationaal Biografisch Woordenboek België. Bruxelles.
Ned. Ceramiek	Vrienden van de Nederlandse Ceramiek. Staatsuitgeverij, Den Haag (The Hague).
Ned. Hist.	Nederlandse Historiën. Populair tijdschrift voor (streek)geschiedenis. Berkel en Rodenrijs.
Ned. Leeuw	Nederlandse Leeuw, maandblad van het Koninklijk Nederlandsch Genootschap voor Geslacht- en Wapenkunde. Den Haag (The Hague).
Ned. MGT	Nederlands Militair Geneeskundig Tijdschrift. Den Haag (The Hague). (Bi-monthly).
Ned. Mndschr. Geneesk.	Nederlandsch Maandschrift voor geneeskunde. Nieuwe reeks van het Maandschrift voor verloskunde en vrouwenziekten en voor kindergeneeskunde. (*1* (1920 – *9* (1931). Continued as: *Maandschrift voor Kindergeneeskunde 21* (1953).
Ned. Mndschr. Verl. Vrouwenz. en kindergeneesk.	Nederlands Maandschrift voor Verloskunde en Vrouwenziekten. Leiden.
Ned. Oogheelk. Bijdr.	Nederlandse Oogheelkundige Bijdragen. Haarlem.
Ned. Spectator	Nederlandse Spectator 1856–1908. Arnhem-Rotterdam-Amsterdam-Den Haag. 4°.
Ned. Theol. T.	Nederlands Theologisch Tijdschrift. Uitgegeven door de Theologische Faculteiten der Rijksuniversiteit Leiden, Groningen, Utrecht en Amsterdam. H. Veenman, Wageningen. From 1966 including: *Reformatorische oriëntatie.*
Ned. T. Hyg. Microbiol. serol.	Nederlands Tijdschrift voor Hygiene en Microbiologie en Serologie. Leiden. Continued as: *Antonie van Leeuwenhoek.*

Ned. T. Natuurk.	Nederlands Tijdschrift voor Natuurkunde. Den Haag (The Hague).
Ned. T. Prakt. Verl.	Nederlandsch Tijdschrift voor Praktische Verloskunde, Zuigelingen-verzorging en praktische hygiëne. Orgaan van de Bond van Nederlandse Vroedvrouwen. Purmerend.
Ned. T. Psychol.	Nederlands Tijdschrift voor de Psychologie en haar grensgebieden. Noord-Hollandse Uitgevers Maatschappij, Amsterdam.
Ned. T. Tandheelk.	Nederlands Tijdschrift voor Tandheelkunde. Amsterdam.
Ned. Zeewezen	Nederlandsche Zeewezen. Den Haag (The Hague).
Neerl. Volksleven	Neerlands Volksleven, uitgave van het Nederlands Volkskundig Genootschap. Meppel.
Neth. J. Med.	Netherland Journal of Medicine. Amsterdam. Continuation of: Folia Medica Neerlandica.
NNBW	Nieuw Nederlandsch Biografisch Woordenboek. 10 vols. 1911–1937. A. W. Sijthoff, Leiden.
NTG	Nederlands Tijdschrift voor Geneeskunde. Bohn, Haarlem (afterwards Amsterdam). (Weekly).
N.T. Med. Stud.	Nederlandsch Tijdschrift voor Medische Studenten. Amsterdam.
NTVerl. Gyn.	Nederlands Tijdschrift voor Verloskunde en Gynaecologie. Haarlem.
Neue Freie Presse	Neue Freie Presse.
Neue Ztschr. ärzt. Fortbild.	Neue Zeitschrift für ärztliche Fortbildung. Berlin.
Neues Wiener Tagebl.	Neues Wiener Tageblatt. Wien.
New Engl. J. Med.	The New England Journal of Medicine. Massachusetts.
Nieuwe Drentse Volksalmanak	Nieuwe Drentse Volksalmanak. Boekerij S. v. d. Burg, Assen.
Nihon Ishigaku Zasshi	Nihon Ishigaku Zasshi. Journal of the Japanese Society of Medical history. Tokyo.
Nijhoffs Bijdr. Vaderl. Gesch. en Oudheidk.	Nijhoffs Bijdragen voor Vaderlandsche Geschiedenis en Oudheidkunde. M. Nijhoff. Den Haag (The Hague).
Nord. Med. Hist. Årsbok	Nordisk Medicin Historisk Årsbok, Yearbook of the medical-historical Museum, Stockholm. Represents also: The Danish Society for Medical History, Copenhagen. The Norwegian Soc. for Medical History, Oslo. Amici Historiae Medicinae, Helsingfors.
Noord-Holland	Noord-Holland. Tijdschrift gewijd aan de Sociaal-culturele situatie in Noord-Holland. Enkhuizen.
Noorden	Het Noorden. Geïllustreerd Tijdschrift voor het Noorden van Nederland. Van Veen & Evers, Groningen.
Not. Rec. Royal Soc. London	Notes and Records of the Royal Society of London. London.
Nosokomos	Nosokomos. Tijdschrift der Nederlandsche Vereeniging tot bevordering der belangen van verpleegsters en verplegers. Amsterdam.
Noury Post	Noury Post. Chemisch en Pharmaceutisch Nieuwsblad. Deventer.
Nouv. Iconogr. de la Salpêtrière	Nouvelle Iconographie de la Salpêtrière. Paris.
NRC	Nieuwe Rotterdamsche Courant. Rotterdam.
Numaga	Numaga. Tijdschrift gewijd aan heden en verleden van Nijmegen en omgeving. Vereniging "Numaga", Nijmegen. (Quarterly).
Obstet. Gynec.	Obstetrics and Gynecology. New York.
Ons Heem	Ons Heem. Tijdschrift ter bevordering van het heemkundig onderwijs. Roermond.
Onze Kunst	Onze Kunst. Formerly: *Vlaamsche School.* Antwerpen.
Onze Neutraliteit	Onze Neutraliteit. Geïllustreerd maandschrift. Schiedam.

Opbouw (1)	De Opbouw. Democratisch Tijdschrift voor Nederland en Indië. Van Gorcum, Assen.
Opbouw (2)	De Opbouw. Orgaan van de Portugees-Israëlitische Gemeente te Amsterdam. Amsterdam.
Ophthalmologica	Ophthalmologica. International Journal of Ophthalmology. Basel-New York.
Ophthal. Opt.	The Ophthalmic Optician. British Optical Association. London.
Opusc.	Opuscula Selecta Neerlandicorum de arte medica, Vol. I–XIX, 1907–1963. Bohn, Haarlem.
Organorama	Organorama. Published in: Dutch, French, English, German and Spanish. Organon, Oss.
Org. Chr. Ver. Nat. Geneesk.	Orgaan van de Christelijke Vereeniging van Natuur- en Geneeskundigen in Nederland. Leiden. Later: Geloof en Wetenschap.
Org. Ver. ter beoef. krijgswtsch.	Orgaan van de Vereniging ter beoefening van de Krijgswetenschappen. Den Haag (The Hague).
Orthodont. franç.	Orthodontie française. Lyon.
Orv. Hetil.	Orvosi Hetilap. Budapest.
Orvostört. Közl.	Orvostörteneti Közlemények communicationes de Historia Artis Medicinae. Formerly: Communicationes ex Bibliotheca Historia medicae Hungarica.
Orv. Szle	Orvosi szemle. Inst. Medico-Farmaceutic. Turgu-Mures R.A.M. Romania.
Osiris	Osiris. Publications of the History of Science Society, till 1962. Cambridge, Massachusetts.
Osped. Ital. Chir.	Ospedali d'Italia; Chirurgia. Firenze.
Österr. Ärzte Ztg.	Österreichische Ärzte Zeitung, Wien.
Österr. Apoth. Ztg.	Österreichische Apotheker-Zeitung, Wien.
Österr. Gemeindezeitung	Österreichische Gemeindezeitung.
Öst. Z. Stomatol.	Österreichische Zeitschrift für Stomatologie. Wien.
Oudhk. Jbk	Oudheidkundig Jaarboek (1921–1946); continued as Bulletin van de Koninklijke Nederlandse Oudheidkundige Bond. Amsterdam.
Oud-Holland	Oud-Holland. Nieuwe bijdragen voor de geschiedenis der Nederlandsche Kunst, letterkunde etc. Later: Orgaan van het Rijksbureau voor Kunsthistorische Documentatie. Staatsuitgeverij, Den Haag (The Hague).
Oud-Utrecht	Oud-Utrecht, maandblad van de Vereniging tot beoefening en tot verspreiding van de kennis der geschiedenis van de stad en provincie Utrecht. Utrecht.
Overijssel	Overijssel. Jaarboek voor Cultuur en Historie. Enschedé.
Pädiat. Pädol.	Pädiatrie und Pädologie. Springer Verlag, Wien.
Pag. Stor. Med.	Pagine di Storia della Medicina. Istituto di Storia della Medicina, Università Roma. (Bi-monthly).
Pap. bibl. Soc. Amer.	Papers of the Bibliographical Society of America.
Parasitology	Parasitology. Cambridge University Press, London-New York. (Bi-monthly).
Periodiek	Periodiek. Maandblad van het Vlaams Geneesherenverbond. Antwerpen.
Perspect. in Biol. Med.	Perspectives in Biology and Medicine. Chicago.
Pharm. J.	Pharmaceutical Journal. London.
Pharm. Rundschau	Pharmazeutische Rundschau. Hamburg.
Pharma-medico	Pharma-medico. Amsterdam.

Phlébologie	Phlébologie. Paris.
Ph. T. België	Pharmaceutisch Tijdschrift voor België. Antwerpen.
PhW	Pharmaceutische Weekblad, orgaan van de Koninklijke Maatschappij der Pharmacie. Erven Bohn, Haarlem; afterwards D. B. Centen, Hilversum.
Ph. Ztg.	Pharmazeutische Zeitung. Frankfurt a/Main.
Physis	Physis. Rivista di Storia della Scienza. Leo S. Olschki, Florence.
Polyt. Wbl.	Polytechnisch Weekblad, Amsterdam.
Popul. Stud.	Population Studies. Cambridge.
Practitioner (The)	The Practitioner. London.
Prakt. Tierarzt	Praktischer Tierarzt. Hannover.
Predikant en Dokter	Predikant en Dokter. G. J. A. Ruis, Zeist (later at Zutphen). (B-monthly, no more published). (*1* = 1931).
Proc. Inst. Med. Chic.	Proceedings of the Institute of Medicine of Chicago. Chicago.
Proc. XXIII Int. Congr. Hist. Med. London. 1972	Proceedings of the XXIII International Congress of the History of Medicine London 2–9 September 1972. 2 Vols. Wellcome Institute of the History of Medicine, London. 1974.
Proc. KNAW	Proceedings of the Koninklijke Nederlandse Akademie van Wetenschappen. Amsterdam.
Proc. Roy. Soc. Med.	Proceedings of the Royal Society of Medicine (Section of the History of Medicine). Royal Soc. of Med., London. (Irregular).
Proc. Staff Meetings Mayo Clinic	Proceedings of the Staff Meetings Mayo Clinic. later: Mayo Clinic Proceedings. Rochester, Minnesota.
Progr. Méd.	Progrès Médical. Paris.
Przegl. lek.	Przeglad Lekarski. Warszawa.
Psych. neurol. Bl.	Psychiatrische en neurologische Bladen (formerly: Psychiatrische Bladen). Dordrecht later (1948): *Folia psychiatrica, neurologica et neurochirurgica neerlandica.*
Psycho-anal. Quart.	Psycho-analytic Quarterly. New York.
Psycho-anal. Rev.	Psycho-analytic Review. formerly: Psychoanalysis and the Psychoanalytic Review. New York.
Psychol. Rep.	Psychological Reports. Louisville, Missoula.
Quad. Storia Univ. Padova	Quaderni di Storia dell'Università Padova.
Quart. Bull. Northw. Univ. Med. Sch.	Quarterly Bulletin of North-Western University Medical School. Chicago.
Rass. Clin. Ter.	Rassegna di Clinica, Terapia e Scienze affini. Roma.
Rass. med. cult.	Rassegna medica e culturale. Milano.
Het Reddingswezen	Het Reddingswezen. Orgaan van de Nationale Bond voor Reddingswezen en Eerste Hulp bij Ongelukken "Het Oranje Kruis". Rotterdam.
Refajah	Refajah. Christelijk Maandblad voor de verpleging van Krankzinnigen, etc. (Not continued).
Reflexen	Reflexen. Uitgave van de Utrechtse Universiteit. Utrecht.
Rehabilitation	Rehabilitation. Journal of the British Council for rehabilitation of the Disabled. London.
Reports Ass. Hist. Eng. Language	Reports of the Association for the History of the English language.
Rev. Anthropol.	Revue Anthropologique. Paris.
Rev. Asoc. med. Argent.	Revista de la Asociacion medica Argentina. Buenos Aires.
Rev. Belge Méd. Dent.	Revue belge de médecine dentaire (Orthodontia Belgica.) Bruxelles.

Rev. Bras. med.	Revista Brasileira de Medicina. Rio de Janeiro.
Rev. Franç. *Odontostomat.*	Revue Française d'Odontostomatologie. Paris.
Rev. Hist. Art. dent.	Revue d'Histoire de l'Art dentaire.
Rev. hist. Méd. *hébraique*	Revue d'histoire de la Médecine hébraique. Organe de la Société d'Histoire de la Médecine hébraique. Paris. (Trimestrielle).
Rev. Hist. Pharm.	Revue d'Histoire de la Pharmacie. Bulletin de la Société histoire de la pharmacie. Paris.
Rev. d'hist. litt. *France*	Revue d'histoire littéraire de la France.
Rev. d'hist. Sci.	Revue d'histoire des Sciences et de leurs applications. Presses Universitaires de France, Paris.
Rev. int. d'Hist. *Militaire*	Revue internationale d'Histoire militaire. Bruxelles.
Rev. Lyon Med.	Revue Lyonnaise de Médecine.
Rev. Med. (Turgu-Mures)	Revista Medicala. Romania.
Rev. neuro-psiquiat.	Revista de Neuro-psiquiatria. Lima.
Rev. Nord	Revue du Nord, revue historique trimestrielle publieé sous les auspices de l'université de Lille et avec le concours du Centre national de la recherche scientifique. Lille.
Rev. phil. Louvain	Revue philosophique de Louvain. Louvain.
Rhumatologie	Rhumatologie. Aix-les-Bains.
R. I. med. J.	Rhode Island Medical Journal. Providence, Rhode Island, USA.
Riv. Stor. crit. *Sci. Med. Nat.*	Rivista di storia critica delle scienze mediche e naturali. Faenza, Italy.
Riv. Stor. Med.	Rivista di storia della Medicina, organo ufficiale della Società Italiana di Storia della Medicina. Roma.
Riv. Stor. Sci. *med. nat.*	Rivista di storia delle Scienze mediche e naturali, organo ufficiale della Società Italiana di storia delle Scienze mediche e Naturali. Leo S. Olschki, Firenze.
Rott. Jbk.	Rotterdams Jaarboekje. Rotterdam.
SA	Sudhoffs Archiv für die Geschichte der Medizin und der Naturwissenschaften. (Formerly: Archiv der Geschichte der Medizin). Franz Steiner Verlag, Wiesbaden.
S. Afr. med. J.	South African medical Journal, Cape Town.
Santa News	Santa News.
Sartonia	Published by "Museum voor de Geschiedenis van de Wetenschappen," Rijksuniversiteit Korte Meer 9, Ghent (België).
Scalpel (Le)	Le Scalpel, Brussels.
School Sci. Rev.	School Science Review. London.
Schweiz. Apoth. Ztg.	Schweizerische Apotheke-Zeitung. Zürich.
Schweiz. med. Wschr.	Schweizerische medizinische Wochenschrift. Basel.
Sci. Hist.	Scientiarum Historia, driemaandelijks tijdschrift voor de geschiedenis van de geneeskunde, wiskunde en natuurwetenschappen. Prinsstraat 5, Antwerpen.
Scot. Soc. Hist. *Med. Proc.*	Scottish Society of the History of Medicine Proceedings. Edinburgh.
Scriptorium	Scriptorium. International Review of Manuscripts Studies. Revue internationale des Etudes relatives aux Manuscrits. Bruxelles.
Slav. east. *Europ. Rev.*	Slavic and east-European Review. Baltimore [?].

660LIST OF SOURCES

Soc. d'hist. Pharm.	*See*: Rev. Hist. Pharm. (Revue d'Histoire de la Pharmacie). Paris.
Soc. d'hist. de la ville d'Ypres	Société d'Histoire de la ville d'Ypres.
Soc. Zorg	Sociale Zorg. later: *Sociaal Bestek*. Den Haag (The Hague).
Soteria	Soteria. Orgaan van de Protestants-christelijke Artsen-Organisatie in Nederland. Published till 1971. Oranje, Zijlstra & Zijlstra. (Monthly).
Soviet. Stud. Philos.	Soviet Studies in Philosophy. International Arts and Science Press, New York.
Specimina Specia	Specimina Specia. Amstelveen.
Spiegel Historiael	Maandblad voor geschiedenis en archeologie. Fibula-Van Dishoeck, Bussum.
Spreekuur Thuis	Maandblad uitgegeven in samenwerking met de Koninklijke Nederlandse Maatschappij tot bevordering der Geneeskunst. Rotterdam.
Stanf. med. Bull.	Stanford medical Bulletin. San Francisco.
Stemmen des Tijds	Stemmen des Tijds. G. J. A. Ruys, Zutphen – (not continued after 1944).
Sterbeeckia	Sterbeeckia. Antwerpen.
Strikel	De Strikel. Frysk Moameblêd. Drachten.
Stud. Mat. Gesch. Philos.	Studien und Materialen zur Geschichte der Philosophie. Olms, Hildesheim.
Stud. Gen.	Studium Generale, Zeitschrift für die Einheit der Wissenschaften in Zusammenhang ihrer Begriffsbildungen und Forschungsmethoden. Springer Verlag, Berlin-Heidelberg-New York.
Studia Rosenthaliana	Studia Rosenthaliana. Tijdschrift voor Joodse wetenschap en geschiedenis in Nederland. Bibliotheca Rosenthaliana, University Library, Amsterdam.
Studien Bibl. Warburg	Studien der Bibliothek Warburg.
Suiker	Suiker. Maandblad van den Anti-suiker Accijnsbond. Breda-Utrecht. 4°.
Surg. Gyn. Obstet.	Surgery, Gynecology and Obstetrics. Chicago.
Sydsvenska medhist. Sällsk. Arsskr.	Sydsvenska Medicin Historiska Sällskapet Arrskrift.
T. Artsenijk.	Tijdschrift voor Artsenijkunde, het Nederlands Apothekersblad (ed. W. F. Daems) 1943–1945 Den Haag (The Hague).
T. Gesch.	Tijdschrift voor Geschiedenis. Wolters-Noordhoff NV, Groningen.
T. Kon. Aard. Gen.	Tijdschrift van het Koninklijk Nederlandsch Aardrijkskundig Genootschap. Amsterdam.
T. Kon. Ned. Gen. Munt- en Penningk.	Tijdschrift van het Koninklijk Nederlandsch Genootschap voor Munt- en Penningkunde, onder de zinspreuk "Concordia res parvae crescunt" te Amsterdam. Amsterdam.
TMA	Tijdschrift voor Medische Analysten. Amsterdam.
T. Ned. Taal en Lett.(erk.)	Tijdschrift voor Nederlandse Taal- en Letterkunde. Leiden.
T. prakt. Verl.	Tijdschrift voor Praktische Verloskunde, hoofdzakelijk ten dienste van Vroedvrouwen. Steensma, Purmerend (continuation of Maandblad voor praktische verloskunde). (Not continued.)
T. Soc. Geneesk.	Tijdschrift voor Sociale Geneeskunde. 14-daags maandblad van de Algemene Nederlandse Vereniging voor Sociale Geneeskunde. Kruyt BV, Bussum.
T. Tandh.	Tijdschrift voor Tandheelkunde. (later: *Nederlands Tijdschrift voor Tandheelkunde*). Utrecht.
T. Veearts.	Tijdschrift voor veeartsenijkunde en veeteelt. Utrecht.
T. Ziekenverpl.	Tijdschrift voor Ziekenverpleging. De Tijdstroom, Lochem.

Taxandria	Taxandria. Tijdschrift voor Noord-Brabantsche geschiedenis en volkskunde. Bergen op Zoom.
Taxon	Taxon. International Association for Plant Taxonomy. Utrecht.
Tegen de Tuberculose	Tegen de Tuberculose. Orgaan van de Nederlandsche Centrale Vereeniging tot Bestrijding der Tuberculose. Den Haag (The Hague).
Thorax	Thorax. Edited for the Thoracic society. British medical association. London.
Tijdspiegel	Tijdspiegel. 1844–1921. Arnhem-Den Haag (The Hague).
Timotheus	Timotheus. Geïllustreerd Weekblad. Den Haag (The Hague). 4°.
Trans. Coll. phys. surg. Gyn. S. Afr.	Transactions of the College of Physicians Surgeons and Gynecologists of South Africa. Cape Town.
Trans. Stud. Coll. Phys. Philad.	Transactions and Studies of the College of Physicians of Philadelphia. Philadelphia.
Triangel/Triangle	Triangel, Triangle. Sandoz Journal of medical Sciences. Basle.
Trib. Med.	Tribuna Medica. Santiago.
Trop. and Geogr. Med.	Tropical and Geographical Medicine. Amsterdam.
Ugeskrift for Laeger	Ugeskrift for Laeger. Copenhagen.
Uitkijk, Op den	Tijdschrift voor het Christlijk gezin. Wageningen. 4°.
Uitzicht	Uitzicht, Onafhankelijk maandblad voor geestelijke stromingen. (*1* (1939) – *4* (1942). Den Haag (The Hague). 8°.
Univ. Mich. med. Bull.	University Michigan medical Bulletin. Michigan.
Vakbl. Biol.	Vakblad voor Biologen. C. de Boer, Hilversum.
Veröff. Int. Gesell. Gesch. Pharm.	Veröffentlichungen der Internationalen Gesellschaft für Geschichte der Pharmazie. Eutin.
Veröff. Schweiz. Gesell. Gesch. Med.	Veröffentlichungen der Schweizerischen Gesellschaft fur Geschichte der Medizin und der Naturwissenschaften. Zürich.
Versl. med. Ver. t. beoef. Overijssels regt en Geschiedenis	Verslagen en Mededelingen van de Vereeniging tot beoefening van Overijsselsch Regt en Geschiedenis. Deventer.
Vest. Akad. med. Nauk.	Vestnik Akademii meditsinsnikh Nauk SSSR, Moskou.
Vlaamsch Geneesk. T.	Vlaamsch Geneeskundig Tijdschrift. Antwerpen.
Vlaamsche Gids	Vlaamsche Gids. Algemeen maandschrift. Bruxelles.
Vlaamsche Kruis, Het	Het Vlaamsche Kruis. Maandschrift tot bevordering van de Volksgezondheid. Antwerpen.
Vlaamse Stam	De Vlaamse Stam [Belgium].
De Vlag	De Vlag. Zeitschrift der Deutsch-Flämischen Arbeitsgemeinschaft.
Vnitrni	Vnitrni Lekarstvi. Praha.
Voeding	Voeding. Maandblad van de Stichting tot wetenschappelijke voorlichting op voedingsgebied. Den Haag (The Hague).
Völk. Beob.	Völkischer Beobachter, Kampfblatt der Nazionalsozialistischen Bewegung Gross-Deutschlands. Norddeutsche Ausgabe. Berlin.
Voortgang	Voortgang. Tijdschrift voor Christendom en Cultuur. Amsterdam. Of this periodical only three issues have appeared: 1946, no 1, 2, 3.
Vox Med.	Vox Medicorum. Orgaan tot het behartigen van de belangen der geneesheeren in Nederland en zijne Koloniën en van allen, die tot de geneeskunde in betrekking staan. Utrecht. (no more published).
Vrag. Dag.	Vragen van den Dag, voor Nederland en Koloniën. A. W. Sijthoff, Leiden. (Monthly).
Vragen des Tijds	Vragen des Tijds. Tjeenk Willink, Haarlem (Monthly).
Vrij Nederland	Vrij Nederland. Amsterdam (Weekly).

Vrijdagavond (De)   De Vrijdagavond. Joodsch weekblad onder redactie van T. Tal, Prins
                         en J. S. da Silva Rosa. 1924–1932. Amsterdam. (Weekly).
Vrije Fries, De   De Vrije Fries. Tijdschrift uitgegeven door het Friesch Genootschap
                         geschied-, oudheid- en taalkunde en de Fryske Akademy. N.V. Han-
                         delsdrukkerij van 1874, Leeuwarden.

Waage, Die   Die Waage. Zeitschrift der Chemie Grünenthal. See: Die Grünenthal
                         Waage. Brimberg, Aachen.
Wapenheraut   Watpenheraut.
Wbl. Winkeliers- en   Weekblad Winkeliers- en Handelsbelangen.
Handelsbel.
Wentia   Wentia. Uitgave van de Koninklijke Nederlandse Botanische Vereni-
                         ging. Noord-Holl. Publ. Cy, Amsterdam.
Westerheem   Westerheem. Tweemaandelijks orgaan van de Archeologische Werk-
                         gemeenschap voor Westelijk Nederland (WAN). Den Haag (The Ha-
                         gue).
West-Vlaanderen   West-Vlaanderen. [Belg.].
Wetensch. Tijdingen   Wetenschappelijke Tijdingen. Orgaan van de Vereeniging voor Weten-
                         schappen. Gent.
Wiad. Lek.   Wiadomosci Lekarskie. Warszawa.
Wiener Klin. Wschr.   Wiener Klinische Wochenschrift. Wien.
Wiener med. Wschr.   Wiener Medizinische Wochenschrift. Wien.
Wijn   Wijn. Uitgeverij M. Wolters, Amsterdam.
Wisc. med. J.   Wisconsin medical Journal. Madison. USA.
WMJ   World Medical Journal. Official journal of the World Medical Asso-
                         ciation. New York.
World Health   World Health. Genève.

Yperman   Yperman. Bulletin de la Société Belge d'Histoire de la Médecine.
                         Bruxelles-Louvain.

Z. Alterforsch.   Zeitschrift für Alterforschung. Dresden, Leipzig.
Z. f. die ges. Neurol. Zeitschrift für die gesamte Neurologie und Psychiatrie. Originalien
  u. Psychiatrie   und Referate. Berlin.
Z. Psychosom. Med.   Zeitschrift für Psychosomatische Medizin. later: *Zeitschrift für psycho-
                         somatische Medizin und Psychoanalyse.* Göttingen.
Zahnärzt. Mitt.   Zahnärztliche Mitteilungen. Köln (Cologne).
Zeeuws T.   Zeeuws Tijdschrift. Middelburg. 4°.
Zh. Nevropat.   Zhurnal Nevropatologii i Psikhiatrii imeni S. S. Korsakova. Moscow.
Psikhiat.
Ziekenfonds, Het   Het Ziekenfonds. Maandblad voor het Ziekenfondswezen in Neder-
                         land later: *Unie,* Utrecht.
Ziekenfondsgids   De Ziekenfondsgids. Maandblad van de Federatie van door Verzeker-
                         den en Medewerkers bestuurde ziekenfondsen V.M.Z. De Bilt.
Het Ziekenhuis   Het Ziekenhuis. formerly: IPZ, officieel orgaan van het Interkerkelijk
                         Protestants Ziekenhuisbureau: "Ons Ziekenhuis", officieel orgaan van
                         de Ver. van Katholieke Ziekenhuizen en "Het Ziekenhuiswezen".
                         Utrecht.
Ziekenhuiswezen   Het Ziekenhuiswezen. Delft.
Ztschr. angew. Chemie Zeitschrift für angewandte Chemie und Zentralblatt für technische
                         Chemie. Leipzig.
Ztschr. diät. u.   Zeitschrift für diätetische und physikalische Therapie. Leipzig.
physik. Therapie

Ztschr. Ges. inn. Med.	Zeitschrift für die gesamte innere Medizin und ihre Grenzgebiete. Leipzig.
Ztschr. Gesch. Naturw. Techn. Med.	Zeitschrift für Geschichte der Naturwissenschaften, Technik und Medizin. B. G. Teubner, Leipzig.
Zur Gesch. Pharm.	Zur Geschichte der Pharmazie, Geschichtsbeilage der Deutschen Apotheker-Zeitung, zugleich Mitteilungsblatt der Internationalen Gesellschaft der Pharmazie; later: *Beiträge zur Geschichte der Pharmazie.* Stuttgart. (Quarterly).

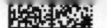